Serum Chemistries

Na⁺ (mmol/L)	135-146
K⁺ (mmol/L)	3.5-5.0
Cl⁻ (mmol/L)	98-109
CO_2 (mmol/L)	24-32
BUN (mg/dL)	12-27
Creatinine (mg/dL)	0.6-1.2
Ca^{2+} (mg/dL)	8.5-10.5
Ionized calcium (mg/dL)	4.5-5.3
Uric acid (mg/dL)	2.2-7 (F); 2.5-8 (M)
Ammonia (µmol/L)	11-35
Glucose, fasting (mg/dL)	50-100
Protein (g/dL)	6-8.5
Albumin (g/dL)	3.3-5.2
Anion gap (mmol/L)	4-16
Phosphate (mg/dL)	2.4-4.5
Magnesium (mEq/L)	1.3-2.1
Prealbumin (mg/dL)	18-38
β-2-microglobulin	1.42-3.41
Bilirubin, total (mg/dL)	0.3-1.1
Bilirubin, direct (mg/dL)	0.1-0.4
Alkaline phosphatase (U/L)	35-150
AST (U/L)	7-42
ALT (U/L)	1-45
LDH (U/L)	110-220
Haptoglobin (mg/dL)	20-165
Iron (µg/dL)	75-175
Iron binding capacity, total (µg/dL)	250-400
Iron saturation (%)	20-50
Ferritin (ng/mL)	20-200
Transferrin (mg/dL)	212-360
B_{12} (pg/mL)	180-900
Folate (ng/mL)	3-18
Red Cell Folate (ng/mL)	140-540
Homocysteine (µmol/L)	5-15
Methylmelonic acid (µmol/L)	0.0-0.4
Tryglycerides (mg/dL)	40-150

Total protein (g/dL)	6.0-8.5
Albumin (g/dL)	3.3-5.2
α-1 globulin (g/dL)	0.1-0.3
α-2 globulin (g/dL)	0.5-0.9
β globulin (g/dL)	0.5-1.2
γ globulin (g/dL)	0.5-1.6
IgG (mg/dL)	723-1685
IgA (mg/dL)	69-382
IgM (mg/dL)	63-277

Serum Free Light Chain Analysis

Free κ (mg/dL)	0.33-1.90
Free λ (mg/dL)	0.57-2.63
κ:λ Ratio	0.26-1.65

Urine Protein Electrophoresis (UPEP)

Urine albumin	<50 %
Urine globulins	60%-67%
Protein:creatinine ratio	<0.2
Total 24-hr protein (mg/total volume)	10-150

Hemoglobin Electrophoresis

Hemoglobin A	>94%
Hemoglobin A2	<3.5%
Hemoglobin F	<2.0%

Case Studies in Hematology and Coagulation

Gene Gulati • Joanne Filicko-O'Hara • John R Krause

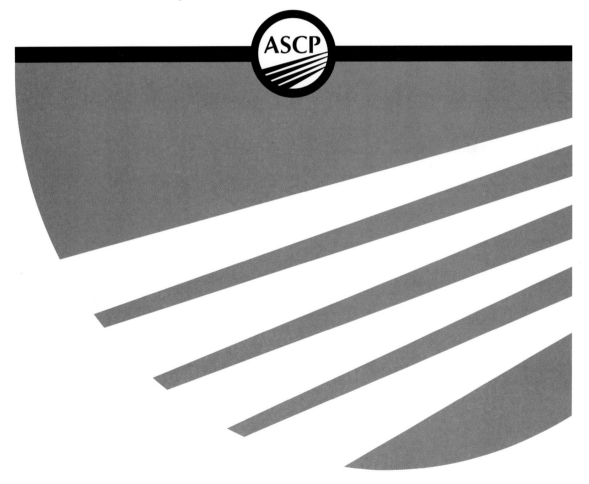

ASCP CaseSet™

Publishing Team
Erik N Tanck (production)
Aimee Algas (editorial/proofreading)
Joshua Weikersheimer (publishing direction)

Notice
Trade names for equipment and supplies described are included as suggestions only. In no way does their inclusion constitute an endorsement of preference by the Author or the ASCP. The Author and ASCP urge all readers to read and follow all manufacturers' instructions and package insert warnings concerning the proper and safe use of products. The American Society for Clinical Pathology, having exercised appropriate and reasonable effort to research material current as of publication date, does not assume any liability for any loss or damage caused by errors and omissions in this publication. Readers must assume responsibility for complete and thorough research of any hazardous conditions they encounter, as this publication is not intended to be all-inclusive, and recommendations and regulations change over time.

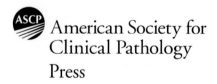

Copyright © 2012 by the American Society for Clinical Pathology. All rights reserved. No part of this publication may be reproduced, stored in a retrieval system, or transmitted in any form or by any means, electronic, mechanical, photocopying, recording, or otherwise, without prior written permission of the publisher.

Developed and designed in Chicago, IL.

Printed in China

16 15 14 13 12

Case Studies in Hematology and Coagulation

ASCP CaseSet™

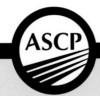

Edited By

Gene Gulati, PhD
Professor of Hematology
Associate Director, Hematology Laboratory
Department of Pathology, Anatomy and Cell Biology
Jefferson Medical College and Thomas Jefferson University Hospital
Thomas Jefferson University, Philadelphia, Pennsylvania

Joanne Filicko-O'Hara, MD
Associate Professor and Attending Hematologist/Oncologist
Director, Fellowship Program in Hematology and Medical Oncology
Department of Medical Oncology
Jefferson Medical College and Thomas Jefferson University Hospital
Thomas Jefferson University, Philadelphia, Pennsylvania

John R Krause, MD
Director of Hematopathology and Hematopathology Fellowship Program
Department of Pathology, Baylor University Medical Center at Dallas
Dallas, Texas
Adjunct Professor of Pathology
Tulane University Health Science Center
New Orleans, Louisiana

Contributors (by last name)

Dorothy Adcock-Funk, MD
Medical/Laboratory Director, Esoterix Coagulation, Englewood, Colorado

Nidhi Aggarwal, MD
*Fellow in Hematopathology, Department of Pathology,
University of Pittsburg Medical Center, Pittsburgh, Pennsylvania*

Essel Dulaimi-Al-Saleem MD
*Fellow in Hematopathology, Department of Pathology,
Drexel University College of Medicine, Philadelphia, Pennsylvania*

Tahseen Al-Saleem, MD
Professor and Director of Hematopathology, Fox Chase Cancer Center, Philadelphia, Pennsylvania

Milon Amin, MD
Resident, Department of Pathology, University of Pittsburg Medical Center, Pittsburgh, Pennsylvania

John Anastasi, MD
Associate Professor of Pathology and Associate Director of Hematopathology, University of Chicago Medical Center, Chicago, Illinois

Babis C Andreadis, MD
*Assistant Clinical Professor of Medicine, University of California, San Franciso, Adult Bone Marrow Transplantation Program,
Helen Diller Family Comprehensive Cancer Center, San Francisco, California*

Helen Bailey, MD
*Staff Pathologist, Department of Pathology and Laboratory Medicine,
Santa Clara Valley Medical Center, San Jose, California*

Alexei Bakhirev, MD
Resident, Department of Pathology, University of New Mexico, Albuquerque, New Mexico

Samir Ballas, MD
*Emeritus Professor of Medicine, Cardeza Foundation,
Honorary Staff member in Internal Medicine/Hematology,
Jefferson Medical College and Thomas Jefferson University Hospital,
Thomas Jefferson University, Philadelphia Pennsylvania*

Adam M Bell, MD
Staff Pathologist, Mercy Medical Center, Des Moines, Iowa

Michael J Berger, MD
*Director of Molecular Diagnostics, Christ Hospital, Cincinnati, Ohio
Staff Pathologist, Molecular Diagnostics and Hematopathology,
Greater Cincinnati Pathologists Inc, Cincinnati, Ohio*

Emmanuel Besa, MD
*Professor of Medical Oncology,
Division of Hematologic Malignancies and Hematopoietic Stem Cell Transplant,
Kummel Cancer Center, Jefferson Medical College and Thomas Jefferson University Hospital, Thomas Jefferson University, Philadelphia, Pennsylvania*

Tawfiqul A Bhuiya, MD
*Associate Professor of Pathology and Vice Chair of Anatomic Pathology,
Department of Pathology & Laboratory Medicine,
Hofstra NS-LIJ School of Medicine, Lake Success, New York*

Franklin A Bontempo, MD
*Associate Professor, Department of Medicine, Division of Hematology/Oncology,
University of Pittsburgh School of Medicine, Pittsburgh, Pennsylvania
Medical Director, Coagulation Laboratory, ITxM Diagnostics, Pittsburgh, Pennsylvania*

Hossein Borghaei, DO
Assistant Professor, Medical Oncology, Fox Chase Cancer Center, Philadelphia, Pennsylvania

David S Bosler, MD
*Head, Cleveland Clinic Laboratories, Attending Pathologist, Hematopathology and Molecular Pathology,
Cleveland Clinic, Cleveland, Ohio*

Scott Bourne, MD
Staff Pathologist, Hematopathology, Physicians Regional Medical Center, Naples, Florida

Matthew C Brennan, MD
*Resident in Internal Medicine, Department of Medicine,
Thomas Jefferson University Hospital, Philadelphia, Pennsylvania*

Carlos Bueso-Ramos, MD
*Professor of Pathology, Department of Hematopathology,
University of Texas MD Anderson Cancer Center, Houston, Texas*

Jaime Caro, MD
*Professor and Attending Hematologist, Department of Medicine and Cardeza Foundation,
Jefferson Medical College and Thomas Jefferson University Hospital,
Thomas Jefferson University, Philadelphia, Pennsylvania*

Dennis A Casciato, MD
Clinical Professor, Department of Medicine, University of California, Los Angeles, Tarzana, California

Devon Chabot-Richards, MD
Resident, Department of Pathology, University of New Mexico, Albuquerque, New Mexico

Karen Chang, MD
*Professor, Department of Pathology and Chief, Division of Clinical Pathology,
City of Hope National Medical Center, Duarte, California*

Mingyi Chen, MD
*Assistant Professor, Department of Pathology and Laboratory Medicine,
UC Davis Health System, Sacramento, California*

John Kim Choi, MD, PhD
*Associate Professor of Pathology & Laboratory Medicine, University of Pennsylvania
Director of Pediatric Hematopathology, Children's Hospital of Philadelphia
Abramson Research Center, Philadelphia, Pennsylvania*

Rushir Choksi, MD
*Fellow in Hematology-Oncology, Division of Hematology-Oncology,
University of Pittsburgh Cancer Institute, Pittsburgh, Pennsylvania*

Adina Cioc, MD
*Assistant Professor of Pathology and Associate Director of Special Hematology,
Department of Laboratory Medicine and Pathology,
University of Minnesota Medical Center, Fairview, Minneapolis, Minnesota*

Lydia Contis, MD
Associate Professor of Pathology, Division of Hematopathology,
Medical Director, Hematology Laboratories, Shadyside and Children's Hospital
Department of Pathology, University of Pittsburg Medical center,
Pittsburgh, Pennsylvania

James D Cotelingam, MD
Professor, Department of Pathology,
Director, Division of Clinical Pathology (Clinical Laboratory)
Louisiana State University Health Sciences Center, Shreveport, Louisiana

Domnita Crisan, MD
Medical Director, Molecular Pathology Laboratory,
Department of Clinical Pathology,
Beaumont Hospitals, Royal Oak, Michigan

Maria Delioukina, MD
Clinical Assistant Professor, Department of Hematology/Hematopoietic Cell Transplantation, City of Hope National Medical Center, Duarte, California

R Patrick Dorion, MD
Associate Pathologist and Doctoral Director of Hematology Laboratory
Pathology Department, Geisinger Medical Center, Danville, Pennsylvania

Douglas Drelich, MD
Instructor and Attending Hematologist, Department of Medicine,
Associate Director, Cardeza Special Hemostasis Laboratory,
Jefferson Medical College and Thomas Jefferson University Hospital
Thomas Jefferson University, Philadelphia, Pennsylvania

Alina E Dulau Florea, MD
Assistant Professor, Hematopathology, Department of Pathology, Anatomy and Cell Biology, Jefferson Medical College and Thomas Jefferson University Hospital, Philadelphia, Pennsylvania

Jennifer Dunlap, MD
Fellow in Hematopathology, Department of Pathology,
Oregon Health and Science University, Portland, Oregon

Cherie H Dunphy, MD
President of North Carolina Society of Pathologists,
Professor of Pathology and Laboratory Medicine,
Director of Hematopathology and Hematopathology Fellowship Program,
Department of Pathology and Laboratory Medicine, University of North Carolina, Chapel Hill, North Carolina

James T Edinger, MD
Fellow in Hematopathology and Dermatopathology
University of Pittsburg Medical Center-Presbyterian, Pittsburgh, Pennsylvania

David Essex, MD
Associate Professor of Medicine,
Section of Hematology and Sol Sherry Thrombosis Research Center,
Temple University School of Medicine, Philadelphia, Pennsylvania

Joan Etzell, MD
Professor, Department of Laboratory Medicine
Director, Clinical Hematology Laboratory, UCSF,
Clinical Hematology Laboratory, University of California at San Francisco,
San Francisco, California

Yuri Fedoriw, MD
Assistant Professor of Pathology and Laboratory Medicine,
Director of Analytical Hematology and Associate Director of Hematopathology,
University of North Carolina, Chapel Hill, North Carolina

Raymond E Felgar, MD
Associate Professor, Department of Pathology,
Director, Hematopathology Fellowship Program,
University of Pittsburgh Medical Center-Presbyterian, Pittsburgh, Pennsylvania

Joanne Filicko-O'Hara
Associate Professor and Attending Hematologist/Oncologist,
Department of Medical Oncology,
Director, Fellowship Program in Hematology and Medical Oncology,
Jefferson Medical College and Thomas Jefferson University Hospital,
Thomas Jefferson University, Philadelphia, Pennsylvania

Alexander Finkelstein, MD
Resident in Laboratory Medicine,
Yale University School of Medicine and Yale-New Haven Hospital,
New Haven, Connecticut

Neal Flomenberg, MD
Professor and Chair, Department of Medical Oncology,
Clinical Deputy Director, Kimmel Cancer Center,
Jefferson Medical College and Thomas Jefferson University Hospital,
Thomas Jefferson University, Philadelphia, Pennsylvania

Kathryn Foucar, MD
Professor, Department of Pathology and Vice Chair of Clinical Affairs,
Medical Director, TriCore Reference Laboratories,
University of New Mexico Health Sciences Center, Albuquerque, New Mexico

Xu Gang, MD
Staff Hematopathologist, Genoptix Medical Laboratory, Carlsbad, California

Ryan Gentzler, MD
Fellow, Hematology/Oncology, Feinberg School of Medicine,
Northwestern University, Chicago, Illinois

Joe K George, DO
Senior Associate, Reading Pediatrics, Wyomissing, Pennsylvania

Melissa R George, DO
Assistant Professor, Division of Clinical Pathology,
Medical Director, Transfusion Medicine & Apheresis,
Penn State Milton S Hershey Medical Center, Hershey, Pennsylvania

Amy S Gewirtz, MD
Associate Professor of Pathology and Vice Chair, Clinical Pathology,
The Ohio State University Medical Center, Columbus, Ohio

Javed Gill, MD
Hematopathologist, Department of Pathology
Baylor University Medical Center, Dallas, Texas

Ryan M Gill, MD
Assistant Professor of Clinical Pathology,
Associate Residency Director, Department of Pathology,
University of California at San Francisco, San Francisco, California

Jerald Z Gong, MD
Associate Professor, Department of Pathology, Anatomy and Cell Biology, Director of Hematopathology and Hematopathology Fellowship Program Jefferson Medical College and Thomas Jefferson University Hospital, Thomas Jefferson University, Philadelphia, Pennsylvania

Mehmet I Goral, MD
Director of Hematology, Department of Pathology and Laboratory medicine, Chester County Hospital, West Chester, Pennsylvania

Bernard Greenberg, MD
Emeritus Professor of Medicine, University of Connecticut Health Center Farmington, Connecticut, Oncologist, Chester County Hematology Oncology, West Chester, Pennsylvania

Dolores Grosso, DPN
Instructor, Department of Medical Oncology, Jefferson Medical College and Thomas Jefferson University Hospital, Thomas Jefferson University, Philadelphia, Pennsylvania

Gene Gulati, PhD
Professor of Hematology, Department of Pathology, Anatomy and Cell Biology, Associate Director of Hematology Laboratory, Jefferson Medical College and Thomas Jefferson University Hospital, Thomas Jefferson University, Philadelphia, Pennsylvania

Jordan M hall, MD
Medical Director of Hematology Section, Department of Pathology and Laboratory Services, Madigan Army Medical Center, Tacoma, Washington

Cheryl Hanau, MD
Professor and Chair, Department of Pathology and Laboratory Medicine, Drexel University College of Medicine, Philadelphia, Pennsylvania

Curtis A Hanson, MD
Professor of Laboratory Medicine and Pathology and Consultant in Hematopathology, Mayo Clinic College of Medicine, Rochester, Minnesota

Jay Herman, MD
Professor of Pathology and Director of Transfusion Medicine, Department of Pathology, Anatomy and Cell Biology, Jefferson Medical College and Thomas Jefferson University Hospital Thomas Jefferson University, Philadelphia, Pennsylvania

Roger H Herzig, MD
Beard Professor of Hematology, Director, University of Louisville Blood & Transplant Program, University of Louisville, Louisville, Kentucky

Katherine High, MD
William H Bennett Professor of Pediatrics, University of Pennsylvania School of Medicine, Investigator, Howard Hughes Medical Institute, Director, Center for Cellular and Molecular Therapeutics, and Attending Physician, The Children's Hospital of Philadelphia and University Pennsylvania Health System, Philadelphia, Pennsylvania

Cheryl Hirsch-Ginsberg, MD
Professor, Department of Pathology, University of Texas MD Anderson Cancer Center, Houston, Texas

Sandra Hollensead, MD
Professor, Department of Pathology, Medical Director of Hematology and Coagulation Laboratory, University of Louisville Hospital and School of Medicine, Louisville, Kentucky

Carol Holman, MD
Associate Professor and Hematopathologist, Department of Pathology, University of Iowa Health Center, Iowa City, Iowa

Steve Hou, MD
Professor, Department of Pathology and Laboratory Medicine, Drexel University College of Medicine Medical Director, Surgical Pathology and Hematopathology, Hahnemann University Hospital, Philadelphia, Pennsylvania

Eric D Hsi, MD
Professor of Pathology, Cleveland Clinic Lerner College of Medicine, Section Head, Hematopathology and Chairman, Department of Clinical Pathology, Cleveland Clinic, Cleveland, Ohio

Yang O Huh, MD
Professor and Attending Pathologist, Department of Hematopathology, University of Texas M D Anderson Cancer Center, Houston, Texas

Matthew T Hurford, MD
Chief of Hematopathology and Director of Hematology, Special Coagulation and Flow Cytometry, Department of Pathology and Laboratory Medicine, Staten Island University Hospital, Staten Island, New York

Gauthami Jalagadugula, MD
Assistant Professor, Sol Sherry Thrombosis Research Center, Temple University School of Medicine, Philadelphia, Pennsylvania

Ajay Kandra, MD
Clinical Hematologist & Medical Oncologist, Carolina Oncology Specialists, PA, Hickory, North Carolina

Margaret Kasner, MD
Assistant Professor, Hematologic Malignancies, Department of Oncology, Jefferson Medical College and Thomas Jefferson University Hospital, Thomas Jefferson University, Philadelphia, Pennsylvania

Craig M Kessler, MD
Professor of Medicine and Pathology and Director, Division of Coagulation, Lombardi Comprehensive Cancer Center, Georgetown University Medical Center, Washington, District of Columbia (DC)

Bhavna Khandpur, MD
Director of Hematology and Associate Director of Blood Bank, Department of Pathology, Norwalk Hospital, Norwalk, Connecticut

Young Kim, MD
Clinical Assistant Professor, Department of Pathology, City of Hope National Medical Center, Duarte, California

Douglas W Kingma, MD
Medical Director of Hematopathology, OncoMetrix, Memphis, Tennessee

Kandice Kottke-Marchant, MD, PhD
Chair, Pathology and Laboratory Medicine Institute, Section Head, Thrombosis and Hemostasis, Cleveland Clinic Lerner College of Medicine, Cleveland, Ohio

Ellen F Krasik, MD, PhD
Fellow in Hematopathology, Departments of Laboratory Medicine and Pathology, Clinical Hematology Laboratory, University of California at San Francisco, San Francisco, California

John Krause, MD
Director of Hematopathology and Hematopathology Fellowship Program, Department of Pathology, Baylor University Medical Center at Dallas, Dallas, Texas, Adjunct Professor, Department of Pathology, Tulane University Health Science Center, New Orleans, Louisiana

Lakshmanan Krishnamurti, MD
Associate Professor of Pediatrics and Director of Hematology, Division of Hematology/Oncology/Bone Marrow Transplant, Director, Comprehensive Hemoglobinopathies Program, Childrens Hospital of Pittsburgh, University of Pittsburgh Medical Center, Pittsburgh, Pennsylvania

Suba Krishnan, MD
Assistant Professor of Pediatrics, Division of Pediatric Hematology, Jefferson Medical College and Thomas Jefferson University Hospital, Thomas Jefferson University, Philadelphia Pennsylvania

Michael Kroll, MD
Professor of Medicine and Chief of Thrombosis and Benign Hematology, University of Texas MD Anderson Cancer Center, Houston, Texas

Nancy Kubiak, MD
Associate Professor, Department of Medicine,
Associate Program Director, Internal Medicine Residency, Luisiana State University Health Sciences Center, Louisville, Kentucky

Janet L Kwiatkowski, MD
Associate Professor of Pediatrics, Director, Thalassemia Program and Attending Hematologist, Children's Hospital of Philadelphia, Philadelphia, Pennsylvania

Robert A Kyle, MD
Professor of Medicine, Laboratory Medicine and Pathology, Consultant, Division of Hematology, Mayo Clinic, Rochester, Minnesota

Joseph Law, MD
Resident, Division of Hematology-Oncology University of Pittsburgh Cancer Institute, Pittsburgh, Pennsylvania

Pei Lin, MD
Associate Professor, Department of Hematopathology, University of Texas MD Anderson Cancer Center, Houston, Texas

Qingyan Liu, MD
Clinical Fellow, National Institutes of Health, Bethesda, Maryland

Mary Lowery-Nordberg, PhD
Professor, Departments of Medicine & Pediatrics,
Director, Hereditary Cancer Risk Assessment Programs, Louisiana State University Health Sciences Center, Feist-Weiller Cancer Center, Shreveport, Louisiana

Ubaldo Martinez-Outschoorn, MD
Assistant Professor, Department of Medical Oncology,
Attending Physician, Hematologic Malignancies and Bone Marrow Transplantation, Jefferson Medical College and Thomas Jefferson University Hospital, Thomas Jefferson University, Philadelphia, Pennsylvania

Robert McKenna, MD
Professor and Director of Hematopathology, Vice Chair for Academic Affairs, Department of Laboratory Medicine and Pathology, University of Minnesota, Minneapolis, Minnesota

Steven E McKenzie, MD
Professor of Medicine and Pediatrics and Attending Physician, Hematology, Cardeza Foundation for Hematological Research, Jefferson Medical College and Thomas Jefferson University Hospital, Thomas Jefferson University, Philadelphia, Pennsylvania

Menchu Ong, MD
Assistant Professor of Pathology and Director of Transfusion Services, Clinical Laboratory, Louisiana State University Health Sciences Center, Shreveport, Louisiana

Michael M Millenson, MD
Director of Hematology, Fox Chase Cancer Center, Philadelphia, Pennsylvania

Ari B Molofsky, MD, PhD
Post-doctoral fellow, Department of Laboratory Medicine, University of California at San Francisco, San Francisco, California

Sara A Monaghan, MD
Assistant professor of Pathology and Medical Director of Hematology Laboratories, University of Pittsburgh Medical Center-Presbyterian and Magee-Womens Hospital, Pittsburgh, Pennsylvania

George Murphy, MD
Professor of Pathology and Dermatopathologist, Brigham and Women's Hospital, Boston, Massachusetts

Melissa Myrsiades, MD
Staff Pathologist, Department of Pathology, Tri-City Medical Center, Oceanside, California

Auayporn Nademanee, MD
Jan and Mace Siegel Professor and Associate Clinical Director,
Director, Matched Unrelated Donor (MUD) Program, Department of Hematology/Hematopoietic Cell Transplantation, City of Hope National Medical Center, Duarte, California

Sujata Narayanan, MD
Resident, Department of Internal Medicine, University of Utah School of Medicine, Salt Lake City, Utah

Beverly P Nelson, MD
Associate Professor of Pathology and Director of Residency Program in Pathology, Northwestern University Feinberg School of Medicine, Chicago, Illinois

Christian P Nixon, MD, PhD
Resident, Department of Laboratory Medicine and Pathology, University of California at San Francisco (UCSF), San Francisco, California

Elise A Occhipinti, MD
Hematopathologist, Ochsner Medical Center, New Orleans, Louisiana

Craig Okada, MD
Assistant Professor, Hematology, Portland VA Medical Center, Oregon Health and Science University, Portland, Oregon

Mihaela Onciu, MD
Director, Hematology and Special Hematology Laboratories,
Department of Pathology, St Jude Children's Research Hospital, Memphis, Tennessee
Current: Pathologist, Oncometrix, Memphis, Tennessee

Menchu Ong, MD
Assistant Professor of Pathology and Director of Transfusion Services,
Clinical Laboratory, Louisiana State University Health Sciences Center, Shreveport, Louisiana

Tal Oren, MD, PhD
Attending Hematopathologist, Emerge Laboratories, Suffern, New York

Stavroula A Otis, MD
Clinical Instructor of Hematology,
Department of Medicine,
Stanford University School of Medicine, Stanford, California

Juan Palazzo, MD
Professor, Department of Pathology, Anatomy and Cell Biology,
Jefferson Medical College and Thomas Jefferson University Hospital
Thomas Jefferson University, Philadelphia, Pennsylvania

Ziad Peerwani, MD
Hematopathologist and Director of Hematology and Coagulation,
Department of Pathology, Baylor All Saints Medical Center, Fort Worth, Texas

Sherrie L Perkins, MD, PhD
Professor of Pathology & Associate Chief, Anatomic Pathology, University of Utah Health Sciences Center
Director, Hematopathology, ARUP Laboratories, Salt Lake City, Utah

Powers Peterson, MD
Associate Professor of Pathology & Laboratory Medicine,
Associate Attending Pathologist, Weill Cornell Medical College in Qatar
New York, New York
Current: Medical Director, Quest Diagnostics Nichols Institute, Valencia, California

Louis Pietragallo, MD
Clinical Associate Professor of Medicine,
Oncologist, Hematology Oncology Division, University of Pittsburgh Medical Center Shadyside Hospital,
Community Cancer Centers, Pittsburgh, Pennsylvania

Raju K Pillai, MD
Clinical Fellow, Division of Hematopathology,
University of Pittsburgh Medical Center-Presbyterian Hospital, Pittsburgh, Pennsylvania

Stefania Pittaluga, MD, PhD
Staff Clinician, National Institutes of Health, Bethesda, Maryland

Josef Prchal, MD
Professor of Medicine, Pathology, and Genetics,
Hematology Division, University of Utah, Salt Lake City, Utah

Margaret V Ragni, MD
Professor of Medicine, University of Pittsburgh Medical School,
Director, Hemophilia Center of Western PA, University of Pittsburgh, c/o Hemophilia Center of Western PA,
Pittsburgh, Pennsylvania

Kanti Rai, MD
Professor of Medicine and Molecular Medicine,
Chief, Division of Hematology-Oncology, Long Island Jewish Medical Center and Hofstra-NS-LIJ School of Medicine, New Hyde Park, New York

Koneti Rao, MD
Sol Sherry Professor of Medicine and Professor of Thrombosis Research and Pharmacology, Chief, Hematology Section and Co-Director, Sol Sherry Thrombosis Research Center, Temple University School of Medicine, Philadelphia, Pennsylvania

Jay S Raval, MD
Clinical Fellow in Transfusion Medicine, The Institute for Transfusion Medicine, Pittsburgh, Pennsylvania

Bill G Richendollar, MD
Staff Pathologist, DeKalb Pathology PC, Decatur, Georgia

Valentin G Robu, MD
Assistant Professor, Department of Pathology,
Fox Chase Cancer Center, Philadelphia, Pennsylvania

Heesun J Rogers, MD
Staff, Section of Hemostasis and Thrombosis,
Department of Clinical Pathology, Cleveland Clinic, Cleveland, Ohio

Marian Rollins-Raval, MD
Clinical Fellow in Hematopathology,
Division of Hematopathology,
University of Pittsburgh Medical Center – Presbyterian Hospital,
Pittsburgh, Pennsylvania

Nancy S Rosenthal, MD
Professor of Pathology and Director of Hematopathology,
Department of Pathology, University of Iowa Hospitals and Clinics,
Iowa City, Iowa

Jascha Rubin, MD
Resident in Internal Medicine, Department of Medicine,
Thomas Jefferson University Hospital, Philadelphia, Pennsylvania

Mohamed E Salama, MD
Associate Professor of Pathology,
Director of Hematopathology Fellowship Training Program,
University of Utah and ARUP Reference Laboratory, Salt Lake City, Utah

Linda M Sandhaus, MD
Associate Professor of Pathology,
Case Western Reserve University School of Medicine,
Medical Director, Hematology Laboratory and Point-of-Care Testing,
University Hospitals of Cleveland Case Medical Center, Cleveland, Ohio

Bertram Schnitzer, MD
Professor of Pathology (Hematopathology), Department of Pathology, University of Michigan, Ann Arbor, Michigan

Cordelia Sever, MD
Clinical Associate Professor, Department of Pathology, University of New Mexico,
Medical Director, Presbyterian Hospital Laboratory, Pathology Associates of Albuquerque Presbyterian Hospital Laboratory, Albuquerque, New Mexico

Ronald Sham, MD
Clinical Professor of Medicine,
University of Rochester School of Medicine and Dentistry,
Medical Director- Mary M Gooley Hemophilia Center,
Hematologist-Rochester General Hospital, Rochester, New York

Imran Siddiqi, MD
Assistant Professor of Clinical Pathology, Department of Pathology, University of Southern California Keck School of Medicine, Medical Director of Clinical Hematology Laboratory, University Hospital and Norris Cancer Center, Los Angeles, California

Alexa J Siddon, MD
Resident in Laboratory Medicine, Yale University School of Medicine and Yale-New Haven Hospital, New Haven, Connecticut

Christine N Sillings, MD
Staff Pathologist, Department of Pathology, Wake Med Health and Hospitals, Raleigh, North Carolina

Brian R Smith, MD
Professor and Chair of Laboratory Medicine, Internal Medicine, and Pediatrics, Chief of Laboratory Medicine, Yale-New Haven Hospital, Yale University School of Medicine, New Haven, Connecticut

Lauren B Smith, MD
Assistant Professor, Department of Pathology, University of Michigan, Ann Arbor, Michigan

Mitchell R Smith, MD
Associate Professor and Director, Lymphoma Service, Fox Chase Cancer Center, Philadelphia, Pennsylvania

Roy E Smith, MD
Professor, Department of Medicine, Division of Hematology-Oncology, University of Pittsburgh Cancer Institute and University of Pittsburgh Medical Center, Pittsburgh, Pennsylvania

David S Snyder, MD
Professor and Associate Chair, Department of Hematology/Hematopoietic Cell Transplantation, City of Hope National Medical Center, Duarte, California

Joo Y Song, MD
Clinical Fellow, National Institutes of Health, Bethesda, Maryland

Tsieh Sun, MD
Professor and Consultant Pathologist, Department of Hematopathology, University of Texas MD Anderson Cancer Center, Houston, Texas

Sara Szabo, MD
Assistant Professor of Pathology, Department of Pathology and Laboratory Medicine, Medical College of Wisconsin, Milwaukee, Wisconsin, Staff Pathologist, Children's Hospital of Wisconsin, Milwaukee, Wisconsin

Edward Thornborrow, MD
Assistant Professor, Department of Laboratory Medicine, Director, Clinical Laboratories at Mt Zion, University of California at San Francisco, San Francisco, California

Adam Toll, MD
Junior Faculty Pathologist, Department of Pathology, Johns Hopkins Hospital, Baltimore, Maryland

Christopher Tormey, MD
Assistant Professor of Laboratory Medicine, Yale University School of Medicine, Attending Clinical Pathologist, VA Connecticut Healthcare System and Yale-New Haven Hospital, New Haven, Connecticut

Elie Traer, MD, PhD
Fellow in Hematology/Oncology, Oregon Health and Science University, Portland, Oregon

An Tran, MD
Fellow in Hematology- Oncology, Division of Hematology-Oncology University of Pittsburgh Cancer Institute, Pittsburgh, Pennsylvania

Elizabeth M Van Cott, MD
Associate Professor, Harvard Medical School, Director, Coagulation Laboratory and Medical Director, Core Laboratory, Massachusetts General Hospital, Boston, Massachusetts

Diana Veillon, MD
Professor of Clinical Pathology, Director, Hematopathology, Flow, Cytometry & Coagulation Clinical Laboratory, Luisiana State University Health Sciences Center, Shreveport, Luisiana

Nicole Verdun, MD
Assistant Professor and Pediatric Hematologist-Oncologist, Children's National Medical Center, Washington, District of Columbia (DC)

Scott Weisenberg, MD
Infectious Disease Physician, Alta Bates Summit Medical Center, Oakland, California

Wendy Wiesend, MD
Chief Resident, Department of Pathology, Beaumont Hospitals, Royal Oak, Michigan

Amanda L Wilson, MD
Staff Pathologist, Monongalia General Hospital, Morgantown, West Virginia

Hassan M Yaish, MD
Professor, Department of Pediatrics, University of Utah, Salt Lake City, Utah

Cecelia Arana Yi, MD
Fellow in Hematology and Medical Oncology, Thomas Jefferson University Hospital, Philadelphia, Pennsylvania

M James You, MD, PhD
Assistant Professor, Department of Hematopathology, Division of Pathology and Laboratory Medicine, University of Texas MD Anderson Cancer Center, Houston, Texas

Jingwei Yu, MD, PhD
Professor, Department of Laboratory Medicine, Director, Cytogenetics Laboratory, University of California at San Francisco, San Francisco, California

James Zehnder, MD
Professor of Pathology and Medicine (Hematology, Director, Coagulation and Molecular Genetic Pathology Laboratories, Department of Pathology, Stanford Hospital and Clinics, Stanford University School of Medicine, Stanford, California

Preface

The case study approach is an invaluable means for gaining practical knowledge of any subject material. Residency and fellowship training programs in various subspecialties often offer a case study approach in their training programs. Most trainees wish to enhance their knowledge base by attending continuing education programs offered by professional organizations. Supplemental materials in the areas of hematopathology and hematology are available, but very limited.

This ASCP CaseSet offers a comprehensive resource for case-based learning in hematology and coagulation for pathology residents and hematopathology and hematology/oncology fellows. We hope it will also serve as a useful reference source for students, mentors, teachers and practitioners of hematology/oncology and hematopathology.

Part I (Sections A through I) presents cases dealing with anemias, acute leukemias, chronic myeloproliferative neoplasms & myelodysplastic syndromes, chronic lymphoproliferative disorders, lymphomas & their mimics, plasma cell disorders, platelet disorders, organisms, and other miscellaneous hematologic conditions.

Part II (Sections J through L) includes cases dealing with bleeding disorders, thrombophilias, and other miscellaneous hemostasis disorders.

Common, uncommon, and some rare entities are included—offering something for everyone from medical students to experienced practitioners. Each case follows a preset format, which includes pertinent findings related to patient's presenting complaint(s), clinical history, family history, medications, physical examination, initial work-up, differential diagnosis, additional work-up, final diagnosis, management approach, and general discussion.

Part III (sections M and N) comprises 27 self-study cases. In Section M, a partial description of each case, which is limited to findings related to patient's presenting complaint(s), clinical history, family history, medications, physical examination, and initial work-up, is followed by a series of 5 questions for the reader to answer, and thereby complete the case as an unknown. Answers to the individual questions are provided in discussions of the individual cases in Section N.

We dedicate this work to all our colleagues and to the many contributors. Without their help, this project would have remained a dream.

We are also grateful to our families for their understanding and support while we spent the many long hours necessary to complete this project.

ASCP Press also deserves a special word of thanks for bringing this publication to fruition.

Gene Gulati
Joanne Filicko-O'Hara
John R Krause

Table of Contents

Section A: Anemias

1	Iron Deficiency Anemia
4	Thalassemia Minor
6	Anemia Associated with Hypotransferrinemia
8	β-Thalassemia Major
10	Anemia Associated with Lead Poisoning
12	Thalassemia Intermedia
15	Anemia Associated with Copper Deficiency
17	Hemoglobin E Disease
19	Congenital Sideroblastic Anemia
22	Macrocytic Anemia Associated with Folate Deficiency
25	Macrocytic Anemia Associated with B_{12} Deficiency
28	Pernicious Anemia
31	Methemoglobinemia
34	Hemolytic Anemia Associated with G6PD Deficiency
36	Anemia Associated with Pyruvate Kinase Deficiency
39	Hemolytic Disease of the Newborn
42	Anemia Associated with Fetomaternal Hemorrhage
45	Autoimmune Hemolytic Anemia, Warm-Reactive
48	Autoimmune Hemolytic Anemia, Cold-Reactive
50	Donath-Landsteiner Hemolytic Anemia (Paroxysmal Cold Hemoglobinuria)
53	Hemoglobin SC Disease
55	Hereditary Spherocytosis
57	Sickle Cell Anemia
60	Hereditary Elliptocytosis
62	Sickle-α-Thalassemia
65	Hereditary Pyropoikilocytosis
68	Anemia Associated with Liver Disease
70	Sickle Cell Anemia with Leg Ulcer
72	Anemia of Chronic Renal Insufficiency
74	Acquired Acanthocytosis
76	Aplastic Anemia
79	Diamond-Blackfan Anemia
82	Congenital Dyserythropoetic Anemia, Type II
84	Fanconi Anemia and Myelodysplastic Syndrome
87	Pure Red Cell Aplasia Associated with Parvovirus Infection
89	Hemochromatosis, HFE-Associated
92	Hemochromatosis, Non-HFE Associated

Preface

Section B: Acute Leukemias

95	Acute Myeloid Leukemia with t(8;21)
98	Acute Myeloid Leukemia with Mutated NPM1
101	Acute Promyelocytic Leukemia with t(15;17)(q22;q12)
104	Acute Myelomonocytic Leukemia
107	Acute Myeloid Leukemia with Myelodysplasia-Related Changes
110	Acute Monoblastic Leukemia
113	Acute Myeloid Leukemia, with inv(3)
116	Acute Megakaryoblastic Leukemia
119	Therapy-Related Acute Myeloid Leukemia
122	Acute Myeloid Leukemia, Acute Panmyelosis with Myelofibrosis Subtype
125	Revised Blastic Plasmacytoid Dendritic Cell Neoplasm
128	Myeloid/Lymphoid Neoplasms with Eosinophilia and PDGFRA Rearrangement
130	Acute Ph– Lymphoblastic Leukemia
133	B-Lymphoblastic Leukemia, Pediatric
136	T-Lymphoblastic Leukemia Pediatric
139	T-Lymphoblastic Leukemia
141	Acute Ph+ Lymphoblastic Leukemia
144	Acute Leukemia of Ambiguous Lineage
146	T-Lymphoblastic Crisis of Chronic Myelogenous Leukemia

Section C: Chronic Myeloproliferative Neoplasms and Myelodysplastic Syndromes

149	Chronic Myelogenous Leukemia
152	Atypical Chronic Myelogenous Leukemia, *BCR-ABL1* Negative
155	Chronic Neutrophilic Leukemia
158	Polycythemia Vera
160	Essential Thrombocythemia
162	Primary Myelofibrosis
165	Systemic Mastocytosis with Associated Clonal Hematologic Non-Mast Cell-Lineage Disease
168	Congenital Polycythemia
170	Myeloproliferative Neoplasm, Unclassifiable
173	Refractory Anemia with Ring Sideroblasts
176	Refractory Anemia with Ring Sideroblasts Associated with Marked Thrombocytosis
178	Refractory Cytopenia with Multilineage Dysplasia
181	Refractory Anemia with Excess Blasts-2
184	Myelodysplastic Syndrome with Isolated del(5q)
187	Myelodysplastic Syndrome, Unclassifiable
189	Chronic Myelomonocytic Leukemia

Section D: Chronic Lymphoproliferative Disorders

192	Chronic Lymphocytic Leukemia
195	Large B-Cell Lymphoma with Underlying Chronic Lymphocytic Leukemia (Richter Transformation)
197	B-Cell Prolymphocytic Leukemia
199	Hairy Cell Leukemia
202	Post-Transplant Lymphoproliferative Disorder
205	T-Cell Prolymphocytic Leukemia
208	T-Cell Large Granular Lymphocytic Leukemia
210	Adult T-Cell Lymphoma/Leukemia
213	Autoimmune Lymphoproliferative Syndrome

Section E: Lymphomas and Their Mimics

216	Classical Hodgkin Lymphoma with Paraneoplastic Neuromyotonia
219	Nodular Lymphocyte-Predominant Hodgkin Lymphoma
222	Lymphocyte-Rich Classical Hodgkin Lymphoma
225	Mixed Cellularity Classical Hodgkin Lymphoma
227	Follicular Lymphoma
230	Mantle Cell Lymphoma
233	Gastric MALT Lymphoma with Associated *H Pylori* Infection
236	Burkitt Lymphoma
239	Diffuse Large B-Cell Lymphoma
241	Double-Hit High-Grade B-Cell Lymphoma
244	T-Lymphoblastic Lymphoma
246	Extranodal NK/T-Cell Lymphoma, Nasal Type
249	Angioimmunoblastic T-Cell Lymphoma
252	Hepatosplenic T-Cell Lymphoma
255	Primary Cutaneous T-Cell Lymphoma, γ-δ Type
258	Nodal Marginal Zone Lymphoma
261	Peripheralization of Follicular Lymphoma
264	Mycosis Fungoides/Sézary Syndrome
266	Follicular Hyperplasia
269	Rosai-Dorfman Disease
271	Kikuchi-Fujimoto Disease (Histiocytic Necrotizing Lymphadenitis)
274	Progressive Transformation of Germinal Centers
277	Castleman Disease

Section F: Plasma Cell Disorders

280	Monoclonal Gammopathy of Undetermined Significance
282	Plasmacytoma
284	Multiple Myeloma
286	IgM-Secreting Myeloma
288	POEMS Syndrome (Polyneuropathy, Organomegaly, Endocrinopathy, Monoclonal Protein and Skin Changes)
291	Primary Amyloidosis
294	Light Chain Deposition Disease
297	Multiple Myeloma and Acquired von Willebrand Disease

Section G: Platelet Disorders

300	Immune Thrombocytopenic Purpura (ITP)
303	Glanzmann Thrombasthenia
305	Gray Platelet Syndrome
307	Wiskott-Aldrich Syndrome
309	δ-Storage Pool Deficiency (Hermansky-Pudlak Syndrome)
311	Inherited Platelet Secretion Defect/Signal Transduction Defect
313	Acquired Platelet Function Defect-Induced by Selective Serotonin-Reuptake Inhibitor

Section H: Hematologic Infectious Diseases

315	Babesiosis
318	Anaplasmosis
320	Malaria (*Plasmodium vivax*)
323	Relapsing Fever Secondary to *Borrelia hermsii*
325	Disseminated *Histoplasma capsulatum*

Section I: Miscellaneous Hematologic Conditions

328	Persistent Polyclonal B-Lymphocytosis
331	Infectious Mononucleosis
334	Alloimmune Neonatal Neutropenia
337	Leukemoid Reaction Associated with Growth Factor Therapy
339	Chronic Benign Neutropenia
342	Acute Graft-vs-Host Disease
346	Chronic Graft-vs-Host Disease
348	Donor Lymphocyte Infusion Therapy
351	Transient Abnormal Myelopoiesis
354	Pelger-Huët Anomaly
357	May-Hegglin Anomaly
359	HIV/Therapy-Related Myelodysplasia
361	Hemophagocytic Lymphohistiocytosis
364	Alveolar Rhabdomyosarcoma of the Bone Marrow
367	Lobular Carcinoma of the Breast, Metastatic to the Bone Marrow
370	Paroxysmal Nocturnal Hemoglobinuria
373	Chédiak-Higashi Syndrome
376	Niemann-Pick Disease
378	Mucopolysaccharidosis Type I (Hurler Syndrome)
380	Primary Hyperoxaluria Involving Bone Marrow

Section J: Bleeding Disorders

382	Factor VII Deficiency
384	Hemophilia A (Factor VIII Deficiency) – Newborn Diagnosis
386	Hemophilia A (Factor VIII Deficiency) Carrier
388	Hemophilia B (Factor IX Deficiency)
390	Hemophilia B (Factor IX Deficiency) Carrier
392	Factor V Inhibitor
394	Factor VIII Inhibitor
396	Acquired Factor X Deficiency
399	Factor XI Deficiency
401	Factor XII Deficiency
403	Factor XIII Deficiency
405	von Willebrand Disease, Variant 2 Normandy
407	Acquired von Willebrand Disease

Section K: Thrombophilias

408	Factor V Leiden
410	Antiphospholipid Antibody Syndrome
412	Prothrombin Gene G20210A Mutation
414	Hereditary Protein C Deficiency, Type I
416	Antithrombin Deficiency
419	Protein S Deficiency

Section L: Miscellaneous Hemostasis Disorders

421	Thrombotic Thrombocytopenic Purpura
423	Heparin-Induced Thrombocytopenia with Thrombosis
425	Disseminated Intravascular Coagulation (DIC)
427	HELLP Syndrome (Hemolysis, Elevated Liver Enzymes, Low Platelets Syndrome)
429	Thrombotic Thrombocytopenic Purpura in a Patient with Sickle Cell Crisis
431	Coagulopathy Associated with Cirrhosis
433	Plasminogen Deficiency, Type 1
435	Congenital Dysfibrinogenemia
437	Ischemic Stroke, Secondary to Atherosclerosis From Elevated Lp(a) Levels
439	CYP2C9 Genotyping for Management of Coumadin Therapy

Self-Study Challenge Cases

Presentation	Case number	Discussion
441	Case 1	468
442	Case 2	469
443	Case 3	471
444	Case 4	473
445	Case 5	474
446	Case 6	476
447	Case 7	477
448	Case 8	479
449	Case 9	481
450	Case 10	482
451	Case 11	484
452	Case 12	486
453	Case 13	487
454	Case 14	488
455	Case 15	490
456	Case 16	492
457	Case 17	494
458	Case 18	496
459	Case 19	498
460	Case 20	500
461	Case 21	502
462	Case 22	503
463	Case 23	504
464	Case 24	506
465	Case 25	508
466	Case 26	510
467	Case 27	514

Iron Deficiency Anemia

Jaime Caro, Ubaldo Martinez-Outschoorn

Patient A 65-year-old female of northern European origin with progressive shortness of breath and fatigue for the past 6 months.

Clinical History The patient had history of hemorrhoids and described occasional bright red blood per rectum after bowel movements, but denied dark stools. Her menopause was at age 50 and her periods were regular without excessive bleeding.

Family History No family history of anemia or other hematologic disorders.

Medications No medications, but takes over-the-counter multivitamins.

Physical Examination Remarkable for pale conjunctiva and skin, no jaundice. Cardiac auscultation revealed a systolic ejection murmur II/VI at the right of upper sternal border. No lymphoadenopathy or hepatosplenomegaly.

Initial Work-Up

CBC		WBC Differential	%	# (×10^3/µL)
WBC (×10^3/µL)	5.6	Neutrophils	70	3.9
RBC (×10^6/µL)	3.55	Bands	0	
HGB (g/dL)	7.4	Lymphocytes	20	1.1
HCT (%)	24.5	Monocytes	5.6	0.3
MCV (fL)	69	Eosinophils	3.4	0.2
MCH (pg)	20.8	Basophils	1	0.1
MCHC (g/dL)	30.2			
PLT (×10^3/µL)	439			
RDW-CV (%)	16.4			

Peripheral blood smear revealed hypochromic, microcytic red cells and no polychromasia (**Figure 1**).

Section A: Anemias
Iron Deficiency Anemia

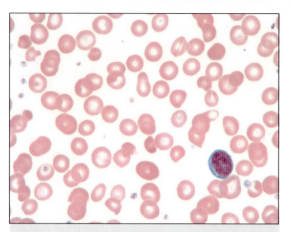

Figure 1 Blood smear (Wright-Giemsa, ×1000) showing microcytic hypochromic red cells.

Differential Diagnosis Clinical conditions associated with a microcytic anemia include iron deficiency with or without concomitant B_{12} or folate deficiency, anemia of chronic inflammatory disease, thalassemia, sideroblastic anemia and lead intoxication. The lack of family history of anemia and her ethnic background makes the diagnosis of thalassemia unlikely. Since there is no history of chronic inflammation, the most likely cause of her anemia is iron deficiency.

Additional Work-Up

Serum chemistries
- Iron saturation 3% (normal 2-50)
- Total iron-binding capacity 513 µg/dL (normal 250-400)
- Ferritin 15 ng/mL (normal 20-200).
- Vitamin B_{12} 250 pg/mL (normal 80-900)
- Folate 6 ng/mL (normal 3-18)

The finding of a high total iron-binding capacity and low ferritin is consistent with iron deficiency. The increased platelet count is a frequent finding in iron deficiency. The evaluation of iron deficiency anemia (IDA) is not complete until the reason for IDA is known. Rectal exam revealed brown stool and fecal occult blood testing was positive. Although our patient had a history of bleeding hemorrhoids, she should have a complete gastrointestinal (GI) work-up including upper GI and colonoscopy to rule-out a concomitant occult malignancy. Indeed, a colonoscopy showed a 3 cm tumor in the transverse colon and she subsequently underwent a surgical resection.

Final Diagnosis Iron deficiency anemia.

Management Approach Treatment of iron deficiency anemia requires administration of iron and correction of the underlying disease(s) that has led to iron deficiency. Iron deficiency anemia can be treated in most cases with oral iron. Intravenous iron is used for those patients that have malabsorption or severe intolerance to oral iron. This patient was started on oral iron (325 mg ferrous sulfate 3 times a day) with complete restoration of hemoglobin. She continued iron supplementation with 1 tablet a day for an extra 3 months to restore her iron deposits.

General Discussion Depending upon severity of anemia, the patients with iron deficiency may present with pallor, weakness, craving for ice and clay etc, dizziness, koilonychia, cheilitis, palpitations, and even dyspnea. The anemia is almost always characterized by microcytic and hypochromic red cells, and a few elliptical cells or so-called "pencil cells" may be evident on the blood smear. Thrombocytosis may accompany iron deficiency anemia in some cases. Total body iron in an adult is 3,000 mg-5,000 mg and most of it is in the circulating red cell compartment. Men and nonmenstruating women lose about 1 mg of iron per day. The liver and kidney do not have a mechanism for excess iron excretion, and iron is only lost through blood loss or exfoliation of skin and mucosal cells. Pregnancy and delivery are associated with a loss of approximately 1,500 mL of blood and 700 mg of iron. Each mL of red cells contains 1 mg of iron; therefore, 500 mL of blood contains 200 mg of iron if the hematocrit is 40%. Iron absorption occurs mostly in the first segment of the duodenum. Heme iron absorption is more efficiently absorbed than inorganic iron. The bioavailability of nonheme iron requires acid digestion and varies by an order of magnitude, depending on the concentration of enhancers (eg, ascorbate, meat) and inhibitors (eg, calcium, fiber, tea, coffee and wine) found in the diet. Copper deficiency is associated with iron deficiency anemia since ferroxidases such as ceruloplasmin and hephaestin act as oxidases of ferrous iron and are required for optimal mobilization of iron from cells to plasma. Only 5%-10% of dietary iron is absorbed if iron stores are normal and can increase to 15%-30% in iron deficiency. However, iron deficiency ensues if the continuous losses of iron through bleeding exceed the increased absorption. Initially, there is lost of storage iron without anemia, a state known as iron depletion. As the losses continue, iron deficiency anemia develops. The most common source of bleeding in the nonmenstruating female is the GI tract. Most nonheme dietary iron is in the ferric (Fe^{3+}) form and is reduced to the ferrous (Fe^{2+}) form by the ferrireductase DCYTB on the enterocyte brush border. Fe^{2+} ions are transported across the apical membrane by DMT1 (divalent metal transporter 1), which also transports divalent forms of manganese, cobalt, copper, zinc, and lead. Metal transport depends on cotransport of protons in the same inward direction, and antacids can interfere with iron absorption. Iron in the ferrous form is exported through the basolateral membrane of enterocytes through ferroportin, which is the only iron exporter in iron-transporting cells. The hepatic peptide hormone hepcidin binds to ferroportin and leads to its degradation, acting as a negative regulator of intestinal iron absorption and macrophage iron recycling. Iron is converted to the ferric state in the basolateral membrane through the action of the copper oxidase protein hephaestin. Ferric iron binds to plasma transferrin with an extremely high affinity. Binding of transferrin to the transferrin receptor on the surface of cells, especially erythroid precursors, allows internalization of iron bound to transferrin, and DMT1 is once again involved in transport of iron-bound transferrin across the endosomal membrane. Within the cytoplasm, iron is sequestered by ferritin, which is a polymeric protein basket. Serum ferritin can be low in hypothyroidism and ascorbate deficiency, and elevated in inflammatory states. However, a plasma ferritin concentration below 12 ng/mL is virtually diagnostic of absent iron stores. Acute and chronic damage to the liver may increase ferritin levels dramatically through inflammatory processes or release of tissue ferritin. The iron supply to tissues can be assessed by plasma iron and total iron-binding capacity. The transferrin saturation is the ratio of serum iron to total iron-binding capacity. Serum iron and transferrin saturation are low with iron deficiency, but both these measurements can be unreliable. Serum iron has large circadian fluctuations and is decreased in the setting of infection, inflammation and malignancy through elevated hepcidin. Serum iron is increased in aplastic and sideroblastic anemias, ineffective erythropoiesis and liver disease. Iron deficiency anemia is not an end diagnosis and the cause must be determined. Patients with IDA may have inadequate dietary intake, hampered absorption, or blood loss.

Section A: Anemias

Thalassemia Minor

Janet L Kwiatkowski

Patient A 9-year-old girl of Italian descent with microcytic anemia noted on routine blood count.

Clinical History The child was brought to her pediatrician for routine well-child care. She had been growing steadily with height at the 3rd percentile and weight at the 10th-25th percentile. Her past history is significant for mild splenomegaly with a hemoglobin level of 9 g/dL. She was found to have acute Epstein-Barr viral infection at that time. She also has reactive airways disease.

Family History Her father is Italian and has known β-thalassemia trait. His height is 5 feet 8 inches. Her mother is ¾ Italian and ¼ German. She has no history of anemia. Her height is 4 feet 11 inches. The family history is otherwise noncontributory.

Medications None.

Physical Examination Very well appearing, interactive child. Vital signs normal. Height 125 cm (3rd %); Weight 27.8 kg (10th %- 25th%). She had no frontal bossing or maxillary hyperplasia. There was no scleral icterus or conjunctival pallor. Her heart exam showed no murmur or gallop. She had no hepatomegaly but her spleen tip was just palpable. The remainder of her examination was normal.

Initial Work-Up

CBC		WBC Differential	%	# (×10³/μL)
WBC (×10³/μL)	5.7	Neutrophils	58	3.3
RBC (×10⁶/μL)	6.36	Bands	0	
HGB (g/dL)	10.2	Lymphocytes	35	2.0
HCT (%)	34.7	Monocytes	5	0.3
MCV (fL)	54.5	Eosinophils	1	0.1
MCH (pg)	16	Basophils	0	
MCHC (g/dL)	29.3	NRBC	1 per 100 WBC	
PLT (×10³/μL)	310	Reticulocyte count (%)	1.6	
RDW-CV (%)	16			
MPV (fL)	6.3			

Peripheral blood smear revealed microcytic red cells, mild hypochromia, and basophilic stippling (**Figure 1**).

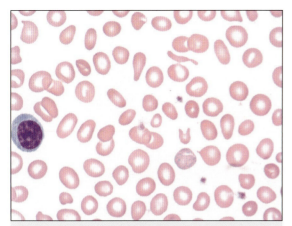

Figure 1 Blood smear (Wright-Giemsa, ×1000) showing anisopoikilocytosis, microcytic red cells, mild hypochromia, and basophilic stippling.

Differential Diagnosis Clinical conditions generally associated with microcytic anemia include β-thalassemia trait, α-thalassemia trait, hemoglobin E disease, hemoglobin E trait, hemoglobin Lepore disease, hemoglobin Lepore trait, iron deficiency anemia, sideroblastic anemia, and lead poisoning. However, microcytic anemia with erythrocytosis, as seen in this case, narrows the differential diagnosis essentially to thalassemia trait (β or α) and hemoglobin E trait/disease.

Additional Work-Up
- Hemoglobin quantitation by high pressure liquid chromatography (HPLC): 91.7% A, 6.3% A_2, 2% F
- β-globin gene analysis: heterozygosity for a nonsense codon 39 mutation of the β-globin gene
- α-globin gene analysis: triplicated α (genotype: α-α/α-α-α)

Iron studies Normal.

Final Diagnosis β-thalassemia trait and α triplication.

Management Approach The most important aspect of the management of β-thalassemia trait involves genetic counseling. When a child is diagnosed with β-thalassemia trait, the parents should be tested to see if they have a risk of having a child with a clinically significant hemoglobinopathy. This testing should include a CBC, with attention to the hemoglobin level, MCV and RBC count, and hemoglobin electrophoresis with HbA_2 and HbF quantitation. It is important to assess for sickle trait and HbE trait as well, to determine if there is a risk of sickle cell disease (S-β-thalassemia) or hemoglobin E-β-thalassemia (a thalassemia syndrome), respectively. In addition, the child will need similar counseling when she is older. Iron supplementation is not necessary and could potentially be detrimental because iron absorption may be slightly increased in β-thalassemia trait, which could lead to iron overload with prolonged iron administration.

General Discussion β-thalassemia trait causes no clinical symptoms. Hematologic findings include microcytosis, an elevated RBC count, and mild or no anemia. Individuals may be misdiagnosed as having iron deficiency anemia, and often receive courses of iron therapy before the diagnosis is made. The correct diagnosis can limit unnecessary diagnostic testing, anxiety, and inappropriate iron supplementation. The diagnosis of β-thalassemia trait is usually made with hemoglobin quantitation that reveals elevated A_2 levels (>3.5%). Hemoglobin F also may be modestly elevated. Less commonly, normal A_2 levels may be present in β-thalassemia trait if iron deficiency coexists and also with certain concomitant δ-globin gene mutations; unexplained microcytosis should be evaluated with α- and β-globin gene testing. In this case, the mild splenomegaly as well as the nucleated red blood cell on white cell differential suggested the possibility of a more significant thalassemia syndrome. This prompted α-globin gene analysis, which revealed an α-globin gene triplication on 1 allele (5 α-genes total). The β-thalassemia phenotype is related to the imbalance of α- and β-globin gene production: excess α chains precipitate causing hemolysis and ineffective erythropoiesis. While in β-thalassemia trait, the globin imbalance is not clinically significant, the concomitant presence of additional α genes worsens this imbalance (higher α to β-globin ratio) and can lead to a β-thalassemia intermedia phenotype. Thus, this child will be monitored periodically to ensure appropriate growth and lack of symptoms related to ineffective erythropoiesis (such as frontal bossing/maxillary hyperplasia, fractures, symptomatic extramedullary hematopoiesis).

Section A: Anemias

Anemia Associated with Hypotransferrinemia

Jaime Caro, Ubaldo Martinez-Outschoorn

Patient A 17-year-old female of northern European ancestry was evaluated because of progressive fatigue and weakness.

Clinical History The patient had been diagnosed with iron deficiency anemia 6 months prior and was started on oral iron therapy with no improvement in symptoms despite being compliant with the oral iron intake. Her internist had recommended intravenous iron infusions and she consulted us for a second opinion. Her menses were regular lasting approximately 2 days to 4 days, and did not require frequent pad changes. There was no history or evidence of gastrointestinal or genitourinary blood loss.

Family History Her mother had been diagnosed with a mild uncharacterized anemia since childhood. Her father had never been tested. Of interest, her parents are first-degree cousins.

Medications Ferrous sulfate.

Physical Examination Her exam was remarkable for pallor and palpable hepatomegaly with liver span of 16 cm in midclavicular line. She did not have jaundice.

Initial Work-Up

CBC		WBC Differential	%	# (×10³/μL)
WBC (×10³/μL)	4	Neutrophils	60	2.4
RBC (×10⁶/μL)	3.9	Bands	0	
HGB (g/dL)	8.2	Lymphocytes	25	1.0
HCT (%)	29.1	Monocytes	10	0.4
MCV (fL)	69	Eosinophils	4	0.2
MCH (pg)	21.0	Basophils	2	0.1
MCHC (g/dL)	28.3	Reticulocytes %	0.6	23.4
PLT (×10³/μL)	397			
RDW-CV (%)	18			

Peripheral blood smear revealed microcytic hypochromic red cells (**Figure 1**).

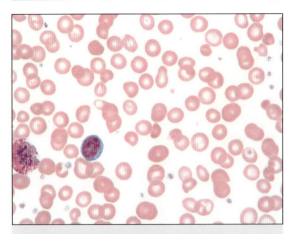

Figure 1 Blood smear (Wright-Giemsa, ×1000) showing microcytic hypochromic red cells.

Differential Diagnosis Conditions associated with hypochromic, microcytic anemia includes iron deficiency, thalassemia, chronic inflammatory diseases and congenital or acquired sideroblastic anemias. In a young female, the most common diagnosis is iron deficiency secondary to increased menstrual bleeding. However, our patient had no history of bleeding and had no response to iron therapy that she took for about 6 months.

Additional Work-Up

Serum iron studies
- Iron 15 μg/dL (normal 75-175)
- Iron-binding capacity 20 μg/dL (normal 250-400)
- Ferritin 2,500 ng/mL (normal 20-200)
- In view of the low iron-binding capacity, a transferrin level by radioimmunoassay (RIA) was obtained
- Serum transferrin 40 mg/dL (normal 204-306)

Liver MRI with iron quantification showed severe iron deposition.

Differential Diagnosis The presence of a very high serum ferritin is not consistent with iron deficiency. Most importantly, the low iron-binding capacity suggests a defect in plasma iron transport. This defect was confirmed by the finding of very low serum transferrin.

Final Diagnosis Anemia associated with hypotransferrinemia.

Management Approach Plasma infusions can replace the missing transferrin and alleviate this condition. Plasma infusions raise the plasma transferrin level for approximately 1 week, which allows erythroblast uptake of iron and maturation with reversal of anemia. This patient was initially started on weekly plasma infusions. Once her hemoglobin level normalized, she was started on a phlebotomy program to remove the excess parenchymal iron stores and then she continued on a monthly plasma replacement.

General Discussion Hypotransferrinemia is a rare hereditary condition where transferrin is low or absent. With insufficient transferrin, most plasma iron cannot be delivered to the maturing erythrocyte and the normal pattern of iron distribution is dramatically altered. This condition is generally inherited in an autosomal recessive pattern. Most individuals with hereditary hypotransferrinemia are diagnosed in childhood, although diagnosis later in life has been reported. The typical presentation is of an iron deficiency anemia unresponsive to iron replacement, even in the intravenous form. Poor response to oral iron therapy is also seen in defects of intestinal iron absorption, but those patients respond to IV iron. In our patient's case, both parents had plasma transferrin levels that were approximately half normal values, suggesting that the patient is either homozygous for a transferrin mutation or, more likely, a compound heterozygote. Hypotransferrinemia can also be acquired and has been described in patients with nephrotic syndrome and patients with erythroleukemia. In atransferrinemia, erythroblasts have decreased iron uptake, leading to a hypochromic microcytic anemia. Importantly, there is also increased intestinal iron absorption and deposition in non-hematopoietic tissues by the non-transferrin-mediated iron uptake system, leading to severe iron overload. The use of IV iron in these patients is greatly contraindicated. Patients with atransferrinemia may have recurrent bacterial infections, which may be related to the presence of free plasma iron that may stimulate bacterial overgrowth. Although rare, the diagnosis should be suspected in cases of hypochromic anemias not responding to oral or IV iron infusions. The diagnosis is established by the finding of low iron-binding capacity and low or absent plasma transferrin. In most cases, plasma or transferrin infusions correct the anemia and the iron overload, suggesting that transferrin allows body iron stores to be reutilized for hemoglobin synthesis.

β-Thalassemia Major

Janet L Kwiatkowski

Patient An 8-month-old girl of Italian descent, who was brought to her pediatrician for routine well-child care.

Clinical History Past history revealed that she was a full-term infant with no complications of the pregnancy or delivery. A complete blood count obtained on first day of her life revealed a hemoglobin level of 14.5 g/dL and an MCV of 102.2 fL. She had no neonatal jaundice. Her newborn screen was "indeterminate" for hemoglobinopathy. The child's diet consisted of breast milk exclusively until age 6 months, with appropriate iron supplementation. Subsequently, iron-fortified formula, infant cereals, and stage 1 foods were added to her diet. She was reported to be a "poor feeder" for at least a few months. The family had not noted any jaundice, pallor, fussiness, or change in activity level. Her stools were normal without evidence of blood. Past history and review of systems were otherwise noncontributory.

Family History Both parents are of Italian descent. The child's mother had been diagnosed with β-thalassemia trait. In addition, there was a history of anemia in multiple family members on the maternal side. There was no history of anemia on the paternal side. The father had undergone testing for hemoglobinopathies in the past and was not diagnosed with β-thalassemia trait. The child has no siblings.

Medications None.

Physical Examination The child appeared pale. Her heart rate was 164 beats per minute. Her weight was 7.1 kg (10th percentile for age), length 67.5 cm (40th percentile for age), and head circumference 42 cm (10th percentile for age). She had subtle frontal bossing. Her sclerae were anicteric and her conjunctivae were pale. Her heart exam showed tachycardia and II/VI systolic ejection murmur. Her spleen was palpable 4 cm beneath the left costal margin. The remainder of her exam was normal.

Initial Work-Up

CBC		WBC Differential	%	# (×10^3/μL)
WBC (×10^3/μL)	18.4	Neutrophils	19	3.5
RBC (×10^6/μL)	2.31	Bands	0	
HGB (g/dL)	5.9	Lymphocytes	76	14.0
HCT (%)	16.0	Monocytes	3	0.6
MCV (fL)	68	Eosinophils	1	0.2
MCH (pg)	25.3	Basophils	1	0.2
PLT (×10^3/μL)	153	NRBC	16 per 100 WBC	
RDW-CV (%)	35.1			

Peripheral blood smear revealed anisocytosis, poikilocytosis, microcytic hypochromic red cells, target cells and nucleated red cells (**Figure 1**).

Section A: Anemias
β-Thalassemia Major

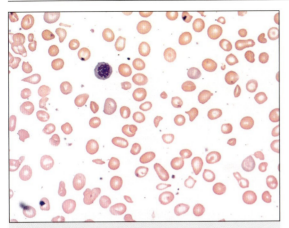

Figure 1 Blood smear (Wright-Giemsa, ×500) showing anisocytosis, poikilocytosis, microcytic red cells, hypochromia, and target cells. A nucleated red blood cell is also present.

Differential Diagnosis Differential diagnosis of microcytic hypochromic anemia typically includes iron deficiency, thalassemia, anemia of chronic disease, and sideroblastic anemia. However, the history and peripheral blood findings are suggestive of thalassemia major or intermedia.

Additional Work-Up
- Hemoglobin quantitation by HPLC: 9.6% A, 2.4% A2, 88% F
- Serum iron 307 μg/dL, iron saturation 84%, and ferritin 146 ng/mL
- Father's CBC: HGB 13.7 g/dL, MCV 61.4 fL, RBC $7.24 \times 10^6/\mu L$
- Hemoglobin quantitation by HPLC: 95.1% A, 3.3% A2, 1.6% F; normal iron studies
- Mother's CBC: HGB 12.5 g/dL, MCV 64.9 fL, RBC $6.2 \times 10^6/\mu L$
- Hemoglobin quantitaion by HPLC: A2 was elevated (complete results not available)

The child's β-globin gene analysis revealed homozygosity for the IVS1, 110 mutation (β^+/β^+). Both parents were heterozygous for this mutation.

Final Diagnosis β-thalassemia major.

Management Approach The only current curative therapy for thalassemia major is hematopoietic progenitor cell transplantation (HPCT). HLA-matched sibling donor HPCT in children is associated with thalassemia-free survival approaching 90%. Unrelated donor HPCT, particularly with extended HLA-haplotype matching has been used with increasingly good results. Reduced intensity conditioning regimens to limit treatment-related toxicity are under study. In the absence of HPCT, management consists of a regular red cell transfusion protocol to maintain the trough hemoglobin level at 9-9.5 g/dL and iron chelation therapy to reduce transfusional iron loading. Genetic counseling must be provided to discuss the risk of future children being affected with β-thalassemia major (25% in this case) as well as options of pre-implantation genetic diagnosis and prenatal testing. Given the lack of a sibling donor, this child was managed with a chronic transfusion program, receiving transfusions every 3-4 weeks. Chelation therapy will be initiated after a couple of years of transfusion.

General Discussion This child's presentation is typical as β-thalassemia major often presents between 3 months and 1 year of age, when γ-globin production wanes and β-globin is instead produced. Signs and symptoms include pallor, poor feeding, poor growth, and fussiness. On physical exam, frontal bossing, maxillary hyperplasia, pallor, tachycardia and hepatosplenomegaly may be present. Thalassemia major refers to a *phenotype* in which chronic transfusions are indicated, and can be seen with β^0, β^+, or a combination of these genotypes. Indications for transfusion therapy include hemoglobin level <7 g/dL and/or clinical symptoms such as poor growth and facial bony changes. The diagnosis of β-thalassemia major may be suggested by newborn screen if no hemoglobin A is present; however, with β^+ mutations, some hemoglobin A may be produced and the diagnosis may only be apparent later. In this child's case, the newborn screen was indeterminant. Her diagnosis was made based on hemoglobin quantitation, with only 9.6% hemoglobin A at 8 months and subsequently confirmed with β-globin gene analysis. Genetic counseling of at-risk families is imperative. In this case, the parents' risk of having a child with β-thalassemia major was not recognized, because the father's hemoglobin A_2 level was normal. However, his red cell microcytosis with an elevated red blood cell count suggests a thalassemia trait (α or β), and β-thalassemia trait was confirmed here with β-globin gene analysis. Normal hemoglobin A_2 levels can be seen with thalassemia trait in the presence of concomitant iron deficiency or δ-globin mutations. Thus, it is important to examine both the CBC and hemoglobin electrophoresis when screening for the carrier state.

Anemia Associated with Lead Poisoning

John R Krause, Gene Gulati, Joanne Filicko O'Hara

Patient A 5-year-old Caucasian male brought to the emergency room with symptoms of vomiting and abdominal pain.

Clinical History The child had been well and growing normally.

Family History Noncontributory.

Medications None.

Physical Examination The child was very restless and irritable. He was responsive to commands. There was mild rebound tenderness on abdominal exam but no organomegaly.

Initial Work-Up

CBC		WBC Differential	%	# (×10³/µL)
WBC (×10³/µL)	7.8	Neutrophils	40	3.12
RBC (×10⁶/µL)	4.04	Bands	10	0.78
HGB (g/dL)	10.3	Lymphocytes	45	3.5
HCT (%)	31.5	Monocytes	5	0.39
MCV (fl)	78			
MCH (pg)	25.5			
MCHC (%)	32.7			
PLT (×10³/µL)	175			
RDW-CV (%)	16			

Peripheral blood smear revealed coarse basophilic stippling (Figures 1 and 2).

Differential Diagnosis There is a slight microcytic anemia. The most impressive finding was the coarse basophilic stippling present in the red blood cells. Coarse basophilic stippling is usually associated with impaired hemoglobin synthesis and may be seen in such conditions as megaloblastic anemia, thalassemias, hemoglobinopathies, sideroblastic anemia, myelodysplastic syndromes and lead poisoning.

Additional Work-Up A blood lead level was significantly elevated at 65 µg/dL.

Final Diagnosis Lead poisoning.

Management Approach Identification and removal of the source of lead exposure is an essential part of the management. Chelation therapy is considered essential for symptomatic patients irrespective of

Section A: Anemias
Anemia Associated with Lead Poisoning

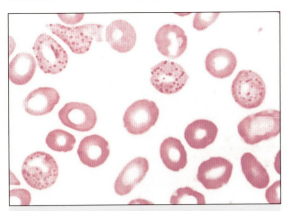

Figure 1 Blood smear (Wright, ×1000) showing coarse basophilic stippling in several red cells.

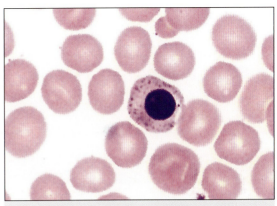

Figure 2 Blood smear (Wright, ×1000) showing coarse basophilic stippling in a nucleated red blood cell.

their blood lead level, and asymptomatic patients with blood level of ≥70 µg/dL, and is recommended also for asymptomatic patients with blood lead levels under 70 µg/dL and over 25 µg/dL. Calcium-disodium EDTA and dimercaptosuccinic acid or DMSA (Succimer) have been used as chelating agents. Supportive therapy is used as needed. Gastric lavage may be necessary to remove soluble lead compounds. This child was treated with intravenous calcium-sodium EDTA. Several cycles of therapy were given before the blood lead values decreased to safe levels.

General Discussion The child was initially thought to have a viral gastroenteritis. The true cause of the gastroenteritis became more apparent upon taking a detailed history that revealed that the child had been living in a 50+-year-old home that was undergoing extensive renovations. This history along with the child's symptoms and presence of coarse basophilic stippling prompted a blood lead level that was elevated. From the hematology aspect, the child did not fit into the category of a hemoglobinopathy or thalassemia, which would be common causes for coarse basophilic stippling in his age group. The anemia was only mildly microcytic whereas thalassemia minor has a much lower MCV and normal or elevated RBC count. Hemoglobinopathies and thalassemia major would show more poikilocytosis including target cells, which were not a feature of this case. The other entities in the differential diagnosis, except for lead poisoning, do not fit with the presentation, physical findings, and CBC findings. Lead poisoning is often associated with a hypochromic microcytic anemia but may present as normocytic hypochromic anemia in some cases. Basophilic stippling is thought to represent aggregates of ribosomes occurring during air drying and staining. Coarse basophlic stippling occurs in the entities listed above. Fine basophlic stipplng, which is much more frequent, is associated with increased red cell production and is commonly seen with increased polychromasia. Fine basophilic stippling is not clinically significant. In children, lead poisoning generally results from ingestion of flaking lead paint or from chewing lead-painted toys. In adults, it results primarily from inhalation of lead compounds used in industrial processes. Other sources of lead exposure include old battery casings, improperly glazed earthenware, gasoline sniffing, etc. Chronic toxicity is more common compared to acute toxicity. Clinical manifestations may include one or more of the following features: encephalopathy, drowsiness, convulsions, stupor, abdominal colic, general malaise, nausea, vomiting, weight loss, anorexia, constipation, apathy, peripheral neuropathy with wrist drop or foot drop, and lead nephrosis resulting in albuminuria, hematuria, and pyuria, gout, and anemia. Acute encephalopathy may be the presenting feature of severe lead poisoning in some cases. Basophilic stippling, when present, represents a strong clue for lead poisoning but its absence can not be used to exclude lead poisoning.

Section A: Anemias

Thalassemia Intermedia

Suba Krishnan

Patient A 7-year-old male, who was referred to a pediatric hematologist for detailed evaluation of his anemia.

Clinical History The patient is of Arab ancestry (parents are recent first generation immigrants from Lebanon) and is known to be anemic since 6 months of age. However, he had no symptoms related to anemia and there was no history of transfusion with whole blood or packed red cells.

Family History He has 1 sibling (5-year-old sister with normal CBC).

Medications None.

Physical Examination Pertinent findings on examination were mild pallor, a grade II/VI systolic ejection murmur over left parasternal edge and soft, nontender spleen tip measuring about 1 cm below left costal margin. Normal dentition and growth parameters: height 50th percentile for age, weight 25th percentile for age.

Initial Work-Up

CBC		WBC Differential	%	# (×10³/μL)
WBC (×10³/μL)	8.1	Neutrophils	46	3.7
RBC (×10⁶/μL)	4.1	Bands	0	
HGB (g/dL)	9.0	Lymphocytes	44	3.6
HCT (%)	28	Monocytees	4	0.3
MCV (fL)	57	Eosinophils	3	0.2
MCH (pg)	24.1	Basophils	3	0.2
PLT (×10³/μL)	161	Reticulocyte count	3.1	
RDW-CV (%)	12.1			

Peripheral blood smear revealed hypochromasia, microcytosis, polychromasia, target cells, and variation in the size of red cells (**Figure 1**).

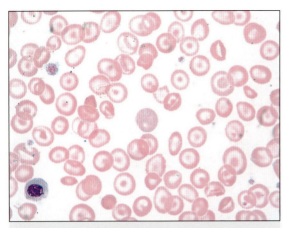

Figure 1 Blood smear (Wright-Giemsa, ×1000) showing microcytic and hypochromic red cells, target cells, polychromasia and a nucleated red cell.

Differential Diagnosis Diagnostic considerations for microcytic hypochromic anemia in a child would include iron deficiency anemia, thalassemia, and the rarer condition of hereditary sideroblastic anemia; presence of reticulocytosis would raise the suspicion of inherited or acquired hemolytic anemias and, more rarely, idiopathic pulmonary hemosiderosis (which would have a picture of iron deficiency with reticulocytosis).

Additional Work-Up
- Normal iron studies, direct antiglobulin test (DAT): negative
- Hemoglobin quantitation by HPLC: HbA: 60.1%, HbA2, 5.3% HbF: 34.6%

In acquired hemolytic anemias such as autoimmune hemolytic anemia, normocytic anemia would be the rule; patient's DAT or direct Coombs test was negative. The anemia associated with most congenital and acquired hemolytic anemias (other than thalassemias) is usually a normocytic anemia, and the hemoglobin electrophoresis (and CBC and mild clinical features) is consistent with a diagnosis of β-thalassemia intermedia. β-globin gene analysis confirmed that the child was homozygous for IVSI-6(T-C) mutation- homozygous β+ mutation without any associated compound heterozygosity. Additionally, his mild splenomegaly and absence of prior need for packed RBC transfusions are also consistent with clinical features of thalassemia intermedia.

Diagnosis Thalassemia intermedia.

Management Approach Mainstay of management involves frequent monitoring of hematologic and clinical status and education of child's family about when to seek emergent medical care. The severity of clinical phenotype is the only differentiation between the 2 main thalassemia subtypes with clinical consequences: thalassemia major and thalassemia intermedia. Even though the IVSI-6(T-C) mutation has the mildest phenotype, it is very difficult, if not impossible, to predict phenotypic expression from genotype in thalassemia intermedia (this patient is homogzygous for this mutation). The onset of thalassemia intermedia is usually later in life with a milder anemia that does not require transfusions to maintain adequate hemoglobin levels during early childhood. As a result most thalassemia Intermedia patients are closely monitored without blood transfusions.

Indications to transfuse in children relate to poor growth, delayed sexual maturation, intercurrent infections, or prior to surgery. Accordingly, if patients are unable to maintain hemoglobin levels >6-7 g/dL, the following interventions can be tried:
- Routine 3-4 week blood transfusions to maintain pretransfusion hemoglobin levels close to 10 g/dL; once commenced on chronic transfusion therapy, iron status must be carefully monitored and iron overload should be aggressively managed with chelation therapy
- Splenectomy
- Hydroxyurea therapy

In some patients, spleen begins to enlarge with progressive anemia. Such patients could respond to splenectomy with intermittent blood transfusion support. However, because of the risk of developing pulmonary hypertension following splenectomy, this option is now uncommon in children and is mainly performed late in life. Some patients with severe thalassemia intermedia may eventually require or opt for allogeneic hematopoietic progenitor cell transplantation (HPCT), similar to that performed in patients with thalassemia major. This is a reasonable alternative to transfusion and chelation if an HLA-matched sibling donor is available. This child will be frequently monitored by CBCs to assess whether he continues to maintain adequate hemoglobin levels and satisfactory growth (by height/weight indices) without transfusion support. He was placed on daily folic acid supplementation to support the increased bone marrow erythropoietic activity. However, he may require transfusion prior to surgeries or while suffering from an infection (patients with congenital hemolytic anemias are susceptible to bone marrow suppression by viral infections including parvovirus B19). The decision to place him on long-term transfusion therapy will be determined by his growth indices and Tanner staging (sexual maturity staging). He will receive all routine childhood immunizations as recommended for his age. In addition, if he is negative for hepatitis A immune status, he will receive anti-hepatitis A vaccine regardless of his infection status with hepatitis C since hepatitis A infections in patients with hepatitis C can lead to fulminant liver disease. Should he require splenectomy, he will be immunized against *Streptococcus pneumoniae* with the 23-valent pneumococcal polysaccharide vaccine prior to splenectomy, and boosters given every 5 years if pneumococcal immunoglobin titers are negative. He should be able to tolerate most daily activities, including as he grows older, participation in gym and physical exercise activities in school. Parents and caregivers should be instructed to be on the lookout for exercise intolerance, which may be a warning signal for worsening anemia and the need for initiation of blood transfusions. They should also be aware that abdominal trauma can cause splenic rupture. Additionally, in some patients, extramedullary hematopoiesis can lead to bony deformities and fractures from mild trauma, particularly if the patient is not on chronic transfusion therapy to suppress bone marrow activity. He will also be closely monitored for the development of gallstones and may require cholecystectomy in the future. The child's parents and extended family will be offered genetic counseling for future pregnancies.

General Discussion Most symptoms of thalassemia intermedia are seen to a greater extent in thalassemia major. However patients with thalassemia intermedia experience a few specific complications that are rare in thalassemia major:

– Cholelithiasis requiring cholecsytectomy
– Extramedullary hematopoiesis leading to the formation of erythropoietic tissue masses that can be detected by magnetic resonance imaging. These masses may cause neurological problems such as spinal cord compression and paraplegia and intrathoracic masses. These masses are radiosensitive and can be managed by radiotherapy, hydroxyurea treatment or chronic transfusion therapy to suppress the extramedullary hematopoiesis
– Leg ulcers are more common in older than in younger patients with thalassemia intermedia and are hard to treat. It has been postulated that poor tissue oxygenation results in formation of these ulcers and also makes them recalcitrant to therapy
– Hypercoagulability: Patients with thalassemia intermedia have an increased risk of thrombosis compared with healthy controls and with thalassemia major patients. Deep vein thrombosis, pulmonary thromboembolism and recurrent arterial occlusion have been described in patients with thalassemia intermedia, occurring in most cases without additional risk factors
– Pulmonary hypertension is a leading cause of congestive heart failure in thalassemia intermedia patients (noted initially in splenectomized patients)

Anemia Associated with Copper Deficiency

Jaime Caro, Ubaldo Martinez-Outschoorn

Patient A 60-year-old female of northern European ancestry was referred from the neurology clinic for evaluation of microcytic anemia accompanied by mild neutropenia and thrombocytopenia.

Clinical History The patient had a history of depression and described progressive fatigue for the past year. She also complained of pain and numbness in the fingertips and she had an unsteady gait with numerous falls. There was no history of bleeding. Gastrointestinal and genitourinary evaluations were negative. A blood count during routine evaluation performed 3 years before was completely normal.

Family History Unremarkable. No family history of anemia.

Medications She had been taking high doses of over-the-counter zinc supplements for several years for the prevention of common colds.

Physical Examination She was a thin female with pallor, poor dentition, but no palpable lymphadenopathy or hepatosplenomegaly, and no jaundice. Neurologic examination was significant for faint tremor, decreased vibration and position sensation, normal strength in all 4 extremities, patellar reflexes 1/4 bilaterally, and downward plantar reflexes bilaterally.

Initial Work-Up

CBC		WBC Differential	%	# (×10^3/µL)
WBC (×10^3/µL)	3.0	Neutrophils	30	0.9
RBC (×10^6/µL)	4.01	Bands	0	
HGB (g/dL)	8.5	Lymphocytes	60	1.8
HCT (%)	28.9	Monocytes	6	0.2
MCV (fL)	72	Eosinophils	3	0.1
MCH (pg)	21.2	Basophils	1	0.0
MCHC (g/dL)	29.4			
PLT (×10^3/µL)	120			
RDW-CV (%)	16			

Peripheral smear showed microcytosis and neutropenia. No abnormal cells or blasts were seen.

Differential Diagnosis The differential diagnosis of pancytopenia includes nutritional deficiencies, toxins and medications, infections, infiltrative processes of the marrow, hypersplenism, and primary bone marrow stem cells disorders. Vitamin B_{12}, folate and copper deficiency, toxins such as ethanol or lead, and medications such as methotrexate and cancer chemotherapy are all associated with pancytopenia. Infections such as EBV infection, viral hepatitis, HIV, and tuberculosis are also frequent causes of pancytopenia. Primary bone marrow disorders that cause pancytopenia include aplastic anemia, paroxysmal nocturnal hemoglobinuria, myelodysplastic syndrome, leukemia and lymphoma. Infiltrative and autoimmune diseases such as metastatic carcinoma with bone

Section A: Anemias
Anemia Associated with Copper Deficiency

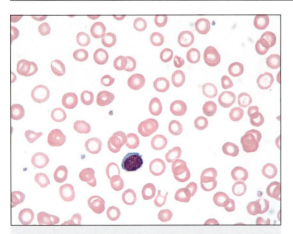

Figure 1 Blood smear (Wright-Giemsa, ×1000) showing microcytic hypochromic red cells.

marrow infiltration, Gaucher disease and autoimmune pancytopenia, as seen in systemic lupus erythematosus, are other well-described causes of pancytopenia. We were concerned about vitamin B_{12} deficiency in this patient with pancytopenia and neuropathy. However, the presence of microcytic anemia made this diagnosis unlikely unless there was a combined B_{12} and iron deficiency.

Additional Work-Up

Serum chemistries:
- Iron 80 μg/dL (normal 75-175)
- TIBC 260 μg/dL (normal 250-400)
- Ferritin 250 ng/mL (normal 20-200)
- Vitamin B_{12} 290 pg/mL (normal 180-900)
- Folate 7 ng/mL (normal 3-18)

The findings of normal serum iron, TIBC and ferritin argue against iron deficiency. Similarly, normal B_{12} and folic acid levels rule out these deficiencies. A bone marrow examination was considered to rule out a primary stem cell disorder or an infiltrative disorder. However, the history of large intake of zinc supplements made us suspicious of an acquired copper deficiency and serum copper studies were ordered.
- Serum copper 1 μmol/L (normal 11-22)
- Ceruloplasmin 5 mg/L (normal 270-370)

Final Diagnosis Pancytopenia related to copper deficiency. The finding of normal blood counts in the past indicates an acquired disorder.

Management Approach The majority of patients show an improvement in their CBC with copper supplements or in mild cases by eliminating excess dietary zinc or zinc supplements. In severe cases, the initial treatment should include intravenous supplementation. The neurological symptoms usually improve but they may persist if significant damage has already occurred. This patient was treated with oral copper supplements (2 mg capsules/day) until her symptoms improved. She was also told to stop using zinc supplements.

General Discussion Copper deficiency is often characterized by a microcytic hypochromic anemia that does not respond to iron therapy. A diagnosis of copper deficiency is usually established by measuring serum copper or ceruloplasmin levels. Acquired copper deficiency most commonly presents with myeloneuropathy that resembles vitamin B_{12} deficiency. Bone marrow findings with copper deficiency include ringed sideroblasts, vacuolization of granulocytic and erythroid precursors, megaloblastic changes, prominent hemosiderin and can be confused with myelodysplasia. The most common causes of copper deficiency are malabsorption and malnutrition. It has been well described in patients undergoing partial gastrectomy for treatment of morbid obesity. Copper deficiency also occurs after chronic use of large doses of zinc. Important copper-binding proteins include ceruloplasmin, cytochrome-c oxidase and superoxide dismutase (SOD). Ceruloplasmin is a ferroxidase that converts ferrous (Fe^{+2}) to ferric (Fe^{+3}) iron, allowing iron to bind to transferrin. Cytochrome-c oxidase is involved in mitochondrial electron flow and ATP production, and is required for the reduction of ferric iron to incorporate it into the heme molecule, and deficiency leads to iron accumulation in mitochondria, which is visible microscopically as ringed sideroblasts. SOD is an antioxidant enzyme important for erythroblast survival. Copper deficiency and deficiency of the previously listed enzymes leads to impaired heme synthesis and decreased RBC survival. Copper deficiency also decreases transferrin concentration in the plasma and facilitates heme degradation secondary to an increase in heme oxygenase. Metallothionein (MTO) is a copper ligand in enterocytes and has a high affinity for transition metals, forming mercaptide bonds. Excess zinc levels induce the synthesis of MTO, which then binds zinc and lead to its excretion in the feces by enterocyte shedding. However, copper, with its higher affinity for MTO, displaces zinc and also is excreted, reducing the amount of copper delivered to the enterocyte. The neurologic damage may be quite significant and is likely secondary to reactive oxygen species (ROS)-related damage of the neurons. Early treatment may result in resolution of symptoms but severe damage may be irreversible.

Hemoglobin E Disease

Suba Krishnan

Patient A 13-month-old male child with hemoglobin E observed on newborn screening.

Clinical History This toddler was born full term by normal delivery. He was hospitalized for 72 hours for neonatal jaundice noted 24 hours after birth, which resolved with 48 hours of phototherapy. There was no history of exchange transfusion. Laboratory data from the newborn period were not available. Parents were instructed by the child's pediatrician to follow-up with a pediatric hematologist for further evaluation and management. He is asymptomatic and in good health.

Family History Both parents are in good health. This is their second child; their first-born son is in good health and has hemoglobin E trait. Both parents are from Laos.

Medications Multivitamin with iron.

Physical Examination Height is 25th percentile for age; weight is 25th percentile for age. No skin or mucosal pallor was noted. His cardiovascular system was normal, and there was no organomegaly. Variant hemoglobin confirmed as hemoglobin E by electrophoresis (i) at alkaline pH on cellulose acetate (hemoglobin E co-migrates with HbC, HbO Arab and HbA_2), and (ii) citrate agar at acid pH (hemoglobin E co-migrates with HbA_2 and is distinct from HbC), and HPLC (hemoglobin E has similar retention times as HbA_2 and Hb Lepore).

Initial Work-Up

CBC

WBC (×10^3/μL)	10.3	Serum Iron (μg/dL)	35
RBC (×10^6/μL)	6.06	Iron-binding capacity (μg/dL)	387
Hgb (g/dL)	10.3	Ferritin (ng/mL)	32
Hct (%)	33.2		
MCV (fL)	67.3	Hemoglobin electrophoresis	
MCH (pg)	20.4	HbE+HbA_2= 92.3%	
MCHC (g/dL)	33.3	HbA_1=5.3%	
Plt (× 10^3/μL)	385	HbF=2.4%	
RDW-CV (%)	16.2		
Retic count (%)	2.6		

Peripheral blood smear revealed microcytic red cells and target cells (**Figure 1**).

Section A: Anemias
Hemoglobin E Disease

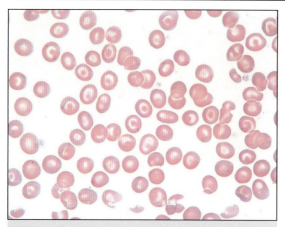

Figure 1 Blood smear (Wright-Giemsa, ×1000) showing microcytic red cells and target cells.

Differential Diagnosis Since newborn screening and hemoglobin electrophoresis have already identified the variant hemoglobin to be HGB E, the differential diagnosis is narrowed to identifying the specific HbE syndrome in this child. Of note, the child's iron studies were not consistent with that of iron deficiency anemia (which must always be considered in the presence of microcytosis in this age group). In this case, the findings of microcytosis with normal hemoglobin, variant hemoglobin being the major hemoglobin present and hemoglobin E + A_2 >90% suggests homozygous hemoglobin E disease.

Additional Work-Up (for confirmation of diagnosis)

Evaluation of Mother's and Father's CBC and Hemoglobin Electrophoresis

Mother		Father	
HGB (g/dL)	11.2	HGB (g/dL)	10.9
MCV (fL)	82	MCV (fL)	84
MCH (pg)	30	MCH (pg)	33
MCHC (g/dL)	33	MCHC (g/dL)	33
HbA_1=72.2%		HbA1=70.7%	
HbF=0.8%		HbF=1.3%	
$HbE+HbA_2$=27%		$HbE+HbA_2$=28%	

Both parents CBC and hemoglobin electrophoresis patterns are consistent with that of HbE trait.

α-globin gene analysis and β-globin gene analysis to rule out compound heterozygosity for α or β-thalassemia
No α gene globin deletions were detected. β-globin gene analysis revealed only the hemoglobin E mutation. DNA sequencing and restriction endonuclease mapping for the β-globin gene cluster failed to reveal the presence of another mutation or a δ β-globin gene mutation. The coinheritance of α-thalassemia often occurs and lowers the percentage of HbE. Iron deficiency also lowers the hemoglobin E percentage. Hemoglobin E β⁺-thalassemia may have an extremely variable laboratory picture. They usually have a mild anemia of approximately 9.5 g/dL. However, significant degree of anemia has been observed, with HGB as low as 5.7 g/dL. The MCV has been approximately 72 ± 6 fL and MCHC has been 29 ± 2 fL.

Final Diagnosis Hemoglobin E disease.

Management Approach Patients with hemoglobin E disease have mild anemia and occasionally may have a slightly enlarged spleen, but are usually asymptomatic and do not require treatment. Most patients are evaluated annually by a haematologist to assess the degree and clinical effects of the mild chronic hemolysis that occurs. This child did not receive any treatment. However, folic acid supplements may occasionally be prescribed to support bone marrow turnover in a subset of patients with reticulocytosis. Interestingly, if a patient with hemoglobin E disease develops diabetes mellitus, HbA_1c cannot be used to monitor their glycemic status because in these patients, the red blood cell lifespan is often variable. In such situations, fructosamine is recommended for monitoring.

General Discussion Due to changing migration patterns of population groups worldwide, the heterogeneous group of HbE disorders is also rapidly increasing in previously unaffected areas of the world. Correct laboratory diagnosis is essential to separate asymptomatic genotypes from severe mutations, and usually necessitates DNA analysis. While the individual with HbE disease is largely unaffected, children of individuals with this condition are at risk of suffering from more serious HbE syndromes that arise from compound heterozygosity involving HbE. Hence genetic counseling of such individuals is crucial. The most serious HbE syndrome is HbE β⁰-thalassemia. The compound heterozygote state of HbE β-thalassemia results in a variable phenotype ranging from a complete lack of symptoms to transfusion dependency. Additional compound heterozygote states include Hb Sickle-E disease (HbSE). SE is also being more frequently diagnosed because of influx of immigrant populations from south east Asian countries in large numbers to areas where sickle cell disease is prevalent. It is important to bear this compound heterozygote state in mind particularly because it can be misdiagnosed as HB SC because of the comigration of C and E patterns on electrophoresis. The clinical phenotype is similar to sickle β⁺-thalassemia. HbE Lepore and HbE δ-β-thalassemia are compound heterozygotes with mild phenotypes. Coinheritance of α-thalassemia often occurs and lowers the percentage of HbE. In summary, care must be taken to accurately differentiate the benign HbE syndromes such as HbEE from those with more serious disorders. Genetic counseling should be offered to all HbEE individuals so they can understand the implications for future offspring.

Congenital Sideroblastic Anemia

John R Krause, Gene Gulati, Joanne Filicko O'Hara

Patient A 12-month-old Caucasian male was found to be anemic at the age of 4 months.

Clinical History The infant had been found to have a hemoglobin of 8.5 g/dL at 4 months of age and was treated with oral and parenteral iron but failed to demonstrate a rise in hemoglobin. He was referred to a pediatric hematologist at a tertiary care hospital for further evaluation.

Family History Both parents and an older male sibling had normal CBC values.

Medications He had been given both oral and parental iron.

Physical examination Normal except for pallor.

Initial Work-Up

CBC		WBC Differential	%	# (×10³/µL)
WBC (×10³/µL)	4.53	Neutrophils	40	1.81
RBC (×10⁶/µL)	3.51	Bands	10	0.45
HGB (g/dL)	6.5	Lymphocytes	33	1.49
HCT (%)	22.4	Monocytes	15	0.67
MCV (fL)	63.8	Eosinophils	2	0.09
MCH (pg)	18.5	Basophils	0	
MCHC (g/dL)	29.0			
PLT (×10³/µL)	259			
RDW-CV (%)	34.0			
MPV (fL)	9.5			

Peripheral blood smear revealed microcytic hypochromic red cells and some anisopoikilocytosis (**Figure 1**).

Section A: Anemias
Congenital Sideroblastic Anemia

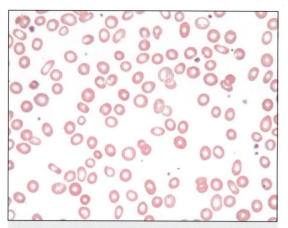

Figure 1 Blood smear (Wright, ×1000) showing anisopoikilocytosis and microcytic and hypochromic red cells.

Differential Diagnosis Clinical conditions associated with microcytic anemia include iron deficiency, thalassemias, certain hemoglobinopathies (eg, hemoglobin Lepore and hemoglobin E), lead poisoning, sideroblastic anemia, and anemia of chronic disease. Peripheral blood findings of microcytc hypochromic anemia with low red cell count and high RDW are suggestive of iron deficiency. However there was no response to oral or parental iron. Further work-up was considered necessary to arrive at the definitive diagnosis.

Additional Work-Up Serum iron was greatly elevated at 262 µg/mL and the total iron-binding capacity was 285 µg/dL. Serum ferritin was very high at 1,200 ng/mL. Bone marrow examination revealed nests of erythroid precursors and increased hemosiderin pigment (**Figures 2** and **3**). In addition to increased iron stores, numerous ring sideroblasts were noted on bone marrow biopsy section and aspirate smears stained with Prussian blue stain (**Figures 4** and **5**). Dysplastic changes were not seen.

Final Diagnosis Congenital sideroblastic anemia.

Management approach Most patients respond to oral pyridoxine therapy in doses of 50 mg-200 mg per day. Some patients may benefit from addition of folic acid to the treatment regimen. Pyridoxine therapy results in an increase in the steady-state hemoglobin level and a decrease in transfusion requirement but it often does not normalize the hemoglobin level and anemia can relapse upon discontinuation of therapy. Iron overload, a common complication of this disorder, may be managed by either phlebotomy or iron-chelation. Marrow transplantation may be considered in the nonresponders. This infant was started on oral pyridoxine, 50 mg/day. The hemoglobin improved to 9.5 g/dL over several months but did not return to normal levels. Red blood cell transfusions continued to be required every 3 months-4 months. Because of the high serum ferritin level, subcutaneous dexferroximine chelation treatment was initiated. The child unfortunately was lost to follow-up.

General Discussion Congenital forms of sideroblastic anemia are rare and constitute a heterogeneous group of disorders. Most individuals are males who develop a hypochromic, microcytic anemia in childhood or early adult years. An X-linked recessive pattern has been described in some families. The underlying pathophysiology is thought to be an impairment of heme biosynthesis. Diminished activity of δ-aminolevulinate synthase (ALA-S), the enzyme catalyzing the first and rate limiting reaction has been found in some cases. A response or partial response to pyridoxine, a cofactor necessary for ALA synthesis, may occasionally occur and is a therapeutic option. However, the prognosis for many of these patients, including the patient described, remains guarded as most individuals eventually succumb to the complications of iron overload.

Section A: Anemias
Congenital Sideroblastic Anemia

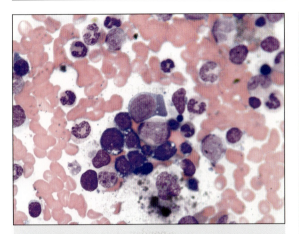

Figure 2 Bone marrow aspirate smear (Wright stain, ×1000) showing cluster of erythroid cells and a histiocyte containing iron pigment.

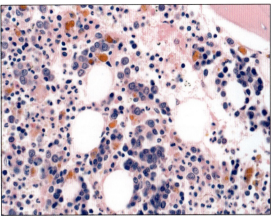

Figure 3 Bone marrow biopsy (H&E, ×500) showing nests of erythroid precursors and increased hemosiderin pigment.

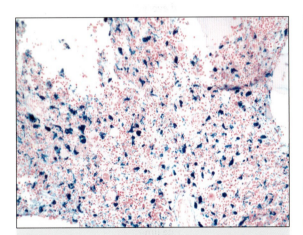

Figure 4 Bone marrow biopsy (Prussian blue, ×200) showing increased iron stores.

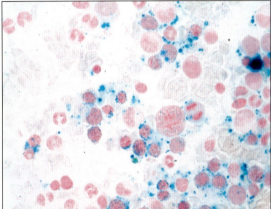

Figure 5 Bone marrow aspirate smear (Prussian blue, ×1000) showing numerous ring sideroblasts.

Section A: Anemias

Macrocytic Anemia Associated with Folate Deficiency

Kathryn Foucar, Melissa Myrsiades

Patient A 31-year-old female presented with fatigue, which had been worsening over the past several months.

Clinical History The patient consumes a fifth of vodka every 2 days-3 days and admits that her diet typically does not include fruits and vegetables, legumes, or fortified cereals or breads.

Family History Unremarkable.

Medications None.

Physical Examination Unremarkable.

Initial Work-Up

CBC		WBC Differential	%	# (×10³/µL)
WBC (×10³/µL)	3.3	Neutrophils	40	1.3
RBC (×10⁶/µL)	1.05	Bands	0	
HGB (g/dL)	4.8	Lymphocytes	59	2.0
HCT (%)	14	Monocytes	1	
MCV (fL)	131	Eosinophils	0	
MCH (pg)	45.7	Basophils	0	
MCHC (g/dL)	34.3			
PLT (×10³/µL)	24			
RDW-CV (%)	29.6			

Peripheral blood smear revealed macrocytic red cells, marked anisopoikilocytosis, rare schistocytes, occasional spherocytes, minimal polychromasia, and occasional circulating megaloblastic nucleated red cells (**Figure 1**). The white blood cells were decreased in number with an absolute neutropenia and monocytopenia. Occasional hypersegmented neutrophils were identified. The platelets were severely decreased with rare giant forms noted.

Section A: Anemias
Macrocytic Anemia Associated with Folate Deficiency

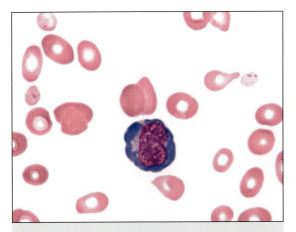

Figure 1 Peripheral blood smear (Wright, ×1000) reveals anisopoikilocytosis, circulating nucleated red blood cell with characteristic megaloblastic change, including "sieve-like" chromatin, pancytopenia and oval macrocytes.

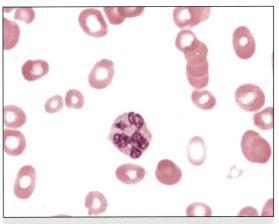

Figure 2 Peripheral blood smear (Wright, ×1000) showing anisopoikilocytosis, polychromatophilic macro-ovalocytes, hypersegmented neutrophil, and red cell fragmentation.

Differential Diagnosis Causes of macrocytic anemia are broad, and include effects from numerous drugs (chemotherapeutic agents, antiretroviral drugs such as zidovudine, antimicrobials such as pyrimethamine, anticonvulsant drugs such as phenytoin, and nitrous oxide). Alcoholism, reticulocytosis, liver disease, hypothyroidism, vitamin deficiencies (vitamin B_{12}, folate), and myelodysplastic syndromes may all cause macrocytosis. Additionally, falsely elevated MCV values may be due to cold agglutinins and hyperglycemia.

Additional Work-Up
- Serum vitamin B_{12} 450 pg/mL (normal 200-1,000)
- Serum folate 4 ng/mL (normal 5-20)

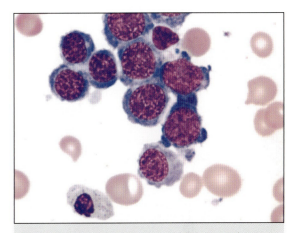

Figure 3 Bone marrow aspirate smear (Wright, ×1000) showing erythroid precursors with megaloblastic change.

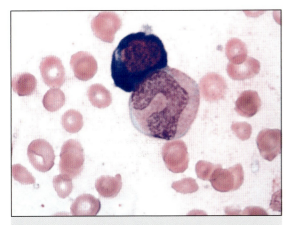

Figure 4 Bone marrow aspirate smear (Wright, ×1000) with giant band.

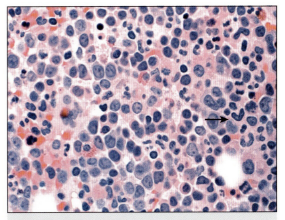

Figure 5 Clot section (H&E, ×400) showing marked hypercellularity with erythroid hyperplasia and megaloblastic changes including giant bands (arrow).

Section A: Anemias
Macrocytic Anemia Associated with Folate Deficiency

Examination of bone marrow aspirate and biopsy revealed a markedly hypercellular marrow (90%) with marked erythroid hyperplasia, and megaloblastic changes in both the erythroid and myeloid lineages. The findings were consistent with megaloblastic anemia.

Final Diagnosis Megaloblastic anemia due to folate deficiency.

Management Approach The cause of the patient's folate deficiency was determined to be related to dietary deficiency. Management included patient education and folate supplementation.

General Discussion Megaloblastic anemia is due to ineffective hematopoiesis from a deficiency of either folate or vitamin B_{12} (cobalamin), or both; there are also very rare hereditary causes. The resulting defective DNA synthesis leads to an asynchrony between nuclear and cytoplasmic maturation because RNA synthesis does not depend on the folate and vitamin B_{12} cofactors. Vitamin B_{12} and folate deficiencies can also cause additional clinical symptoms, the most significant being neurologic manifestations. The characteristic megaloblastic morphologic changes in the bone marrow include a marked hypercellularity with both erythroid and myeloid hyperplasia, and increased apoptosis. The erythroid precursors have large nuclei with finely dispersed ("sieve-like") chromatin with more mature cytoplasm, as the hemoglobinization remains intact. The myeloid precursors often show giant forms and large megakaryocytes may be seen. It should be noted that the megaloblastic changes in erythroid precursors may be masked if there is concomitant iron deficiency or other causes of anemia; however, the characteristic changes in the myeloid precursors should still be evident. The CBC data usually shows cytopenias. The MCV values range from 100 fL-150 fL. Blood smear usually reveals oval macrocytes, red cell fragments (due to increased fragility of the abnormal cells), and nucleated red cells with megaloblastic changes. Hypersegmented neutrophils are also characteristic, but not specific; this is often an early event and may be seen before anemia develops. Deficiency of vitamin B_{12} can occur through several mechanisms, the most common of which is defective absorption related to decreased intrinsic factor, while folate deficiency is generally due to dietary deficiency or increased requirement. In adults, total body stores of vitamin B_{12} are significant enough to last 2 years-5 years on a deficient diet but folate stores last only 3 months-5 months. Deficiencies in infants occur in a much shorter time frame due to decreased storage levels, and are often the result of inadequate maternal intake. Dietary deficiency of folate may be seen in patients from low socioeconomic backgrounds, chronic alcoholics, and drug addicts who consume inadequate amounts of folate-rich food. Excessive cooking of food also destroys folate. Increased folate requirements can occur in settings of increased cell turnover or growth, including infants, pregnant and lactating women, and in patients with malignancies or chronic hemolytic anemia or blood loss. Additional laboratory testing for serum vitamin B_{12} and folate is usually needed to determine the cause of the megaloblastic anemia. Documentation of folate deficiency in serum can be difficult because serum folate levels fluctuate with diet, and should be tested on a fasting serum sample. Red cell folate levels give a better reflection of the folate status at the time of cell formation, as red cells are metabolically inactive. Serum homocysteine level may also be useful because it will be increased in both vitamin B_{12} and folate deficiencies. In addition, an increased methylmalonic acid level is a highly sensitive and specific marker for vitamin B_{12} deficiency.

Macrocytic Anemia Associated with B$_{12}$ Deficiency

Cordelia Sever

Patient A 58-year-old male, who presented with weakness and paresthesias of fingers and toes.

Clinical History The patient has long history of schizophrenia, controlled with medication. He had poor eating habits, in part because of paranoia about certain foods.

Family History Noncontributory.

Medications Clozapine.

Physical Examination The patient appeared underweight and had a pale waxy pallor. He complained of general weakness and difficulty in walking.

Initial Work-Up

CBC		WBC Differential	%	# (×10^3/μL)
WBC (×10^3/μL)	7.2	Neutrophils	64	4.6
RBC (×10^6/μL)	2.02	Bands	0	
HGB (g/dL)	9.5	Lymphocytes	32	2.3
HCT (%)	29	Monocytes	3	0.2
MCV (fL)	142	Eosinophils	1	0.1
MCHC (g/dL)	33.2	Basophils	0	
PLT (×10^3/μL)	91			
RDW-CV (%)	18.5			

Peripheral blood smear revealed macrocytic red cells, macroovalocytes, and hypersegmented neutrophils (**Figures 1** and **2**).

Section A: Anemias
Macrocytic Anemia Associated with B_{12} Deficiency

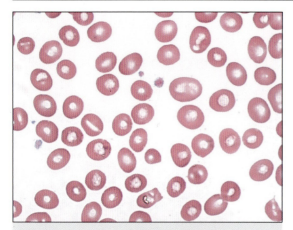

Figure 1 Blood smear (Wright-Giemsa, ×1000) showing macrocytic red cells and macro-ovalocytes.

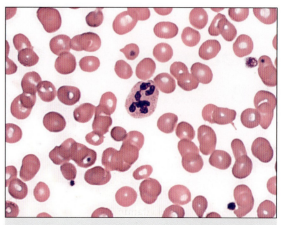

Figure 2 Blood smear (Wright-Giemsa, ×1000) showing a hypersegmented neutrophil.

Differential Diagnosis The patient's emaciated appearance and the high MCV immediately brought to mind nutritional deficiencies. With vitamin B_{12} deficiency high on the list, pernicious anemia with autoantibodies needed to be ruled out. In addition, an adverse drug reaction entered the differential diagnosis since clozapine is associated with cytopenias in about 1% of patients, which however is predominantly neutropenia, agranulocytosis and aplastic anemia. The neutrophil count was preserved in this patient.

Additional Work-Up

Vitamin B_{12} level was low at 133 pg/mL (normal 200-1,100), methylmalonic acid was increased at 7.76 µmol/L (normal 0.00-4.00). Serum and red cell folate levels were normal; there was no evidence of anti-parietal or anti-intrinsic factor blocking antibodies. Examination of bone marrow aspirate smears showed giant bands, metamyelocytes, and megaloblastic and dyspoietic erythroid precursors (**Figures 3** and **4**).

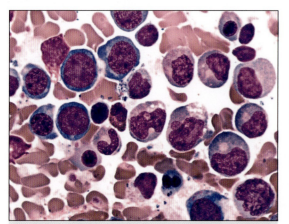

Figure 3 Bone marrow aspirate smear (Wright-Giemsa, ×500) showing giant bands, metamyelocytes, megaloblastic and dyspoietic erythroid precursors.

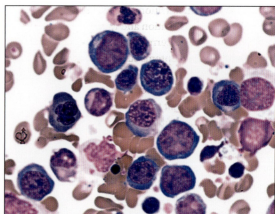

Figure 4 Bone marrow aspirate smear (Wright-Giemsa, ×500) showing megaloblastic and dyspoietic erythroid precursors.

Final Diagnosis Anemia (megaloblastic) and thrombocytopenia secondary to nutritional vitamin B_{12} deficiency.

Management Approach Once symptomatic vitamin B_{12} deficiency is documented, replacement therapy needs to be initiated to reverse the peripheral blood cytopenias and neurologic symptoms (they may be irreversible). A number of publications including randomized controlled trials have shown that high-dose oral supplementation of 1 mg (or 2 mg) every day is as effective as intramuscular injections since approximately 1% of oral vitamin B_{12} is absorbed by passive diffusion independent of intrinsic factor availability. Nevertheless, most hematologists still prefer to start daily treatment with 1 mg vitamin B_{12} (cyanocobalamin) intramuscularly for 3 days-5 days to assure immediate high-dose bioavailability in patients with florid symptoms. Long-term administration depends on the underlying etiology and is life long for patients with antibodies to intrinsic factor or parietal cells. Most patients are eligible for daily oral treatment; however, a subgroup of patients with cognitive impairment or psychosocial issues may be better served with monthly 1 mg intramuscular injections to assure compliance. This patient received 1 mg vitamin B_{12} intramuscular injections daily for 5 days, followed by once weekly injections until normalization of blood counts. He received nutritional counseling, further oral vitamin B_{12} supplementation and psychiatric evaluation to determine whether current medication was keeping the schizophrenic symptoms sufficiently under control.

General Discussion The concurrent schizophrenia made it initially difficult to distinguish between psychotic symptoms and neurologic symptoms secondary to vitamin B_{12} deficiency. The latter are characterized by paresthesias, numbness in legs or less commonly arms, difficulty walking as well as memory loss and disorientation. Although antibodies to intrinsic factor and parietal cells remain important etiologies for pernicious anemia, a significant number of patients develop vitamin B_{12} deficiency without demonstrable antibodies. In particular, atrophic gastritis is a frequent underlying cause and has a high prevalence in the elderly population, estimated as high as 10%-30% of people over 60 years of age. Associated conditions include *Helicobacter pylori* infection, peptic ulcer disease and long-term treatment with proton pump inhibitors that should be questioned or investigated when taking a clinical history. Other causes of malabsorption such as prior surgery with removal of small bowel, in particular terminal ileum, should be kept in mind. Purely nutritional deficiencies are infrequent, associated with purely vegetarian diets without appropriate vitamin B_{12} supplementation and, as in this case, other psychosocial factors influencing unusual dietary habits. In the laboratory evaluation, it should be kept in mind that low serum vitamin B_{12} levels are not completely diagnostic for true vitamin B_{12} deficiency and should always be further supported with high serum methylmalonic acid levels. A complete blood count demonstrating the classic findings of peripheral cytopenias with macrocytic red cells (macro-ovalocytes in particular) and hypersegmented (5- and 6-lobed) neutrophils are important additional findings for providing further evidence of true vitamin B_{12} or folate deficiency. Macrocytosis exceeding an MCV of 120 fL-130 fL is rarely seen in myelodysplastic syndromes or drug induced macrocytosis, which are important causes of cytopenias to rule out, especially in the elderly population. A thorough clinical history and laboratory evaluation of peripheral blood and serum allow a definitive diagnosis of vitamin B_{12} deficiency in most patients. Therefore, bone marrow examination is needed infrequently and reserved for patients with multiple medical conditions or the possibility of concurrent other hematologic abnormalities, such as a myelodysplastic syndrome. When evaluating those bone marrows, it is important to keep in mind that vitamin B_{12} deficiency can cause fairly severe dyspoiesis, but usually the telltale megaloblastic chromatin of erythroid precursors, giant bands, and metamyelocytes point to the benign etiology. Megaloblastic changes associated with B_{12} or folate deficiency often involve all proliferating cells of the body including all hematopoietic cell lineages and epithelial cells.

Pernicious Anemia

Elise A Occhipinti, John R Krause

Patient A 25-year-old African-American male presented to the emergency department with a 2-week history of vomiting and diarrhea

Clinical History The patient also reported numbness and tingling in hands and feet, along with darkening of the skin in those areas. He has had an unintentional 50 kg weight loss during the past year. Three months prior to presentation, the patient received 5 units of packed red blood cells at an outside institution for "low blood counts." Folic acid supplementation was also instituted at that time.

Family History Noncontributory.

Medications Folic acid, esomeprazole.

Physical Examination Vital signs were normal. His heart rate was 88 with a 2/6 systolic ejection murmur. Pertinent findings included pale conjunctivae, left upper quadrant tenderness with a palpable spleen tip, hyperpigmentation of the palms and soles, and no vibratory or touch sensation on palmar surfaces bilaterally. He refuses to ambulate.

Initial Work-Up

CBC		WBC Differential	%	# (×10³/µL)
WBC (×10³/µL)	1.7	Neutrophils	38	0.6
RBC (×10⁶/µL)	2.4	Bands	0	
HGB (g/dL)	7.6	Lymphocytes	60	1.0
HCT (%)	22.2	Monocytes	1	
MCV (fL)	94.2	Eosinophils	1	
MCH (pg)	32.4	Basophils	1	
MCHC (g/dL)	34.4			
PLT (×10³/µL)	151			
RDW-CV (%)	31.5			
MPV (fL)	9.4			

The peripheral blood smear revealed anisocytosis, macrocytes, and occasional ovalocytes (**Figure 1**).

Section A: Anemias
Pernicious Anemia

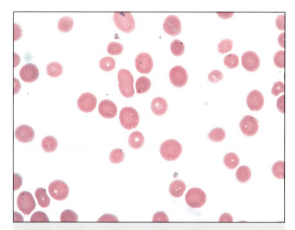

Figure 1 Blood smear (Wright-Giemsa, ×1000) showing anisocytosis, macrocytes and ovalocytes.

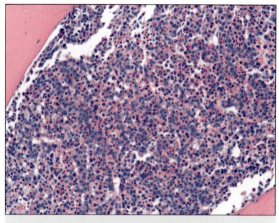

Figure 2 Bone marrow biopsy (H&E, ×20) showing hypercellular marrow.

Differential Diagnosis Clinically the diagnostic considerations included a hematologic malignancy, systemic lupus erythematosis, autoimmune vasculitis, and vitamin B_{12} deficiency.

Additional Work-Up
- LDH 1,471 units/L (normal 110-220)
- Serum B_{12} 319 pg/mL (normal: 214-865)
- RBC folate 720 ng/mL (normal 140-540)
- Plasma homocysteine 188 µM/L (normal: 4 -12)
- Methylmalonic acid 24.10 µM/L(normal: 0-0.4)
- Intrinsic factor blocking antibody positive
- Anti nuclear antibody (ANA) within normal limits.
- Antineutrophil cytoplasmic antibodies-classical (ANCA-C) within normal limits
- Antineutrophil cytoplasmic antibodies-protoplasmic (ANCA-P) within normal limits

Stomach, Proximal Body, Biopsy Severe chronic gastritis with focal mild activity and intestinal metaplasia. An immunohistochemical stain for *H pylori* was negative.

Bone Marrow Aspirate and Biopsy Hypercellular marrow with megaloblastic features (**Figures 2-4**).

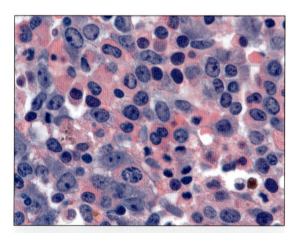

Figure 3 Bone marrow biopsy (H&E, ×1000) showing hypercellular marrow with increased immaturity and florid megaloblastic change in the erythroid series.

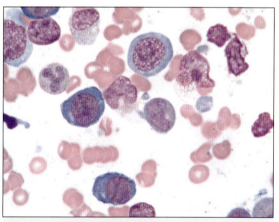

Figure 4 Bone marrow aspirate smear (Wright-Giemsa, ×1000) showing erythroid hyperplasia and marked megaloblastic changes including giant bands.

Section A: Anemias
Pernicious Anemia

Final Diagnosis B_{12} deficiency secondary to atrophic gastritis (pernicious anemia).

Management Approach The patient received 2 units of packed red blood cells upon admission to the hospital. During his 5-day hospital stay he received daily filgrastim, folic acid and intramuscular B_{12}. Upon discharge, the patient's CBC was within normal limits. The patient did not return for follow-up appointments.

Discussion This case illustrates a common scenario in diagnostic hematopathology in which previous therapy interferes with critical laboratory tests. In this presentation, the patient's prior red blood cell transfusion and folic acid therapy served to normalize the MCV, folate and B_{12} levels despite profound megaloblastoid changes in the bone marrow. Previous transfusion also resulted in a confusing peripheral blood smear in which a heterogenous population of oval macrocytes and spherocytes was admixed with normochromic, normocytic cells. Hypersegmented neutrophils were not seen in the peripheral smear. The patient's pancytopenia, elevated LDH and atypical peripheral smear morphology combined with the normal MCV and serum B_{12} levels initially skewed the diagnosis toward a myelodysplastic or leukemic process. However, evaluation for nausea, vomiting and diarrhea prompted an endoscopic procedure that revealed severe atrophic gastritis suggestive of pernicious anemia. The diagnosis was confirmed by markedly elevated methylmalonic acid and homocysteine levels in conjunction with the presence of autoantibodies against intrinsic factor.

Methemoglobinemia

Kathryn Foucar, Devon Chabot-Richards

Patient A 57-year-old Navajo male, who presented to the emergency department with chest pain and shortness of breath.

Clinical History The patient reported 3 weeks of worsening chest pain with associated dyspnea. The pain was 7-8/10 and was worse with deep breaths. He felt like his chest "would explode." The pain was centrally located and did not radiate. There was no associated nausea or vomiting. He complained of headache and felt lightheaded with exertion. He is a jewelry maker, and primarily works with silver. He has not had any new environmental exposures. Past history is significant for hypertension and arthritis.

Family History Both his parents died when he was quite young of unknown cause. His sister died 6 years ago after receiving dapsone for pemphigus.

Medications Metoprolol and aspirin. He has not taken any new medications, including over-the-counter or herbal remedies.

Physical Examination He was afebrile, tachycardic (heart rate 112), and tachypneic (respiratory rate 22-24). His oxygen saturation was 90% on 5 L O_2. Initially, he was unable to speak in full sentences; this improved with supplemental oxygen. There was bluish discoloration around his lips and of the mucous membranes and tongue, which did not resolve with oxygen. His respirations were labored, but lung sounds were clear.

Initial Work-Up

CBC		WBC Differential	%	# (×10³/μL)
WBC (×10³/μL)	9.3	Neutrophils	74	6.9
RBC (×10⁶/μL)	7.0	Bands	3	0.3
HGB (g/dL)	19.9	Lymphocytes	14	1.3
HCT (%)	62	Monocytes	7	0.6
MCV (fL)	87	Eosinophils	2	0.2
MCH (pg)	28.4	Basophils	0	
MCHC (g/dL)	32.3			
PLT (×10³/μL)	152			
RDW-CV (%)	16.4			

Peripheral blood smear revealed red cell crowding consistent with the CBC finding of elevated HGB, RBC and HCT (**Figure 1**).

Section A: Anemias
Methemoglobinemia

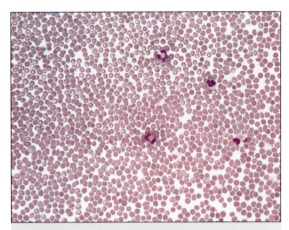

Figure 1 Peripheral blood smear (Wright, ×400) showing red cell crowding.

Additional Work-Up		
Methemoglobin	25.8%	Normal 0%-3%
Methemoglobin reductase activity	Undetectable	Normal 8.2-19.2 IU/g HGB

Arterial Blood Gas	
pH	7.14 (normal 7.35-7.45)
pCO$_2$	40 (normal 32-40)
pO$_2$	95 normal (65-75)
HCO$_3$	25 normal (18-26)
Measured O$_2$ sat	96

Other tests and imaging studies were unremarkable.

Differential Diagnosis The differential diagnosis includes disease processes causing insufficient oxygen delivery to the tissues, including cardiovascular conditions, pulmonary conditions, hematologic conditions, infectious processes, and toxic exposure. Cyanosis that persists after administration of oxygen with normal oxygen saturation, along with a gap between oxygen saturation measured by pulse oximetry and arterial blood gas is highly specific for methemoglobinemia.

Final Diagnosis Congenital methemoglobinemia with acute exacerbation of unknown etiology.

Management Approach It is generally recommended that treatment of methemoglobinemia be based on symptoms rather than levels of methemoglobin. In mild cases, high-flow oxygen and removal of any known oxidizing agents may be all that is required. Treatment with methylene blue is used in cases with significant clinical manifestations. Methylene blue acts as an electron donor in the NADPH-dependent reductase pathway. In extreme cases, hyperbaric oxygen therapy to increase dissolved plasma oxygen and exchange transfusion to increase levels of normal hemoglobin may be used. Because the patient responded well to supplemental oxygen, treatment with methylene blue was not necessary. A unit of blood was phlebotomized to prevent complications of erythrocytosis. The patient was admitted for observation.

General Discussion Methemoglobinemia is a disorder in which there are increased levels of methemoglobin found in red blood cells. In normal hemoglobin, the oxygen-carrying iron ion exists in a reduced (Fe^{2+}) state.

In methemoglobin, the iron has been oxidized (Fe^{3+}) and cannot carry oxygen. This results in a functional anemia in which there is normal red blood cell mass; however, the cells are unable to carry and deliver oxygen to the tissues. Blood with elevated levels of methemoglobin appears brown in color, lending a gray-blue cast to the skin of affected individuals. Normally, methemoglobin accounts for <1% of total hemoglobin. Small amounts of methemoglobin are formed over the course of the day, but these are rapidly reduced under normal circumstances. There are multiple enzymatic pathways for reduction of methemoglobin. The major pathway relies on cytochrome b5 reductase (methemoglobin reductase), which transfers electrons from NADH to methemoglobin. This pathway accounts for 95% of the reduction of methemoglobin. There are several alternate pathways, most importantly the NADPH-dependent methemoglobin reductase pathway.

Methemoglobinemia is most commonly acquired and is found in cases of exposure to oxidizing drugs or chemicals resulting in increased production of methemoglobin. The list of known agents is extensive; however, the classical associations are with nitrates and nitrites, local anesthetics such as benzocaine, and antibiotics such as dapsone. The increased oxidation of hemoglobin seen with these drugs can overwhelm the endogenous reductase pathways, resulting in symptomatic disease. Patients with acquired methemoglobinemia often experience hemolytic anemia. This does not occur in patients with congenital disease and the etiology is unknown. Congenital methemoglobinemia is an autosomal recessive disease caused by mutations in the cytochrome b5 reductase gene. It is divided into 2 categories. Patients with type 1 disease usually have missense mutations, causing decreased enzyme stability. The enzyme deficiency only manifests in erythrocytes because the anucleate, mature cells cannot manufacture proteins. These patients have methemoglobin levels >20% but only occasionally experience symptoms. They may have constitutional cyanosis. As a result of chronic, mild hypoxia, patients have increased levels of erythropoietin and polycythemia. They have a normal life span. Type 1 disease is most often sporadic, but is endemic in Athabascan, Navajo, and Yakutsk populations. Type 2 disease is caused by nonsense mutations, with absence of the reductase enzyme. These patients have systemic symptoms, including severe neurologic deterioration, and rarely live into adulthood. Although it has not been conclusively demonstrated, it is generally believed that patients who experience acquired methemoglobinemia may be heterozygous for cytochrome b5 reductase deficiency. Most individuals are asymptomatic with methemoglobin levels up to 15%. Between 15%-30%, patients begin experiencing symptoms of hypoxia including headache, dizziness, fatigue, and exercise intolerance. As the methemoglobin continues to rise, symptoms worsen with levels of 50% associated with arrhythmias, seizures, coma, and death. Patients with underlying pulmonary, cardiac, or hematologic disease; infants; and the elderly experience worse symptoms at lower levels. Patients with congenital disease can tolerate higher levels without symptoms.

Hemolytic Anemia Associated with G6PD Deficiency

Cheryl Hirsch-Ginsberg, Michael Kroll

Patient A 62-year-old African-American man was admitted to a local hospital following a seizure.

Clinical History A destructive lesion was found on the patient's left shoulder, with metastases to the liver. A biopsy revealed aggressive large cell lymphoma with high-grade features. PET CT showed extensive disease in both kidneys, brain and liver. He was transferred to our institution for evaluation and treatment of his lymphoma. Pertinent past medical history includes longstanding hypertension, chronic renal insufficiency and pancreatitis. There was no history of any blood disorder. The patient was begun on treatment with hyper-CVAD (cyclophosphamide, vincristine, doxorubicin and dexamethasone). Hyperuricemia (15 mg/dL) was treated with 1 dose of rasburicase. Shortly thereafter he was noted to have an oxygen saturation of 80% while on 2 liters of oxygen via nasal cannula. There was no improvement in oxygen saturation following administration of 100% O_2 with a non-rebreather mask. When an arterial blood gas was drawn, the blood looked venous with a dark maroon-brown color. A diagnosis of methemoglobinemia was made and the patient was started on methylene blue.

Family History Positive for hypertension and chronic renal disease in parents and siblings. There was also a possible history of thalassemia trait and sickle cell disease.

Medications The patient's home medications included clonidine, hydralazine, hydrocodone and metoprolol tartrate.

Physical Examination Notable for cyanosis, a palpable left shoulder mass and left axillary adenopathy.

Initial Work-Up

CBC		WBC Differential	%	# (×10³/µL)
WBC (×10³/µL)	6.1	Neutrophils + bands	55.0	33
RBC (×10⁶/µL)	4.64	Immature granulocytes	0.2	0.1
HGB (g/dL)	11.0	Lymphocytes	34.6	2.1
HCT (%)	34.6	Monocytes	9.6	0.6
MCV (fL)	75	Eosinophils	0.3	0.0
MCH (pg)	23.7	Basophils	0.2	0.0
MCHC (g/dL)	31.8			
PLT (×10³/µL)	298			
RDW-CV (%)	15.3			
MPV (fL)	9.7			

Following rehydration the HGB dropped slightly to 9.7 g/dL and was 9.2 g/dL following rasburicase administration. However, following methylene blue administration the Hgb dropped to 6.5 g/dL, and the haptoglobin level was <8 mg/dL (normal 30-200). Peripheral blood smear revealed numerous blister and hemighost cells with retracted hemoglobin, coarse basophilic stippling, and nucleated red cells (**Figure 1**).

Section A: Anemias
Hemolytic Anemia Associated with G6PD Deficiency

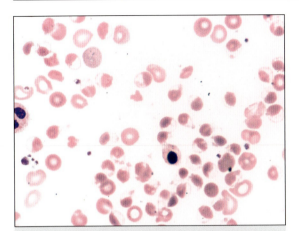

Figure 1 Peripheral blood smear (Wright-Giemsa, ×1,000) showing many hemighost cells, nucleated red cell and basophilic stippling.

Differential Diagnosis The methemoblobinemia was considered to be due to rasburicase. It was confirmed 2 days later, when 1.3 % methemoglobin was measured (reference range of 0.0-1.0). Hemolysis was considered to be due to glucose 6-phosphate dehydrogenase (G6PD) deficiency because of the patient's gender and race, and the clinical course of hemolysis following methylene blue administration. Peripheral blood smear was consistent with the diagnosis. The general differential diagnoses of hemolysis are based on age and the rapidity of hemolysis. In newborns, alloimmune-based hemolytic disease is included in the differential diagnosis. In children and adults, autoimmune and nonimmune causes of nonspherocytic hemolytic anemia should be considered, including pyruvate kinase deficiency and other much less common deficiencies in glycolytic pathway enzymes, such as hexose monophophate shunt pathway enzyme deficiency and deficiencies or excesses in enzymes involved in nucleotide metabolism. For cases of intermittent hemolysis, oxidant-induced hemolytic anemia can occur in the absence of enzyme deficiencies if the offending agent is potent enough and exposure is in sufficient quantities. The major offending substances are dapsone, sulphasalazine, and nitrate contamination of drinking water (agriculture or industrial chemical causes). Finally, as far as the morphology of the peripheral blood smear is concerned, unstable hemoglobins can give a similar picture of "bite cells," basophilic stippling and polychromasia.

Additional Work-Up Reticulocyte count 3.9% (reference range 0.5-1.5); G-6-PD 3.1 IU/g Hb (reference range 8.6-18.6).

Final Diagnosis G6PD deficiency in a patient with aggressive large cell lymphoma.

Management Approach Following withdrawal of the offending oxidative agent, acute episodes of G6PD deficiency are usually self limited, because reticulocytes contain more enzyme than older red cells and so are able to better withstand oxidative stress. The long-term strategy is to avoid oxidant chemicals, drugs (rasburicase and methylene blue) and foods (ie, fava beans). Much of acute management consists of maintenance of adequate urine flow, especially if there has been a significant hemoglobinuria. Although usually not required, anemia can be managed with red cell transfusion. As was the case with this patient, anti-oxidant medication, (ascorbic acid 300 mg 3 times a day by mouth for 3 days for the methemoglobinemia) can be given to hasten recovery.

General Discussion Methemoglobinemia is characterized by abnormal hemoglobin reduction in which the iron in the hemoglobin molecule cannot remain in the normal ferrous state (Fe^{2+}) but with oxidative stress it moves in to ferric state (Fe^{3+}). Congenital causes include hemoglobin variants (M or H, etc) that prevent reduction of iron, and conditions that impair the production of NADH or NADPH, which are critical for keeping heme iron in the ferrous state. Among these conditions is G6PD deficiency, which causes impaired NADPH production used in the methemoglobin reductase pathway and in the glutathione reductase pathway, and which is critical to maintain the cell membrane. The G6PD gene is located on the X-chromosome, leading to a sex-linked inheritance pattern in which hemizygous men and homozygous women are fully affected and heterozygous women are variably affected depending on their pattern of X inactivation. There are over 400 variants of G6PD proteins present in different ethnic groups and with varying degrees of enzyme impairment. G6PD A⁻ is the most common type affecting the African-American populations. All G6PD-deficient patients have shortened red cell survival that is often well compensated. Many patients are without anemia unless stressed. However, infection or ingestion of an oxidant drug or food (ie, fava beans), can produce severe intravascular hemolysis leading to hemoglobinemia, hemoglobinuria (with risk of renal failure) and jaundice. Methylene blue should never be given to African-American men until G6PD deficiency is ruled out. This is because G6PD deficiency affects at least 10% of African-American men and methylene blue reduces Fe^{3+} by transferring the hydrogen ion from red cell NADPH, which can not be resynthesized adequately by G6PD in those who have a deficiency of the enzyme. Peripheral blood smear often reveals blister or bite cells that are the result of Heinz body formation where the oxidized hemoglobin precipitates, migrates to the unstable membrane, and is then torn away from the rest of the cell by phagocytic macrophages in the spleen. Our case also shows many hemighost cells, where the hemoglobin is condensed and retracted to half of the cell. Basophilic stippling may be present in G6PD, although in this patient the cause may be related to possible mild thalassemia. Also present in our case are occasional nucleated red cells, which are not a usual feature of G6PD deficiency, but may be due to this patient's underlying lymphoma with a myelophthisic picture, due to bone marrow involvement.

Anemia Associated with Pyruvate Kinase Deficiency

Sherrie L Perkins, Hassan M Yaish, Mohamed E Salama

Patient A 2-week-old girl of healthy parents was referred to hematology clinic because of anemia and jaundice.

Clinical History The baby was found to be anemic (hemoglobin 10.6 g/dL) and jaundiced at birth. Her hemoglobin levels remained stable for next 10 days, then fell to 6.4 g/dL, which required transfusion.

Family History Noncontributory.

Medications None.

Physical Examination Notable for pallor, jaundice, and hepatosplenomegaly.

Initial Work-Up

CBC			WBC Differential	%	# (10^3/μL)
WBC (×10^3/μL)	16.4		Neutrophils	60	9.8
RBC (×10^6/μL)	3.3		Bands	5	0.8
HGB (g/dL)	10.6		Lymphocytes	30	4.9
HCT (%)	29		Monocytes	4	0.6
MCV (fL)	100		Eosinophils	1	0.2
MCH (pg)	30		Basophils	0	
MCHC (g/dL)	29		**Chemistry**		
PLT (×10^3/μL)	190		Serum LDH (U/L)	1,700	
RDW-CV (%)	17		Haptoglobin (mg/dL)	<8	
MPV (fL)	11		Direct bilirubin (mg/dL)	0.9	
Reticulocyte, count	4.6%		Indirect bilirubin (mg/dL)	4	

Peripheral smear showed normocytic, normochromic red blood cells, significant polychromasia and numerous echinocytes (**Figure 1**).

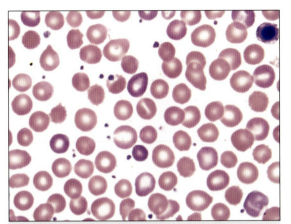

Figure 1 Blood smear (Wright stain, ×1000) showing contracted/dehydrated cells with circumferential sharp spicules and significant polychromasia.

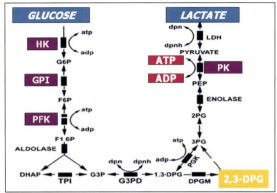

Figure 2 Embden-Myerhof pathway; recognized enzyme defects are indicated by the rectangular bars. HK=hexokinase, GPI=glucose 6-phosphate isomerase, PFK=6-phsophofructokinase, PTI=triose phosphate isomerase, G3PD=glyceraldehyde-3-phosphate dehydrogenase, PGK=phosphoglycerate kinase, DPGM=2-3 diphosphoglycerate mutase, PK=pyruvate kinase, LDH=lactate dehydrogenase.

Differential Diagnosis Anemia with reticulocytosis and these abnormal findings on peripheral blood smear are suggestive of hemolytic anemia. Echinocytes and/or acanthocytes are encountered in several clinical conditions in the newborn, including enzyme deficiencies in the glycolytic pathway, such as pyruvate kinase deficiency (PKD), and severe G6PD deficiency, vitamin E deficiency, ATP depletion, accumulation of calcium and infantile pyknocytosis. In both ABO incompatibility and hereditary spherocytosis, the presence of a large number of spherocytes is striking. α-thalassemia (hemoglobin H disease) may also be associated with distorted and contracted cells.

Additional Work-Up The direct antiglobulin test and osmotic fragility were both normal. At 6 months of age, pyruvate kinase activity was assayed in the parents and child, revealing moderate deficiency in both parents at 5.6 and 4.7 IU/gHGB and clear deficiency in the girl at 1.8 IU/gHGB (normal 5.9-8.1 IU/gHGB). Molecular analysis indicated that the girl was a compound heterozygote.

Diagnosis Pyruvate kinase deficiency.

Management Approach Some patients with PK deficiency do not require therapy whereas other may require blood or red cell transfusion and/or splenectomy. Folic acid supplementation may be prescribed in cases with increased bone marrow activity. Hematopoietic progenitor cell transplantation, at least in theory, is the only possible curative treatment. This patient's hemoglobin level was stable during infancy and she did not require any further blood transfusions. Follow-up at 2 years of age revealed a child with appropriate growth for age and slight compensated anemia. Splenectomy was not required.

General Discussion The mature red cell lacks mitochondria and completely depends on glucose metabolism as a source of energy. Glucose is catabolized to pyruvate and lactate mostly via the anaerobic glycolytic (Embden-Myerhof) pathway (**Figure 2**). In the process, ATP is generated and plays a major role in maintaining a cation gradient in the red cells, thus protecting them from premature death. Deficiencies in glycolytic pathway enzymes result in congenital nonspherocytic hemolytic anemia (CNSHA), which is initially observed during infancy or childhood. Although CNSHA may result from a heterogeneous group of disorders, glycolytic pathway enzyme deficiencies are the most clinically important group of which pyruvate kinase (PK) is most prevalent. In patients with PK deficiency, a metabolic arrest occurs in the pathway at the level of the deficient enzyme. Intermediate byproducts and various glycolytic metabolites proximal to the metabolic block accumulate in the red cells. Red cells become depleted of the distal products (eg, lactate and ATP) in the pathway. High levels of 2,3-diphosphoglycerate (2,3-DPG) accumulation act to increase the patient's exercise tolerance despite severe anemia by shifting the hemoglobin-oxygen dissociation curve. However, the lack of ATP disturbs the cation gradient across the red cell membrane, resulting in loss of potassium and water. This disruption of the cation gradient leads to red cell dehydration, contraction, crenation and premature destruction. PK-deficient reticulocytes can circumvent this defect by using the oxidative phosphorylation

Section A: Anemias
Anemia Associated with Pyruvate Kinase Deficiency

pathway to produce ATP. However, this compensatory ability is diminished when the reticulocytes are exposed to hypoxia or as red cells age. Although uncommon, PK deficiency accounts for approximately 90% of cases of glycolytic pathway enzyme deficiency-associated anemia. Similar to most other glycolytic pathway deficiencies, PK deficiency is inherited as an autosomal recessive trait. Most cases manifest in infancy or early childhood with anemia secondary to chronic hemolysis, which worsens with infections or other stresses. Newborns with PK deficiency commonly present with anemia, jaundice, and splenomegaly. In severe cases the hemolytic anemia results in fetal hydrops. In older children, adolescents, and adults with PK deficiency, anemia may range from transfusion dependent to asymptomatic, even among patients with the same level of deficiency. This variability occurs because of differential effects of mutations. Depending on the mutation type, effects may range from a minimal effect to symptomatic homozygotes with changes in both enzyme levels and/or activity. In addition, compound heterozygotes with 2 different mutations (1 can be qualitative and the other quantitative) also vary symptomatically. Congenital nonspherocytic hemolytic anemia (CNSHA) is usually suspected when there is chronic hemolysis in a child with normal red cell morphology and osmotic fragility. Given the autosomal recessive inheritance, the family history is usually negative unless other siblings are affected.

The first step in evaluating an affected child involves a direct antiglobulin test (Coombs test) to rule out an immune-mediated hemolytic process and a sucrose lysis test to rule out paroxysmal nocturnal hemoglobinuria, a condition very rarely seen in children. If the hemolytic anemia is thought to be hereditary, it is usually classified as either a nonspherocytic (when no spherocytes are seen on blood smear) or spherocytic (when spherocytes are encountered on blood film examination). CNSHA requires further work-up to identify patients with hemoglobinopathy or unstable hemoglobins. Hemoglobin evaluation/electrophoresis may help in the first category while isopropanol stability test may identify patients with unstable hemoglobins. Finally, screening tests for deficiencies of specific RBC enzymes such as G6PD and PK may be performed, followed by quantitative red cell enzyme assays to determine the specific nature of the enzymatic defect, if appropriate. Fluorescence of nicotinamide adenine dinucleotide (NADH) is a useful screening test for the detection of red cell enzyme deficiencies. In practice, it is often enough to know whether the activity of the enzyme in question is markedly deficient. The first spot should fluoresce brightly. With the normal sample, fluorescence disappears after 15 minutes of incubation. In contrast, in pyruvate kinase–deficient samples, fluorescence fails to disappear even after 45 minutes or 60 minutes of incubation, as there is no oxidation of the fluorescent NADH molecule. False-negative results may be observed if the patient has recently received a transfusion and large numbers of transfused cells containing normal levels of pyruvate kinase are still circulating. There may be little relationship between the severity of hemolysis and the measured level of pyruvate kinase activity due to different stabilities of the pyruvate kinase variants or the degree of reticulocyte response. Some patients with high reticulocyte counts may have normal screening tests. Quantitative red cell enzyme assays give definitive confirmation of screening test results. Molecular analysis will also confirm an enzymatic defect and may provide information useful in genetic counseling. Pyruvate kinase is derived from 2 genes that can give rise to 4 distinct isoforms of the enzyme. More than 50 different mutations have been identified as causes of hemolytic anemia. Most are missense mutations giving rise to abnormal proteins. Some nonsense or splicing mutations also have been identified.

In summary, PK deficiency may present with variable clinical features that may overlap with other CNSHA. Persistent anemia and/or jaundice, even in the absence of reticulocytosis, in the first months of life should be investigated. Definitive diagnosis is often delayed due to limitations in interpreting enzymatic activities in newborns, reticulocytosis, or the confounding effects of transfusion. Information obtained from the blood smear examination is frequently helpful in making the diagnosis early in life. The degree and course of anemia associated with PK deficiency varies widely from mild or compensated to life threatening, requiring exchange transfusion. Severe pyruvate kinase deficiency may require splenectomy early in life.

Section A: Anemias

Hemolytic Disease of the Newborn

Jay H Herman, Melissa R George, Joe K George

Patient A 38-week gestational-age Caucasian male baby born via spontaneous vaginal delivery to a 30-year-old G4P3 mother.

Clinical History The mother received adequate prenatal care and the pregnancy was uneventful. The mother's prenatal testing revealed her to be HBV, HIV, Group B *Streptococcus*, and VDRL negative. Her blood type was O, Rh positive.

Family History Mother has asthma and father is healthy.

Medications Mother had taken prenatal vitamins.

Physical Examination The baby's APGARs were 9 and 9 at 1 minute and 5 minutes, respectively. He had a nuchal cord; however, the delivery was otherwise uneventful. Vital signs: temperature 98.2°F, heart rate 152/min, and respiration rate 42/min. The infant displayed slight jaundice, but was otherwise awake, alert, and well-perfused.

Initial Work-Up (at 4 Hours of Life)

CBC		WBC Differential	%	# (×10³/μL)
WBC (×10³/μL)	21.6	Neutrophils	55	11.9
RBC (×10⁶/μL)	2.9	Bands	7	1.5
HGB (g/dL)	11.6	Lymphocytes	29	6.3
HCT (%)	32.5	Monocytes	6	1.3
MCV (fL)	115	Eosinophils	2	0.4
MCH (pg)	40	Basophils	1	0.2
MCHC (g/dL)	35.7	NRBC	60/100 WBC	
PLT (×10³/μL)	300			
RDW-CV (%)	16.7	**Bilirubin**	**mg/dL**	
MPV (fL)	9.5	Direct	0.2	
		Indirect	8.0	
		Total	8.2	

Bilirubin (mg/dL): total 8.2, direct 0.2 and indirect 8.0.
Peripheral blood smear revealed increased polychromasia, many spherocytes and normoblastemia (**Figure 1**).

Section A: Anemias
Hemolytic Disease of the Newborn

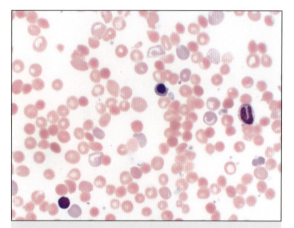

Figure 1 Blood smear (Wright-Giemsa, ×500) showing spherocytes, polychromasia and a nucleated red cell.

Differential Diagnosis The differential diagnosis of an anemic newborn with hyperbilirubinemia can be sorted based on the results of the direct antiglobulin test. Isoimmunization (ABO, Rh) gives a positive result with direct antiglobulin test (DAT or Coombs). Conditions with a negative DAT/Coombs include enclosed hemorrhage, increased enterohepatic circulation, twin-twin transfusion, delayed cord clamping, asphyxia, bowel obstruction, hypothyroidism, breastfeeding, Gilbert syndrome, Crigler-Najjar syndrome, enzyme deficiencies (eg, G6PD), hereditary spherocytosis, and disseminated intravascular coagulation. However, peripheral blood smear findings of spherocytes, polychromasia and normoblastemia narrowed the likely diagnoses to hereditary spherocytosis and hemolytic disease of the newborn (HDN) due to ABO incompatibility. HDN due to Rh incompatibility is not associated with the presence of spherocytes in the blood smear. Hereditary pyropoikilocytosis (HPP) and G6PD deficiency under acute oxidant stress may be associated with spherocytes in the peripheral blood smear but were considered unlikely due to the absence of significant poikilocytosis associated with the former and blister cells and bite cells associated with the latter. Autoimmune hemolytic anemia will be another consideration if the patient was an adult but it rarely, if ever, occurs in a newborn.

Additional Work-Up Bilirubin results at 8 hours of life were: total 9.9 mg/dL, direct 0.3 mg/dL and indirect 9.6 mg/dL. The reticulocyte count was 18.6%.

Blood type A, Rh positive, direct antiglobulin test (Coombs): positive for IgG, negative for C3d. Elution studies showed reactivity against Group A cells.

Final Diagnosis Hemolytic disease of the newborn (HDN) secondary to ABO incompatibility.

Management Approach In general, treatment of hyperbilirubinemia in an infant is based upon a standard nomogram that takes into account gestational age, postnatal age, and total and indirect bilirubin levels. This nomogram stratifies infants into high, intermediate and low-risk groups. Phototherapy is used to detoxify bilirubin and convert it to products that can be excreted without further conjugation or metabolism. In severe cases, phototherapy may fail and exchange transfusion must be implemented to remove bilirubin from the infant's circulation. For this infant, triple phototherapy alone was ineffective and exchange transfusion was implemented. The infant had a 2-volume exchange, which removes about 85% of red cells and up to 45% of serum bilirubin. Exchange transfusion coupled with continued phototherapy brought his bilirubin down to a safe level.

General Discussion Hyperbilirubinemia can be categorized based on the type of bilirubin that is elevated, which also elucidates its pathophysiology. Causes of direct or conjugated hyperbilirubinemia include conditions in which there is decreased excretion of bilirubin, a blockage to hepatic excretion or impaired bilirubin transport mechanism. Such conditions include: sepsis, severe hemolysis, biliary atresia, hepatitis, and enzyme deficiencies such as galactosemia, tyrosinemia or α-1-antitrypsin deficiency. Indirect hyperbilirubinemia is generally associated with conditions that cause excess production of bilirubin, reduced hepatic uptake, and impaired bilirubin conjugation. Excess production of bilirubin is generally the result of hemolytic anemias. In this case, the cause of the indirect hyperbilirubinemia was hemolytic disease of the newborn. Hemolytic disease of the newborn occurs when maternal antibodies to fetal red blood cell antigens, cross the placenta and cause hemolysis and anemia. It can occur as a result of Rh or ABO incompatibility between the mother and the fetus. Rarely, other antigen (such as K1 [Kell], Fy^a [Duffy]) incompatibilities may also cause HDN. The widespread use of Rho(D) immune globulin (RhIG) as a preventive measure over the past several years has markedly reduced the incidence of HDN due to Rh-incompatibility, specifically HDN due to anti-D. RhIG does not prevent formation of antibodies against minor antigens in the Rh system such as C and E, which can also cause HDN. HDN due to ABO incompatibility may affect first-born infants since antibodies against

ABO antigens that are not present in a person form naturally in response to antigenic substances in our environment. The mothers are generally Group O, because the lack of any A or B antigen preferentially permits their immune system to hyper-respond, leading to an IgG component of anti-A or anti-B. This is in addition to the normally occurring IgM component. In addition, Group O individuals can also make a composite antibody that reacts with either A or B antigens as part of their alloantibody called anti-A,B, which may also be IgG in nature. IgG antibodies can readily cross the placenta and this results in ongoing hemolysis. The resultant anemia is generally mild. HDN due to anti-D, though seen infrequently at least in the United States, can be quite severe, and may lead to fetal demise. Peripheral blood smear has a high degree of circulating normoblasts, leading to its other name, erythroblastosis fetalis. In HDN due to ABO antibodies, the anemia may be milder, and spherocytes are the most common abnormality on smear, with relatively fewer normoblasts.

Section A: Anemias

Anemia Associated with Fetomaternal Hemorrhage

Jay H Herman, Melissa R George

Patient A 22-year-old G2P1 at 28 weeks gestation was transferred from an outside hospital to a maternal fetal medicine practice group at a tertiary care hospital for decreased fetal movement for 24 hours.

Clinical History The patient had had a primary low transverse C-section because of fetal distress at term 3 years prior. The pregnancy was otherwise uneventful and the baby was born healthy. A repeat C-section was planned for this delivery. She has no significant medical conditions.

Family History The patient's mother is 47-years-old and has hypertension and asthma. The patient's father is 49 years old and has hypertension and diabetes.

Medications Prenatal vitamins.

Physical Examination The mother has no pallor, tachycardia or hypotension. There is no hepatomegaly or lymphadenopathy.

Initial Work-Up (Mother)

CBC		WBC Differential	%	# (×10³/μL)
WBC (×10³/μL)	4.0	Neutrophils	60	2.4
RBC (×10⁶/μL)	4.2	Bands	9	0.4
HGB (g/dL)	11.5	Lymphocytes	20	0.8
HCT (%)	34.5	Monocytes	8	0.3
MCV (fL)	79	Eosinophils	2	0.02
MCH (pg)	26	Basophils	1	0.04
MCHC (g/dL)	32			
PLT (×10³/μL)	150			
RDW-CV (%)	15.5			
MPV (fL)	9			

Her ABO type was O, Rh positive, antibody screen negative, syphilis negative, rubella immune, group B streptococcus negative, HIV 1/2 antibody negative. Ultrasonography: Mild fetal hydrops, without hepatosplenomegaly. Estimated fetal weight was 1,600 g.

Section A: Anemias
Anemia Associated with Fetomaternal Hemorrhage

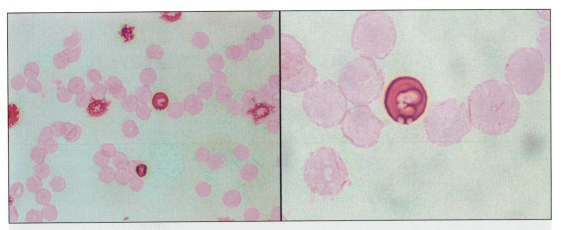

Figure 1 Kleihauer-Betke (left ×400, right ×1000). Darkly-stained fetal red cells in a background of pale-staining maternal cells ("ghost cells").

Additional Work-Up

Fetal laboratory results from prenatal umbilical blood sampling:
- Hemoglobin: 4.0 g/dL
- Hematocrit: 13%
- Blood type: A, Rh positive

Kleihauer-Betke (K-B) testing performed on a maternal blood sample on the day of the umbilical sampling showed 1.1% of red cells positive for the presence of fetal hemoglobin. (Normally there are no detectable fetal cells).

Differential Diagnosis Diagnostic considerations included fetomaternal hemorrhage, false-positive K-B due to increased maternal hemoglobin F, with fetal anemia, hemolytic disease of the newborn, thalassemia major, or marrow aplasia.

Final Diagnosis Anemia associated with fetomaternal hemorrhage causing nonimmune hydrops.

Management Approach In general, fetomaternal hemorrhage is managed based on the quantification of fetal blood loss into maternal circulation, using a Kleihauer-Betke stain or flow cytometry. The fetus is also assessed for middle cerebral artery peak systolic velocity. If the fetal blood loss is <20 percent of fetal volume, and there are no signs of fetal compromise, the fetus can be observed with close ultrasound monitoring. If the fetal blood loss is >20% and the gestational age is under 32 weeks, intravascular intrauterine transfusion is considered. If the fetus is over 32 weeks gestational age and shows lung maturity, early delivery may be considered. In this case, umbilical blood sampling performed at 28 weeks gestational age demonstrated fetal anemia to correlate with the evidence of decreased fetal movements and low fetal hemoglobin. The fetus was treated with intrauterine transfusion using 40 mL of CMV-safe, <5 day old, irradiated, Group O, Rh compatible CPDA-1 red cells packed to a higher than usual hematocrit just before transfusion. The fetal hemoglobin rose to 7.0 after the first transfusion. The fetus was monitored with daily fetal heart monitoring. Ultrasound was performed every other day. One week later, the fetus still appeared mildly hydropic by ultrasound, so another transfusion of 40 mL was given, raising the fetal hemoglobin to 10.1 mg/dL. By ultrasound, the fetal hydrops appeared to resolve. Concern over potential chronic fetomaternal bleeding prompted weekly cordocentesis, but no further transfusion was required. Timing of delivery was dictated by amniocentesis, which showed fetal lung maturity. A cesarian delivery was performed at 32 weeks. Examination of the placenta showed a small subchorionic hematoma. No arteriovenous malformation or other atypical vascular malformation of the placenta could be detected. At delivery the male infant weighed 2.2 kg. He was slightly pale, but vigorously crying. Apgars were 7-8 at 1 minute-5 minutes, respectively. At delivery, fetal hemoglobin was 10.5 mg/dL. The infant was treated with surfactant. He was discharged after 5 days in the hospital. The reticulocyte count at birth was elevated with NRBC evident on the infant's smear and the bilirubin level was mildly elevated. However, it did not rise higher and phototherapy was not required. The direct antiglobulin test (DAT) on the cord sample was negative for IgG.

Section A: Anemias
Anemia Associated with Fetomaternal Hemorrhage

General Discussion Normally, the placenta acts as a barrier between the maternal and fetal circulatory systems. Any derangement to this barrier, such as trauma or structural insufficiency of the blood vessels, can allow fetal cells into maternal circulation. Fetomaternal hemorrhage complicates 1-3 per 1,000 births, although few large series have actually studied the incidence. Fetomaternal hemorrhage is diagnosed by detection of hemoglobin F-positive cells in a maternal blood sample. This is accomplished in 1 of 2 ways, the Kleihauer-Betke test or flow cytometry. To perform the Kleihauer-Betke test, a technologist treats a maternal blood smear with an acidic solution. At low pH conditions, the hemoglobin A of adult red cells elutes across the cell membrane and causes them to stain pale pink. The adult cells are termed "ghost cells" because of their pale color. Fetal red cells retain their color because hemoglobin F is stable at low pH. A minimum of 2,000 red cells are counted at ×1000 magnification and the number of fetal cells is reported as a percentage. Some suggest routine Kleihauer-Betke screening of Rh-negative women after 20 weeks gestation, since a diagnosis of massive antenatal fetal maternal hemorrhage would guide dosage of prophylactic anti-Rh immune globulin during pregnancy. The volume of fetal blood in maternal circulation is determined by the following formula, which assumes an average maternal blood volume of 5,000 mL):

$$\text{Volume of fetal RBCs} = \frac{\text{fetal cells (\%) on Kleihauer-Betke smear} \times 5{,}000 \text{ mL}}{100 \text{ (correction for percentage)}}$$

Multiplying the above number by a factor of 2 will yield the volume in mL of fetal whole blood in maternal circulation, assuming an expected fetal hematocrit close to the mean of 50%. In this case, the volume of fetal blood loss at the time of the fetomaternal hemorrhage was 110 mL, $(1.1 \times 5{,}000/100) \times 2$. This was approximately 2/3 of the fetal blood volume at the time, assuming that at 28 weeks fetal blood volumes are 90-105 mL/kg. Although there was an ABO incompatibility between mother and infant that could have resulted in HDN if the mother was hyperimmune with IgG anti-A, the lack of evidence of ongoing hemolysis or worsening jaundice argues against this. A positive DAT is not always present in HDN due to ABO compatibility owing to decreased antigen density but the negative DAT is also evidence against HDN. The lack of worsening fetal anemia over the 4 weeks of in utero follow-up and the evidence of red cell production at birth argues against thalassemia or a marrow disorder.

Autoimmune Hemolytic Anemia, Warm-Reactive

John Krause, Gene Gulati, Joanne Filicko-O'Hara

Patient A 45-year-old woman, who was found to be anemic on a routine visit to her physician.

Clinical History The patient has a history of systemic lupus erythematosus (SLE). She reports photosensitivity and years of joint pains in hands and wrists.

Family History Both parents have hypertension.

Medications She has been treated with nonsteroidal anti-inflammatory agents (NSAIDs) and intermittent corticosteroids.

Physical Examination Remarkable only for a facial "butterfly" rash and signs of arthritis involving both hands and wrists.

Initial Work-Up

CBC		WBC Differential	%	# (×10³/µL)
WBC (×10³/µL)	5.2	Neutrophils	62	3.2
RBC (×10⁶/µL)	2.44	Bands	4	0.2
HGB (g/dL)	8.0	Lymphocytes	20	1.0
HCT (%)	24.5	Monocytes	12	0.6
MCV (fl)	100.2	Eosinophils	2	0.1
MCH (pg)	32.1			
MCHC (g/dL)	36.9			
RDW-CV (%)	18.5			
PLT (×10³/µL)	190			

Peripheral blood smear revealed numerous spherocytes and marked polychromasia (**Figures 1** and **2**).

Section A: Anemias
Autoimmune Hemolytic Anemia, Warm-Reactive

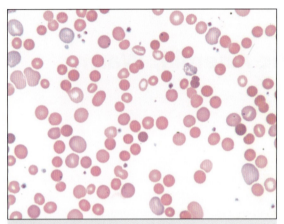

Figure 1 Blood smear (Wright, ×400) showing spherocytes, polychromasia, and anisocytosis.

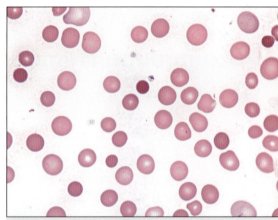

Figure 2 Blood smear (Wright, ×1000) showing spherocytes, polychromasia, and anisocytosis.

Differential Diagnosis Clinically, diagnostic considerations included blood loss secondary to NSAID induced gastritis, anemia of chronic disease, and autoimmune hemolytic anemia. However, the blood smear findings were compatible with either autoimmune hemolytic anemia or hereditary spherocytosis in hemolytic crisis.

Additional Work-Up
- Reticulocyte count: 13%
- Reticulocyte # 317.2 ×10³/µL (normal 20-76)
- Serum haptoglobin 10 mg/dL (normal 20-165)
- LDH 460 U/L (normal 100-190)
- Total bilirubin: 3.2 mg/dL
- Direct bilirubin: 0.2 mg/dL

A direct antiglobulin test (DAT or Coombs test) was positive. A bone marrow examination, though not indicated, was done and it revealed a normoblastic erythroid hyperplasia (**Figures 3, 4** and **5**).

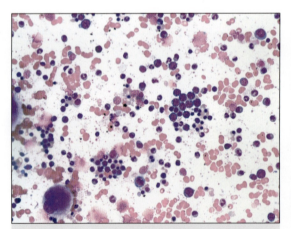

Figure 3 Bone marrow aspirate smear (Wright, ×400) showing erythroid hyperplasia with normoblastic maturation and reversal of the ME ratio.

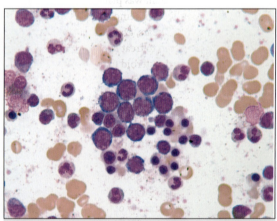

Figure 4 Bone marrow aspirate smear (Wright, ×1000) showing erythroid hyperplasia with normoblastic maturation and reversal of the ME ratio.

Section A: Anemias
Autoimmune Hemolytic Anemia, Warm-Reactive

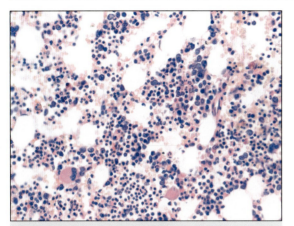

Figure 5 Bone marrow biopsy (H&E, ×400) showing trilineage maturation with erythroid hyperplasia.

Final Diagnosis Autoimmune hemolytic anemia, warm-antibody reactive.

Management Approach Besides supportive care with red cells or blood transfusion as needed, the therapeutic modalities include glucocorticoids, rituximab, plasma exchange, plasmapheresis, and splenectomy. Cytotoxic drugs such as cyclophosphamide, azathioprine and 6-mercaptopurine have also been used in patients unresponsive to other therapies. Most patients with SLE respond favorably to treatment with corticosteroids. Folate supplementation is recommended to meet the increased demand for the vitamin because of increased erythropoiesis. This patient was placed on prednisone at varying doses to keep her hemoglobin levels above 8 g/dL. Over the past 2 years, azathioprine and methotrexate were given to treat her lupus symptoms and to replace her corticosteroid therapy, but her hemoglobin levels would decrease whenever daily doses of prednisone were <15 mg/day.

Discussion Autoimmune hemolytic anemia (AIHA) occurs whenever an individual produces antibodies directed against antigens on their own red blood cells resulting in decreased red blood cell survival. These autoantibodies are classified as warm or cold depending on the optimal thermal activity of the antibody. Warm autoantibodies react best at 37°C and are usually IgG. Hemolysis occurs secondary to extravascular removal of the antibody coated red cells by macrophages in the reticuloendothelial system or by intravascular hemolysis by activation of the complement system. Warm autoantibodies in the adult population are commonly associated with underlying autoimmune disorders such as SLE (as in this patient) and malignances such as lymphoma. Cold autoantibodies are usually IgM and are present when testing is done at 4°C. Cold autoantibodies can have a thermal range that extends to room temperature. Pathologic cold autoantibodies may be associated with lymphomas, but are more commonly associated with *Mycoplasma pneumoniae* and Epstein-Barr infections. Other viral infections can be associated with AIHA in both adults and children. Typical peripheral blood findings in warm-reactive AIHA include spherocytes resulting from red cell membranes being partially removed by macrophages in the reticuloendothelial system, anisocytosis, and polychromasia. Nucleated red blood cells may also be seen. Hereditary spherocytosis (HS) and hemolytic disease of the newborn due to ABO incompatibility (HDN-ABO) are also associated with peripheral blood findings of spherocytosis and polychromasia. However, the DAT test is negative in HS and positive in HDN-ABO and AIHA. In cold agglutinin disease, there may be similar peripheral blood findings but an additional feature will be the presence of red cell agglutination. A bone marrow examination is usually not required to make a diagnosis of AIHA. However, if performed, the marrow is usually hypercellular with an erythroid hyperplasia. Marrow iron is usually present or even increased. If the hemolysis is severe and prolonged, a relative deficiency of folic acid or even vitamin B_{12} may occur resulting in a megaloblastic/megaloblastoid maturation. AIHA occurs in approximately 10% of patients with systemic lupus erythematosus. It may be the sole presenting sign of the disease and may predate the appearance of disease manifestations by several years. Many of the SLE patients with AIHA have elevated titers of IgG cardiolipin antibodies. It is not certain whether SLE patients with AIHA will exhibit a more benign or more severe overall prognosis for their primary disease.

Autoimmune Hemolytic Anemia, Cold-Reactive

Jay H Herman, Melissa R George

Patient A 38-year-old African-American woman, who presented to the emergency department with shortness of breath.

Clinical History The patient had been hospitalized with an upper respiratory infection at another hospital 3 weeks before this admission. She presented at the time of the current admission with dyspnea, wheezing, cough, fatigue and feeling like her "heart was racing." She had a history of diabetes, hypertension, and hyperlipidemia.

Family History Noncontributory.

Medications Insulin, metformin, simvastatin, enalapril, carvedilol, acetaminophen/oxycodone.

Physical Examination Unremarkable. There was no pallor, no ecchymoses or obvious bleeding. Her vital signs were: temperature 98.3°F, heart rate 110/min, blood pressure 127/74.

Initial Work-Up

CBC (post-incubation at 37°C)		WBC Differential	%	# (×10³/µL)
WBC (×10³/µL)	7.6	Neutrophils	51	3.9
RBC (×10⁶/µL)	3.5	Bands	2	0.2
HGB (g/dL)	8.2	Lymphocytes	36	2.7
HCT (%)	24.6	Monocytes	8	0.6
MCV (fL)	99	Eosinophils	3	0.2
MCH (pg)	33.1	Basophils	0	
MCHC (g/dL)	33.3	Reticulocytes	2.1	
PLT (×10³/µL)	223	Immature reticulocyte fraction	26.2	
RDW-CV (%)	24.4	Absolute reticulocytes (normal 25-75)		60
MPV (fL)	10.8			

Erythrocyte sedimentation rate = 85. PT and PTT results were within normal limits.
Peripheral blood smear revealed red cell agglutination and occasional spherocytes. No significant anisopoikilocytosis was appreciated, nor were any abnormal cells or intracellular or extracellular organisms seen (**Figure 1**).

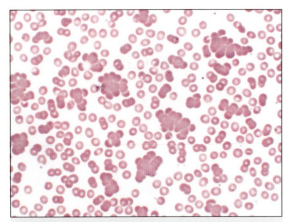

Figure 1 Blood smear (Wright-Giemsa, × 500) showing red cell agglutination (several clumps/aggregates of red cells are present).

Differential Diagnosis Peripheral blood smear findings are suggestive of a hemolytic process. Diagnostic considerations included autoimmune hemolytic anemia (cold-reactive or mixed cold and warm-reactive), alloimmune hemolytic anemia and cold agglutinin disease.

Additional Laboratory Work-Up
- Haptoglobin <6 mg/dL, LDH 663 U/L.
- Direct antiglobulin test (DAT or Coombs) negative for IgG and negative for C3d
- A serum antibody screen showed reactivity against all cells tested at room temperature but was negative when the sample was prewarmed to 37°C
- Urine hemoglobin positive.
- Total bilirubin 2.2 mg/dL, direct 0.9 mg/dL, indirect 1.3 mg/dL
- G6PD screen 10.3 (normal range: 4.6-13.5).
- Hemoglobin electrophoresis: no abnormal hemoglobins detected

Specific thermal amplitude studies demonstrated the cold reactivity was absent above 30°C, but became positive at increasing titer as the reaction approached room temperature. The cold agglutitin titer at room temperature was >1:1,024.

Final Diagnosis Autoimmune hemolytic anemia due to cold agglutinins.

Management Approach The management of autoimmune hemolytic anemia (AIHA) secondary to cold agglutinins depends largely on the severity of the hemolysis and the duration of disease. A key component of management is avoidance of cold. Patients must dress warmly even in the summer, and avoid ambient cold temperatures. If transfusion is required the blood should be given through a warming device. If the patient has an underlying hematologic malignancy, treating that condition will generally improve the cold agglutinin disease. Plasmapheresis may be useful as an adjunctive treatment, especially in the initial stages of hemolysis. However, the half-life of protein replacement is 5 days, so chronic maintenance is not very practical. In the common form of the disease from infection-associated cold agglutinins, hemolysis is self-limited as the titer spontaneously diminishes. In this case, once hemodynamic stability was achieved, the patient was discharged to home and managed through routine hematology follow-up as an outpatient.

General Discussion The clinical presentation of cold agglutinin autoimmune hemolytic anemia is similar to any other anemia with dyspnea, fatigue and rapid pulse being among the presenting symptoms. Additionally, these patients may also experience symptoms related to red cell agglutination upon exposure to cold, such as acrocyanosis of the fingertips, toes, nose and ears. Rarely, ulceration of the skin may develop. Cold agglutinins may lead to scleral icterus and splenomegaly from chronic hemolysis. Cold agglutinins are almost always IgM antibodies, explaining the negative direct antiglobulin test (DAT) against IgG and C3 in this patient. They are often produced in response to an infection or malignancy. The infections most commonly associated with cold agglutinins are *Mycoplasma pneumoniae* in adults and mononucleosis in children. In the case of *M pneumoniae*, the antibody has specificity for the I antigen and in mononucleosis, the specificity is for the i antigen. Cold agglutinins may sometimes be associated with other bacteria and viral infections. An unusual strain of *Listeria monocytogenes* has been associated with anti-I antibodies. Molecular mimicry may be the explanation for why these infectious agents cause antibodies of these specificities to form. Given the patient's presenting symptoms, history of respiratory infection and immune compromise secondary to diabetes, an infection such as *M pneumonia* or some other organism that causes high-titer anti-I would be the most likely cause of her cold agglutinin hemolysis. Aside from infectious etiologies, cold agglutinin disease may also be associated with hematologic malignancies such as chronic lymphocytic leukemia, lymphomas and Waldenström macroglobulinemia. In these cases, cold agglutinins with other specificities, often monoclonal in nature, are seen.

Significant red cell agglutination caused by cold agglutinins generates erroneous automated CBC results. Specifically, it produces falsely low RBC count and HCT and falsely high MCH and MCHC. The MCV may be falsely high if tiny clumps of red cells are counted as single cells. When larger clumps of red cells are not counted, the RBC count is erroneously low. Although generally not affected, hemoglobin result may be falsely low in some cases, presumably due to incomplete lysis of large red cell clumps in the hemoglobin measurement process. Incubating the blood specimen at 37°C for 10 minutes-15 minutes prior to reanalyzing for CBC usually resolves this problem and generates reliable results.

Section A: Anemias

Donath-Landsteiner Hemolytic Anemia (Paroxysmal Cold Hemoglobinuria)

Sherrie L Perkins, Hassan M Yaish, Mohamed E Salama

Patient A 6-year-old, previously healthy boy, who was brought to the emergency department with a sample of dark-colored urine.

Clinical History The child had a 2-week history of upper respiratory tract infection. The parents indicated that the child had not ingested any harmful agents. The child had played outside in the snow 1 day before admission. He then developed dark-colored urine, dysuria and emesis.

Family History Noncontributory.

Medications None.

Physical Examination Unremarkable. Dark-colored urine was noted.

Initial Work-Up

CBC		WBC Differential	%	# (×10³/µL)
WBC (×10³/µL)	11	Neutrophils	75	8.3
RBC (×10⁶/µL)	2.3	Bands	2	0.2
HGB (g/dL)	7	Lymphocytes	18	2.0
HCT (%)	21.4	Monocytes	5	0.6
MCV (fL)	82	Eosinophils	0	
MCH (pg)	28	Basophils	0	
MCHC (g/dL)	35.7	Reticulocytes	5.5 %,	
PLT (×10³/µL)	312	Nucleated RBCs	11/100 WBC	
RDW-CV (%)	18			
MPV (fL)	10.3			

Peripheral blood smear examination showed large numbers of atypical lymphocytes suggestive of viral process, slight to moderate spherocytosis, numerous nucleated red cells and polychromasia (**Figure 1**).

Serum: haptoglobin <8 mg/dL, LDH 2,331 U/L, BUN 38, creatinine 0.65 mg/dL, potassium 1.3 mg/dL.
Urine: creatinine 48.4 mg/dL, Urine protein 1,741 mg/dL, heme positive.

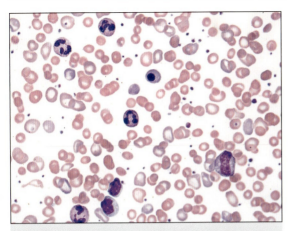

Figure 1 Blood smear (Wright, ×1000) showing anisocytosis, mild poikilocytosis, significant polychromasia with occasional spherocytes, and a nucleated red cell.

Differential Diagnosis Peripheral blood smear findings, hemoglobin in urine, low haptoglobin and high LDH are suggestive of intravascular hemolysis. The conditions associated with intravascular hemolysis include autoimmune hemolytic anemia, hemoglobinopathies, red cell enzyme deficiencies (such as G6PD deficiency), mechanical destruction as in burns, microangiopathic hemolytic anemia, and paroxysmal nocturnal hemoglobinuria.

Additional Work-Up
- Renal ultrasound with Doppler: normal study with bilaterally enlarged kidneys consistent with acute glomerulonephritis or acute tubular necrosis
- Direct antiglobulin test (DAT) was positive
- Urine test was positive for hemoglobin
- Serum hemoglobin 170 mg/dL
- Donath-Landsteiner test was positive

Final Diagnosis Donath-Landsteiner hemolytic anemia (DLHA)

Management approach The mother was told to avoid cold exposure. The patient was treated with steroids. On follow-up, the patient's anemia has responded to steroids with a normalizing reticulocyte count and hemoglobin level.

General discussion Donath-Landsteiner hemolytic anemia (previously referred to as paroxysmal cold hemoglobinuria) is the least common subtype of autoimmune hemolytic anemia, accounting for 1%-7% of cases and is most commonly seen in children, where it may comprise up to 40% of acute transient hemolytic anemia cases. It is an intravascular hemolytic anemia caused by a cold-reacting immunoglobulin IgG antibody directed specifically against the P antigen on the red cell surface and is usually triggered by a viral infection. It is usually a self-limited disorder; however, there may be severe hemolysis with intermittent episodes that occur upon exposure to cold, manifesting by episodes of hemoglobinuria or dark urine and associated systemic symptoms of fever, chills, malaise, cramping, nausea or pain. The hemolysis often leads to severe anemia with attendant signs of intravascular hemolysis including polychromasia, circulating nucleated red cells, and spherocytes. Splenomegaly may be encountered. Patients may also develop renal insufficiency as a result of the overwhelming hemoglobinuria and renal tubular damage. Intravascular hemolysis can be related to both immune and nonimmune mechanisms. Among immune-mediated causes are incompatible transfusion, autoimmune hemolytic anemia and drug-antibody mediated complexes. Nonimmune causes of hemolysis include hemoglobinopathies, red cell enzyme deficiencies such as G6PD deficiency, mechanical destruction (burns), microangiopathic hemolytic anemia, malaria and paroxysmal nocturnal hemoglobinuria. The direct globulin test (DAT) is useful for separating immune and nonimmune mechanisms. A positive DAT is generally indicative of immune-related hemolysis. DAT detects in vivo sensitization of erythrocytes by bound immunoglobulin. An autoimmune hemolysis is the most probable etiology of this child's positive DAT, since he was neither transfused nor given drugs implicated in immune-mediated hemolysis. Autoimmune hemolysis can be classified into warm reactive antibodies, cold reactive antibodies and Donath-Landsteiner hemolytic anemia. Donath-Landsteiner hemolytic anemia is characterized by an IgG autoantibody (Donath-Landsteiner antibody) that binds to red cells in the cold, but hemolysis occurs only after warming to 37°C. This is a polyclonal antibody that acts as an autohemolysin by binding to the P antigen on the patient's red cells at lower temperatures. After warming, the autohemolysin fixes complement, leading to hemolysis. In contrast, cold agglutinin disease is due to a cold-reacting IgM antibody where antibody affinity decreases upon warming, leading to red cell agglutination with mild to moderate hemolysis. The Donath-Landsteiner test is performed to confirm a Donath-Landsteiner hemolytic anemia diagnosis by demonstrating the characteristic biphasic nature of the autohemolysin. Donath-Landsteiner antibody fixes complement to erythrocyte membranes. The antibody has the greatest avidity for its antigen

Section A: Anemias
Donath-Landsteiner Hemolytic Anemia (Paroxysmal Cold Hemoglobinuria)

in the cold; therefore, complement is bound during 4°C incubation. The enzymatic steps in complement activation are completed only during the subsequent warm incubation at 37°C. The test involves splitting an aliquot of blood and incubating one sample at room temperature and one at 4°C and then exposing both samples to 37°C. If the Donath-Landsteiner antibody is present, centrifugation will demonstrate hemolysis in the cooled sample but not the sample kept at 37°C. It is thought that the patient's extremities, especially the distal digits when exposed to cold, cause the antibody to attach to red cells, and once the cells circulate to warmer body temperature areas the complement attached to the cells will be activated, resulting in hemolysis. The low avidity of the Donath-Landsteiner antibody (at room temperature) allows antibody dissociation from its antigen, resulting in a negative direct antiglobulin test with monospecific anti-IgG. Since the antibody readily elutes from warm red cells, crossmatching is generally not a problem. Donath-Landsteiner hemolytic anemia is usually a self-limited disorder that will resolve spontaneously with resolution of the associated viral illness. Protection from the cold is key to preventing severe hemolysis during the disease course. Treatment of AIHA in general (including DLHA) is directed by the severity of the patient's symptoms and the hemoglobin level. Patients who are stable with mild anemia (Hgb of 9-12 g/dL) should be observed closely. Those with lower levels of hemolysis (6-9 g/dL) could also be observed, or if highly symptomatic then should receive blood transfusions. Knowing the difficulty in obtaining matched blood in this setting, the least incompatible units should be given with the aim to improve the patient's symptoms temporarily while waiting for the other treatment measures to work. Corticosteroids are effective in warm-reacting AIHA as well as Donath-Landsteiner hemolytic anemia (80% of the time). They should be given in a dose of 1-2 mg/kg IV initially, then PO for 3 weeks-4 weeks, followed by slow taper. This modality is less effective in pure IgM cold agglutinin disease, which is treated in the severe forms by plasmapheresis. The role of high-dose IgG treatment is not as well defined. It is given as 1 g/kg IV daily for 5 days. It is reported to be effective in only 1/3 of the cases. Splenectomy, when all treatments fail may offer a temporary or permanent solution in >2/3 of the cases. In recent years, rituximab, a monoclonal antibody directed against CD20 on the B lymphocytes, has shown significant efficiency and immunosuppressive activity and should probably be tried before splenectomy.

Hemoglobin SC Disease

Samir Ballas

Patient A 24-year-old African-American man known to have sickle cell disease was admitted to the hospital with a recurrent acute painful crisis. He tried to manage his pain at home but failed to achieve adequate pain relief.

Clinical History The pain involved his anterior chest wall, right upper extremity (from shoulder to hand), left knee and left leg. The throbbing pain had an intensity score of 9 on a verbal scale from 0 (no pain) to 10 (worst pain). He had no fever, cough or dyspnea. The diagnosis of sickle cell disease was made during infancy. During childhood and adolescence he had relatively few acute painful episodes. During the 4 years to 6 years prior to admission he started to have frequent painful crises. He was admitted to the hospital 10 times and treated in the emergency department 24 times during the previous year. DNA analysis revealed that he had hemoglobin SC disease with deletion of 1 α gene. His hemoglobin genotype was β^s/β^c; -α/αα. Other complications of his disease included avascular necrosis of hips and shoulders and multiple bone infarcts in the right humerus, left femur, knee, tibia and ribs both anteriorly and posteriorly.

Family History One parent had sickle trait and the other had hemoglobin C trait.

Medications Folic acid, diazepam and acetaminophen/oxycodone.

Physical Examination Vital signs were within normal limits. The sclerae were not icteric. The lungs were clear and the heart revealed a Grade II/VI systolic murmur with no arrhythmias. A nontender spleen tip was felt in the left upper quadrant. The liver was not palpable and he had no lymphadenopathy. There was diffuse tenderness to palpation over the right shoulder, hips, knees and left leg. Allodynia over the left leg was noted. There was also tenderness over the rib cage and throughout the spine, mostly in the cervical and lumbosacral regions, with no gross body deformities. The rest of the physical exam was unremarkable.

Initial Work-Up

CBC		Differential	%	# (×10³/μL)
WBC (×10³/μL)	9.6	Neutrophils	55	5.3
RBC (×10⁶/μL)	3.45	Bands	3	0.3
HGB (g/dL)	9.1	Lymphocytes	36	3.5
HCT (%)	26.6	Monocytes	4	0.4
MCV (fL)	77	Eosinophils	1	0.1
MCH (pg)	26.5	Basophils	1	0.1
MCHC (g/dL)	34.4	Reticulocyte count	1.2	
PLT (×10³/μL)	250			
RDW-CV (%)	15.6			

The original diagnostic hemoglobin electrophoresis results were hemoglobin S 51% and hemoglobin C 49%. Examination of the peripheral smear showed target cells, hemoglobin SC crystalloids, blister-like cells, and "boat-shaped" cells (**Figures 1** and **2**).

Section A: Anemias
Hemoglobin SC Disease

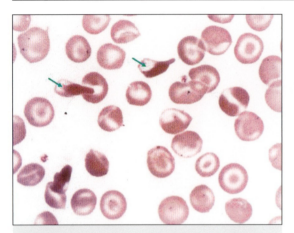

Figure 1 Blood smear (Wright-Giemsa, ×1000) showing target cells, boat-shaped cells, SC crystalloids and blister-like cells (arrows).

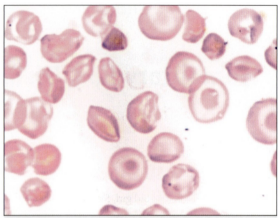

Figure 2 Blood smear (Wright-Giemsa, ×1000) showing target cells, boat-shaped cells and Howell-Jolly bodies.

Differential Diagnosis The patient already carried a specific diagnosis of hemoglobin SC disease and heterozygous α-thalassemia.

Additional Work-Up Total bilirubin 2.2 mg/dL, alkaline phosphate 458 IU/L, AST 258 IU/L and ALT 74 IU/L. X-rays of hips and long bones confirmed the presence of avascular necrosis and multiple bone infarcts.

Final Diagnosis Hemoglobin SC disease with acute painful crisis, avascular necrosis, multiple bone infarcts and heterozygous α-thalassemia.

Management Approach His clinical condition was initially stabilized with symptomatic and supportive care, which included hydration and parenteral meperidine (150 mg every 2 hours as needed) and parenteral diphenhydramine (50 mg every 4 hours as needed). However, a few days later, while still in the hospital, he became increasingly agitated, his mental status deteriorated acutely and he complained of severe pain. His temperature increased to 103.6°F, pulse 135/min and respiratory rate 32/min. HGB decreased to 6.0 g/dL, WBC count increased to $27 \times 10^3/\mu L$ with 50 NRBC per 100 WBC. Numerous blister cells were seen on the smear (**Figure 1**), platelet count decreased to $50 \times 10^3/\mu L$, serum creatinine increased to 3.0 mg/dL, potassium to 5.5 mm/L and SpO_2 decreased to 71 mmHg on room air. He was transferred to the cardiac care unit and intubated. Despite all heroic measures, his condition continued to deteriorate with a fatal outcome. Autopsy showed evidence of multiorgan involvement with sickled cells mostly in the lungs, kidneys and liver. Marrow emboli were noted in both lungs (**Figure 3**). The liver was enlarged to 2,400 g with cholestasis, the heart was enlarged to 450 g with left ventricular hypertrophy and right atrial dilatation with mural thrombi. The kidneys were congested with acute tubular necrosis and fibrin deposits in the large vessels. The final diagnosis was acute multiorgan failure due to fat/bone marrow embolization complicating an acute sickle cell painful crisis.

General Discussion Patients with hemoglobin SC disease usually have milder anemia, less painful crises, less priapism, and fewer leg ulcers than patients with SS. Retinopathy, blindness, splenomegaly and thromboembolic complications; however, occur more frequently in hemoglobin SC disease. This patient is unusual in having frequent acute painful crises. Patients with sickle cell disease of any type who experience frequent and severe painful crises seem to have poor prognosis and increased morbidity and mortality. Moreover, acute multiorgan failure and acute chest syndrome (ACS) are serious complications of painful crises. About 50% of ACS and almost all multiorgan failure with fat embolism occur during the evolution of a painful crisis. The onset of multiorgan failure in this patient was so sudden and severe that appropriate management with blood exchange transfusion could not be done in due time.

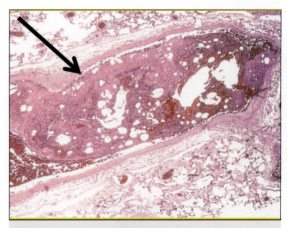

Figure 3 Autopsy specimen of lung (H&E, × 200) showing a large bone marrow embolus.

Hereditary Spherocytosis

Gene Gulati, Joanne Filico O'Hara, John Krause

Patient An 18-year-old girl, 5 months pregnant (G1 P0), came into an obstretician's office for a prenatal check-up.

Clinical History Noncontributory.

Family History Her mother had undegone splenectomy approximately 10 years ago for a condition unknown to the patient.

Medications None.

Physical Examination The patient appeared pale and jaundiced. Her abdomen is gravid with an enlarged uterus palpable in the lower abdomen/pelvis.

Initial Work-Up

CBC	
WBC (×10³/µL)	10.6
RBC (×10⁶/µL)	2.58
HGB (g/dL)	8.7
HCT (%)	23.5
MCV (fL)	91
MCH (pg)	33.7
MCHC (g/dL)	37.1
PLT (×10³/µL)	242
RDW-CV (%)	16.1
MPV (fL)	8.7

WBC Differential	%	# (×10³/µL)
Neutrophils	76	8.1
Bands	4	0.4
Lymphocytes	11	1.2
Monocytes	8	0.8
Basophils	1	0.1

Peripheral blood smear revealed spherocytes and polychromasia (**Figure 1**).

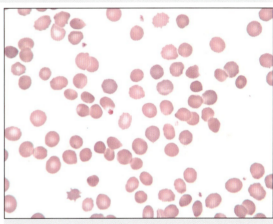

Figure 1 Blood smear (Wright, ×1000) showing spherocytes and polychromasia. An acanthocyte and a few echinocytes are also present.

Differential Diagnosis Two clinical conditions typically associated with normocytic normochromic or hyperchromic anemia with the blood smear revealing spherocytes and polychromasia in an adult are hereditary spherocytosis and immune hemolytic anemia (warm antibody-mediated). A small number of spherocytes, particularly microspherocytes are also often seen in the blood smear of patients with severe burns over ⅔ of the body. In a newborn baby, hemolytic disease of the newborn, ABO-incompatibility type may also be included in the differential diagnosis. Before additional work-up towards reaching a final diagnosis is performed, it is important to confirm the presence of true spherocytes, as opposed to pseudospherocytes, in the blood smear by an experienced hematomorphologist. A true spherocyte is characterized by its round shape, slightly reduced diameter, slightly increased thickness, normal volume, absence of central pallor, and dense staining in the readable area away from the feather edge of the blood smear. In contrast, a pseudospherocyte is a round cell with normal or slightly increased diameter, normal thickness, normal volume, and no central pallor, and it stains like a normal red cell. While examining the blood smear for the presence of spherocytes, 1 should be alert to the fact that transfused red cells at times may also mimick true spherocytes. The Coombs test is helpful in the differential diagnosis between hereditary spherocytosis and immune hemolytic anemia.

Additional Work-Up
- Coombs test: negative
- Reticulocyte % 7.0
- Reticulocyte 180.6 (10^3/μL)
- Serum.
- Bilirubin: total 3.1, direct 1.1
- LDH: 310
- Haptoglobin <20

Final Diagnosis Hereditary spherocytosis.

Management Approach The clinical course of hereditary spherocytosis is variable among patients. Some have an asymptomatic course with mild anemia or no anemia whereas others may have a life-threatening course marked by severe anemia, marked jaundice, bone marrow expansion and extramedullary hematopoiesis. The majority of patients; however, fall in between these extremes and require individualized symptomatic treatment that may include blood transfusion(s), splenectomy, folate supplementation for chronic erythroid hyperplasia, folate administration to ward off megaloblastic crisis, packed red cell transfusion for aplastic crisis, and cholecystectomy for biliary lithiasis. Splenectomy ameliorates hemolysis and consequently reduces the transfusion requirements but does not eliminate the spherocytic defect. Vaccination against *S pneumoniae* is recommended prior to splenectomy. Most patients with little or no hemolysis follow a benign clinical course and require no treatment. It is recommended that the children of families with a history of spherocytosis should be screened for this disorder. This patient was transfused with whole blood and given folate supplementation.

General Discussion Hereditary spherocytosis is a red cell membrane disorder that is most prevalent among people of northern European ancestry. The usual mode of inheritance is autosomal dominant with variable expression but autosomal recessive pattern has also been reported in some studies. Spontaneous mutations have also been noted. A variety of molecular defects in genes encoding for a number of red cell membrane proteins, including spectrin, ankyrin, protein 3, and protein 4.1 have been noted. Among these, defective/dysfunctional ankyrin and/or spectrin is/are responsible for the lack of deformability of red cells in most cases. Clinical manifestations are variable but include pallor, fatigue, anemia, jaundice, splenomegaly, and shortness of breath in some cases. The chronic hemolytic state varies widely in severity from no apparent anemia (compensated hemolysis) to severe anemia, with red cells being normocytic and either normochromic or hyperchromic. Peripheral blood smear may reveal only a few spherocytes that may be easily missed on routine microscopic examination or easily discernible with many spherocytes. Depending upon the degree of anemia, a variable degree of polychromasia is also noted. Howell-Jolly bodies, target cells, and thrombocytosis are additional findings noted often in the blood smears of patients who have undergone splenectomy in the course of the management of the disease. Complications that may arise include gallstones, hemolytic crisis, megaloblastic crisis, and aplastic crisis, the latter often triggered by a viral infection or some sort of stress. Iron overload may also become a problem in patients who receive repeated blood transfusions and iron supplementation as part of the management of their severe disease. The laboratory findings often reveal increased reticulocyte count (except in aplastic crisis), bilirubin, and LDH. The Coombs test is negative. The osmotic fragility test, often performed in the past for the laboratory diagnosis of hereditary spherocytosis, is now neither available nor considered necessary for the diagnosis. The primary diagnostic tools include careful clinical history of the patient and his/her family and peripheral blood smear examination.

Sickle Cell Anemia

Lakshmanan Krishnamurti, Jay Raval, Raymond E Felgar

Patient A 2-week-old female infant with an abnormal newborn screen.

Clinical History The child was born normal at term. Newborn screen revealed the presence of hemoglobins F and S, suggestive of sickle cell disease.

Family History Noncontributory.

Medications None.

Physical Examination Well-nourished infant, sleeping comfortably, no icterus or hepatosplenomegaly.

Initial Work-Up

CBC	Value	Normal Range
WBC (×10³/μL)	9.0	5.0-20.0
RBC (×10⁶/μL)	4.89	3.10-5.30
HGB (g/dL)	16.5	12.5-20.5
HCT (%)	49.4	39.0-63.0
MCV (fL)	97.5	86.0-124.0
MCH (pg)	32.7	31.0-39.0
MCHC (g/dL)	33.5	31.0-35.0
RDW-CV (%)	16.1	11.8-15.2
PLT (×10³/μL)	423	156-369
Newborn screen	FS (indicating that hemoglobins identified in the patient in decreasing order of estimated concentration are fetal hemoglobin and hemoglobin S).	FA (indicating that hemoglobins identified in the patient in decreasing order of estimated concentration are fetal hemoglobin and the normal adult hemoglobin, hemoglobin A).

Peripheral blood smear revealed target cells and occasional, partially sickled red cells (**Figure 1**).

Section A: Anemias
Sickle Cell Anemia

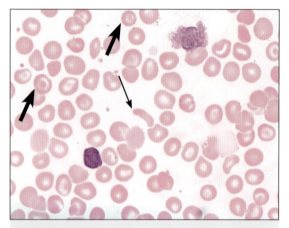

Figure 1 Blood smear (Wright-Giemsa, ×1000) showing target cells (thick arrows) and partially sickled red cells (thin arrow).

Differential Diagnosis Newborn with an electrophoretic pattern of FS is suspected to have homozygous sickle cell disease (SS) or a double heterozygote for sickle and β^0-thalassemia.

(HbS/β^0-thalassemia). The 2 are similar in clinical severity. HbS/β^0-thalassemia is suspected when there is microcytosis and can be confirmed by β-globin gene sequencing studies or by parental studies. Hemoglobin electrophoresis should be repeated at age 6 months-1 year, by when it is anticipated that the globin gene switching will be complete and level of fetal hemoglobin is expected to be minimal.

Additional Work-Up

Hemoglobin electrophoresis revealed hemoglobin A_1 0.0%, hemoglobin A 2 0.3%, hemoglobin F 75.5% and hemoglobin S 24.2%. No hemoglobin A was present. By high-performance liquid chromatography (HPLC), in addition to HbF (expected at this age), there was an abnormal peak in the S window. These results are consistent with homozygous S disease (SS or βS/βS or sickle cell anemia) or compound heterozygous S and β^0-thalassemia (HbS/β^0-thalassemia). However, these results along with normal MCV favor the former.

Final Diagnosis Sickle cell anemia.

Management Approach Comprehensive care and supportive care have increased life expectancy and decreased morbidity in sickle cell disease (SCD). Neonatal screening programs enable early identification of patients and early institution of preventive antibiotics and pneumococcal vaccination. Screening of the cerebral arteries by transcranial Doppler ultrasound (TCD) can identify high-risk patients for stroke. Intervention with regular erythrocyte transfusions for patients found to be at high risk has been shown to diminish the risk of stroke. Chronic transfusions carry the risk of iron overload syndrome, alloimmunization and hyperhemolysis syndrome. Hydroxyurea has been shown to induce the synthesis of HbF and decrease sickle cell crises, acute chest syndrome and prolong survival. Exchange transfusion in multiorgan failure syndrome, acute stroke or severe acute chest crises can be life saving. This patient was enrolled in comprehensive care, and started immediately on penicillin prophylaxis and received pneumococcal vaccine.

General Discussion Sickle cell anemia is a hemolytic disease characterized by abnormally sickle shaped red blood cells, which are removed from the circulation and destroyed at increased rates, leading to anemia. Sickle cell hemoglobin is composed of 2 normal α chains with 2 mutated β chains. The most common mutation is the replacement of the β6 glutamic acid for valine (HbS). This mutation occurs as homozygous (HbSS) or in combination with different β chain gene mutations like β^0 (HbS/β) or HbSC (β6 glutamic acid for leucine). In deoxygenated conditions, hydrophobic interactions of the separate hemoglobin molecules results in polymerization of the hemoglobin with resultant deformation of the erythrocyte. Normal passage of erythrocytes through small blood vessels requires flexibility of the cell, which is severely hampered by the sickled state. Activation of adhesion molecules on the erythrocyte and endothelial cells results in increased adherence of the erythrocytes to the vascular lining and contributes to obstruction. Intravascular hemolysis releases free hemoglobin, which binds with high affinity to nitric oxide, disturbing the normal vascular homeostatic function of nitric oxide. The resulting vasoconstriction further compromises the transit time of erythrocytes and contributes to vaso-occlusion. Functional asplenia due to multiple infarctions has been found before the age of 1 year. At age 5 years, 94% of the sickle patients will be asplenic and more susceptible for sepsis caused by encapsulated bacteria. Virtually every organ can be affected by microinfarctions. Small occlusive events are very painful if occurring in bone or lungs. Painful vaso-occlusive crisis are the hallmark of sickle cell disease. Repeated pain crisis has affects quality of life severely. Hand-foot syndrome is a painful swelling of hands and feet due to dactylitis and usually the first manifestation of SCD in children under 3 years of age. Approximately 10% of patients will develop stroke, typically between the ages of 2 and 6 years and 22% have changes in cerebral parenchyma on MRI that suggest a silent stroke. Repeated painful bone crises result in bone sequesters and growth disturbances, osteonecrosis and increased susceptibility for *Salmonella* or *Staphylococcus aureus* osteomyelitis. Avascular necrosis of the femoral and humeral head can cause destruction of joints and lead to pain and immobility. Renal medullary microinfarctions may result in renal papillary necrosis with loss of nephrons and kidney function. Hyposthenuria as a result of repetitive microinfarctions of in the renal medulla will give uncontrolled loss of water and nocturnal enuresis. Approximately 30%-45% of male sickle cell patients will have at least 1 episode of priapism during their lifetime.

Irreversible ischemic penile injury may result in fibrosis and erectile dysfunction. Acute chest syndrome (ACS) is the combination of fever, chest pain and respiratory distress with new pulmonary consolidations on chest X-ray. Initially ACS can be difficult to differentiate from pneumonia and both can exist at the same time. Clinical symptoms of ACS however are far more severe than of pneumonia. Chronic pulmonary insults either infarctions or repeated infections results in pulmonary fibrosis and pulmonary hypertension. Additionally the binding of nitric oxide by free hemoglobin can lead to acute cardiac death, which can also be attributed to right ventricular hypertrophy with dysfunction. The presence of pulmonary hypertension is highly associated with increased mortality.

Hereditary Elliptocytosis

Gene Gulati, Joanne Filicko O'Hara, John Krause

Patient A 10-year-old boy, who was brought to the emergency room with a laceration on his head as a result of a fall at home.

Clinical History He has a history of seizure disorder.

Family History Both parents known to be mildly anemic throughout life.

Medications Valproic acid.

Physical Examination Normal except for the open wound on left side of the head.

Initial Work-Up

CBC	
WBC (×10³/μL)	6.5
RBC (×10⁶/μL)	4.04
HGB (g/dL)	11.5
HCT (%)	33.8
MCV (fL)	84
MCH (pg)	28.4
MCHC (g/dL)	33.9
PLT (×10³/μL)	250
RDW-CV (%)	12.7
MPV (fL)	10.4

WBC Differential	%	# (×10³/μL)
Neutrophils	16	1.1
Bands	1	0.0
Lymphocytes	71	4.6
Monocytes	4	0.3
Eosinophils	7	0.5
Basophils	1	0.0

Peripheral blood smear revealed marked elliptocytosis (**Figure 1**) and occasional schistocytes.

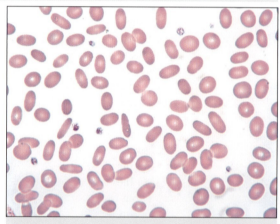

Figure 1 Blood smear (Wright, ×1000) showing marked elliptocytosis.

Differential Diagnosis Although a slight to moderate degree of elliptocytosis may be observed in a number of disorders including hereditary elliptocytosis, iron deficiency anemia, thalassemias, anemia of renal disease, megaloblastic anemia, myelodysplastic syndrome, and chronic myeloproliferative neoplasms, marked elliptocytosis, as noted in this case, is seen essentially only in hereditary elliptocytosis. Theoretically, the hereditary nature of this diagnosis can be confirmed by finding elliptocytosis in the blood smears of other family members, particularly the patient's parents. However, when the family members are not available for study, the diagnosis of hereditary elliptocytosis may still be made with reasonable certainty as long as the degree of elliptocytosis is marked (3+ or 4+, ie, over 50% of red cells are elliptical or oval in shape). Up to 5% of elliptocytes may be seen in the blood smear of healthy persons. Pseudoelliptocytosis, an uncommon artifact of blood smear preparation, should not be mistaken for true elliptocytosis.

Additional Work-Up No additional laboratory work-up was done and none is usually necessary. Significant hemolysis, seen in some cases, results in a high reticulocyte count, increased serum bilirubin (primarily indirect) and lactic dehydrogenase (LDH), and decreased serum haptoglobin. Red cell membrane studies and elucidation of molecular defect in individual cases remain in the realm of research oriented medical centers and are not considered essential.

Final Diagnosis Hereditary elliptocytosis.

Management Approach A large majority of patients are asymptomatic with little or no anemia and require no treatment. Folate supplementation may be recommended to prevent folate deficiency in a hemolytic state. A few patients, who reveal moderate or severe hemolysis may require supportive measures including blood transfusions and may benefit from splenectomy. This patient did not require any therapy.

General Discussion Hereditary elliptocytosis is a heterogeneous group of disorders that share the common characteristic finding of elliptical erythrocytes in the peripheral blood smear. The proportion of red cells that are elliptical varies from 25%-100%. The elliptocytes are usually normocytic and normochromic. It must be noted that the degree of hemolysis does not correlate with the number of elliptocytes present. The prevalence in the United States is reported to be 3-5 per 10,000. It is usually inherited as an autosomal dominant trait and is relatively more common in African-Americans. A wide variety of mutations in several different genes that encode proteins of the red cell membrane skeleton have been identified, including deficient or defective spectrin, protein 4.1, protein 3, and glycophorin C. Deficient or defective spectrin (failure of self-association of heterodimers into heterotetramers) is the most common abnormality. Genetic testing and/or biochemical analysis of individual membrane proteins help identify the underlying defect but are neither routinely available nor required for diagnosis and management. Rather, a positive family history and/or the presence of elliptocytes in the blood smears of other family members (parents, siblings, and children) is/are more important for the diagnosis. Over 85% of cases are asymptomatic and reveal no anemia or mild anemia and are diagnosed by chance when a blood smear is examined as a part of the complete blood count for a non-related condition. Approximately 10% to 15% of cases may reveal moderate to severe anemia as a result of uncompensated hemolysis. Peripheral blood smears of such cases often reveal a significant number of red cell fragments (schistocytes), variable degree of poikilocytosis, variable degree of polychromasia, and/or a variable number of spherocytes, in addition to the prominent elliptocytosis. Elliptocytes, like spherocytes are less deformable compared to the normal red cells. Patients with clinically significant uncompensated hemolysis often reveal pallor, fatigue, sceleral icterus, splenomegaly, and in rare cases, leg ulcers. Complications, such as cholecystitis and cholelithiasis may also occur. Three morphologic subtypes of hereditary elliptocytosis include common hereditary elliptocytosis (HE), spherocytic elliptocytosis (SE), and southeast Asian ovalocytosis (SAO) or stomatocytic elliptocytosis. Additionally, a severe variant of common HE, known by the names of hereditary pyropoikilocytosis (HPP) has also been recognized, though primarily in individuals of African ancestry. Peripheral blood smears of HPP are characterizd by the presence of microspherocytes, elliptocytes, red cell fragments and poikilocytosis. The red cells of HPP are prone to severe fragmentation at temperatures above 37°C. Spherocytic elliptocytosis is seen primarily in individuals of European ancestry, and their peripheral blood smear reveals elliptocytes and spherocytes but not poikilocytosis. The SAO is commonly found in malaria-endemic southasian countries, such as Malaysia, Melanesia, Indonesia, New Guinea, and the Philippines and the blood smear often reveals ovolocytes with 1 or 2 transverse slits giving them the appearance of stomatocytes.

Section A: Anemias

Sickle-α-Thalassemia

Samir Ballas

Patient A 22-year-old Hispanic woman known to have sickle cell disease transferred her care to our sickle cell program.

Clinical History The patient reported that when she was 3 years old she had an episode of dactylitis in both hands and hematologic work-up revealed a diagnosis of sickle cell disease. Past medical history included frequent acute painful episodes, several episodes of pneumonia, 1 episode of acute chest syndrome that required treatment in the intensive care unit including red cell exchange transfusion and avascular necrosis of the right hip. She received an estimated 50 red cell transfusions since early childhood. She is G0 P0 A0.

Family History Her father and 1 sister have sickle cell trait and 2 brothers have no abnormal hemoglobins. The patient did not recall if her mother was ever tested.

Medications Folic acid and acetaminophen/oxycodone.

Physical examination Normal vital signs with no scleral icterus, hepatosplenomegaly or lymphadenopathy.

Initial Work-Up

CBC		WBC Differential	%	# (×10^3/µL)
WBC (×10^3/µL)	12.0	Neutrophils	46	5.5
RBC (×10^6/µL)	4.17	Bands	0	
HGB (g/dL)	9.2	Lymphocytes	44	5.3
HCT (%)	30.0	Monocytes	8	1.0
MCV (fL)	72	Eosinophils	2	0.2
MCH (pg)	22.1	Basophils	0	
MCHC (g/dL)	30.7	Reticulocyte count	8	
PLT (×10^3/µL)	464	Nucleated red cells	5/100WBC	
RDW-CV (%)	19.3			

Peripheral blood smear revealed polychromasia, microcytic hypochromic red cells, sickle cells, occasional target cells, and a few nucleated red cells (**Figure 1**).
Serum ferritin was 1,820 ng/mL.
Hemoglobin electrophoresis showed hemoglobin S 88%, F 6% and A$_2$ 6%.

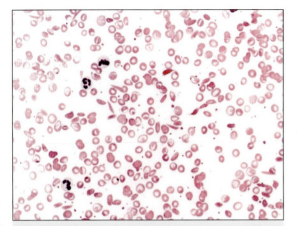

Figure 1 Blood smear (Wright-Giemsa, ×500) showing sickle cells, target cells and microcytic hypochromic red cells.

Differential Diagnosis
- Microcytic hypochromic anemia: Iron deficiency is unlikely in view of the clinical history and the multiple blood transfusions.
- Sickle cell anemia (SS): This is the most common type of sickle cell disease in the USA. Except for the microcytic hypochromic indices the clinical picture and the CBC are consistent with sickle cell anemia. The coexistence of α-thalassemia with SS may explain the red cell indices.
- Sickle-β^+-thalassemia: The relatively mild anemia and the red cell indices are in favor of this diagnosis. One would expect; however, to see more target cells in the peripheral smear and the MCV is usually in the 60s. The fact that the hemoglobin electrophoresis showed no hemoglobin A is against this diagnosis.
- Sickle-β^0-thalassemia: The relatively mild anemia and the paucity of target cells are against this diagnosis. Also the MCV is usually in the 60s. Nevertheless it is a possible diagnosis.
- Hemoglobin SC disease: This diagnosis is easily ruled out due to the description of the peripheral smear that, usually, shows numerous target cells, microspherocytes and boat-shaped sickle cells, also referred to as fat sickle cells. Avascular necrosis is known; however, to occur in young patients with hemoglobin SC disease due to the hyperviscosity associated with mild anemia. Moreover, hemoglobin electrophoresis showed no hemoglobin C.
- Avascular necrosis: As mentioned above this diagnosis occurs in young patients with those sickle cell syndromes associated with mild anemia, including, usually, hemoglobin SC disease or sickle-β^+-thalassemia but could occur in other types

albeit less often. In general avascular necrosis occurs in relatively older patients, except in the conditions mentioned.
- Transfusional hemosiderosis: This is a possible diagnosis because of the history of multiple blood transfusions.

Additional Work-Up In order to confirm the diagnosis her medical records from pediatrics were obtained. Surprisingly those records indicated that she has sickle-β^0-thalassemia. The high level of hemoglobin A_2 is consistent with the diagnosis of sickle-β^0-thalassemia. In order to determine the nature of the thalassemic mutation she had, molecular diagnostics were performed. To that end, DNA was extracted from peripheral leukocytes by PCR and tested by reverse dot hybridization that detects over 90% of the known thalassemic mutations in Hispanics. Surprisingly, no mutation was detected by this technique. Because of this, the diagnosis of sickle-β^0-thalassemia was questioned. In order to resolve the issue her mother was tested and she had sickle trait indicating that the patient had SS. Finally her α genotype was determined and she was found to be homozygous for the 3.7 kb α-globin gene deletion: $-\alpha^{3.7}/-\alpha^{3.7}$ (normal α genotype: aa/aa). The α-globin genotype of the parents was not done.

Final Diagnosis Sickle-α-thalassemia ($\beta s/\beta s; -\alpha 3.7/-\alpha 3.7$).

Management Approach She was kept on folic acid and acetaminophen/oxycodcone. Supportive/symptomatic therapies included vaccination as needed, blood transfusion for symptomatic anemia. Confirming the diagnosis of iron overload by repeating iron studies in the steady state treatment with hydroxyurea to decrease the frequency of painful crises and Exjade for iron overload (if confirmed) were discussed with the patient for consideration. Her actual diagnosis and its impact on family planning were also discussed.

General Discussion Sickle cell anemia with coexistent α-thalassemia is a unique entity and is associated with certain features as shown in **Table 1**. It occurs in about 5% of patients with SS. It is almost always confused with sickle-β^0-thalassemia because both have microcytic hypochromic indices and both have increased levels of hemoglobin A_2. The MCV in sickle-α-thalassemia is usually in the 70s whereas that of sickle-β^0-thalassemia is in the 60s. Target cells are more abundant in the latter. The reason why hemoglobin A_2 is increased in "SS and $-\alpha/-\alpha$" seems to be due to a greater posttranslational affinity of the limited α-globin chains for δ chains rather than for the β^s globin chains resulting in preferential production of Hb A$_2$.

Table 1. Sickle-α-thalassemia (β^s/β^s; −α$^{3.7}$/−α$^{3.7}$) compared with SS without a gene deletion (β^s/β^s; αα/αα)

Milder anemia
Microcytic hypochromic red cell indices
High hemoglobin A$_2$ level
Controversial effect on HbF level
Splenomegaly in adults
Increased prevalence of avascular necrosis
Increased prevalence of retinopathy
Decreased prevalence of strokes
Decreased prevalence of leg ulcers
No effect of frequency of painful crises
Less tissue damage

Hereditary Pyropoikilocytosis

John Kim Choi

Patient A 13-year-old African-American female with mild anemia.

Clinical History She had had anemia diagnosed at birth, had a splenectomy at age 5 for refractory anemia and now presented for routine follow-up with mild anemia.

Family History Mother and 3 siblings with anemia.

Medications Penicillin, folic acid.

Physical Examination Patient's vital signs were normal. Remarkable were only the pallor, mild scleral icterus, and surgical scar in the left upper quadrant of her abdomen. She had no palpable liver or adenopathy, and there was no evidence of bleeding or ecchymoses.

Initial Work-Up

CBC		Normal	WBC Differential	%	# ($\times 10^3$/μL)
WBC ($\times 10^3$/μL)	19.8	(6.0-17.5)	Neutrophils	55.1	10.9
RBC ($\times 10^6$/μL)	5.46	(4.1-5.1)	Bands	0	
HGB (g/dL)	10.0	(12.0-16.0)	Lymphocytes	31.5	6.2
HCT (%)	33.4	(36.0-46.0)	Monocytes	7.9	1.6
MCV (fL)	61.1	(78.0-102.0)	Eosinophils	5.0	1.0
MCH (pg)	18.4	(25.0-35.0)	Basophils	0.4	0.1
MCHC (g/dL)	30.1	(31.0-37.0)			
PLT ($\times 10^3$/μL)	728	(150-400)			
RDW-CV (%)	31.2	(11.5-14.5)			
MPV (fL)	6.2	(7.4-10.4)			

Peripheral blood smear revealed profound poikilocytosis and red cell fragments (**Figure 1**) with normal estimated numbers of platelets.

Section A: Anemias
Hereditary Pyropoikilocytosis

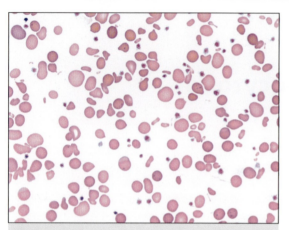

Figure 1 Blood smear (Wright-Giemsa, ×500) showing marked poikilocytosis and red cell fragmentation (image kindly provided by Marybeth Helfrich of Children's Hospital of Philadelphia).

Differential Diagnosis Although the differential diagnosis of mild anemia is quite extensive, after review of the peripheral smear, the differential becomes more limited and includes hereditary pyropoikilocytosis, severe thermal burn, autoimmune hemolytic anemia, and artifactual heat exposure of drawn peripheral blood.

Additional Work-Up Reticulocyte count 3.3% (normal: 0.5%-1.5%), Coombs test (direct and indirect) negative, lactate dehydrogenase 340 mg/dL (normal: 100-200), bilirubin 2.1 mg/dL (normal: 0.3-1.3). Flow cytometry showed reduced eosin-5'-maleimide binding to red cells (**Figure 2**).

Final Diagnosis Hereditary pyropoikilocytosis.

Management Approach Treatment is supportive transfusions and if necessary, splenectomy at ages 5-9. Patients who receive multiple transfusions must be monitored for need for iron chelation therapy to avoid the long-term complications of iron overload. Patients who undergo splenectomy should be immunized against encapsulated organisms (pneumococcus, hemophilus influenza and meningococcus prior to splenectomy). While there is general agreement in using prophylactic antibiotics for 1 year to 2 years post-splenectomy and in asplenic children <5 years of age, continued use beyond this time is controversial. Some guidelines recommend no additional prophylactic antibiotic coverage while others recommend coverage until 16 years of age, as in this case. Most patients are prescribed folic acid therapy to compensate for the overwhelming hemolysis and erythrocytosis.

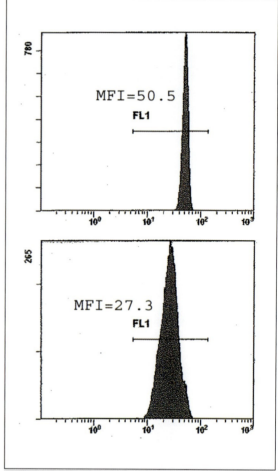

Figure 2 Flow cytometry histograms of peripheral blood stained with EMA. Upper histogram represents normal sample. Lower histogram represents the patient sample. MFI = mean fluorescent intensity resulting from EMA binding.

General Discussion The profound poikilocytosis seen in the peripheral blood smear has a relatively small differential as noted above. The CBC indices indicate microcytic anemia. The increased red cell count and the blood smear with many spherocytes and no hypochromic cells argue against severe iron deficiency. While the indices are consistent with thalassemia, the paucity of target cells would argue otherwise. The elevated platelet is a false thrombocytosis resulting from the automated machine counting small red cells and red cell fragments as platelets. Hereditary pyropoikilocytosis (HPP) is an inherited hemolytic anemia characterized by defects in the red cell cytoskeleton, profound poikilocytosis, and red cell fragmentation at a reduced thermal temperature. Peripheral blood smear is morphologically similar to that seen in patients with severe thermal burns.

Although initially classified separately from hereditary elliptocytosis (HE), HPP shares the same molecular and biochemical findings and is considered a more clinically severe subset of HE. Furthermore, while HE typically has heterozygous mutations, HPP has homozygous or compound heterozygous mutations leading to more severe cytoskeletal defects. The patient typically presents with hyperbililrubinemia, hemolytic anemia and splenomegaly within the first few months of life. Patients with prolonged and severe anemia will present with growth retardation and/or gallbladder disease. Peripheral blood smear demonstrates anisopoikilocytosis consisting predominantly of microspherocytes and micropoikilocytes with occasional elliptocytes. Microcytosis is usually severe with MCV of 50 fL-60 fL. Fragmentation of the red cells in HPP may occur at temperature over 37°C compared to 49°C for normal red cells. Peripheral blood smears can have artifactual pyropoikilocytosis, for example, unrefrigerated peripheral blood heated during transportation on a hot day from a satellite hospital. Rapid flow cytometry analysis shows decreased binding of eosin-5′-maleimide (EMA) to RBC in HPP and in a subset of HE. EMA is a fluorescent dye that binds specifically to the RBC anion transport protein (band 3), permitting rapid quantitation of band 3 using flow cytometry. This test also reliably detects specific reduced EMA binding in hereditary spherocytosis, congenital dyserythopoietic anemia-type 2, southeast Asian ovalocytosis, and cytohydrocytosis. In contrast, normal EMA binding is seen with autoimmune hemolytic anemia, sickle disease, G6PD deficiency, and thalassemia. Missense and nonsense mutations have been identified in α-spectrin, β-spectrin, and protein 4.1; these mutations disrupt the horizontal interactions of the cytoskeleton. In contrast, different mutations in α-spectrin, β-spectrin, protein 4.1, protein 4.2, ankyrin, and band 3 are seen in hereditary spherocytosis; these mutations disrupt the vertical interactions of the cytoskeleton.

Anemia Associated with Liver Disease

Yuri Fedoriw, Cherie H Dunphy

Patient A 65-year-old Laotian woman, who presented with right upper quadrant pain and for a follow-up from a recent hospitalization.

Clinical History The patient had a longstanding history of schistosomiasis-induced liver cirrhosis and reported a month-long history of progressive right upper quadrant pain and associated shortness of breath and cough. She was recently hospitalized for similar symptoms and was found to have a large left pleural effusion. The effusion was drained with partial resolution of the respiratory symptoms. However, the patient was extensively diuresed during her hospitalization, subsequently developing renal insufficiency. Prior to discharge, a right upper quadrant ultrasound demonstrated a possible hepatic mass.

Family History Unremarkable.

Medications Spirololactone, propranolol, prilosec, lactulose, glipizide, and lantus.

Physical Examination Vital signs were normal. Her exam was remarkable for bradycardia, jaundice, ecchymoses, 3+ pitting edema of the lower extremities, and palpable liver edge (2 cm below the costal margin). Her lung examination revealed mild crackles at the left base.

Initial Work-Up

CBC		WBC Differential	%	# ($\times 10^3/\mu L$)
WBC ($\times 10^3/\mu L$)	6.0	Neutrophils	70	4.2
RBC ($\times 10^6/\mu L$)	3.8	Lymphocytes	25	1.5
HGB (g/dL)	9.5	Monocytes	3	0.2
HCT (%)	31.0	Eosinophils	2	0.1
MCV (fL)	82	Basophils	0	
MCH (pg)	25.0			
MCHC (g/dL)	30.6			
PLT ($\times 10^3/\mu L$)	176			
RDW-CV (%)	23.0			

Peripheral blood smear revealed significant anisopoikilocytosis with numerous target cells, and rare acanthocytes and echinocytes (**Figure 1**).

Anemia Associated with Liver Disease

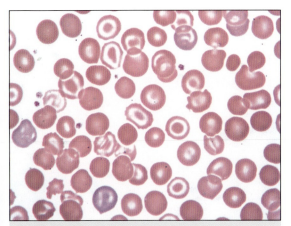

Figure 1 Blood smear (Wright-Giemsa, ×1000) showing anisopoikilocytosis, several acanthocytes, and occasional echinocytes.

Differential Diagnosis Anemia secondary to liver cirrhosis, anemia secondary to renal insufficiency, drug/toxin effect, nutritional deficiency, and hemodilution.

Additional Work-Up
- PT 16.2 sec (normal 10.2-12.8)
- INR 1.4 (normal 0.8-1.2)
- PTT 33.2 sec (normal 17.7-37.9)

Chemistry panel
- Urea nitrogen 106 mg/dL
- Creatinine 3.7 mg/dL
- Glucose, random 118 mg/dL
- Estimated glomerular filtration rate (eGFR) (mL/min/1.73 m^2) 13.1
- Total protein 5.6 g/dL
- Albumin 2.2 g/dL
- AST 158 U/L
- ALT 76 U/L
- Bilirubin(total) 6.1 mg/dL

MRI of the abdomen revealed a 15 × 14 × 10 cm mass in the right hepatic lobe and evidence of portal hypertension. Subsequent biopsy of the hepatic mass confirmed hepatocellular carcinoma.

Diagnosis Anemia associated with liver cirrhosis/failure secondary to schistosomiasis.

Management Approach The management for this patient is largely palliative. Therapy is targeted towards the underlying cause of hepatic failure and supportive measures (ie, blood component transfusions) are instituted when clinically applicable.

General Discussion Peripheral blood findings are not entirely specific, and only a subset of patients has the classic morphologic changes of liver insufficiency. Classically, target cells and acanthocytes predominate, the latter 2 notably associated with alcoholic liver disease and abetalipoproteinemia respectively. The primary and longstanding diagnosis in this patient is progressive liver failure due to infection by the parasitic fluke, *Schistosoma*. Patients with this degree of hepatic insufficiency usually demonstrate a mild to moderate anemia associated with shortened red cell survival and abnormal/ineffective erythropoiesis. Abnormal lipid processing and an aberrant cytokine milieu may be mechanistically important. The development of bone fide cirrhosis results in additional phenomenon, including coagulopathies and renal insufficiency that ultimately contribute to the anemia. The marginally increased prothrombin time with normal activated partial thromboplastin time suggests that synthetic function is partially preserved in this patient.

Sickle Cell Anemia with Leg Ulcer

Samir Ballas

Patient A 37-year-old African-American man with sickle cell anemia, who presented with pain in both knees and ankles.

Clinical History The patient was diagnosed with sickle cell anemia in early childhood. Major complications of his disease included frequent acute painful crises, chronic pain syndrome, blindness in the right eye due to sickle retinopathy, pulmonary hypertension, cholelithiais for which he had laparoscopic cholecystectomy, recurrent leg ulcers, and priapism. He now presented with new leg ulcers on the lateral aspect of both ankles during his routine follow-up visit in the sickle cell clinic. His pain scored 5 on a scale of 10.

Family History Both parents have sickle cell trait. He has 1 sister with normal HGB.

Medications Folic acid, methadone, and allopurinol.

Physical examination Vital signs were normal, sPO$_2$ on room air varied between 88 and 90%, sclerae were intensely icteric, Grade III/VI systolic murmur over the precordium, liver span of 14 cm, tenderness over the low back and over both knees. There was a 3 × 2 cm leg ulcer on the lateral side of each ankle (see **Figure 1**); both ulcers were not deep, erythematous, and clean with no fibrinous exudates, purulent material or other evidence suggestive of infection.

Initial Work-Up

CBC		WBC Differential	%	# (×10^3/μL)
WBC (×10^3/μL)	12.0	Neutrophils	45	5.4
RBC (×10^6/μL)	1.96	Bands	0	
HGB (g/dL)	6.4	Lymphocytes	42	5.0
HCT (%)	18.0	Monocytes	9	1.1
MCV (fL)	92.0	Eosinophils	3	0.4
MCH (pg)	32.7	Basophils	1	0.1
MCHC (g/dL)	36.6	Nucleated red cells	4 per 100 WBC	
PLT (×10^3/μL)	365			
RDW-CV (%)	18.1	Reticulocyte count	26.9%	520.0

Peripheral blood smear revealed anisopoikilocytosis, polychromasia, numerous sickle cells, occasional target cells, Howell-Jolly Bodies and a few nucleated red cells.

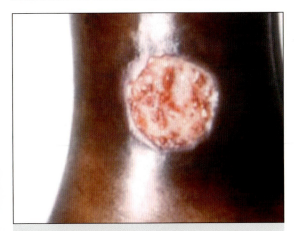

Figure 1 Leg ulcer in a patient with sickle cell anemia.

Differential Diagnosis Diagnostic considerations included Sickle cell anemia (SS), hemoglobin SC Disease. sickle-β^+-thalassemia and sickle-β^0-thalassemia.

Additional Work-Up Hemoglobin electrophoresis results obtained at the time of initial diagnosis were 91% S, 3% A_2 and 6% F. Urinalysis showed specific gravity of 1.007, pH 8.0, and 3+ urobilinogen with no proteinuria or hematuria. Pertinent findings in the comprehensive metabolic panel showed total bilirubin of 7.1 mg/dL, direct bilirubin 2-2 mg/dL, AST 59 IU/L, Alk Phos 124 IU/L, LD 553 IU/L, urate 9.0 mg/dL and serum ferritin 265 ng/mL. His α genotype was normal with 4 α genes present thus confirming the diagnosis of typical SS with no α gene deletion.

Final Diagnosis Sickle cell anemia.

Management Approach Hydroxyurea therapy is currently the only approved therapy for patients with sickle cell anemia to decrease the complications related to this disease, particularly severe pain crisis. Despite his severe anemia and low oxygen saturation, he had no signs or symptoms of anemia and no dyspnea or difficulty breathing. His clinic file showed that these numbers were his usual steady state parameters and he is being followed by a pulmonologist. Accordingly no blood transfusion or oxygen administration was planned. He received appropriate therapy for the leg ulcers at our wound center. His ulcers were debrided to the superficial fascial level with a surgical curet. Regranex topical gel (recombinant human platelet-derived growth factor) was then applied over the ulcers. The patient was instructed to clean the ulcers and apply a thin layer of Regranex over the ulcer avoiding covering skin beyond the edge of the ulcer once daily. He was followed by the wound center every 2 weeks, and as the ulcer started to heal, the amount of the ointment was decreased. About 3 months after initiating this treatment the ulcers healed.

General Discussion Leg ulceration is a common complication of sickle cell anemia. It is less common in hemoglobin SC disease and sickle-β^+-thalassemia. Leg ulcers are more common in males and adults and less common in patients with α-gene deletion, high total HGB level and high level of hemoglobin F. Standard treatments for leg ulcers are appropriate for the treatment of superficial ulcers as described in this patient. However, blood transfusion, exchange transfusion, or hyperbaric oxygen may be beneficial if more severe in these patients. Deep ulcers may be associated with osteomyelitis. Leg ulcers constitute a contraindication for the use of hydroxyurea, which may cause leg ulceration, worsen existing leg ulcers or reopen healed ulcers. It is for this reason that this patient was not started on hydroxyurea.

Anemia of Chronic Renal Insufficiency

Yuri Fedoriw, Cherie H Dunphy

Patient A 71-year-old African-American female, who presented for routine follow-up of longstanding diabetes and hypertension.

Clinical History The patient initially presented to her primary care physician 5 years prior to this visit with asymptomatic hyperglycemia and hypertension. She was treated on an outpatient basis, but was generally noncompliant with her medications. Two years prior, she was admitted for a cerebral vascular accident (CVA); however, she has minimal sequelae after extensive rehabilitation. Since initial diagnosis, she has had slowly progressive renal insufficiency and anemia. Within the past few months, the patient was admitted again to the hospital with hypertensive emergency and new onset seizure necessitating prolonged stay in the intensive care unit. A hemodialysis catheter was placed in her right groin; however, her kidney function somewhat improved without dialysis. She secondarily developed an arteriovenous fistula from the catheter, requiring a vascular stent.

Family History The patient is a Jehovah's Witness and denies smoking or alcohol use. She lives with her husband and is cared for daily by a home health aid.

Medications Aspirin/extended-release dipyridamole, baby aspirin, carvedilol, conjugated estrogens, simvastatin, folic acid, furosemide, iron supplement, vitamins, recombinant insulin, acetaminophen.

Physical Examination Unremarkable.

Initial Work-Up

CBC		WBC Differential	%	#($\times 10^3/\mu$L)
WBC ($\times 10^3/\mu$L)	7.1	Neutrophils	59.2	4.2
RBC ($\times 10^6/\mu$L)	3.03	Lymphocytes	31.0	2.2
HGB (g/dL)	8.5	Monocytes	5.6	0.4
HCT (%)	26.9	Eosinophils	4.2	0.3
MCV (fL)	92	Basophils	0	
MCH (pg)	29	Reticulocyte count	1.5	
MCHC (g/dL)	32			
PLT ($\times 10^3/\mu$L)	437			
RDW-CV (%)	20.0			

Peripheral blood smear demonstrated numerous echinocytes or burr cells (red cells with multiple projections on their surfaces) (**Figure 1**).

Chemistry panel
- Sodium 145 mmol/L
- Potassium 4.9 mmol/L
- Chloride 114 mmol/L
- CO_2 20 mmol/L
- Urea nitrogen 105 mg/dL
- Creatinine 2.6 mg/dL
- Glucose, random 204 mg/dL
- Estimated glomerular filtration rate (eGFR) 19.83 mL/min/1.73m^2

Section A: Anemias
Anemia of Chronic Renal Insufficiency

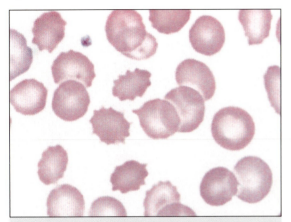

Figure 1 Blood smear (Wright-Giemsa, ×1000) showing numerous echinocytes or burr cells (red cells with numerous evenly distributed projections and relatively preserved central pallor).

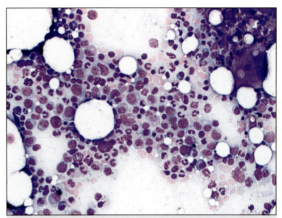

Figure 2 Bone marrow aspirate smear (Wright-Giemsa, ×400) showing a slightly hypercellular marrow with preserved trilineage hematopoiesis. Erythroid series showed no significant dyspoietic changes.

Additional Work-Up Serum iron studies demonstrated borderline low iron and iron-binding capacity, with a transferrin saturation of 12%. The ferritin level was mildly increased. The bone marrow aspirate was performed to exclude other causes of persistent anemia. Bone marrow evaluation demonstrated a slightly hypercellular bone marrow with preserved trilineage hematopoiesis and no dyspoietic changes (**Figure 2**). Iron stain demonstrated abundant storage iron (**Figure 3**); however, decreased iron was present in the red cell precursors.

Differential Diagnosis Anemia of chronic disease, anemia of renal insufficiency, drug effect, and possible primary hematolymphoid neoplasms, including lymphoma, plasma cell myeloma, and myelodysplasia.

Final Diagnosis Anemia of chronic renal insufficiency.

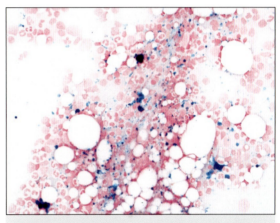

Figure 3 Bone marrow aspirate smear (Prussian blue, ×400) showing increased storage iron.

Management Approach The goal of therapy in this patient is prevention of further renal dysfunction by careful control of the underlying diabetes and hypertension. Erythropoietin replacement is necessary, as the synthetic function will likely not dramatically improve.

General Discussion Anemia is an invariable manifestation of progressive renal insufficiency/failure, owing primarily to the decreased production of erythropoietin by renal peritubular cells. Most patients present with symptoms corresponding to the etiology underlying their renal disease, and the hypoprolifertaive anemia manifests late in their clinical course. As the synthetic function most often parallels the glomerular filtration, the anemia corresponds to the degree of renal insufficiency measured by creatinine clearance. Moreover, accompanying azotemia and fluid overload worsen the anemia by direct suppression of erythropoiesis and dilutional effect, respectively. Although not unique, echinocytes (burr cells) are the classic morphologic finding in uremic patients. Changes in the bone marrow may also be nonspecific; however, such evaluation may be necessary to exclude other possible causes of peripheral blood cytopenias.

Acquired Acanthocytosis

Gene Gulati, Joanne Filicko O'Hara, John Krause

Patient A 46-year-old male, who was admitted to the hospital with liver failure.

Clinical History The patient had been a heavy drinker and smoker until about 2 weeks prior to this admission. He was previously diagnosed with insulin-dependent diabetes complicated by peripheral neuropathy, hypertension, and end-stage liver disease secondary to alcoholic cirrhosis (itself complicated by hepatic encephalopathy). He is now admitted with end-stage liver disease and evaluated for orthotopic liver transplantation.

Family History His father has coronary artery disease and an aunt has diabetes and systemic lupus erythematosus.

Medications He is on a number of medications for his multiple problems (including insulin, rifaximin, furosemide, spironalactone, hydroxizine, magnesium oxide, multivitamin tablets, etc).

Physical Examination Gross jaundice. He is drowsy but arousable, and has 1+ edema of right lower extremity.

Initial Work-Up

CBC		WBC Differential	%	# (×10^3/μL)
WBC (×10^3/μL)	5.9	Neutrophils	75	4.4
RBC (×10^6/μL	2.08	Bands	3	0.2
HGB (g/dL)	7.6	Lymphocytes	13	0.8
HCT (%)	21.1	Monocytes	7	0.4
MCV (fL)	101.4	Eosinophils	2	0.1
MCH (pg)	36.5	Reticulocyte count	6.7	140
MCHC (g/dL)	36.0	IRF (%)	11.1	
PLT (×10^3/μL)	34			
RDW-CV (%)	26.2			
MPV (fL)	9.6			

Peripheral blood smear revealed acanthocytes and echinocytes along with moderate degree of polychromasia (**Figure 1**).

Differential Diagnosis Normocytic or slightly macrocytic anemia and thrombocytopenia are common findings in patients with liver disease. Clinical conditions associated with acanthocytosis include severe liver disease (spur cell anemia), abetalipoproteinemia (Bassen-Kornzweig syndrome), hypobetalipoproteinemia, McLeod syndrome, In (Lu) Lu (a–b–) phenotype, severe malnutrition (anorexia nervosa), certain neurologic diseases such as chorea-acanthocytosis syndrome and HARP syndrome, hypothyroidism, panhypopitutarism, myelodysplasia, chronic myeloproliferative neoplasms, hyposplenism or status post splenectomy. A small number of acanthocytes may also be seen in the blood smears of premature infants. Echinocytosis is often associated with severe uremia but is not an infrequent finding

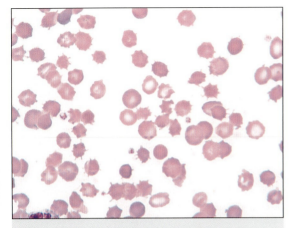

Figure 1 Blood smear (Wright, ×1000) showing acanthocytes and echinocytes.

in severe liver disease. Echinocytes are also common artifacts of blood smear preparation, drying and/or staining process. A small number of echinocytes may also be seen in the blood smears of patients with hypomagnesemia, hypophosphatemia, and pyruvate kinase deficiency.

Additional Work-Up Additional abnormal laboratory findings included the following:
Serum
- Bilirubin (mg/dL): total = 25.5, direct = 6.1
- Protein (g/dL): total = 5.5, albumin = 2.9
- Alkaline phosphatase (U/L) = 158 (normal 29-92)
- Ammonia (mcmol/L) = 63 (normal 11-35)
- Glucose (mg/dL) = 122 (normal 50-100)

Plasma
- PT (sec) 45.6 (normal 11-15)
- PTT 64 sec (normal 20-35)

Final Diagnosis Acanthocytosis and echinocytosis associated with severe liver disease.

Management Approach Treatment of disorders with acanthocytosis depends on the underlying condition(s). Management of abetalipoproteinemia includes dietary restriction of long-chain fatty acids and supplementation with medium-chain triglycerides and lipid-soluble vitamins A, D, E, and K. Iron and folate supplementation may also be needed in some cases. Occupational and physical therapy may be helpful in managing neurologic manifestations. Appropriate care of severe liver disease often necessitates careful fluid management, correction of metabolic disturbances, treatment of hypoglycemia, and careful nutritional management. This patient, while on the waiting list for liver transplant, was maintained on supportive care with multiple agents including packed red cells, albumin, fresh frozen plasma, and vitamin K.

General Discussion Acanthocytosis may be inherited (eg, homozygous autosomal recessive abetalipoproteinemia and homozygous autosomal dominant familial hypobetalipoproteinemia) or acquired (eg, associated with severe liver disease and severe malnutrition). Clinical manifestations are variable depending upon the underlying condition and may involve more than one organ or system. Lymphadenopathy, hepatomegaly and splenomegaly may be present in some cases. Presenting symptoms may include diarrhea, slow weight gain, pallor, jaundice, abdominal pain, ataxia, tremors, visual abnormalities, and dyskinesias. A number of mutations in the microsomal triglyceride transfer protein (MTP) gene located on chromosome 4 are capable of causing congenital absence of β-apolipoprotein in the plasma, as well as decreased levels of cholesterol, low-density lipoprotein (LDL), and very-low-density lipoprotein (VLDL). Mutations in the APOB gene located on chromosome 2 have been implicated in cases of familial hypobetalipoproteinemia, which is characterized by reduced synthesis of β-apoprotein in the liver and decreased levels of LDLs in plasma. A variety of other gene mutations have also been described in disorders grouped under the name of neuroacanthocytosis, in which the plasma lipoprotein levels are; however, normal and the acanthocyte pathophysiology varies with the underlying condition. The number of acanthocytes seen in the blood smear is variable from a few to many among the clinical conditions associated with acanthocytosis. Acanthocytes, sometimes also referred to as spur cells, are spherocytic red cells with a variable number of spiny projections irregularly distributed over the surface. These cells are hyperchromic and stain densely with Romanowsky stain, like spherocytes. Accumulation of either sphingomyelin or cholesterol in excess, primarily in the outer half of the red cell membrane, is often the cause of acanthocyte formation in many cases. Laboratory findings are also variable depending upon the underlying condition, but may include mild to moderate normocytic anemia, reticulocytosis, increased serum bilirubin and lactate dehydrogenase (LDH), and abnormal serum lipid profile (absent or decreased betalipoproteins) and decreased plasma levels of fat soluble vitamins particularly in cases of abetalipoproteinemia, hypobetalipoproteinemia, and malnutrition. Liver function tests and total protein and albumin levels are abnormal in liver disease.

Aplastic Anemia

Carol Holman, Robert McKenna

Patient A 3-year-old girl with increased bruising, petechiae, and nose bleed.

Clinical History The patient was born at 38 weeks gestation after a normal uncomplicated pregnancy. Her birth weight was 7 pounds, 8 ounces. She was slightly jaundiced at birth, but this resolved spontaneously. At 1 year of age, she experienced her first episode of epistaxis and has had several episodes since. Her left naris was cauterized 3 times, most recently 2 months prior. She has had a few episodes of otitis media, but not recently. There have been no other significant infections. She has not traveled outside of the United States. She is developmentally normal.

Family History Noncontributory.

Medications None.

Physical Examination The patient appeared pale, but otherwise well. Head and neck examination revealed no notable dysmorphic features. She had a small resolving petechial lesion on the right side of her tongue. There was no palpable adenopathy. Her abdomen was soft, and nontender, with no hepatosplenomegaly or masses palpable. There were scattered resolving superficial bruises, but no skin lesions were noted.

Initial Work-Up

CBC		WBC Differential	%	# (×10³/µL)
WBC (×10³/µL)	2.9	Neutrophils	1	0.03
RBC (×10⁶/µL)	2.24	Bands	0	
HGB (g/dL)	6.5	Lymphocytes	99	2.87
HCT (%)	18.7	Monocytes	0	
MCV (fL)	84.0	Eosinophils	0	
MCH (pg)	29.0	Basophils	0	
MCHC (g/dL)	34.7	Reticulocyte count	0.1	
PLT (×10³/µL)	6			

Reticulocyte count 0.1%.

Differential Diagnosis The differential diagnosis of pancytopenia in a young child is quite broad. Possible etiologies include acquired aplastic anemia (due to radiation, drugs/chemicals, viruses, or immune diseases, or idiopathic), inherited bone marrow failure syndromes (most commonly Fanconi anemia), myelodysplastic syndrome, paroxysmal nocturnal hemoglobinuria, systemic lupus erythematosis, Sjogren syndrome, vitamin B_{12}/folate deficiency, infection, and storage disease. The bone marrow may also be infiltrated, as in acute leukemias, hemophagocytic lymphohistiocytosis, metastatic solid tumors, and osteopetrosis.

Additional Work-Up
- Diepoxybutane (DEB) testing for Fanconi anemia was negative
- Hepatitis serology was negative
- Autoimmune serology was negative
- Bone marrow examination revealed hypocellular marrow with essentially no hematopoiesis (**Figures 1** and **2**)
- Cytogenetic analysis revealed normal female karyotype

Final Diagnosis Aplastic anemia, probably idiopathic.

Management Approach Matched sibling progenitor cell transplantation is the best available therapy. Medical management with immunosuppressive agents (antithymocyte globulin, or ATG, cyclosporine, etc) is the alternative treatment if a suitable match cannot be found. If there is no response to immunosuppressive therapy, hematopoietic progenitor cell transplant using an alternative donor (matched or mismatched unrelated donor, mismatched related donor) should be considered. In this patient, initial treatment was supportive, with red blood cell and platelet transfusions. Febrile illnesses were carefully monitored, and blood cultures performed. Episodes of bacteremia were treated with intravenous antibiotics. The patient was immediately referred for transplant evaluation, and was found to have an HLA-matched sibling. The transplant was successful. Post-transplant, she had an extended period of mixed chimerism (**Figure 3**), and she received cyclosporine for a year due to concern for graft failure. Her peripheral counts improved gradually. She maintained a normal absolute neutrophil count by 60 days post-transplant, and a normal platelet count by 140 days post-transplant. She did have low-grade, ongoing hemolysis that resolved by 1 year post-transplant. At 2 years post-transplant, the patient had marrow cellularity

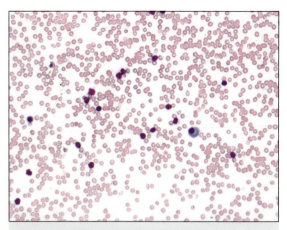

Figure 1 Bone marrow aspirate concentrate smear (Wright-Giemsa, ×200).

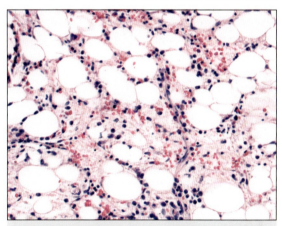

Figure 2 Biopsy (H&E, ×200) pre-transplant essentially no hematopoiesis is identified.

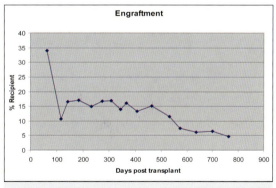

Figure 3 Post-transplant chimerism data (RFLP analysis by PCR was performed on the blood monomuclear fraction).

Section A: Anemias
Aplastic Anemia

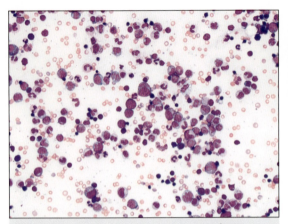

Figure 4 Bone marrow aspirate concentrate smear (Wright-Giemsa, ×200).

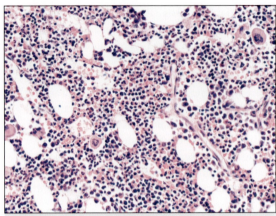

Figure 5 Biopsy (H&E, ×200) at 2 years post-transplant trilineage hematopoiesis is seen with overall cellularity of 60%-70%.

of 60%-70% with trilineage hematopoietic maturation (**Figures 4** and **5**), with normal hemoglobin, platelet, and neutrophil counts. Evidence of graft-vs-host disease was not present and the patient is currently doing well, 5.5 years post-transplant.

General Discussion Depending on its severity, clinical presentation of hypoplastic or aplastic anemia may include general weakness, fatigue, tachycardia, petechiae, and fever. Usually, there is no organomegaly. There is no single diagnostic test for acquired aplastic anemia.

The minimal diagnostic criteria are pancytopenia in the setting of a hypocellular/acellular bone marrow without infiltration, fibrosis, or dysplasia. Bone marrow examination may reveal lymphocytosis and many hematogones, particularly in children. Congenital marrow failure syndromes, such as Fanconi anemia, should be excluded. The red cells are generally normocytic and normochromic but may be slightly macrocytic in some cases. The reticulocyte count is markedly reduced, even to a level of zero in some cases.

Diamond-Blackfan Anemia

John Kim Choi

Patient An 11-month-old female presented by the family with the complaint of failure to thrive.

Clinical History Noncontributory.

Family History Unremarkable.

Medications None.

Physical Examination The patient was underweight and in the <5th percentile for height for her age. She was pale and tachycardic with a faint murmur. She has a cleft lip and palate. Her parents report that she is very irritable.

Initial Work-Up

CBC Normal		Normal	WBC Differential	%	# (×10³/μL)
WBC (×10³/μL)	5.8	(6.0-17.5)	Neutrophils	24	1.4
RBC (×10⁶/μL)	1.27	(3.7-5.3)	Bands	0	
HGB (g/dL)	3.8	(10.5-13.5)	Lymphocytes	74	4.3
HCT (%)	12.3	(33.0-39.0)	Monocytes	2	0.1
MCV (fL)	96.9	(70.0-86.0)	Eosinophils	0	
MCH (pg)	30.1	(23.0-31.0)	Basophils	0	
MCHC (g/dL)	31.2	(30.0-36.0)			
PLT (×10³/μL)	330.0	(150-400)			
RDW-CV (%)	21.2	(11.5-14.5)			
MPV (fL)	7.8	(7.4-10.4)			

Peripheral blood smear revealed macrocytic red cells but was otherwise unremarkable.

Differential Diagnosis In a pediatric patient with severe and isolated anemia, the main differentials are Diamond-Blackfan anemia, transient erythroblastopenia of childhood, and parvovirus infection.

Additional Work-Up Reticulocyte: 3.7% (normal 0.5-1.5). Molecular test of the bone marrow was negative for parvovirus DNA. Hemoglobin F was elevated. Cytogenetic test for Fanconi anemia (diepoxybutane-induced chromosomal breakage test) was negative. Bone marrow aspirate smear revealed normal cellularity (**Figure 1**) and erythroblastopenia (**Figure 2**).

Section A: Anemias
Diamond-Blackfan Anemia

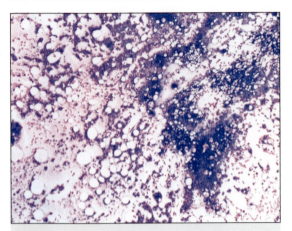

Figure 1 Bone marrow aspirate smear (Wright-Giemsa, ×20) showing normal cellularity.

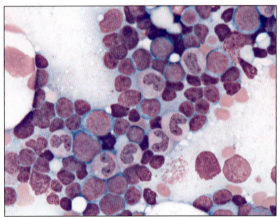

Figure 2 Bone marrow aspirate smear (Wright-Giemsa, ×500) showing erythroblastopenia.

Final Diagnosis Diamond-Blackfan anemia.

Management Approach Most DBA patients (62.6%), particularly those presenting at older age, with family history of DBA and normal platelet count, respond to steroid therapy. Because of the morbidity associated with early steroid exposure, the current recommendation is to delay the use of steroid during the first year of life. Transfusion is used during the first year of life and in those that do not initially respond or become nonresponsive to steroids. Approximately 40% of patients will remain steroid-dependent, 40% will remain transfusion dependent, and 20% will be in remission without medication or transfusion. Although controversial, allogeneic hematopoietic progenitor cell transplant (HPCT) has been used successfully to treat DBA. This patient was transfused and treated with steroids with good response.

General Discussion Diamond-Blackfan anemia (DBA) is a rare congenial anemia with an incidence of 5-7 per million births and no gender predominance. Most patients present in early infancy (2 months-4 months) with isolated severe macrocytic anemia. Approximately 40% of the patients have other congenital anomalies such as renal defects, cardiac defects, craniofacial abnormalities, or radial ray abnormalities. There is an increased risk of developing acute myeloid leukemia and other malignancies, but the exact risk remains undefined. The diagnostic criteria for classical DBA include anemia before age 1, reticulocytopenia, macrocytosis, normal marrow cellularity, markedly decreased erythroid precursors, and normal to mild neutropenia. More recent criteria have been established for nonclassical DBA that incorporate recent molecular findings and their variable penetrance.

The patient with classic DBA typically presents with macrocytic anemia (MVC around 110 fL-140 fL) and reticulocytopenia. The WBC count, differential, and platelet counts are usually normal, although some patients can present or develop neutropenia, as in this case. Peripheral blood smear shows normal red cell morphology except for the macrocytosis. Other laboratory findings include elevated hemoglobin F, red cell adenosine deaminase, i antigen expression, and erythropoietin. The bone marrow demonstrates decreased erythroid precursors with maturation arrest at the proerythroblast and basophilic normoblast stages. There is an absence of giant pronormoblasts with nuclear inclusion that can be seen with parvovirus infection and transient erythroblastopenia of childhood (TEC). The myeloid and megakaryocytic cells are usually normal. Normal maturing B cells (hematogones) are increased. The morphologic findings in TEC are similar to those in DBA and their distinction is best done on clinical history and natural course of the disease. Similar to DBA, TEC can present with isolated macrocytic anemia and variable neutropenia. Unlike DBA, TEC does not have elevated hemoglobin F and red cell adenosine deaminase. Furthermore, TEC typically presents at an age >1 year and without associated physical anomalies. Most importantly, TEC, unlike DBA, spontaneously resolves in 5 weeks-10 weeks. Approximately 75%-90% of DBAs are sporadic, with the remainder being inherited in an autosomal recessive, autosomal dominant, and

X-linked patterns. Approximately, 25% of DBAs have heterozygous mutations in the ribosomal protein S19 (RPS19) located on chromosome 19q13. RPS19 is a protein component of the 40S ribosomal subunit and mutations cause DBA with mostly autosomal dominant pattern of inheritance. Other identified DBA mutations involve genes encoding for other ribosomal subunits (**Table 1**). These mutations lead to intrinsic defects in erythroid precursors leading to apoptosis.

Table 1. Genetic mutations in DBA

DBA subtype	Chromosome locus	Gene-reference
1	19q13	RPS19 [11-13]
2	8p23	Not identified
3	10q22	RPS24 [15]
4	15q	RPS17 [16]
5	3q29	RPL35A [17]
6	1p22	RPL5 [18]
7	1p36	RPL11 [18]
8	2p25	RPS7 [18]

Congenital Dyserythropoetic Anemia, Type II

James Cotelingam, Menchu Ong, Diana Veillon

Patient A 16-year-old female with mild anemia.

Clinical History The patient was referred to our institution after being followed up at an outside hospital with mild anemia for 2 years. Her hemoglobin levels ranged between 11-12 g/dL. Her menstrual periods were regular and not excessive in amount. Past medical history was significant for recurrent streptococcal pharyngitis, tonsillectomy, adenoidectomy and infectious mononucleosis. She complained of tiredness and was afebrile. There was no weight loss or jaundice.

Family History Mild anemia was reported in the father, but was never subclassified. No maternal history of anemia was elicited.

Medications None.

Physical Examination Afebrile, well-developed female with no dysmorphic features. There was no jaundice or pallor. Small, jugulodigastric nodes were palpable. The spleen tip was also palpable. The remainder of the physical examination was unremarkable.

Initial Work-Up

CBC		WBC Differential	%	# (×10³/µL)
WBC (×10³/µL)	4.6	Neutrophils + Bands	59.2	2.7
RBC (×10⁶/µL)	2.85	Lymphocytes	31.4	1.4
HGB (g/dL)	10.0	Monocytes	5.2	0.2
HCT (%)	28.1	Eosinophils	4.2	0.2
MCV (fL)	98.7	Basophils	0.0	0.0
MCH (pg)	35.1	Reticulocyte count	1.3	30
MCHC (g/dL)	35.5			
PLT (×10³/µL)	298			
RDW-CV (%)	15.4			
MPV (fL)	8.1			

Peripheral blood smear revealed anisopoikilocytosis with occasional basophilic stippling. Total bilirubin 1.0 mg/dL (normal 0.2-1.2); LDH 739 U/L (normal 125-243); direct antiglobulin test: negative.

Differential diagnosis Diagnostic considerations included thalassemia, autoimmune hemolytic anemia, megaloblastic anemia, red cell enzyme deficiencies (G6PD and pyruvate kinase), myelodysplasia, PNH, disorders of unstable hemoglobin, and congenital dyserythropoietic anemia.

Additional Work-Up
- Bone marrow biopsy showed a hypercellular, erythroid predominant bone marrow with marked dyserythropoietic changes in erythroid precursors including large and multinucleate forms involving the early and late normoblastic series (**Figure 1**).

Section A: Anemias
Congenital Dyserythropoetic Anemia, Type II

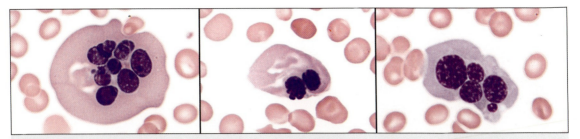

Figure 1 Bone marrow aspirate smear (Wright-Giemsa, ×400) showing a spectrum of nuclear abnormalities in erythroblasts: multinuclearity (left), symmetric binuclearity (center), and multinuclearity with dyskinesis (right).

Pronormoblasts appeared conspicuous. Basophilic stippling was evident in erythroid elements including multinucleate forms. Erythropoiesis was normoblastic and megaloblastoid. Myeloid maturation was orderly. Megakaryocytes were present and maturing. Lymphocytes and plasma cells were not increased. Reticulin was not increased. Stainable iron was absent. Laboratory studies included a normal female karyotype 46, XX, negative Ham test; positive antigen i hemeagglutination; serum ferritin: 27.5 ng/mL (normal 4.6-204); serum iron: 120 μg/dL (normal 25-156); serum transferrin saturation: 35% (normal 20-50); serum folate: 17.2 ng/mL (normal 7.2-15.4); serum vitamin B_{12}: 999.7 pg/mL (normal 208-954) normal PNH test on blood by flow cytometry; G6PD (U/10 × 12 RBC): 401 (normal 146-376); pyruvate kinase (IU/g); HGB: 12.2 (normal 9-22); no abnormal hemoglobin identified on electrophoresis
- CT abdomen: splenomegaly and cholelithiasis observed

Final Diagnosis Congenital dyserythropoietic anemia (CDA), type II.

Management Approach The treatment of CDA II is supportive and consists of monitoring hematologic parameters and iron status. Progressive iron accumulation has been reported, and phlebotomy may be performed if there is evidence of iron overload. Chelation is recommended when ferritin levels are repeatedly above 1,000 ng/L. Splenectomy may normalize red cell survival and increase hemoglobin levels, thereby decreasing transfusion requirements and allowing regular phlebotomy. Severe cases may benefit from allogeneic bone marrow transplant. This patient received supportive treatment with periodic evaluation of CBC and iron studies. Her lowest documented hemoglobin was 10.6 g/dL. Oral iron supplement was given with close clinical follow-up because of the predisposition for iron overload.

General Discussion CDAs are rare hereditary hematopoietic disorders primarily affecting erythropoiesis. Four criteria need to be present to diagnose CDA:
1. Hereditary nature of an anemia.
2. Evidence of ineffective erythropoiesis.
3. Characteristic appearance of bone marrow erythroblasts.
4. Exclusion of other causes of congenital anemia.

Additionally, molecular techniques have recently identified the gene associated with CDA, type I. There are 3 major subtypes of CDA. Our patient's results were most compatible with CDA II. Clinically, there is mild anemia with jaundice and splenomegaly. Basophilic stippling and suboptimal reticulocyte response for the degree of anemia are suggestive of disordered erythropoiesis. The bone marrow reveals erythroid hyperplasia with dyserythropoiesis and binuclearity in 10%-35% of erythroblasts. Multinucleate forms are rarely observed. On electron microscopy, a double membrane parallel to the cytoplasmic membrane of erythroblasts is present. This is believed to be the peripheral cisternae of smooth endoplasmic reticulum. The acidified serum test (Ham test) is positive and this is why the condition is also-called hereditary erythrocyte multinuclearity with positive acidified serum (HEMPAS). Herein, patient's red cells will lyse only in acidified normal serum, but not in the patient's own acidified serum. The red blood cells of CDA II contain i antigen and show agglutination with sera containing anti-i. The red blood cells of this patient had both I, which was expected, and i, which was not. Erythrocyte membrane analysis by sodium dodecyl sulfate polyacrylamide gel electrophoresis (SDS-PAGE) shows a narrower and faster moving band 3, a finding linked to a disturbance in the biosynthesis of N-linked oligosaccharides. It is believed that this abnormality contributes to premature red cell destruction.

Fanconi Anemia and Myelodysplastic Syndrome

Adina Cioc, Robert McKenna

Patient A 10-year-old boy with a 3-month history of easy bruising and hematomas.

Clinical History The patient was the product of an uncomplicated pregnancy and was born full-term weighing 7 pounds 2 ounces. At birth an abnormality of the right thumb was noted, which was surgically corrected at 6 months of age. Until his current presentation, he was healthy with no major infections or hospitalizations.

Family History The patient's parents are of western European descent. They are third or fourth cousins to each other. He has 3 siblings who are healthy. There is no known family history of blood dyscrasias or hematologic malignancies.

Medications None.

Physical Examination The patient's height and weight were both at the 10th percentile while both his parents are tall. There were multiple scattered café-au-lait spots. Surgical correction was noted on his right hand. The rest of the physical exam was normal.

Initial Work-Up	
CBC	
WBC (×10³/μL)	5.7
RBC (×10⁶/μL)	2.95
HGB (g/dL)	10.4
HCT (%)	30.3
MCV (fL)	103
MCH (pg)	35.5
MCHC (g/dL)	34.5
PLT (×10³/μL)	110
RDW-CV (%)	18.5
Absolute neutrophil count	1.1×10³/μL

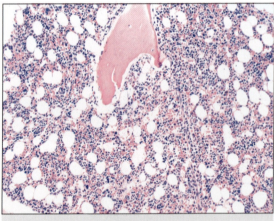

Figure 1 Bone marrow biopsy (H&E, ×100) essentially normocellular for age.

Differential Diagnosis The differential diagnosis of a child with pancytopenia (neutropenia, anemia, and thrombocytopenia) includes acquired aplastic anemia (either idiopathic, or induced by drugs/chemicals, viruses, or immune diseases), inherited bone marrow failure syndromes (of which Fanconi anemia is the most common), paroxysmal nocturnal hemoglobinuria, vitamin B_{12}/folate deficiency, myelodysplastic syndromes, acute leukemias, hemophagocytic lymphohistiocytosis, metabolic storage diseases, metastatic tumors, etc.

Additional Work-Up In this case the clinical suspicion of Fanconi anemia was high, due to the patient's

Section A: Anemias
Fanconi Anemia and Myelodysplastic Syndrome

physical stigmata of abnormal thumb, café-au-lait spots, and low height and weight for age. Chromosomal breakage analysis was performed and showed that both spontaneous and diepoxybutane (DEB)-induced chromosomal breakage were highly elevated and consistent with a diagnosis of Fanconi anemia. Bone marrow biopsy and aspiration were performed. The marrow cellularity was variable, 70%-90% (**Figure 1**). Dyserythropoiesis was observed in >10% of the erythroid precursors, and was characterized mainly by megaloblastoid features, irregular nuclear contours, and binucleation (**Figure 2**). Granulocytic maturation did not show evidence of dysplasia, but there was a slight increase in blasts at 3%. Numerous small hypolobated megakaryocytes were present (**Figure 3**). Chromosomal studies showed complex clonal abnormalities, including a duplication of the long arm of chromosome 1, an extra copy of the distal long arm of chromosome 3, and a loss of the distal long arm of chromosome 11.

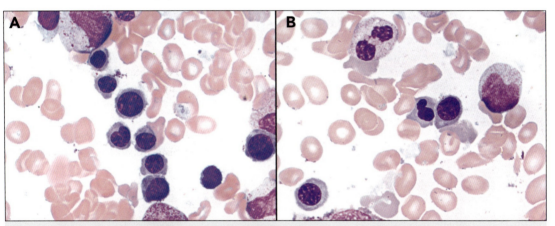

Figure 2 Bone marrow aspirate smear (Wright-Giemsa, **A** ×1000, and **B** ×500) showing dyserythropoiesis characterized by irregular nuclear contours and megaloblastoid features.

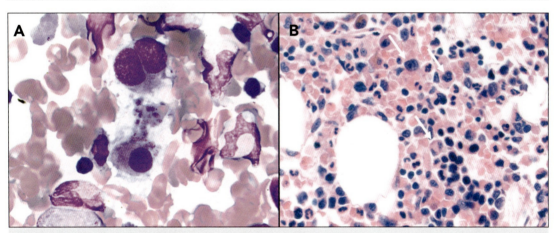

Figure 3 Bone marrow; **A** aspirate smear (Wright-Giemsa, ×1000) and **B** biopsy (H&E, ×500) in which megakaryocytes appear dysplastic showing small hypolobated nuclei.

Section A: Anemias
Fanconi Anemia and Myelodysplastic Syndrome

Final Diagnosis Myelodysplastic syndrome (MDS), refractory cytopenia with multilineage dysplasia (RCMD), arising in the background of Fanconi anemia.

Management Approach Hematopoietic progenitor cell transplantation (HPCT) is the only current curative treatment for the bone marrow failure. Outcome is better with HLA-identical sibling donors (who do not have FA as verified by DEB or mitomycin C [MMC] testing) and in younger patients who have not yet developed complications from their bone marrow failure. Patients who cannot undergo HPCT can be treated with androgens (oxymetholone), growth factor, or can be supported with red blood cell and platelet transfusions. This patient underwent 8/8 matched unrelated HPCT since none of his siblings were HLA-identical. His post-transplantation course was uneventful. A bone marrow biopsy performed at 2 years post-HPCT showed 60%-65% cellularity, no evidence of dysplasia, and 100% donor engraftment.

General Discussion Fanconi anemia (FA) is an inherited disorder associated with genomic instability, bone marrow failure (BMF) and predisposition to hematologic malignancies (myelodysplastic syndrome and acute myeloid leukemia) and/or solid tumors (squamous cell carcinomas of the head and neck). Most patients show an autosomal dominant pattern of inheritance. Characteristic congenital malformations are present in up to 60%-70% of affected children and include short stature, hypopigmented spots and café-au-lait spots, abnormality of thumbs, microcephaly, and hypogonadism. Patients often present with mild to moderate thrombocytopenia. Anemia, when detected, is often macrocytic. Hemoglobin electrophoresis usually shows increased concentrations of hemoglobin F, and serum α-fetoprotein (sAFP) levels are usually elevated. The diagnosis is made by the presence of increased chromosomal breakage in lymphocytes cultured in the presence of DNA cross-linking agents such as mitomycin C (MMC) or diepoxybutane (DEB). Prenatal testing can be performed for known affected families. MDS is a particularly challenging diagnosis in FA due to the frequent presence of dysplastic features in the bone marrows of these patients, especially dyserythropoiesis characterized by nuclear/cytoplasmic dyssynchrony, binucleated or multinucleated erythroid cells, and fragmented erythroid nuclei. When dyserythropoiesis is accompanied by at least 10% dysplastic cells in 1 or 2 other myeloid cell lines, a morphologic diagnosis of MDS, RCMD, can be made in FA marrows by following the current WHO criteria. Similarly, in the presence of increased bone marrow blasts, a diagnosis of MDS, refractory anemia with excess blasts (RAEB) is warranted. Relevant to the development of MDS in FA is the emergence of abnormal cytogenetic clones in the bone marrows of these patients. Frequently observed in these cases are gain of 1q, gain of 3q, and losses of 7 or 7q.

Pure Red Cell Aplasia Associated with Parvovirus Infection

Cherie H Dunphy, Yuri Fedoriw

Patient A 36-year-old African-American female, who presented with a 4-day history of progressive fatigue.

Clinical History The patient presented to the emergency room approximately 5 months prior to this presentation and was diagnosed with HIV infection, AIDS (CD4 count 68/µL) and severe *Pneumocystis* pneumonia. Her hospitalization was complicated by bilateral pneumothoraces requiring prolonged ventilatory support. She was eventually extubated and transferred to a rehabilitation facility. Approximately 1 month ago, the patient was discharged home with good weight gain and functional recovery. The patient now presents again with 4 days of progressive fatigue, loss of appetite, nausea and vomiting. She denied fevers, chills, and night sweats and had not noticed blood in her stool or urine.

Family History Unremarkable.

Medications The patient was discharged from the most recent hospitalization with the following medications: azithromycin, dapsone, ritonavir, tenofovir, valacyclovir, fosamprenavir, lamivudine, metoclopromide, efomeprazole, metoprolol, recombinant erythropoietin, paroxetine, and potassium.

Physical Examination Vital signs were normal. Lung exam showed distant breath sounds. Her examination was otherwise unremarkable.

Initial Work-Up

CBC		WBC Differential	%	# (×10³/µL)
WBC (×10³/µL)	6.6	Neutrophils	59.6	3.9
RBC (×10⁶/µL)	0.77	Bands	0	
HGB (g/dL)	2.2	Lymphocytes	31.3	2.1
HCT (%)	6.6	Monocytes	8.1	0.5
MCV (fL)	87	Eosinophils	1.0	0.1
MCH (pg)	29	Basophils	0	
MCHC (g/dL)	33	Reticulocyte count	0	
PLT (×10³/µL)	612			
RDW-CV (%)	13.7			

Peripheral blood smear examination revealed no morphologic abnormalities.
Creatinine 0.8 mg/dL, lactate dehydrogenase (LDH) 583 U/L, haptoglobin 184 mg/dL, billirubin 0.3 mg/dL.

Differential Diagnosis The finding of isolated anemia without evidence of hemolysis or overt renal failure in a patient with HIV infection/AIDS should raise the possibility of pure red cell aplasia (PRCA), most notably caused by parvovirus B19 infection. Other contributing or causative etiologies include antiretroviral effects, renal insufficiency, and/or nutritional deficiencies. Less commonly, thymoma, early myelodysplastic syndrome, or large granular lymphocytic (LGL) leukemia may also present with PRCA.

Section A: Anemias
Pure Red Cell Aplasia Associated with Parvovirus Infection

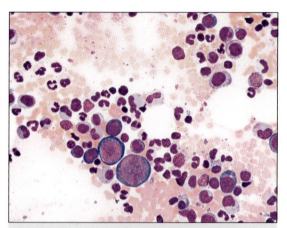

Figure 1 Bone marrow aspirate smear (Wright, × 400) showing giant early erythroid precursors (proerythroblasts) with distortion of the nuclei by large intranuclear viral inclusions.

Figure 2 Bone marrow biopsy (H&E, × 400) showing a large intranuclear inclusion (center of field).

Additional Work-Up Bone marrow aspirate smear demonstrated large early erythroid precursors containing nuclear viral inclusions of parvovirus B19 (**Figure 1**). Bone marrow biopsy section also revealed enlarged cells with nuclear viral inclusions, consistent with parvovirus B19 (**Figure 2**). Parvovirus B19 serology (IgM and IgG) was negative. However, polymerase chain reaction (PCR) analyses of the bone marrow aspirate and of the peripheral blood (serum) both detected parvovirus DNA.

Final Diagnosis Marked anemia due to pure red cell aplasia caused by parvovirus B-19 in the setting of HIV infection.

Management Approach PRCA of autoimmune origin was first treated successfully with intravenous immunoglobulins (IV Ig) >20 years ago. Since then, B19-associated PRCA in solid-organ transplant recipients and in human immunodeficiency virus (HIV)-infected patients has also been successfully treated with IV Ig. This patient was started on IV Ig therapy at 0.5 g/kg IV × 2 days. She was also transfused with 5 units of red blood cells. Her hemoglobin and hematocrit response was excellent after transfusion, and the patient's peripheral blood counts stabilized.

General Discussion This patient presented with pure red cell aplasia (PRCA) due to parvovirus B19 infection, which was diagnosed based primarily on bone marrow examination and subsequent confirmation by PCR analysis of the bone marrow aspirate. The bone marrow aspirate smear revealed numerous giant early erythroid precursors (proerythroblasts) with distortion of the nuclei by the large intranuclear viral inclusions, a feature typical of parvovirus-induced PRCA. These intranuclear inclusions were also appreciated in the H&E-stained bone marrow sections. Initial serologic testing for parvovirus B19 was negative; however, subsequent PCR analyses of both serum and bone marrow aspirate were positive. This phenomenon reflects the inherent higher sensitivity of molecular assays in confirming the initial pathologic diagnosis of the bone marrow examination and a common phenomenon of negative (noncontributory) serologic results in a severely immunocompromised patient. Anemia is a common finding in the HIV-positive population and the etiology is often multifactorial. As concurrent pathology contributing to anemia is not uncommon in these patients, a thorough investigation is necessary to exclude other causes. Therefore, the diagnosis of parvovirus-induced PRCA is made with morphologic evidence of red cell aplasia in the bone marrow biopsy or aspirate, confirmation by either serologic or molecular testing and exclusion of other potentially treatable etiologies.

Hemochromatosis, HFE-Associated

Ronald Sham

Patient A 63-year-old white male, who was originally evaluated for hemochromatosis 18 years earlier.

Clinical History His family is of European descent and the original evaluation was prompted by a family history of possible hemochromatosis. Screening iron studies performed at the age of 45 were suggestive of hemochromatosis. His history otherwise was unrevealing and his review of systems was notable for the absence of any history of liver disease, cardiac symptoms, hyperpigmentation of the skin, diabetes, arthropathy or impotence. His review of systems for disorders unrelated to hemochromatosis was also negative.

Family History It was reported that patient's father had diabetes and hemochromatosis with liver disease and died at the age of 48. The patient's paternal grandfather had diabetes but lived into his 70s. A maternal grandmother died at a young age of unknown cause. A number of other paternal relatives died without clear features suggesting hemochromatosis. The patient has 2 siblings who are not known to have hemochromatosis, although one used alcohol excessively and is known to have liver disease.

Physical Examination At the time of his initial evaluation he was healthy appearing with normal blood pressure. His head, eyes, ears, nose, and throat (HEENT) exam was unremarkable. His cardiac and pulmonary exam was normal. His abdominal exam was notable for the absence of any hepatosplenomegaly. Musculoskeletal exam was notable for the absence of any signs of joint damage. Skin exam was notable for the absence of stigmata of liver disease or signs of hyperpigmentation.

Initial Work-Up
- WBC $4.7 \times 10^3/\mu L$, HCT 44%, PLT $198 \times 10^3/\mu L$
- Serum iron 236 µg/dL (normal 75-175)
- Total iron-binding capacity 253 µg/dL (normal 250-400)
- Transferrin saturation 93% (normal 20-50)
- Ferritin reported >1,000 ng/mL (normal 20-200)
- AST and ALT were normal

Differential Diagnosis The differential diagnosis for an elevated ferritin in this range (>1,000) includes iron overload (due to hereditary hemochromatosis or other iron overload states), as well as inflammatory states where there may be an elevated ferritin as an acute phase reactant. Since the patient was clinically stable and not acutely or chronically ill, it seemed unlikely that the ferritin elevation was reactive and more likely that this represented iron overload.

Additional Work-Up At the time of original presentation, the patient underwent a liver biopsy that showed increased iron consistent with early hemochromatosis. The liver architecture was intact with no signs of inflammation, fibrosis or fatty change. The iron stain showed a striking increase in iron in the hepatocytes. The quantitative iron was 184 µmol and the hepatic iron index was 4.09. Years later, in 1998, he had HFE genotyping performed. His HFE genotype showed that he is a C282Y homozygote.

Section A: Anemias
Hemochromatosis, HFE-Associated

Final Diagnosis Hereditary hemochromatosis with HFE genotyping showing a homozygous state for C282Y. This is the classic genotype for hereditary hemochromatosis. Patients with a serum ferritin <1,000 are very unlikely to have liver disease associated with hemochromatosis. Patients with a ferritin >1,000 and patients with liver enzyme abnormalities should have a liver biopsy to assess for any significant pathologic findings such as cirrhosis.

Management Approach After the liver biopsy and the clinical/pathologic diagnosis of hemochromatosis was established, the patient was begun on a phlebotomy regimen. He was originally phlebotomized weekly as tolerated until his ferritin value was in the normal range. He was subsequently placed on maintenance phlebotomy, and to this day he continues on phlebotomy approximately every 2 months. His ferritin is maintained at approximately 100 ng/mL. He has never developed clinical features of organ dysfunction secondary to hemochromatosis, and for many years has maintained his ferritin in the normal range.

General Discussion Hemochromatosis is one of the most common hereditary disorders in Caucasians. It must be distinguished from other disorders associated with an elevated ferritin as well as from other forms of iron overload including transfusion iron overload. This distinction is important both in terms of mechanism and clinical management. Some individuals may be suspected of iron overload based on an elevated ferritin; however, it must be recognized that ferritin and serum iron values are altered by acute or significant chronic illnesses or liver diseases and therefore iron status is best evaluated in a patient who is clinically stable. The pathophysiology of the different forms of iron overload is quite distinct. Patients with ineffective erythropoiesis with subsequent anemia may have enhanced intestinal absorption of iron resulting in iron overload. Their iron overload may be exacerbated by red blood cell transfusion support that results in iron accumulation in the Kupffer cells in the liver as opposed to the hepatocytes, which is distinct from the pattern seen in most forms of hereditary hemochromatosis. Furthermore, many patients with iron overload and an underlying hematologic disorder cannot receive phlebotomy as a therapy due to their anemia, and rely on iron chelators to manage their iron overload. Patients with chronic liver disease associated with alcohol excess or other etiologies also have iron overload, which is distinct from hereditary hemochromatosis. Hereditary hemochromatosis includes a number of distinct disorders including most commonly HFE-related hemochromatosis and less commonly ferroportin disease, 2 forms of juvenile hemochromatosis, and hemochromatosis associated with transferrin receptor 2 mutations. The current classification scheme divides hereditary hemochromatosis into 5 genetically distinct subtypes show in **Table 1**. HFE-related (Type 1) hemochromatosis accounts for the great majority of patients with hereditary hemochromatosis. HFE-associated hemochromatosis is autosomal recessive and there are 3 mutations that are most commonly associated with the disorder. There is some geographic variability in regard to these mutations, but the C282Y mutation is associated with the most significant clinical course. There are a number of postulated pathophysiologic mechanisms for HFE-associated hemochromatosis, but the exact mechanism is not fully defined. The HFE mutation was first reported in 1996 and genotyping became commercially available shortly thereafter. Prior to the availability of genotyping, the diagnosis was based on clinical and laboratory features. Laboratory testing other than genotyping still plays a major role in diagnosis and management. Screening for hemochromatosis has become an important, and controversial part of clinical practice. Most patients with HFE mutations that may result in iron overload will have enhanced absorption of iron lifelong. They will therefore have an elevated transferrin saturation even at a young age; however, iron stores, as measured by ferritin, do not typically become increased until later in life. There is often a difference between males and females as females will have blood loss with menstrual periods as well as childbirth and therefore women with genetic hemochromatosis do not develop significant iron overload until later in life. Many patients may have hemochromatosis gene mutations but not have iron overload biochemically. Furthermore, of those with biochemical iron overload, only a subset are likely to develop clinically significant organ dysfunction. This point has resulted in some uncertainty regarding management of patients with hemochromatosis and how to distinguish between "genetic hemochromatosis" and "clinical hemochromatosis." This is not dissimilar to other genetic disorders where the genetic disorder predisposes one to the condition, but not all individuals develop evidence of the disease. Because the prevalence of the gene is high, but the penetrance of the disease is fairly low, the value of screening remains controversial. The other subtypes of hemochromatosis are considerably less common. Currently, commercial testing for these other subtypes of hemochromatosis is not readily available. If a patient is felt to have hemochromatosis yet has no HFE mutations or does not fit clinically with the pattern seen in HFE-related hemochromatosis, the diagnosis often requires referral to a specialized center. In that setting empiric phlebotomy treatment is often started to ensure the safety of the patient.

Table 1. Hereditary hemochromatosis types

	HFE	Juvenile	Juvenile	TfR2	Ferroportin
Type	1	2A	2B	3	4
Gene	HFE	HJV	HAMP	TfR2	FPN1
Protein	HFE	Hemojuvelin	Hepcidin	Transferrin receptor 2	Ferroportin
Inheritance	Autosomal recessive	Autosomal recessive	Autosomal recessive	Autosomal recessive	Autosomal dominant
Iron depostion	Hepatocyte	Hepatocyte	Hepatocyte	Hepatocyte	Macrophage (usually)
Clinical points	Great majority of all patients with hereditary hemochromatosis	Early age of onset	Early age of onset		"Hepcidin resistance" is another rare subtype

Note that with the exception of type 4, most do well with phlebotomy and do not develop anemia. Juvenile forms are most likely to result in significant organ damage. The "hepcidin resistance" form of type 4 disease can have hepatocyte iron deposition and an earlier age of onset.

Hemochromatosis, Non-HFE Associated

Ronald Sham

Patient A 69-year-old white male, who had been evaluated for hemochromatosis 35 years earlier.

Clinical History The patient's family is of European descent. He relates that when he was in his late 20s he began feeling sluggish. He had no prior medical history at that point in time. Following a series of diagnostic evaluations he was ultimately noted to have liver enzyme abnormalities that led to a liver biopsy. The liver biopsy revealed that he had hemochromatosis. He was started on a phlebotomy regimen and has continued for approximately 35 years. Years after his diagnosis he had bilateral hip replacements, which were done when he was in his early 50s. He had developed degenerative arthritis that was fairly severe, likely as a complication of iron overload. He fortunately never developed diabetes, cardiac dysfunction, or overt clinical evidence of liver dysfunction, nor has he developed hyperpigmentation.

Family History The patient has 4 adult children who have been evaluated; 3 of the children also have hemochromatosis. These family members are all being treated with regular phlebotomy. He has 5 granddaughters, 3 of whom also have hemochromatosis, and they are also on regular phlebotomy regimens. To the best of his knowledge there was no family history of hemochromatosis in earlier generations of family members. The family pedigree is displayed in **Figure 1**.

Physical Examination He was healthy appearing. His head, eyes, ears, nose, and throat (HEENT) exam was unremarkable, and his cardiac and pulmonary exams were normal. His abdominal exam was notable for minimal hepatomegaly with a liver edge felt 2 cm below the right costal margin. He did not have splenomegaly or stigmata of chronic liver disease. Musculoskeletal exam was notable for some minimal problems with his gait secondary to his bilateral hip replacement. He also had arthritic changes in the wrists and finger joints. His skin was notable for the absence of hyperpigmentation.

Initial Work-Up The decades-old initial laboratory studies were not available. However, he was known to have had a markedly elevated ferritin with an elevated transferrin saturation. His ferritin on maintenance phlebotomy has been in the low normal range, and his transferrin saturation remains approximately 80%-90% despite the low iron stores.

Differential Diagnosis The differential diagnosis for an elevated ferritin in this range includes iron overload as well as inflammatory states where the elevated ferritin may be present as an acute phase reactant. At the time of his initial evaluation, he had liver enzyme abnormalities, which can also account for an elevated ferritin. Once the diagnosis of hemochromatosis was established, the differential diagnosis included the multiple subtypes of hemochromatosis described below.

Additional Work-Up The patient had a liver biopsy at approximately age 35. The biopsy showed a strongly positive iron stain with granular hemosiderin deposits within hepatocytes. There was moderate portal fibrosis but no necrosis or inflammation. Subsequently, in more recent years when the entire family was under evaluation, additional studies were done, which included HFE genotyping. The patient and other family members did not possess HFE mutations suggesting

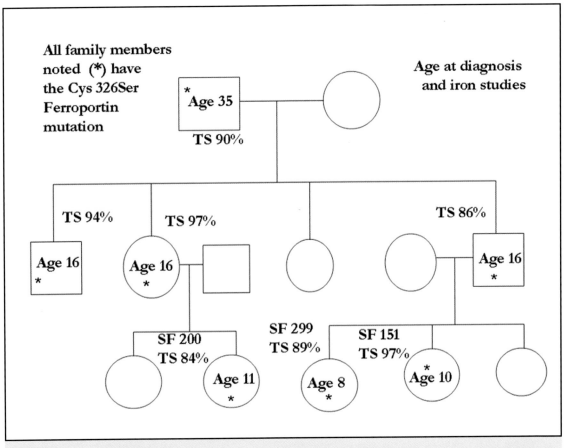

Figure 1 Family pedigree showing the inheritance pattern, age at diagnosis and laboratory features of the individuals with the Cys326Ser mutation in the ferroportin gene. TS = transferrin saturation; SF= serum ferritin.

this was hereditary hemochromatosis that was not HFE-related. The great majority of patients with familial hemochromatosis have HFE mutations. There are a number of less common disorders associated with familial iron overload that can occur; therefore, in collaboration with a hematology research center additional molecular diagnostic studies were performed. Ultimately the patient and his family were shown to have a mutation in the ferroportin gene (Cys326Ser) proving they have a subtype of ferroportin disease (type 4 hemochromatosis).

Diagnosis Ferroportin disease (type 4 hemochromatosis) with a Cys326Ser mutation.

It should be noted that this genotypic and phenotypic subtype is distinct from the more common forms of "ferroportin disease." The unique features associated with this genotype are discussed below. The more common forms of ferroportin disease has an older age of onset and is associated with iron accumulation in the macrophages as opposed to hepatocytes as seen in this form. This subtype has feature more akin to juvenile hemochromatosis.

Management Approach The patient has been on maintenance phlebotomy for 35 years. He and the rest of his family are now managed with maintenance phlebotomy in an effort to keep their iron stores in the normal range. He is the only individual in the family with organ damage (arthritis) and therefore he has some additional care for that aspect of his medical condition. He has had periodic assessment of liver function as well given the initial liver biopsy findings. He will be maintained on lifelong phlebotomy.

General Discussion Ferroportin disease is also referred to as type 4 hemochromatosis. Type 1 hemochromatosis is the most common type of genetic hemochromatosis that is associated with HFE

Section A: Anemias
Hemochromatosis, Non-HFE Associated

mutations. Type 2 hemochromatosis is also referred to as juvenile hemochromatosis and there are 2 subtypes resulting from mutations in either the hemojuvelin gene or hepcidin gene. Type 3 hemochromatosis is due to a mutation in the transferrin receptor 2 gene. Ferroportin disease is an autosomal dominant disorder that is distinct from the other subtypes of hemochromatosis that are autosomal recessive. Ferroportin disease can be associated with various mutations in the ferroportin gene. Ferroportin is the main iron exporter in humans. It is present on hepatocytes, enterocytes and macrophages. Ferroportin is modulated by the action of hepcidin, a key iron regulatory protein. Patients with ferroportin disease have abnormal responses to the normal regulatory effects of hepcidin. This family has a mutation in ferroportin such that they are resistant to the normal effects of hepcidin. In normal individuals, hepcidin will bind to ferroportin on the basolateral aspect of enterocytes resulting in internalization and degradation of the protein. That enables iron export to proceed in a regulated manor. With this specific mutation, the affected family members are resistant to the regulatory effects of hepcidin and therefore the ferroportin is not internalized and they continue to absorb iron exceeding that necessary for erythropoiesis and other daily iron needs. These individuals develop iron overload with a phenotype showing an elevated transferrin saturation level and elevated ferritin. There are a number of distinct subtypes of ferroportin disease and this family has a subtype that is clinically more severe than other individuals described in the literature. These family members developed iron overload at a younger age; the 3 granddaughters had relatively high ferritin values by age 10. They have some pathologic features similar to that seen in the other subtypes of hemochromatosis in that the iron accumulates in the hepatocytes; however, the pathophysiology as noted is quite distinct. Management is similar in that they require phlebotomy to maintain their iron stores in a safe range. The more common types of ferroportin disease are distinct from other hemochromatosis subtypes in that affected individuals are more likely to have difficulty with phlebotomy and develop anemia. That has not been an issue with this family. In the future it is likely that other variants of ferroportin disease will be described as well as mutations in other iron regulatory proteins resulting in hemochromatosis.

Section B: Acute Leukemias

Acute Myeloid Leukemia with t(8;21)

R Patrick Dorion

Patient A 32-year-old man, who presented with low back pain and feeling tired for a few weeks.

Clinical History He has had an appendectomy, tonsillectomy and adenoidectomy in the past. He also has a history of alcohol, cocaine and marijuana abuse. He smokes half a pack of cigarettes a day.

Family History His father died of cirrhosis at age 30. His mother has had 2 hip replacements.

Medications Lorazapam and acetaminophen/oxycodone.

Physical Examination Healthy-appearing male with no adenopathy, organomegaly, petechiae or ecchymoses.

Initial Work-Up

CBC		WBC Differential	%	# (×10³/μL)
WBC (×10³/μL)	6.2	Neutrophils	7	0.4
RBC (×10⁶/μL)	3.8	Bands	0	
HGB (g/dL)	13.5	Lymphocytes	40	2.5
HCT (%)	38.4	Monocytes	3	0.2
MCV (fL)	99.6	Eosinophils	2	0.1
MCH (pg)	35.0	Basophils	0	
MCHC (g/dL)	35.1	Myelocyte	1	0.1
PLT (×10³/μL)	91	Blasts	47	2.9
RDW-CV (%)	16.3			

Results of serum chemistries and PT and PTT were within normal ranges.
Peripheral blood smear revealed several blasts with occasional Auer rods (**Figure 1**).

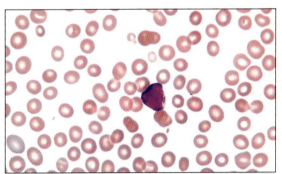

Figure 1 Blood smear (Wright-Giemsa, ×1000) showing a blast with an Auer rod.

Differential Diagnosis With the findings of 47% blasts in the peripheral blood, the differential diagnosis is narrowed to an acute leukemic process. The presence of Auer rods further narrows the differential diagnosis to an acute myeloid leukemia. The critical point is differentiating between acute promyelocytic leukemia (APL) and other myeloid leukemias since the therapy is different and APL can have severe disseminated intravascular coagulopathy (DIC).

Additional Work-Up Bone marrow was hypercellular with a prominent increase in blasts (**Figure 2**). The aspirate smear yielded 46% blasts, some of which had azurophilic granules and a few showed Auer rods (**Figure 3**). Flow cytometry performed on the bone marrow aspirate revealed a blast population that was positive for the following markers: CD45 (low intensity), CD34, MPO, CD117, CD71 (moderate intensity), CD13, CD33, HLA-DR, CD15, and TDT. The blasts were negative for: CD14, CD64, CD24, CD2, CD3, CD4, CD8, CD5, cytoplasmic CD3, CD19, CD20, cytoplasmic CD79a, surface immunoglobulins, CD10, and κ and λ light chains. Classic cytogenetic studies revealed an abnormal karyotype with 46, XY, t(8;21)(q22;q22) in all the metaphases analyzed (**Figure 4**). PML/RARA FISH probe was negative. FISH probe for ETO/RUNX1 was; however, positive (**Figure 5**).

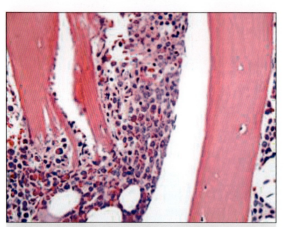

Figure 2 Bone marrow biopsy (H&E, ×200) showing hypercellular marrow with prominent increase in blasts.

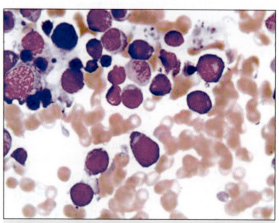

Figure 3 Bone marrow aspirate smear (Wright-Giemsa, ×1000) showing increased number of blasts.

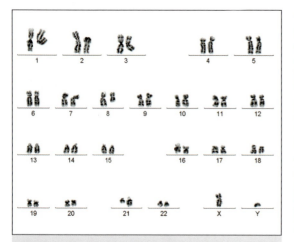

Figure 4 Bone marrow karyotype showing t(8;21).

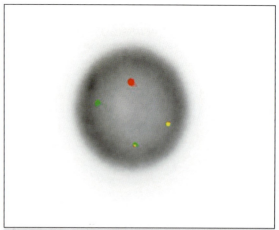

Figure 5 Bone marrow (FISH probe for ETO/RUNX1) showing positivity.

Final Diagnosis Acute myelogenous leukemia with t(8;21) translocation.

Management Approach All acute myeloid leukemias except acute promyelocytic leukemia (APL) are given an induction regimen with chemotherapy that usually includes cytarabine and daunorubicin/idarubicin (anthracyclines). The goal is to achieve a complete remission. In newly diagnosed adults, it is possible to achieve a 50%-75% remission status. Without consolidation therapy, almost all patients will relapse. The goal of consolidation therapy is to remove undetectable disease. Consolidation therapy is tailored to individual patients depending on the prognostic factors found. In high-risk patients, if tolerated, an allogeneic hematopoietic progenitor cell transplant (HPCT) is recommended. This patient was induced with cytarabine and daunorubicin and achieved a complete remission. He was consolidated with high-dose cytarabine (HiDAC). Approximately 2½ years after consolidation he had a cytogenetic relapse and received salvage chemotherapy with etoposide and cyclophosphammide and achieved a complete remission again. He then underwent an allogeneic HPCT from a male sibling and achieved 100% chimerism. He did have grade 1 graft-vs-host disease, which responded to steroids. He remains disease free; however, in the interval since HPCT, he has had 2 episodes of gram-negative sepsis and a pulmonary embolism.

General Discussion Acute myelogenous leukemia (AML) is fairly uncommon. It is reported to cause 1.2% of cancer deaths in the United States. It has a 5-year survival of 17%-70% depending on the subtype. AML with a more favorable prognosis include acute promyelocytic leukemia with the t(15;17) PML/RARA translocation, acute myelomonocytic leukemia with eosinophilia with inversion of chromosome 16 (inv 16) and translocation t(8;21). High-risk factors with poor prognosis include a previous myelodysplastic syndrome or myeloproliferative neoplasm, secondary AML arising after previous chemotherapy, no remission after induction, relapse of disease and an older age. High-risk cytogenetic abnormalities include abnormalities in chromosomes 5, 7 and FLT 3 gene. Translocation t(8;21) is reported to be the most frequently encountered chromosomal abnormality in AML especially in the acute myeloid leukemia with maturation subtype. It may be associated with eosinophilia in the marrow but not as commonly as in those patients with inv16. It has a high rate of complete remission on conventional chemotherapy. It is also frequently associated with other chromosomal abnormalities such as a loss of a sex chromosome. The genes involved in t(8;21) are the ETO from chromosome 8 q22 and AML1 from chromosome 21 q22. The translocation results in a hybrid gene. The resulting gene is 5'AML-ETO with breakpoints at the very 5' end of ETO between exons 5 and 6 in AML1. The oncogenesis is probably from an altered transcriptional regulation of normal AML1 target genes.

Acute Myeloid Leukemia with Mutated NPM1

Joan E Etzell, Ellen F Krasik

Patient A 68-year-old man, who presented with a complaint of dyspnea on exertion for the past 2 months.

Clinical History The patient is a retired engineer, who used to be an avid runner and swimmer. He reported noticing a decrease in exercise tolerance over the past few months.

Family History No family history of hematopoietic malignancies. Father died at age 70 from colon cancer.

Medications Hydrochlorothiazide, lisinopril, lovastatin, doxazosin.

Physical Examination The patient was tired-appearing but in no acute distress. Vital signs included temperature 98.1°F, blood pressure 123/68 mmHg, heart rate 86 beats/min, and respiratory rate 19 breaths/minute. Head and neck, chest, and cardiac exams were unremarkable. His abdomen was soft, nontender, without hepatosplenomegaly, and his extremities and skin were unremarkable.

Initial Work-Up

CBC		WBC Differential	%	# ($\times 10^3/\mu L$)
WBC ($\times 10^3/\mu L$)	6.1	Neutrophils	20	1.2
RBC ($\times 10^6/\mu L$)	2.29	Bands	0	
HGB (g/dL)	7.8	Lymphocytes	38	2.3
HCT (%)	22.9	Monocytes/promonocytes	26	1.6
MCV (fL)	100	Eosinophils	2	0.1
MCH (pg)	34.3	Basophils	0	
MCHC (g/dL)	34.2	Immature granulocytes	11	0.7
PLT ($\times 10^3/\mu L$)	167	Blasts	3	0.2

*Peripheral blood smear revealed circulating immature granulocytes including blasts and monocytosis. Blasts accounted for <5% of the white cells while promonocytes (blast equivalents) accounted for approximately 10% (**Figure 1**).*

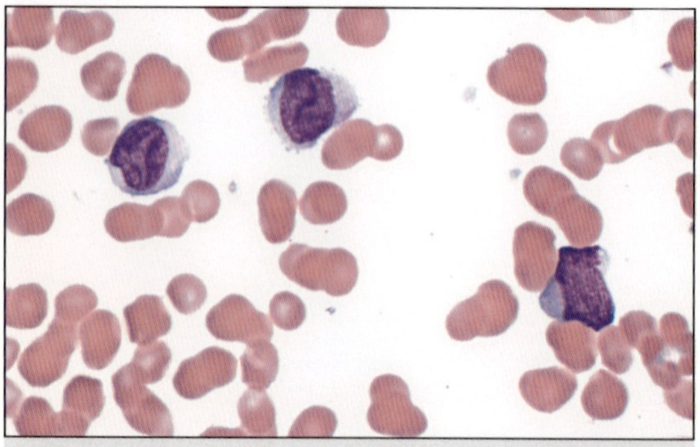

Figure 1 Blood smear (Wright-Giemsa, ×1000) showing a blast on the right and 2 promonocytes in the upper left.

Differential Diagnosis The CBC and peripheral smear findings are concerning for an underlying hematopoietic disorder. The presence of neutropenia, marked anemia, and monocytosis (>1 × $10^3/\mu L$) with ~15% blasts and promonocytes (blast equivalents) raises the possibility of a myelodysplastic/myeloproliferative neoplasm such as chronic myelomonocytic leukemia-2 or acute leukemia (if bone marrow blasts/promonocytes are >20%). The monocytosis argues against refractory anemia with excess blasts (RAEB), and the peripheral blast count precludes the diagnosis of other myelodysplastic syndromes (MDS). Bone marrow biopsy examination with concurrent flow cytometric immunophenotyping and cytogenetic studies are required for definitive characterization of the patient's disease.

Additional Work-Up The bone marrow biopsy sections were hypercellular (90% cellularity) and showed diffuse sheets of immature cells consistent with blasts and immature monocytes, together representing 80% of the marrow cellularity (**Figure 2**). A few cells with fine nuclear grooves or mildly indented nuclear contours resembling promonocytes and immature monocytes were seen (**Figure 3**, arrowhead). Flow cytometric immunophenotyping performed on the aspirate identified a myeloid blast population (50% of cells) that expressed weak CD4, weak CD11c, weak CD33, bright MPO, and CD117 with weak-to-absent coexpression of CD13. There was no coexpression of CD34, TdT, CD14, B-cell markers, or other T-cell markers on this population. A second population (48% of cells) expressed weak CD4, variable CD11c, CD33, weak MPO, and variable CD15 with subset coexpression of CD14, an immunophenotype consistent with maturing monocytic precursors. Cytogenetic studies revealed a normal male karyotype, 46, XY. Additional testing for NPM1 and FLT3-ITD mutations showed that this patient's leukemia harbored an NPM1 mutation but lacked mutation of FLT3-ITD.

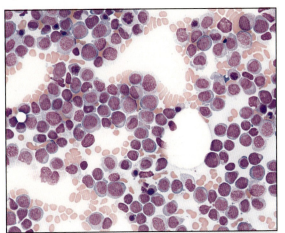

Figure 2 Bone marrow aspirate smear (Wright-Giemsa, ×400) showing many large blasts that, with fine chromatin and moderately abundant lightly basophilic cytoplasm, are compatible with monoblasts.

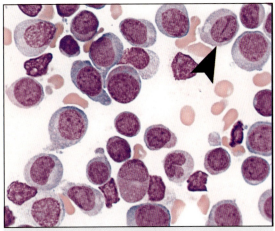

Figure 3 Bone marrow aspirate smear (Wright-Giemsa, ×1000) showing many blasts that are large with fine chromatin and moderately abundant lightly basophilic cytoplasm, compatible with monoblasts. Occasional promonocytes with nuclear folds or grooves (arrowhead) are also noted.

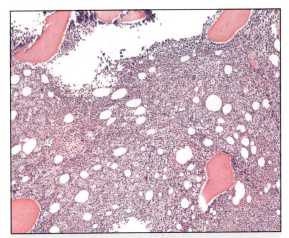

Figure 4 Bone marrow (H&E, ×100) showing hypercellular marrow with effacement by blasts and occasional promonocytes.

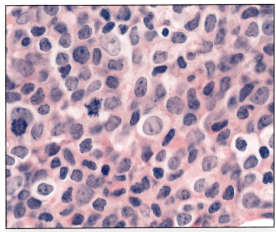

Figure 5 Bone marrow (H&E, ×1000). Hypercellular marrow reveals effacement by blasts and occasional promonocytes. Mitotic figures are noted.

Section B: Acute Leukemias
Acute Myeloid Leukemia with Mutated NPM1

Final Diagnosis Acute myeloid leukemia (AML) with mutated NPM1. This AML shows monocytic differentiation, a normal karyotype, and is FLT3-ITD negative.

Management Approach The standard approach to induction chemotherapy includes cytarabine given in a continuous infusion over 7 days along with an anthracycline such as daunorubicin or idarubicin for 3 days (ie, 7+3 regimen). Incorporation of high-dose cytarabine, or addition of other agents such as etoposide, fludarabine, or cladribine may be included as part of a clinical investigation. Consolidation therapy for acute myeloid leukemia generally includes high-dose cytarabine. The number of cycles of high-dose cytarabine and the use of hematopoietic progenitor cell transplantation (HPCT) in consolidation is based on the patient's risk of relapse. Patients with "good risk" disease usually receive 3-4 cycles of high-dose cytarabine; whereas those with "high risk" disease are usually offered HPCT in first remission if a donor is available. Risk has been stratified based on cytogenetics, with normal cytogenetics in the intermediate risk category. Allogeneic HPCT has been the treatment of choice after achieving the first remission for intermediate-risk AMLs, including those with a normal cytogenetics. However, the benefit of allogeneic HPCT in patients with NPM1-positive/FLT3-negative AML (favorable prognosis) has not been well established, and alternative approaches, such as autologous stem cell transplant, may be considered in these patients. This patient was started on allopurinol for prevention of tumor lysis syndrome. He subsequently underwent induction chemotherapy with cytarabine and idarubacin. A bone marrow examination on day 21 of his chemotherapy cycle showed complete remission, but his induction course was complicated by renal insufficiency, tumor lysis, intubation for respiratory failure secondary to leukemic infiltrates, possible transfusion-related lung injury (TRALI), episodes of massive hemoptysis, and hypernatremia. He later underwent consolidation chemotherapy with high-dose cytarabine and etoposide and subsequently received an autologous HPCT after a preparatory regimen of busulfan and etoposide. At 8 months post-HPCT he was doing well with no signs of relapse.

General Discussion While the identification of karyotypic abnormalities in AML can provide prognostic information, only 55%-60% of AML cases demonstrate clonal chromosomal abnormalities. In patients with AML with normal cytogenetic studies, testing for mutations of NPM1 and FLT3 can provide information for risk classification. Mutation of NPM1 is found in 1/3 of all AML and in 45%-64% of AML with normal karyotype. It is more common in women, and the prevalence increases with age. Patients often present with a high white blood cell count (not seen in this case) and high bone marrow blast count. There is strong association with morphologic features resembling acute myelomonocytic leukemia (FAB M4) and acute monocytic leukemia (FAB M5), with mutated NPM1 seen in 80%-90% of the latter.

Mutant NPM1 is also seen in AML with prominent nuclear invaginations. In AML with NPM1$^+$, blasts usually do not express CD34 (as in this case) but do typically express monocytic markers (CD14, CD11b). NPM1, located at chromosome 5q35, encodes nucleophosmin, a nucleolar phosphoprotein that shuttles between the nucleus and cytoplasm. Nucleophosmin's functions include promotion of ribosome formation, control of centrosomal duplication, modulation of tumor-suppressor transcription factors, and regulation of nuclear proteins. Mutations usually occur in exon 12 of NPM1 and result in alterations in tryptophan residues at the C-terminus of the nucleophosmin protein. A nuclear export signal is generated and results in aberrant cytoplasmic localization of the protein. One mutation, designated mutation A, accounts for 70%-80% of all NPM1 mutations in adult AML. Mutations can be detected by PCR-based assays, and immunohistochemical staining for nucleophosmin can identify aberrant cytoplasmic localization. In fact, immunohistochemical stains have demonstrated that often more than one bone marrow lineage carries the NPM1 mutation. In AML with normal karyotype, NPM1 mutation confers a favorable prognosis, with good response to induction chemotherapy and higher complete remission rates, longer event-free survival, and longer overall survival compared to AML with wild-type NPM1. Of note, 35%-40% of NPM1$^+$ AML also carries the FLT3-ITD mutation. Such dual mutant AMLs have a prognosis intermediate between the unfavorable NPM1$^-$/FLT3-ITD$^+$ group and the favorable NPM1$^+$/FLT3-ITD$^-$. NPM1 mutations appear to be very stable, and quantitative PCR assays may be used in the future to monitor and quantify minimal residual disease.

Acute Promyelocytic Leukemia with t(15;17)(q22;q12)

Lydia Contis

Patient A 55-year-old male, who presented to the emergency room complaining of epistaxis over a 3-day period.

Clinical History After evaluation, the nasal blood vessels were cauterized, and the patient sent home. Approximately 2 weeks later, he again presented to the emergency room with gingival bleeding. Laboratory values showed a WBC of $53.2 \times 10^3/\mu L$ and a platelet count of $133 \times 10^3/\mu L$. He was admitted to the hospital for further evaluation.

Family History Noncontributory.

Medications None.

Physical Examination Notable only for an erythematous oropharynx with small ulcers and gingival hyperplasia. Scattered ecchymoses were noted over the arms and lower legs.

Initial Work-Up

CBC	WBC	Differential	%	# ($10^3/\mu L$)
WBC ($\times 10^3/\mu L$)	60.1	Neutrophils	2	1.2
RBC ($\times 10^6/\mu L$)	2.94	Bands	3	1.8
HGB (g/dL)	9.4	Lymphocytes	4	2.4
HCT (%)	26.3	Monocytes	3	1.8
MCV (fL)	89.6	Eosinophils	0	
MCH (pg)	32.1	Basophils	0	
MCHC (g/dL)	35.8	Myelocytes	24	14.4
PLT ($\times 10^3/\mu L$)	97	Metamyelocytes	16	9.6
RDW-CV (%)	20.3	Blasts/Promyelo	48	28.9

Peripheral blood smear demonstrated blasts and abnormal promyelocytes with nucleoli, bilobed or rounded nuclei or sliding plate nuclei and with granulated cytoplasm (**Figure 1**).

- PTT 46 seconds (normal 22.7-35.6)
- PT 24.1 seconds (normal 11.7-15.3)
- INR 2.1 (normal 0.8-1.2) fibrinogen 79 mg/dL (normal 205-508)

Differential Diagnosis Acute myeloid leukemia, promyelocytic vs nonpromyelocytic.

Additional Work-Up Bone marrow biopsy was hypercellular (95% cellular) with an extensive infiltrate of abnormal leukemic promyelocytes (**Figure 2**). Manual differential of the bone marrow aspirate demonstrated: blasts 7.3%, abnormal promyelocytes 62.3%, myelocytes 6.3%, metamyelocytes 5.3%, bands 3.3%, neutrophils 0.3%, eosinophils 1.3%, monocytes 1.0%, normoblasts 9.3%, lymphocytes 3.3%. Abnormal

Section B: Acute Leukemias
Acute Promyelocytic Leukemia with t(15;17)(q22;q12)

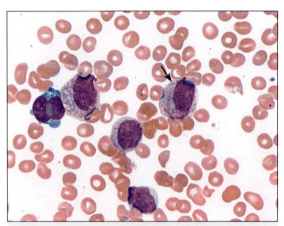

Figure 1 Peripheral blood smear (Wright-Giemsa, ×1000) showing leukemic hypergranular promyelocytes with multiple Auer rods (arrow).

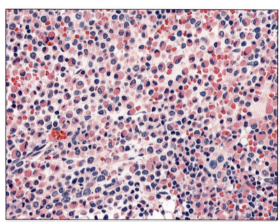

Figure 2 Bone marrow biopsy (H&E, ×400) showing hypercellular marrow with numerous promyelocytes.

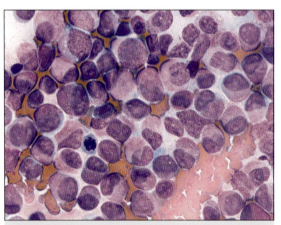

Figure 3 Bone marrow aspirate smear (Wright-Giemsa, ×1000) showing leukemic hypergranular promyelocytes.

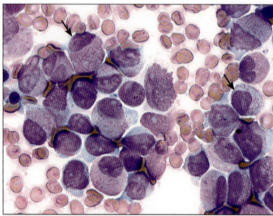

Figure 4 Bone marrow aspirate smear (Wright-Giemsa, ×1000) showing leukemic hypergranular promyelocytes and blasts with multiple Auer rods (arrows).

promyelocytes demonstrated dense cytoplasmic granulation and (**Figure 3**). A number of blasts contained multiple Auer rods (**Figure 4**).

Flow cytometry studies performed on the bone marrow demonstrated a leukemic cell population with the following phenotype: dim CD45+, CD33+, CD15+, HLA-DR–, CD56+, partial CD4+, CD13–, strongly myeloperoxidase positive and CD34–.

Cytogenetics 47, XY, +8, t(11;22)(q23;q11.2), t(15;17)(q22;q21)[20]. The presence of t(11;22)(q23;q11.2) in all cells was thought to represent a constitutional abnormality. FISH studies performed on the bone marrow were positive for PML/RARA gene rearrangement in 209/220 interphase cells examined (95.0%).

Molecular Analysis PML-RARα fusion transcript from intron 3 or exon breakpoint was detected at a relative expression level of 99.4% compared to the reference cell line RNA. PML-RARα fusion transcript was not detected by quantitative real-time PCR at exon/intron 6 breakpoint regions.

Final Diagnosis Acute promyelocytic leukemia with t(15;17)(q22;q12); PML-RARA.

Management Approach The current standard approach to therapy is with the concomitant administration of targeted terminal granulocytic differentiation therapy with all-trans retinoic acid (ATRA), and anthracycline based chemotherapy. Complete remission can be achieved in 90%-95%

of patients. Patients must be monitored closely for disseminated intravascular coagulation (DIC) as intracerebral and pulmonary hemorrhages can occur prior to and during induction of therapy. This patient initially received idarubicin and ATRA therapy with resolution of his coagulopathy. He achieved remission and remains clinically stable.

General Discussion Acute promyelocytic leukemia (APL) is characterized by the t(15;17)(q22;q21) translocation resulting in the fusion of the promyelocytic leukemia gene (PML) and retinoic acid receptor α (RARα) gene (PML/RARα). The fusion product PML-RARα homodimerizes, binds to DNA and works as a transcriptional repressor which inhibits expression of target genes necessary for granulocytic differentiation. Variant chromosomal translocations, such as t(11;17), t(5;17), can be detected in up to 2% of APL cases. This leukemia accounts for approximately 10%-15% of acute myeloid leukemia cases in the United States. APL is very uncommon in children <10 years of age. The 2 main morphologic types of APL are the classic hypergranular variant, as in this case, comprising the majority of APL cases, and the microgranular or hypogranular variant, comprising approximately 15%-20% of APL cases. Leukopenia is typically seen in association with the hypergranular variant, while leukocytosis is more commonly seen in the microgranular variant. The microgranular subtype is also associated with the short bcr 3-type PML-RARA fusion gene and FLT3 mutations. The leukemic promyelocytes of the hypergranular variant demonstrate nuclear variability with reniform or bilobed nuclei.

Nucleoli are variably prominent. A perinuclear hof, seen in normal promyelocytes, is usually not present in the abnormal promyelocytes of (APL). The cytoplasm is abundant with numerous large azurophilic cytoplasmic granules that can often obscure the nucleus. Blasts can also contain single or bundles of Auer rods (faggot cells). The Auer rods of the hypergranular variant are usually larger than in other types of AML. The microgranular variant blast is smaller with a bilobed or folded nucleus with agranular or finely granular cytoplasm. APL blasts can express bright CD33, variable CD13, CD117 and are largely negative for HLA-DR and CD34 expression. CD56 expression, as in this case, has been associated with a less favorable clinical course. Blasts of the hypogranular variant frequently express HLA-DR as well as CD2, a finding which has been associated with a less favorable prognosis. Very strong myeloperoxidase expression is seen in the abnormal promyelocytes by cytochemistry and by flow cytometry. Sudan black B and chloroacetate esterase are also strongly positive in the blasts of the hypergranular variant. Minimal residual disease (MRD) monitoring can be performed by sequential quantitative reverse transcription polymerase chain reaction (RT-PCR). Relapse can occur in 10%-20% of patients. Patients at high risk for relapse include those with elevated WBC (>10,000/μL) at diagnosis, age over 55 years, expression of CD56 on the blasts, internal tandem duplications of the FLT3 gene mutation as well as the predominance of the PML-RARAbcr3 isoform. Complete remission can be achieved in 90%-95% of patients. Overall survival is approximately 80%.

Acute Myelomonocytic Leukemia

Margaret Kasner, Cecilia Arana Yi

Patient A 56-year-old European-American woman, who was admitted to the hospital because of fatigue, decreased energy and lightheadedness.

Clinical History The patient had been well until 2 weeks earlier when she began to experience symptoms of fatigue, decreased energy, poor appetite and feeling faint. She denied presence of fever, chills, bleeding or easy bruising, chest pain, respiratory or digestive complaints.

Family History Father died of "leukemia." She had 3 brothers and 2 sisters, 1 of whom died from brain cancer at age 63.

Medications None.

Physical Examination She appeared pale and fatigued. Oral examination revealed gingival hypertrophy. She had no petechiae, bruising or adenopathy. There was no palpable splenomegaly.

Initial Work-Up

CBC		WBC Differential	%	# (×10³/µL)
WBC (×10³/µL)	30.4	Neutrophils	39	11.9
RBC (×10⁶/µL)	2.4	Bands	5	1.5
HGB (g/dL)	6.3	Lymphocytes	7	2.1
HCT (%)	19.8	Monocytes	20	6.1
MCV (fL)	83	Eosinophils	1	0.3
MCH (pg)	26.3	Basophils	1	0.3
MCHC (g/dL)	31.8	Metamyelocytes	3	0.9
PLT (×10³/µL)	274	Myelocytes	2	0.6
RDW-CV (%)	16.5	Promyelocytes	1	0.3
MPV (fL)	10.3	Blasts	21	6.4
		Reticulocytes	4.1	

Peripheral blood smear review revealed several blasts, a few immature myeloid cells and monocytes (**Figure 1**).

Section B: Acute Leukemias
Acute Myelomonocytic Leukemia

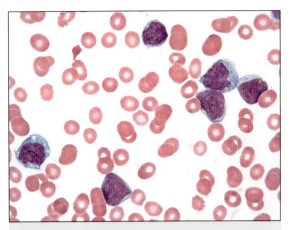

Figure 1 Blood smear (Wright-Giemsa, ×1000) showing 3 blasts, 2 monocytes and a lymphocyte.

Results of chemistry panel were within normal limits	
PT (seconds)	19.7 (normal 11-15)
PTT (seconds)	34 (normal 20-35)
Fibrinogen (mg/dL)	223
D-Dimer (µg/mL)	>20
Iron (µg/dL)	83
IBC (µg/dL)	290
Iron saturation (%)	39
Ferritin (ng/mL)	503
Haptoglobin (mg/dL)	69
LDH (U/L)	616
Folate (ng/mL)	16
Vitamin B_{12} (pg/mL)	286

Differential Diagnosis Acute myeloid leukemia (de novo or evolving from myelodysplastic syndrome or myeloproliferative neoplasm), acute lymphoid leukemia and cellular phase of myelofibrosis. Peripheral blood findings and clinical presentation made acute myeloid leukemia, particularly monocytic and myelomonocytic subtypes more likely.

Additional Work-Up Bone marrow biopsy was hypercellular with granulocytic hyperplasia (**Figure 2**). Many cells appeared large and immature containing irregular nuclei with fine chromatin and some with nucleoli, and moderate amount of cytoplasm. The aspirate smear showed increased number of blasts, immature granulocytes and monocytic cells in proportions consistent with acute myelomonocytic leukemia (**Figure 3**). Occasional dysplastic megakaryocytes and atypical erythroid precursors were also noted. Flow cytometry performed on bone marrow aspirate identified a population of cells that were positive for CD117, CD13, CD33, CD34, CD38, CD52, CD64, and HLA-DR but negative for CD118, CD4 and CD15, a phenotype suggestive of acute myeloid leukemia with myelomonocytic differentiation. Cytogenetics: 47, XX, +8[3]/46, XX[18]. Molecular Studies: negative for RARA gene rearrangement, BCR/ABL1, AML1/ETO, FLT3 receptor, and FLT 3 ITD and positive for nucleophosmin.

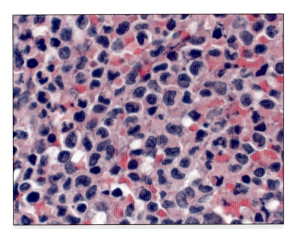

Figure 2 Bone marrow biopsy (H&E, ×500) showing hypercellular marrow with immature myeloid and monocytoid cells including some blasts.

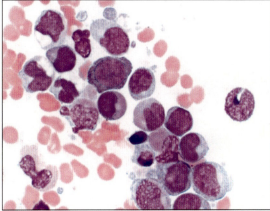

Figure 3 Bone marrow aspirate smear (Wright-Giemsa, ×1000) showing blasts, other immature myeloid cells and monocytes.

Final Diagnosis Acute myelomonocytic leukemia (AML-M4).

Management Approach Standard treatment of acute myeloid leukemia, including acute myelomonocytic subtype, consists of induction therapy with high-dose cytarabine and an anthracycline. This is followed by consolidation therapy using various doses and sequences of similar agents with or without stem cell transplantation. This patient was treated with idarubicin and cytarabine. Bone marrow at day 14+ showed aplasia and no evidence of residual or recurrent leukemia. Repeated bone marrow at 45 days showed hyperplastic bone marrow with no evidence of acute leukemia. Patient was thought to be in complete remission. Therefore standard consolidation therapy with high-dose cytarabine was initiated. She was also evaluated for potential hematopoietic stem cell transplant, which would be considered if she relapses in the future.

General Discussion Acute myelomonocytic leukemia, (AMML or AML-M4) is defined by the presence in the blood and/or marrow of myeloblasts, monoblasts and promonocytes that together make up 20%-79% of all nucleated cells. The monocytic lineage must be confirmed by immunophenotyping (CD64, CD14, CD11b, CD11c, etc) and/or cytochemical stains (nonspecific esterase). The myeloid markers such as CD13 and CD33 and myeloperoxidase, sudan black, and specific esterase) will help confirm the granulocytic lineage if so needed. The sum of granulocytic cells at various stages of maturation including blasts is also usually 20% or greater. If the monocytic population exceeds 80% of the marrow nucleated cells, the diagnosis of acute monocytic or monoblastic is entertained. If monocytes make-up <20% of marrow cells, the diagnosis of AMML can still be made if the peripheral blood monocyte count equals or exceeds $5 \times 10^3/\mu L$. Auer rods may be present in some cells in some cases. There are no defining cytogenetic characteristics; however, some cases that are associated with inv(16) present favorable prognosis. Typical laboratory findings include normocytic normochromic anemia, thrombocytopenia and leukocytosis. Patients often present with extramedullary disease including gingival hypertrophy, leukemia cutis and meningeal leukemia. This subtype is common in older patients (median age 50 years). Prognosis in acute myelomonocytic leukemia is variable. The presence of nucleophosmin mutation and the absence of FLT 3-ITD and FLT 3 receptor mutation are associated with good prognosis.

Acute Myeloid Leukemia with Myelodysplasia-Related Changes

Brian R Smith, Tal Oren, Christopher A Tormey

Patient A 70-year-old man with 1-month history of weakness, fatigue, and lethargy.

Clinical History Past medical history is significant for smoking (20 packs a year but quit 42 years ago), alcohol abuse, hypertension, and macrocytic anemia. The patient denied significant nausea, vomiting, chills, night sweats, or significant recent weight loss.

Family History Noncontributory.

Medications Amlodipine, atenolol, clonidine, hydrochlorothiazide, losartan.

Physical Examination An elderly man appearing pale and fatigued, but otherwise in no apparent distress. There were no abnormal findings. Temperature 97.6°F, blood pressure 143/97, pulse 87 and respiratory rate of 25. His SpO_2 was 99% on room air.

Initial Work-Up

CBC	
WBC (×10^3/μL)	4.4
RBC (×10^6/μL)	0.95
HGB (g/dL)	3.6
HCT (%)	10.5
MCV (fL)	110
MCH (pg)	37.7
MCHC (g/dL)	34.3
PLT (×10^3/μL)	25
MPV (fL)	9.1

WBC Differential	%	# (×10^3/μL)
Neutrophils	60	2.6
Lymphocytes	25	1.1
Monocytes	10	0.4
Eosinophils	1	0.0
Basophils	0	
Blasts	3	0.1

Peripheral blood smear revealed dysplastic neutrophils and occasional blasts (**Figure 1**).

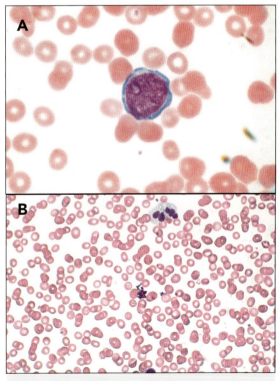

Figure 1 Blood smear **A** (Wright-Giemsa, ×1000) showing a large, agranular, circulating blast with 1 prominent nucleolus; **B** (Wright-Giemsa, ×400) showing a hypogranular neutrophil.

Section B: Acute Leukemias
Acute Myeloid Leukemia with Myelodysplasia-Related Changes

Differential Diagnosis Diagnostic considerations included myelodysplastic syndrome and acute leukemia (myeloid, lymphoid, mixed lineage).

Additional Work-Up
- Direct Coombs test: negative
- Lactate dehydrogenase (U/L): 181 (normal 125-250)
- Vitamin B_{12} (pg/mL): 1,516 (normal 200-900)
- Reticulocyte count (%): 2.5 (normal 0.5-2.0)

Bone marrow was hypercellular (**Figure 2**) and revealed atypical megakaryocytosis (**Figure 3**), immature dysplastic granulocytes and blasts (**Figure 4**). The erythroid precursors were markedly reduced in number. Immunophenotyping by flow cytometry on marrow aspirate identified a population of cells that had intermediate forward scatter and low side scatter and were CD45dim+, myeloperoxidase +, CD13+, CD33+, CD64+, CD14subset+, and CD11b+. HLA-DR was uniformly negative in this population. A subset of these cells were CD34+ CD117+. Rapid PCR-based screen for recurrent AML translocations [t(9;22), t(15;17), t(8;21), and inv16] was negative for all these genetic abnormalities.

Conventional karyotype 45, XY, –5 –11 –12, add(17)(p11.2), –22, +3mar [13]/46, XY [2].

FISH nuc ish (MLL × 7-10) [193/200/ish 3 mar (MLL+)].

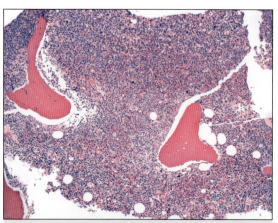

Figure 2 Bone marrow biopsy (H&E, ×100) demonstrating hypercellularity, increased immature elements, and atypical megakaryocytes.

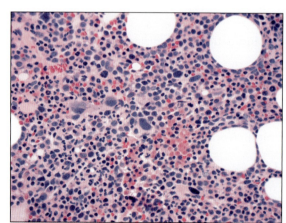

Figure 3 Bone marrow biopsy (H&E, ×400) demonstrating increased immature elements and atypical megakaryocytes.

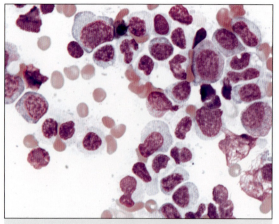

Figure 4 Bone marrow aspirate smear (Wright-Giemsa, ×400) showing blasts and dysplastic myeloid cells.

Final Diagnosis Acute myeloid leukemia with myelodysplasia-related changes (MDS-associated cytogenetic abnormality) including amplification of MLL.

Management Approach Treatment for patients with this form of acute myelogenous leukemia lacks a specific molecular target. Thus, therapies are aimed at cytoreduction, typically using a combination of chemotherapeutic drugs such as an antimetabolite (eg, cytarabine) and an anthracycline (eg, idarubicin). For patients achieving a sustained remission, hematopoietic progenitor cell transplantation (HPCT) is also an option. As a general rule, AML with myelodysplastic features has a poor prognosis.

This patient was treated with induction chemotherapy (idarubicin and cytarabine). The patient's induction course was severely complicated by cytopenias that required substantial red blood cell and platelet transfusion support. The patient also encountered frequent infectious complications. The patient ultimately expired secondary to sepsis and multiorgan failure, attributable to his underlying disease and concomitant chemotherapy.

General Discussion Due to the lack of HLA-DR and the hypogranular, bilobed myeloid elements, a diagnosis of hypogranular acute promyelocytic leukemia was entertained; molecular testing for the t(15;17) translocation was negative, arguing against this possibility. HLA-DR- AML is unusual, but has been described. When the results of the karyotype became available, in conjunction with the morphologic features, a diagnosis of AML with myelodysplasia-related changes was rendered. AML with myelodysplasia-related changes is a heterogeneous category in the 2008 WHO classification that represents approximately 24%-35% of all cases of AML. Initially reserved for cases of AML in which there is multilineage dysplasia or a clear antecedent diagnosis of an MDS (or MDS/MPD), this category has now been expanded in the 2008 WHO category to include cases with a "myelodysplastic syndrome-related cytogenetic abnormality." Accordingly, there are 3 possible reasons for which a case could be assigned to this category, and a given case could meet 1, 2, or all 3 criteria to qualify for inclusion. The 3 reasons are (a) previous history of MDS, (b) an MDS-related cytogenetic abnormality, and (c) multilineage dysplasia. This case demonstrated at least 1 feature that warrants its inclusion in this WHO category. The karyotype contained at least one unbalanced abnormality (monosomy 5) that is sufficient for a diagnosis of AML with myelodysplastic-related changes. The presence of a complex karyotype with at least 3 cytogenetic abnormalities, none of which are within the AML with recurrent genetic abnormalities subgroup, as seen in this case, is also sufficient for inclusion in this category. In addition to the increased number of blasts, there was a significant amount of dysplasia at least in the myeloid lineage, although the observed numbers did not strictly meet the imposed WHO criteria of 50% of cells in a particular lineage. Finally, although an antecedent diagnosis of myelodysplastic syndrome was not technically present in this patient, the clinical history of a sustained macrocytic anemia in the years prior to presentation may be considered consistent with that hypothesis. In the cytogenetic work-up of this patient's bone marrow sample, a FISH probe for the mixed lineage leukemia (MLL) gene demonstrated amplification of this locus on 3 marker chromosomes. This secondary finding should not be confused with the often discussed recurrent genetic *translocations* of MLL, in which the MLL gene is fused to a variety of different partner gene. In the vast majority of these translocation cases, the disease gets recognized as a distinct entity within the broader category of AML with recurrent genetic abnormalities and is classified as such. However, there are 2 prominent exceptions to this rule. Cases with the t(11;16)(q23;p13.3) and t(2;11)(p21;q23) cytogenetic abnormalities, although they do involve the MLL locus, should be classified within the AML with myelodysplasia-related changes category rather than the variant MLL translocations category since these 2 genetic abnormalities are often seen in MDS-related leukemias.

Acute Monoblastic Leukemia

Margaret Kasner, Matthew Brennan, Scott Bourne

Patient A 59-year-old female complaining of generalized weakness and dyspnea on exertion.

Clinical History The patient also complained of blurred vision, diarrhea and a 10-pound weight loss over a few weeks. 2 days prior to presentation she had increasing dizziness with near falls in the shower.

Family History Mother died of an unknown cancer, 3 sisters had breast cancer.

Medications Citalopram, amlodipine, metoprolol, folic acid, nicotine patch, lisinopril, glipizide.

Physical Examination Her oral exam was remarkable for gingival hyperplasia, but no thrush. She had cervical, submandibular, and left axillary lymphadenopathy that was hard, nontender, but mobile. Her cardiac exam was normal but pulmonary exam showed coarse breath sounds, decreased at the bases.

Initial Work-Up

CBC		WBC Differential	%	# ($10^3/\mu L$)
WBC ($\times 10^3/\mu L$)	178.5	Neutrophils	1	1.8
RBC ($\times 10^6/\mu L$)	2.42	Bands	1	1.8
HGB (g/dL)	6.7	Lymphocytes	7	12.5
HCT (%)	20.7	Monocytes	8	14.3
MCV (fL)	86	Eosinophils	2	0.1
MCH (pg)	27.7	Basophils	0	
MCHC (g/dL)	32.4	Metamyelocyte	1	1.8
PLT ($\times 10^3/\mu L$)	84	Myelocyte	1	1.8
RDW-CV (%)	17.4	Blasts	81	144.6

Peripheral blood smear examination revealed many large immature cells with large round or some what folded nuclei, fine chromatin, high N:C ratio and abundant bluish or blue-gray cytoplasm. A majority of these cells were considered to be monoblasts and promonocytes (**Figures 1** and **2**).

Section B: Acute Leukemias
Acute Monoblastic Leukemia

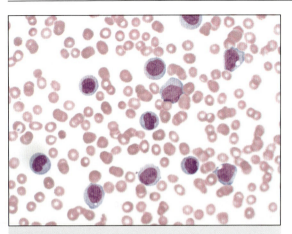

Figure 1 Blood smear (Wright-Giemsa, ×500) showing several monoblasts (round nuclei) and promonocytes (indented, lobated nuclei).

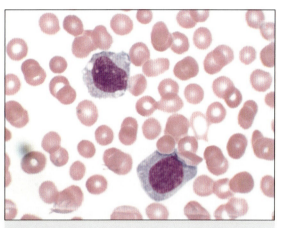

Figure 2 Bone marrow biopsy (H&E, ×200) showing hypercellular marrow with prominent increase in blasts.

Differential Diagnosis Diagnostic considerations based on clinical presentation and peripheral blood findings included acute myeloid leukemia, acute lymphoid leukemia, acute biphenotypic leukemia, and blast crisis of chronic myelogenous leukemia.

Additional Work-Up Bone marrow biopsy was hypercellucellular (90%-95%) and diffusely infiltrated by a population of immature blastic cells (**Figure 3**). The immature blastic cells accounted for >95% of the cells seen in the aspirate smear (**Figure 4**). Some of these cells had irregular indented nuclei as well as cytoplasmic vacuolization, suggestive of monocytic differentiation (**Figure 5**).

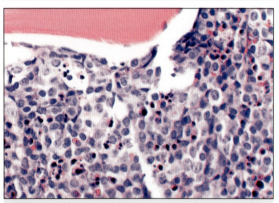

Figure 3 Bone marrow biopsy (H&E, ×400) showing hypercellular marrow with sheets of large, monotonous, monomorphic cells with fine powdery chromatin and inconspicuous nucleoli. The normal bone marrow architecture is completely effaced. Tingible body macrophages with karyorrhetic debris are also seen.

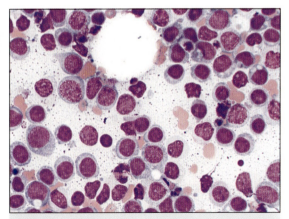

Figure 4 Bone marrow aspirate smear (Wright-Giemsa, ×500) showing diffuse infiltrate of blastoid cells. Normal hematopoeisis is markedly reduced.

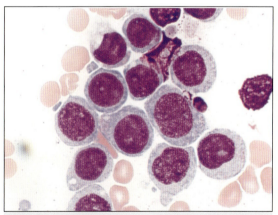

Figure 5 Bone marrow aspirate smear (Wright-Giemsa, ×1000) showing a cluster of blasts (most likely monoblasts).

Section B: Acute Leukemias
Acute Monoblastic Leukemia

Flow Cytometry (Bone Marrow and Blood)
Leukemic cells were CD45+, CD4+, CD64+, CD15+, CD38+, CD56+, HLA-DR+, CD11b±, CD33±, CD56−/+, CD117−/+, CD13−, CD34−, CD52−, MPO−, and TDT−.

FISH Cytogenics (Bone Marrow) t(9;11)(p22;q23) positive but t(9;22)(q34;q11) BCR/ABL1 and t(8;21)(q22;q22) AML1/ETO negative.

Diagnosis Acute monoblastic leukemia.

Management Approach Induction therapy is given to reduce the tumor burden to a level that leukemic cells are no longer detectable in the blood or bone marrow. In patients <60 years old and with no antecedent hematologic disease, induction with 7+3 (7 days continuous infusional cytarabine at 100-200 mg/m^2/d and 3 days of either daunorubicin 60-90 mg/m^2 or idarubicin 12 mg/m^2) is frequently utilized. The addition of etoposide has shown an improved disease-free, but not overall survival advantage. Postremission chemotherapy is given to reduce the residual undetectable leukemic burden to a level compatible with cure. The major options that exist for intermediate risk AML (including t(9;11)) are 3-4 cycles of high-dose cytarabine (HiDAC), high-dose chemotherapy with autologous stem cell rescue, allogeneic transplant from a histocompatible sibling or unrelated donor, or a clinical trial. This patient received standard induction chemotherapy with cytarabine and idarubicin, and a day +32 bone marrow biopsy showed the patient to be in morphologic remission. She then received 1 cycle of high-dose cytarabine consolidation. Prior to further consolidation treatment, she suffered cardiac arrest and died.

General Discussion Acute myeloid leukemia is a clonal expansion of nonlymphoid hematopoietic progenitors. The leukemia suppresses normal hematopoiesis resulting in symptoms secondary to cytopenias. The monocytic subtype of AML may be associated with extramedullary involvement resulting in gingival hyperplasia, pulmonary infiltrates, hepatomegaly, splenomegaly, lymphadenopathy, leukemia cutis, myeloid sarcoma, and CNS involvement. Increased intracranial pressure results in headaches, blurred vision, and vomiting. Acute monocytic leukemia may also be associated with hyperleukocytosis (a blast count can reach over $100 \times 10^3/\mu L$), which in turn leads to leukostasis and thrombosis from inelastic monocytic cells plugging blood vessels, which can then lead to shortness of breath, hypoxia, diffuse pulmonary infiltrates, headache, blurred vision, heart failure, MI, and priapism. Diagnosis of AML is made when at least 20% of nucleated cells in the bone marrow or peripheral blood are myeloid blasts. The diagnosis of acute monoblastic/monocytic leukemia is made when 80% or more of the leukemic cells are of monocytic lineage (monoblasts + promonocytes + monocytes) and a neutrophil component is minor (<20%). In acute monoblastic leukemia, monoblasts predominate, whereas in acute monocytic leukemia, promonocytes and monocytes predominate. Cells of monocytic lineage usually display nonspecific esterase (NSE) activity and may show some scattered myeloperoxidase (MPO) activity. By flow cytometry, there is variable expression of CD13, CD33, and CD117. CD4, CD14, CD11b, CD11c, CD36. CD64, CD68 and/or lysozyme may be expressed, while CD34 is often negative. FISH can be used to evaluate for 11q23 mutations, which involves the myeloid/lymphoid or mixed-lineage leukemia (MLL) gene, including t(9;11)(p22;q23). MLL gene aberrations are associated with both de novo and therapy-related AML secondary to topoisomerase inhibitors, occurring 1 year to 3 years post exposure. AML with MLL abnormalities often have monocytic features, are often diagnosed with soft tissue infiltration, and have a poorer prognosis than other cytogenetic types of AML.

Acute Myeloid Leukemia, with inv(3)

Raymond E Felgar, Milon Amin

Patient A 61-year-old female, who presented with low-grade fevers and a 1-day history of abdominal pain.

Clinical History The patient had recently developed an upper respiratory infection. She also had a history of hypertension and hypothyroidism.

Family History One brother with diabetes.

Medications Felodipine, simvastatin, levothyroxine, and furosemide.

Physical Examination No lymphadenopathy or splenomegaly noted on physical examination. No petechiae or ecchymoses are noted. Liver enzymes, amylase, and lipase levels were within normal ranges. Computed tomography scan of the abdomen and chest X-ray were unremarkable.

Initial Work-Up

CBC

WBC (×10³/µL)	27.1
RBC (×10⁶/µL)	3.67
HGB (g/dL)	10.0
HCT (%)	29.7
MCV (fL)	80.8
MCH (pg)	27.3
MCHC (g/dL)	33.8
PLT (×10³/µL)	189
RDW-CV (%)	22.7

WBC Differential	%	# (10³/µL)
Neutrophils	4	1.1
Bands	5	1.4
Lymphocytes	18	4.9
Monocytes	11	3.0
Eosinophils	1	0.3
Basophils	0	
Metamyelocytes	2	0.5
Blasts	59	16.0

Peripheral blood smear revealed many blast cells (**Figure 1**).

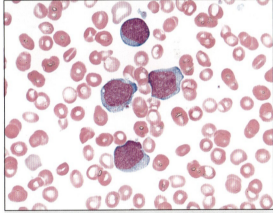

Figure 1 Blood smear (Wright-Giemsa, ×1000) showing several blasts.

Differential Diagnosis Although an infectious process could be considered, the elevated blast count in the peripheral blood smear would be unusual and indicates a leukemic process. The differential diagnosis based on blood smear examination includes acute myeloid leukemia, blastic transformation of chronic myelogenous leukemia, and (less likely) acute lymphoblastic leukemia.

Additional Work-Up Blood cultures were negative. Bone marrow aspirate smear showed 74% blasts on the manual differential count. Small, monolobate and apparently dysplastic megakaryocytic forms were also noted (**Figures 2** and **3**), which prompted the addition of CD41a (platelet glycoprotein IIb/IIIa) and CD61 (platelet glycoprotein IIIa) markers to the flow cytometric analysis of the bone marrow aspirate. In addition, immunohistochemistry staining for CD61 and CD34 was performed on the bone marrow biopsy (**Figures 4** and **5**). Flow cytometric immunophenotypic studies performed on the aspirate showed an abnormal myeloblast population (approximately 60% of all cells by CD34 staining). The blasts were positive for CD34, CD13, CD33, CD117, and HLA-DR, with a subset was positive for CD15. The blasts showed dim expression of CD45 and CD4, and were negative for CD8, CD7, CD56, TdT, MPO, and cytoplasmic CD3. Specific gating on the CD34+ population alone showed that approximately 7% of the blasts may also be positive for CD41a and/or CD61; however, the pattern of CD41a and CD61 staining was heterogeneous, such that the possibility of platelet satellitism (giving falsely positive staining) could not be entirely excluded. Immunohistochemical stains on biopsy showed that the blasts were positive for CD117 (c-kit). 50%-60% of blasts were positive for CD34 and 20% were positive for myeloperoxidase. An immunostain for CD61 highlighted abnormal megakaryocytes, but did not show definitive staining of blasts. Cytogenetic evaluation demonstrated a mosaic karyotype with an abnormal clone with the following karyotype: 45, XX, inv(3)(q21q26), del(5)(q13q33), –7, del(11)(p11.2p15), –17, add(21)(q22), add(22)(q13.3), +mar[19] (**Figure 6**).

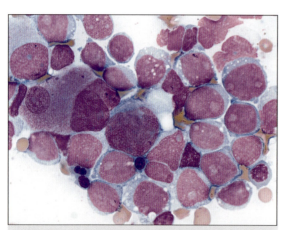

Figure 2 Bone marrow aspirate smear (Wright Giemsa, ×1000) showing blasts and a dysplastic megakaryocyte.

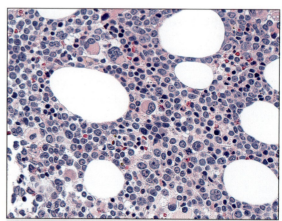

Figure 3 Bone marrow biopsy (H&E, ×400) showing many blasts.

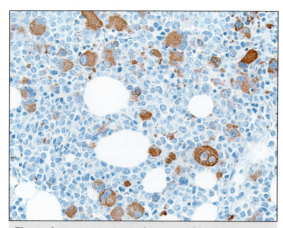

Figure 4 Bone marrow biopsy (CD61, ×400) highlighting megakaryocytes.

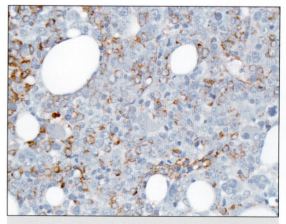

Figure 5 Bone marrow biopsy (CD34, ×400) highlighting blasts.

Section B: Acute Leukemias
Acute Myeloid Leukemia, with inv(3)

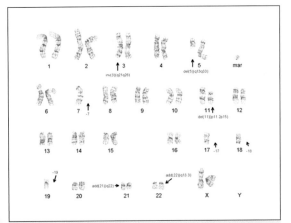

Figure 6 Karyotype: showing inv(3) in addition to several additional cytogenetic abnormalities (see text) [note: missing chromosomes 18 and 19 are a result of random loss in this cell].

Final Diagnosis Acute myeloid leukemia with inv(3)(q21q26).

Management Approach The current therapeutic approach is chemotherapy, followed by hematopoietic progenitor cell transplantation (HPCT). Data on treatment outcomes with specific chemotherapeutic regimens for this subtype of AML are quite limited. Possible chemotherapy agents include those for other subtypes of acute myeloid leukemia (AML), including anthracyclines (daunorubicin or idarubicin) and cytarabine. 2 patients have had documented response to a combination of thalidomide and arsenic trioxide. This patient was treated with 3 re-induction regimens to achieve a remission, followed by consolidative chemotherapy. She then underwent a peripheral blood, allogeneic HPCT approximately 4 months after initial diagnosis. At day 30, post-allogeneic HPCT, a marrow evaluation showed recurrent AML with 24% blasts in the bone marrow. She was then discharged to home hospice care.

General Discussion AML with inv(3)(q21q26) is a specifically recognized subtype of AML with recurrent cytogenetic abnormalities in the 2008 World Health Organization classification of hematogic malignancy. These cases show somewhat characteristic morphologic and cytogenetic findings and an adverse clinical prognosis. Cases with t(3;3)(q21;q26.2) are also included within this category. The critically affected genes involve disruptions in the RPN and EVI1 genetic loci. AML with inv(3)(q21q26) or t(3;3)(q21;q26.2); *RPN1-EVI1* represents 1%-2% of all AML cases. It is most commonly found in adults, with no gender predilection. This form of AML may be associated with normal or increased platelet counts. Atypical, dysplastic megakaryocytes, especially small, monolobate forms, are often present, with associated multilineage dysplasia. It often shows overlapping morphologic features with acute megakaryoblastic leukemia (AML-M7), but does not generally have a distinct megakaryoblast population. This form of AML lacks a specific set of immunophenotypic features: blast cells are typically positive for CD13, CD33, HLA-DR, CD34 and CD38. Aberrant expression of CD7, CD41 and CD61 may occur in some cases, but this is found only in a subset of the blast population. Common secondary cytogenetic abnormalities associated with AML with inv(3)(q21q26) include a complex karyotype, del(5q) and monosomy 7 (seen in 50% of patients), all of which were identified in this particular case. It is believed that the critical oncogenes involved in the pathogenesis of this AML subtype are *EVI1* and *RPN*, located on 3q26.2 and 3q21, respectively. It is postulated that abnormalities in chromosome 3 cause *RPN1* to enhance *EVI1* expression, which causes increased cell proliferation with impaired differentiation. This is in contrast to leukemias harboring the t(3;21)(q26.2;q22) abnormality, which is typically found in therapy-related AML. Patients previously diagnosed with AML may acquire an inv(3)(q21q26.2) or t(3;3)(q21;q26.2), which may indicate accelerated or aggressive blast phases of their clinical courses. In a study of 18 patients, 15 died within 10 months of diagnosis. 3 of 3 patients suffered early relapses, despite both bone marrow transplantation and aggressive chemotherapy. Ultimately, this form of AML carries a poor prognosis and a shorter survival.

Acute Megakaryoblastic Leukemia

Margaret Kasner, Ajay Kandra

Patient An 81-year-old female, who presented to the hospital with fatigue and dyspnea.

Clinical History The patient was treated 3 years earlier with melphalan and prednisone for IgG λ myeloma. Upon relapse 18 months prior, she was treated with lenalidomide and dexamethasone. She has been in remission from her myeloma for the past 12 months, but has had persistent anemia. Evaluation 8 months prior including bone marrow aspirations showed no evidence of myeloma but she did have findings consistent with myelodysplastic syndrome. She has had intermittent transfusions since that time. She also has a history of hypertension, diabetes and DVT.

Medications Lenalidomide, aldactone, hydrochlorothiazide, mirtazapine, warfarin, and valacyclovir.

Family History Unremarkable.

Physical Examination Appeared fatigued but in no real distress. Her exam in general was unremarkable. In particular, she had no adenopathy, splenomegaly, rashes or petechiae.

Initial Work-Up

CBC		WBC Differential	%	# ($\times 10^3/\mu L$)
WBC ($\times 10^3/\mu L$)	7.5	Neutrophils	49	3.7
RBC ($\times 10^6/\mu L$)	3.44	Bands	7	0.5
HGB (g/dL)	9.8	Lymphocytes	22	1.7
HCT (%)	30.8	Monocytes	6	0.5
MCV (fL)	90.0	Eosinophils	0	
MCH (pg)	28.5	Basophils	0	
MCHC (g/dL)	31.8	Metamyelocytes	2	0.1
PLT ($\times 10^3/\mu L$)	519	Myelocytes	2	0.1
RDW-CV (%)	19.2	Blasts	12	0.9

*Peripheral blood smear revealed several blasts, a few other immature myeloid cells and occasional giant platelets. Blasts were characterized by medium to large size, fine chromatin, one or more nucleoli, small amount of basophilic cytoplasm with blebbing and/or pseudopod formation, and high N:C ratio (**Figure 1**).*

Section B: Acute Leukemias
Acute Megakaryoblastic Leukemia

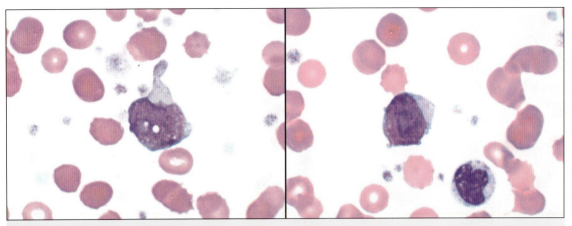

Figure 1 Blood smear (Wright-Giemsa, ×1000) showing 2 blasts, 1 with cytoplasmic blebs and 1 with pseudopod. A giant platelet is also present.

Differential Diagnosis Myeloproliferative disorder, myelodysplastic syndrome, acute myeloid leukemia, recurrent/relapsed myeloma.

Additional Work-Up (Bone Marrow Biopsy) The overall cellularity was increased (60%-70%) with increased number of megakaryocytic cells. Normal hematopoietic elements were significantly decreased. The storage iron was markedly increased. The aspirate smear revealed left-shifted megakaryocytopoiesis and some dysplastic megakaryocytes (**Figure 2**). By immunohistochemistry, the blast cells, which accounted for nearly 60% of marrow cells, stained weakly with CD34 and strongly with CD61. Cytogenetic analysis of bone marrow demonstrated a normal female karyotype in all cells analyzed. Flow cytometry of bone marrow identified an atypical population of CD45–negative megakaryoblasts, which constituted 89% of all analyzed cells (90% of the non-erythroid cells) and had the following antigenic pattern: CD61+, CD34–/+, CD38–/+ (**Figure 3**).

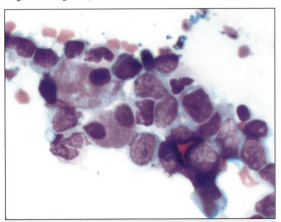

Figure 2 Bone marrow aspirate smear (Wright-Giemsa, ×1000) showing blasts and dysplastic megakaryocytes.

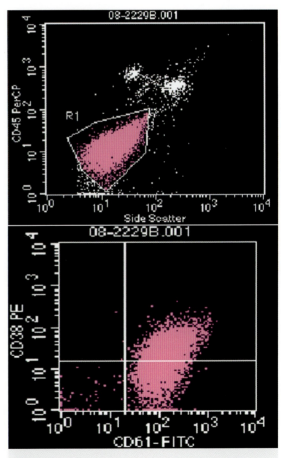

Figure 3 Flow cytograms showing nearly entire gated blast population expressing CD61 with a subset expressing both CD38 and CD61.

Section B: Acute Leukemias
Acute Megakaryoblastic Leukemia

Final Diagnosis Acute megakaryoblastic leukemia (AML-M7).

Management Approach Treatment of acute megakaryoblastic leukemia (AMKL) has been similar to other sub types of AML, using contemporary induction regimens containing anthracycline and cytarabine. Eligible patients should be considered for allogeneic stem cell transplantation. Clinical experience with AMKL has been rather limited. This patient was started on azacitidine (DNA hypomethylation agent) in consideration of her age. She received azacytidine 75 mg/m^2 daily for 5 days every 4 weeks. She was treated with hydroxyurea in between cycles to keep her platelet counts under control. She went on to receive about 5 cycles of treatment with azacitidine. After the 5th cycle she developed febrile neutropenia requiring hospitalization. She eventually succumbed to septic shock from MRSA. A peripheral blood flow cytometry few days prior to her death did not reveal any evidence of leukemia.

General Discussion Acute megakaryoblastic leukemia (AMKL) is a rare subtype of acute myelogenous leukemia (AML), which is also known as AML-M7. It has a bimodal age distribution with one peak in early childhood (age <3 years) and another peak in the middle-aged adults. It accounts for up to 15% of childhood AML and up to 5% of newly diagnosed adult AML. In children, it is frequently seen in association with cytogenetic abnormalities, t(1;22)(p13; q13) or numeric abnormalities of chromosome 21, especially trisomy 21. In adults it has been associated with variable and complex (multiple) cytogenetics. It has been found to be the most common form of AML in children with Down syndrome, and its prognosis is excellent in this group of patients. AMKL can arise de novo or as a secondary malignancy. Idiopathic myelofibrosis or essential thrombocythemia may sometimes progress to AMKL. The prognosis in children without Down syndrome or in adults is poor. Patients usually present with cytopenias, particularly thrombocytopenia. However, some cases may present with thrombocytosis, as in this case, and/or leucocytosis and/or circulating blasts. Dysplastic features may be present in one or more cell lineages in the blood and/or marrow. An increased numbers of large and atypical platelets may be seen due to shedding of the megakaryoblast cytoplasmic blebs. Lymphadenopathy and hepatosplenomegaly are uncommon. AMKL may be underestimated or misdiagnosed as there is a difficulty of obtaining ("dry tap") and interpreting bone marrow specimens. Megakaryoblasts represent the prominent or the dominant leukemic cell population. Marrow fibrosis, as demonstrated by reticulin stain, is frequently present but is not an invariant finding. The diagnosis of AMKL is based on presence 20% or more blasts of which 50% or more are of megakaryocytic lineage. The latter is confirmed by immunophenotyping using antibodies against glycoprotein (GP) IIb/IIIa (CD41a), von Willebrand factor, (vWF), GP Ib (CD42), and/or GP IIIa (CD61). Other less often used methodologies include detection of cytoplasmic factor VIII expression, and electron microscopy demonstration of platelet peroxidase (PPO) activity. Leukocyte common antigen (CD45) is negative.

Therapy-Related Acute Myeloid Leukemia

John Anastasi

Patient A 58-year-old male, who presented with fatigue and nose bleeds.

Clinical History The patient had a history of non-small cell lung cancer diagnosed 2 years prior to the current presentation. The lung cancer was treated with radiation therapy, VP-16 (a topoisomerase II inhibitor) and daunorubicin, and the patient apparently did well. However, the patient now presents with pancytopenia.

Family History There is no pertinent family history.

Medications No current medications (see above for past therapies).

Physical Examination Unremarkable.

Initial Work-Up

CBC	
WBC (×10³/μL)	4.3
RBC (×10⁶/μL)	2.90
HGB (g/dL)	8.6
HCT (%)	25.6
MCV (fL)	88.3
MCH (pg)	29.7
MCHC (g/dL)	33.6
PLT (×10³/μL)	25
RDW-CV (%)	14.9

WBC Differential	%	# (×10³/μL)
Neutrophils	2	0.1
Bands	2	0.1
Lymphocytes	49	2.1
Monocytes	23	1.0
Eosinophils	0	
Basophils	0	
Myelocytes	1	0.0
Blasts	23	1.0

Peripheral blood smear revealed blasts and increased number of monocytes, some of which were immature (**Figure 1**).

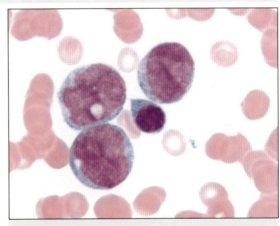

Figure 1 Blood smear (Wright, ×1000) showing blasts with nuclear folding, and moderately abundant cytoplasm characteristic of monoblasts.

Differential Diagnosis Diagnostic considerations based on peripheral blood findings of pancytopenia (neutropenia, anemia, and thrombocytopenia), circulating blasts, and monocytosis included therapy-related MDS/AML (probably with 11q23 involvement) and other causes of marrow failure including metastatic tumor.

Section B: Acute Leukemias
Therapy-Related Acute Myeloid Leukemia

Additional Work-Up Bone marrow examination revealed extensive replacement of normal marrow elements by blasts (**Figure 2**) similar to those seen in the blood. The blasts had large nuclei, fine chromatin, variable nucleoli, some nuclear folding and abundant cytoplasm (**Figure 3**). Phagocytic activity by blasts noted on the Wright-stained aspirate smear (**Figure 4**) and their positivity with α-naphthyl acetate (ANA) esterase stain (**Figure 5**) were indicative of monocytic differentiation.

Flow Cytometry Acute Leukemia Panel Blasts from the marrow aspirate were shown to be CD34–, DR+, CD33+, CD15+, CD13 weak+, CD11b partially +, CD56+, CD4+, CD14–.

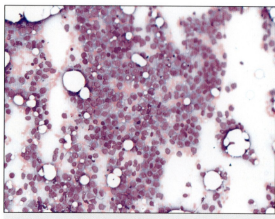

Figure 2 Bone marrow aspirate smear (Wright, ×400) showing extensive replacement of normal marrow elements by blasts.

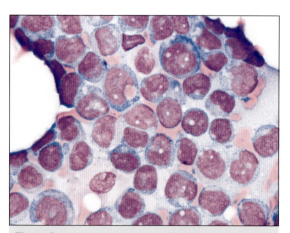

Figure 3 Bone marrow aspirate smear (Wright, ×1000) showing many blasts with feature of monoblasts (slight nuclear folding).

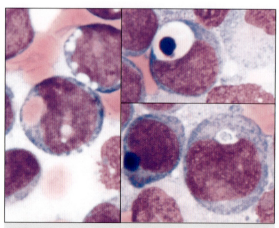

Figure 4 Bone marrow aspirate smear (Wright, ×1000) showing blasts engulfing erythrocytes, nucleated red cell precursors, and platelets.

Cytogenetic Analysis Karyotype 46XY, t(8;16)(p11;p13)[20].

Diagnosis Therapy-related acute myeloid leukemia with monoblastic features, hemophagocytic activity and associated t(8;16)(p11;p13).

Management Approach Patients with therapy-related acute myeloid leukemia (t-AML) generally undergo the same induction chemotherapy as patients with de novo AML, including an anthracycline (idarubicin or daunorubicin) and cytarabine. However, these patients often do not achieve remission—or if they do achieve remission, relapse within a short time. It is therefore reasonable that all eligible patients be evaluated for (1) enrollment in clinical trials of induction therapy

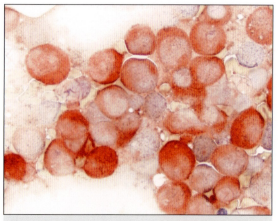

Figure 5 Bone marrow aspirate smear (nonspecific α-naphthyl acetate [ANA] esterase, ×1000) showing positive reaction in most cells.

and (2) allogeneic hematopoietic progenitor cell transplantation (HPCT) as part of consolidation therapy. This patient was treated with on an investigational treatment protocol for patients with therapy-related acute myeloid leukemia. He had a prolonged course of pancytopenia requiring multiple packed red blood cell and platelet transfusions. Although his marrow eventually was cleared of the leukemia, and his counts improved, he relapsed 7 months after the initial diagnosis. He died from respiratory failure and pulmonary hemorrhage without receiving further treatment of his t-AML.

General Discussion The initial impression was that the patient had developed a therapy-related AML (t-AML) that had features of acute monoblastic leukemia, so it was speculated in the bone marrow report that the case might have an abnormality involving chromosome 11q23 (MLL). Translocations involving 11q23 after topoisomerase II inhibitor therapy are common [t(9;11)(p21;q23) being most frequent], and are typically seen a year or so after the initial treatment. They also are associated with leukemias that have monocytic differentiation. However, the cytogenetic studies showed no 11q23 abnormality but revealed t(8;16)(p11;p13). This translocation is rare but has also been reported after topoisomerase II inhibitor therapy in t-AML. It involves the MOZ gene on chromosome 8 and the CBP gene on chromosome 16. The translocation has been noted to be associated with hemophagocytic activity of the leukemic monocytic blasts. Review of the aspirate revealed the expected findings (**Figures 3** and **5**). The neoplastic monocytes are seen ingesting erythrocytes, nucleated red cells and sometimes platelets. t-AML with t(8;16) can have features of monoblastic or myelomonocytic leukemias and the phagocytic activity can sometimes be seen in the blood as well as in the aspirate. The phagocytosis may not be entirely diagnostic as it can be seen in other leukemias and may sometimes be difficult to see in this entity. Cytogenetic analysis is crucial in making the diagnosis of this specific leukemia. t-AML routinely carries a poor prognosis and patients should be offered therapy on investigational studies if available. Although many patients will respond to induction therapy, long-term survival is poor. Consolidation therapy in first remission may include investigational allogeneic transplant options for eligible patients as well.

Acute Myeloid Leukemia, Acute Panmyelosis with Myelofibrosis Subtype

M James You, Carlos Bueso-Ramos

Patient A 66-year-old man, who sought care because of progressive fatigue, weakness, bone pain and fever for approximately 3 months prior to his check-up.

Clinical History The patient was found to be anemic and received a short trial of Procrit without much of an improvement in his blood counts.

Family History Noncontributory.

Medications Simvastatin.

Physical Examination Minimal splenomegaly was identified. There was no palpable liver.

Initial Work-Up		
CBC		
WBC (×10^3/μL)	3.2	
RBC (×10^6/μL)	3.13	
HGB (g/dL)	9.3	
HCT (%)	27.8	
MCV (fL)	89	
MCHC (g/dL)	33.5	
PLT (×10^3/μL)	38	
RDW-CV (%)	15.2	
MPV (fL)	9.8	
WBC Differential	**%**	**# (×10^3/μL)**
Neutrophils	58	1.9
Bands	5	0.2
Lymphocytes	31	1.0
Monocytes	3	0.1
Eosinophils	1	0.0
Blasts	1	0.0

*Peripheral blood smear revealed dysplastic granulocytes and occasional blasts (**Figure 1**).*

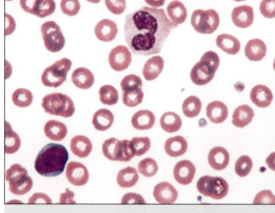

Figure 1 Blood smear (Wright, ×1000) showing a dysplastic neutrophil and a blast. Note minimal erythrocyte poikilocytosis and absence of teardrop cells

Differential Diagnosis Diagnostic considerations included myelodysplastic syndrome, including refractory anemia with excess of blasts in transformation and acute myeloid leukemia.

Additional Work-Up Bone marrow biopsy was hypercellular (80%) and showed increased number of megakaryocytes, many of which were dysplastic. Fibrosis and increased immature cells were also noted (**Figures 2** and **3**). Reticulin stain demonstrated marked fibrosis, 3+ on a 0-3 scale (**Figure 4**). There was no significant collagen fibrosis. Immunohistochemical staining showed increased CD34+ immature cells (**Figure 5**) and CD61 highlighted increased megakaryocytes with hypolobation (**Figure 6**). Bone marrow aspirate smears were suboptimal, showing rare particles. Bone

Section B: Acute Leukemias
Acute Myeloid Leukemia, Acute Panmyelosis with Myelofibrosis Subtype

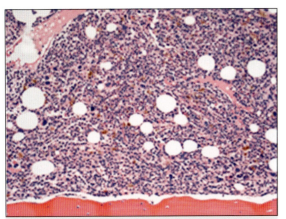

Figure 2 Bone marrow biopsy (H&E, ×100) showing hypercellularity.

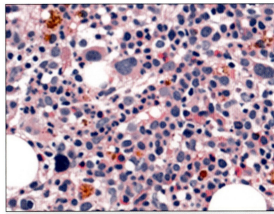

Figure 3 Bone marrow biopsy (H&E, ×400) showing hypercellularity.

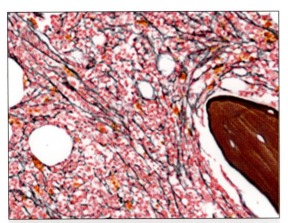

Figure 4 Bone marrow biopsy (reticulin stain, ×400) showing markedly increased reticulin fibrosis.

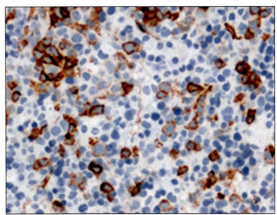

Figure 5 Bone marrow biopsy (CD34, ×400) showing CD34+ blasts.

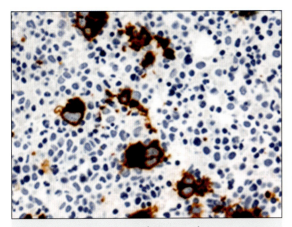

Figure 6 Bone marrow biopsy (CD61, ×400) showing CD61+ megakaryocytes.

marrow touch preparations revealed increased number of blasts (24%), atypical hypolobated megakaryocytes, and left-shifted dysplastic granulocytes (**Figure 7**). Flow cytometric analysis of the bone marrow aspirate demonstrated a population of blasts, positive for CD34, CD117, HLA-DR, CD13, CD33, CD38 and MPO (subset). The blasts were negative for CD10, TdT, and B- and T-cell markers. Cytogenetic studies demonstrated a complex karyotype, 44-49, XY, del(2)(p15p23), add(11)(q25), −12, add(12)(p13), −17, −18, +19, +21, +22, +1-6mar[cp18].

Section B: Acute Leukemias
Acute Myeloid Leukemia, Acute Panmyelosis with Myelofibrosis Subtype

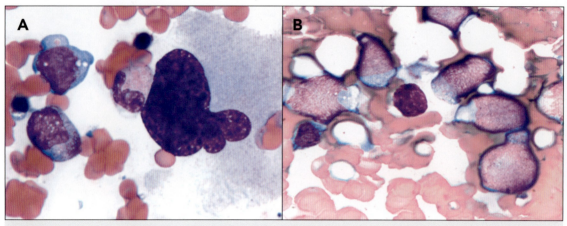

Figure 7 Bone marrow aspirate smear (Wright-Giemsa, ×1000) **A** showing atypical megakaryocytes, dysplastic granulocytes and a blast, and **B** showing increased blasts.

Final Diagnosis Acute myeloid leukemia, acute panmyelosis with myelofibrosis subtype.

Management Approach Treatment of acute panmyelosis with myelofibrosis may include supportive care with blood and platelet transfusion, corticosteroids, chemotherapy, imatinib, bone marrow transplant, and splenectomy for symptoms associated with splenomegaly. This patient received induction chemotherapy on an investigational study using idarubicin, cytarabine, and sorafenib but the disease was persistent. Subsequently, the patient underwent bone marrow transplant, and has been well.

General Discussion Acute panmyelosis with myelofibrosis is a rare subtype of acute myeloid leukemia, not otherwise specified. It is characterized by pancytopenia with minimal poikilocytosis and absence of dacrocytes (teardrop erythrocytes). There is no or minimal organomegaly. The bone marrow aspirate smears are frequently suboptimal, hypocellular due to marrow fibrosis. The blasts are 20% or more of all the bone marrow cells but are difficult to quantify accurately due to the poor quality of the aspirate smears. Touch imprints may help in identifying foci of blasts. It is important to indicate in the diagnosis that this is a subtype of acute myeloid leukemia for purposes of clinical management. Finally, morphologic distinction between acute panmyelosis with myelofibrosis, high-grade myelodysplastic syndrome, acute megakaryocytic leukemia, acute myeloid leukemia with myelodysplasia-related changes and myelofibrosis may be difficult. Acute megakaryoblastic leukemia exhibits at least 20% blasts, at least 50% of the blasts are megakaryoblasts. In contrast, blasts in acute panmyelosis with myelofibrosis are more heterogenous and typically express CD34, as shown in this case. Distinction between acute panmyelosis with myelofibrosis and acute myeloid leukemia with myelodysplasia-related changes and myelofibrosis can be very challenging. Acute panmyelosis with myelofibrosis presents with more abundant atypical megakaryocytes, and proliferation of granulocytic and erythroid cells. Clinically, acute panmyelosis with myelofibrosis shows a more abrupt onset and ominous course. The presence of marked trilineage dysplasia and cytogenetic findings of del(5q) and/or del(7q) favors acute myeloid leukemia with myelodysplasia-related changes and myelofibrosis. Younger patients should be treated aggressively with induction therapy followed by consolidation therapy. If an eligible donor can be found, allogeneic hematopoietic progenitor cell transplantation may be offered as the only therapy to provide the potential for long-term disease-free survival.

Blastic Plasmacytoid Dendritic Cell Neoplasm

Tahseen Al-Saleem, Hossein Borghaei, Valentin G Robu

Patient A 55-year-old male, who presented with erythematous to violaceous skin lesions.

Clinical History The first skin lesion appeared 6 months prior on his upper arm. Currently they are increased in number and involve his face and back. He also complained of increasing fatigue and night sweats for the past few weeks.

Family History Not significant for any cancers.

Medications Esomeprazole, naproxen, aspirin, lisinopril.

Physical Examination He was afebrile and in no apparent distress. The skin examination revealed numerous erythematous to violaceous 3 cm-4 cm domed nodules involving the upper arm, face and back. There was no lymphadenopathy or organomegaly present.

Initial Work-Up The results of all laboratory investigations, including CBC with differential, were within normal limits. CT scans showed no lymphadenopathy or hepatosplenomegaly. Sections of a skin biopsy showed an infiltrate of primitive hematopoietic cells arranged as nodular aggregates in the entire dermis and extending into the subcutaneous fat (**Figure1A**). The epidermis was spared. The malignant cells had a monotonous, blast-like appearance (**Figure1B**) and were medium size with scant agranular blue-gray cytoplasm, irregular nuclei with fine chromatin and 1 or several small nucleoli.

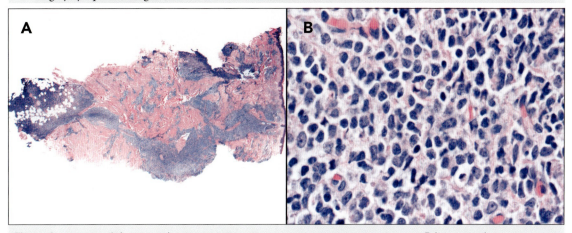

Figure 1 Skin biopsy **A** (H&E, ×100) showing a diffuse infiltrate in the dermis with epidermal sparing; **B** (H&E ×1000) showing intermediate-sized neoplastic cells with irregular nuclei, fine chromatin, and scant cytoplasm.

Differential Diagnosis Based on morphologic features, the usual differential diagnosis would include benign nodules/aggregates of plasmacytoid dendritic cells, cutaneous T-cell lymphoma, nasal-type NK-cell lymphoma and leukemia cutis.

Section B: Acute Leukemias
Blastic Plasmacytoid Dendritic Cell Neoplasm

Additional Work-Up By immunohistochemical stains, the tumor cells stained diffusely positive for CD56 (**Figure 2A**), CD4 (**Figure 2B**), CD43, CD123 and TCL-1, the findings consistent with a blastic plasmacytoid dendritic cell neoplasm (BPDCN). Many cells stained for CD68 (with a dot-like pattern) and TdT (approximately 60% cells positive). They were negative for CD3, CD7, CD20, CD34, CD117, TIA-1, myeloperoxidase and lysozyme. A staging bone marrow biopsy was negative for involvement by BPDCN, but interestingly showed a possible related myeloid neoplasm, systemic mastocytosis (**Figures 3A** and **3B**).

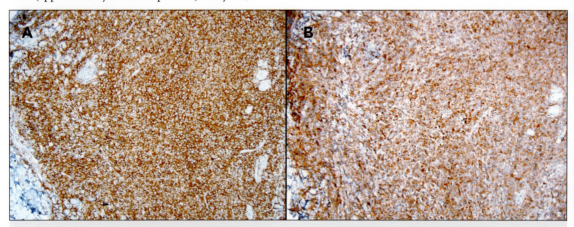

Figure 2 Skin biopsy **A** (CD56, ×200) showing the tumor cells are positive, and **B** (CD4, ×200) showing the tumor cells are positive.

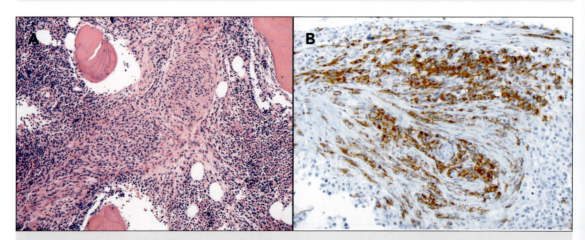

Figure 3 Bone marrow biopsy **A** (H&E, ×200) showing spindle cell infiltrates, and **B** (CD117, ×400) showing the infiltrates are positive.

Diagnosis Blastic plasmacytoid dendritic cell neoplasm.

Management Approach Despite a somewhat indolent initial presentation in some cases, the clinical course is aggressive, with a median survival of 12 months-14 months. Given the rarity of this disease there are no standard treatment regimens. New evidence suggests better outcomes for the patients receiving protocols based on treatment of acute lymphoblastic leukemia followed by allogeneic stem cell transplantation in first complete remission. This patient underwent induction chemotherapy with an acute myeloid leukemia regimen that led to the resolution of his initial skin lesions. 3 months after completion of the chemotherapy, he had developed multiple new skin lesions all over his body that on biopsy proved to be recurrent BPDCN. At this time the bone marrow biopsy showed minimal disease involvement and persistent systemic mastocytosis. He underwent reinduction chemotherapy followed by allogeneic bone marrow transplant. However, 13 months after the transplant, he passed away from transplant-related complications with no evidence of the disease.

General Discussion Blastic plasmacytoid dendritic cells neoplasm is a disease of many names. It has been called blastic NK-cell lymphoma, CD4+CD56+ hematodermic neoplasm, agranular CD4+ natural killer cell leukemia and other variations. Recent advances in understanding the putative cell of origin of this neoplasm lead to the change of the name and also the chapter location in the new WHO classification of tumors of hematopoietic and lymphoid tissue. This entity is no longer considered a lymphoma and it is currently classified under the more appropriate chapter of acute myeloid leukemia and related precursors neoplasms. BPDCN is more common in elderly patients (median age of 65 years), but 30% of patients are younger than 50 years, including children. An approximate 3:1 male predominance holds. The initial presentation can be asymptomatic with solitary or multifocal skin lesions that vary in appearance form bruise-like areas to violaceous patches and tumor nodules. The disease appears to be limited to the skin in approximately half of the cases. Minimal involvement of the bone marrow and peripheral blood is commonly present. Rare cases have overt leukemia at the onset without evidence of skin disease. Other common sites of involvement at presentation are lymph nodes (40% of cases), spleen, liver and tonsils. Cytopenias (especially thrombocytopenia) are commonly present, whereas systemic B symptoms are rare. The usual skin lesions show a diffuse pattern of dermal involvement with sparing of the epidermis. The malignant cells have a monotonous, blast-like appearance. Angioinvasion and necrosis are characteristically absent, whereas occasional mitotic figures are present. Bone marrow involvement varies from a mild interstitial infiltrate usually identified by immunohistochemistry to a diffuse total replacement of the marrow elements. The BPDCN is defined as typically expressing CD4 and CD56 in the absence of lineage-specific markers for B, T or NK cells and myelomonocytic cells. They also express the plasmacytoid dendritic cell-associated antigens CD123 (interleukin-3 α-chain receptor), TCL1, BDCA-2/CD303, CD2AP, BDCA-4, CLA (cutaneous lymphocyte-associated antigen) and the interferon-α-dependent molecule MxA. Some other markers commonly expressed are CD43, CD45RA, CD68 (50% of cases with a dot-like Golgi pattern), CD7, CD33, CD2 (rare cases) and TdT (approximately 30% of cases). Markers such as CD3, CD5, CD8, CD13, CD16, CD19, CD20, CD34, CD79a, PAX5, T-cell receptor, myeloperoxidase and lysozyme are consistently negative, and expression of such markers should question the diagnosis of BPDCN. EBV is negative both by immunohistochemical and in situ hybridization methods. Stains for cytotoxic molecules such as perforin and TIA-1 are negative; however, granzyme B can be detected on flow cytometry but usually not in paraffin sections.

Myeloid/Lymphoid Neoplasms with Eosinophilia and PDGFRA Rearrangement

Young Kim, David S Snyder, Maria Delioukina

Patient A 43-year-old Filipino man presented with complaints of fever, pruritus, and urticaria-like skin lesions.

Clinical History Following chemotherapy for an initial diagnosis of NK/T-cell lymphoma, the patient was transferred to our institution for evaluation for autologous hematopoietic progenitor cell transplantation (HPCT) in first remission. He also reported a 2-year history of eosinophilia.

Family History Diabetes mellitus.

Medications Glyburide and januvia, both for diabetes.

Physical Examination Revealed right axillary, right posterior cervical, and right groin lymphadenopathy.

Initial Work-Up A CBC at initial presentation showed anemia and leukocytosis, with 65% eosinophils. An excisional biopsy of a right axillary lymph node revealed diffuse replacement of the normal nodal architecture by a monotonous population of immature cells with blastic chromatin and scattered macrophages (**Figure 1**). A staging bone marrow biopsy revealed hypercellular marrow with left-shifted granulopoiesis and multiple clusters of immature cells (**Figure 2**).

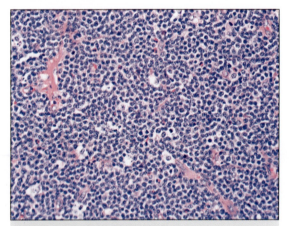

Figure 1 Lymph node biopsy (H&E, ×40) showing a monotonous population of blastic cells with scattered histiocytes.

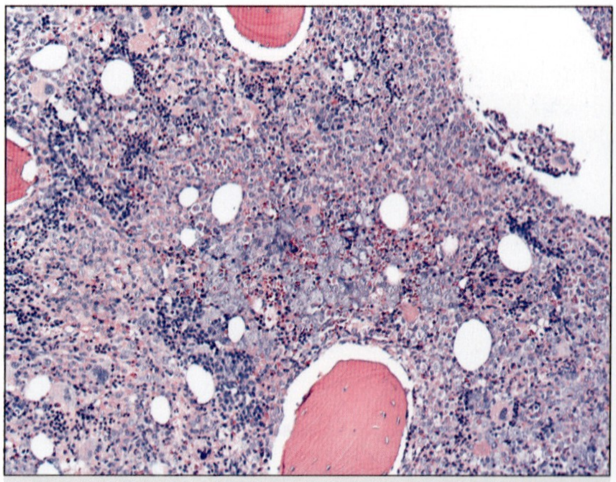

Figure 2 Bone marrow biopsy (H&E, ×20) showing hypercellular marrow with myeloid hyperplasia.

Differential Diagnosis The differential diagnosis of the lymph node included peripheral T-cell lymphoma, NK/T-cell lymphoma, and lymphoblastic lymphoma. The differential diagnosis of the bone marrow included the chronic myeloproliferative neoplasms. Also, because of the unusual association of 2 neoplasms and the presentation with eosinophilia, the differential diagnosis should include an entity designated as "myeloid and lymphoid neoplasms with eosinophilia and abnormalities of PDGFRA, PDGFRB, or FGFR1" in the WHO 2008 classification.

Additional Work-Up Immunohistochemistry on the right axillary lymph nodes showed positive staining with CD3 and TdT (**Figure 3**) but not with BCL2, CD7, CD8, CD56, CD57, or CD20. Immunohistochemistry on the bone marrow showed increased numbers of cells staining for CD33 (**Figure 4**) and CD117 but not for CD3 or TdT. Classic cytogenetic studies performed on bone marrow aspirate sample showed no abnormalities. There was no evidence of t(9;22) or deletion of derivative of chromosome 9 in the bone marrow. 3-color FISH studies on bone marrow sample and paraffin sections of the lymphoma showed CHIC2 deletion in 46.4% and 87.0% of cells, respectively, resulting in FIP1L1/PDGFRA fusion.

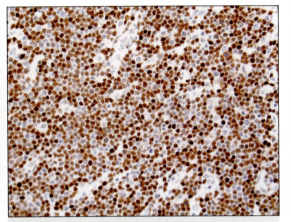

Figure 3 Lymph node biopsy (TdT, ×40) in which the tumor cells show strong nuclear positivity for TdT.

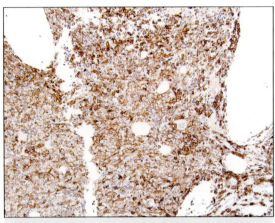

Figure 4 Bone marrow biopsy (CD33, ×20) in which the majority of cells are positive and consequently of myeloid lineage.

Final Diagnosis Myeloid and lymphoid neoplasms with eosinophilia and abnormalities of PDGFRA.

Management Approach These patients generally respond to treatment with tyrosine kinase inhibitors. This entity was formally recognized in 2003 and thus long-term prognosis is not known.

This patient received cyclophosphamide, doxorubicin, vincristine and prednisone (CHOP) chemotherapy at the initial diagnosis of lymphoma. Upon transfer to our institution, where we issued the diagnosis listed above, the patient was started on decitabine, with a good clinical response, but with short follow-up time. The patient's dose was gradually adjusted from 100 mg daily to 40 mg daily because of cardiac intolerance (paroxysmal atrial fibrillation).

General Discussion Myeloid and lymphoid neoplasm with eosinophilia and rearrangements of PDGFRA, PDGFRB or FGFR1 are a group of rare entities that results from formation of a fusion gene encoding an aberrant tyrosine kinase. Patients with PDGFRA rearrangement usually present with fatigue or pruritus, and are more commonly men than women. Most patients have splenomegaly and some have hepatomegaly. There is marked eosinophilia and the cells are mostly mature. The bone marrow biopsy also shows marked eosinophilia and sometimes shows an increase in mast cells and/or reticulin fibrosis. A minority of patients may present as acute myeloid leukemia or T-lymphoblastic lymphoma with concurrent eosinophilia. Recognition of this entity is important, because the disease has been shown to be very responsive to tyrosine kinase inhibitors. The PDGFRA rearrangement is not identified by conventional cytogenetic studies. The main method for the detection of this abnormality is 3-color fluorescence in situ hybridization (FISH) method to detect a CHIC2 deletion (FIP1L1/PDGFRA translocations).

Acute Ph– Lymphoblastic Leukemia

R Patrick Dorion

Patient A 29-year-old male presented for evaluation of a low platelet count.

Clinical History He visited his primary care physician because he felt a decrease in energy and had had intermittent nausea for 8 months. The patient reported an intentional weight loss of 12 pounds over the past few months. He worked in an office and had no exposure to chemicals. Lab work revealed elevated liver function test results and a low platelet count. He was referred to hematology for further work-up and care.

Family History A grandfather, who was a heavy smoker, died of lung cancer. Both parents are alive and have no significant medical history.

Medications None.

Physical Examination He appeared well and had normal vital signs. He had no palpable lymph nodes. His liver and spleen were not palpable. He was mildly jaundiced and had scleral icterus.

Initial Work-Up

CBC		WBC Differential	%	# (×10³/μL)
WBC (×10³/μL)	4.3	Neutrophils	5	0.2
RBC (×10⁶/μL)	3.52	Bands	0	
HGB (g/dL)	10.8	Lymphocytes	78	3.4
HCT (%)	30.9	Monocytes	0	
MCV (fL)	87.8	Eosinophils	1	0.0
MCH (pg)	30.7	Basophils	0	
MCHC (g/dL)	35.0	Metamyelocyte	1	0.0
PLT (×10³/μL)	27	Blasts	15	0.6
RDW-CV (%)	18.2	Nucleated red cell (#/100 WBC)	1	

Peripheral blood smear review revealed a few small to medium blasts characterized by fine chromatin, scant basophilic cytoplasm and high N:C ratio (**Figure 1**).
Lactic dehydrogenase 383 U/L; alkaline phosphatase 340 U/L; total bilirubin 3.3 mg/dL.

Section B: Acute Leukemias
Acute Ph– Lymphoblastic Leukemia

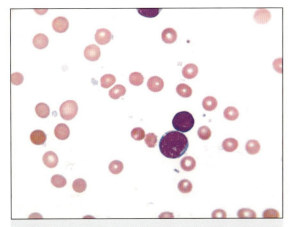

Figure 1 Blood smear (Wright-Giemsa, ×1000) showing representative blasts.

Differential Diagnosis Pancytopenia with circulating blasts in a young adult led us to consider acute myeloid leukemia, acute lymphoid leukemia and peripheralization/leukemic phase of lymphoma in the differential diagnosis.

Additional Work-Up Bone marrow biopsy was hypercellular and virtually replaced by blasts (**Figure 2**). Myelopoiesis, megakaryopoiesis and erythropoiesis were markedly decreased. The aspirate smear showed preponderance of blasts (97%) that were small to medium size and had fine chromatin and scant basophilic cytoplasm with very high N:C ratio (**Figure 3**). No Auer rods were appreciated.

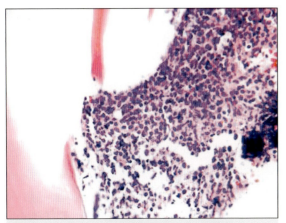

Figure 2 Bone marrow biopsy (H&E, ×200) showing hypercellular marrow with preponderance of blasts and marked reduction of normal hematopoietic elements.

Figure 3 Bone marrow aspirate smear (Wright-Giemsa, ×1000) showing numerous blasts with very few normal hematopoietic elements.

By flow cytometry the blasts in the aspirate were positive with CD19, CD10, CD24, HLA-DR, CD34 and TDT. There was low density CD33 and CD11b. MPO was negative. Markers for T cells were negative. Classic cytogenetics demonstrated no Philadelphia chromosome t(9;22) (**Figure 4**). There were however other chromosomal abnormalities in 45% of the metaphases analyzed: 46, XY, del(4)(q31), dup (6)(p21.1p21.3), t(12;14)(p13;q11.2). FISH studies for BCR/ABL were negative.

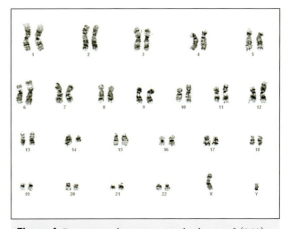

Figure 4 Bone marrow karyotype; note the absence of t(9;22).

Section B: Acute Leukemias
Acute Ph– Lymphoblastic Leukemia

Final Diagnosis B-cell acute lymphoblastic leukemia, Ph–.

Management Approach The treatment of pediatric acute lymphoblastic leukemia (ALL) has been quite successful with a survival rate of 78%-85%. In adults, the diagnosis of ALL carries a more dismal prognosis. Before therapy, baseline laboratory studies such as liver and renal function tests, electrolytes, glucose, LD, uric acid, albumin and total protein are recommended. Cytogenetic studies are imperative since it is important prognostically to determine the presence of Philadelphia chromosome or other chromosomal abnormalities that have bearing in the prognosis. If the patient is young, HLA typing for potential marrow transplant can be done. EKG and cardiac function studies should also be done if cardiotoxic drugs are being considered. A lumbar puncture should be done in all patients to exclude leukemic involvement of the cerebrospinal fluid. Combination chemotherapy is the primary mode of treatment for adult ALL. Multiple different regimens exist and depending on which trial, if any, the patient is placed on, will determine the chemotherapeutic agent. Anthracyclines such as daunorubicin, in combination with cyclophosphamide, L-asparaginase, vincristine, prednisone and methotrexate can be utilized. If L-asparaginase is given, the fibrinogen level should be monitored closely as some adults with ALL can have a precipitous drop in fibrinogen levels. This patient was treated on a protocol that included induction with vincristine, daunorubicin, prednisone and L-asparaginase. He tolerated chemotherapy well but did develop mild paresthesias in the fingers and hyperglycemia. He went into remission but relapsed shortly afterwards and expired approximately 6 months after diagnosis.

General Discussion Adult ALL is not common. It accounts for 20% of all adult leukemias, acute myeloid leukemias being more common. The incidence increases after age 50. The prevalence is higher in Caucasians; however Hispanics have a poorer prognosis. Typical laboratory findings include thrombocytopenia and/or anemia and/or neutropenia. The WBC count may be elevated, normal or decreased. A leukoerythroblastic picture with nucleated red blood cells and immature cells including blasts is also a frequent finding in leukemic/infiltrative processes. Other laboratory findings can include an elevated lactic dehydrogenase due to lysis of the tumor cells. Liver function test results can be elevated for multiple reasons such as liver failure, hepatitis or leukemic infiltration. Clinical features may include bone pain, arthralgias, splenomegaly, hepatomegaly and/or lymphadenopathy. Cytogenetics plays a very important role in prognosis. The most common translocation is t(12;21) followed by t(1;19), t(9;22), t(4;11), t(7;14) and t(11;14). Hyperdiploidy with >50 chromosomes and t(12;21) TEL-AML1 fusion seem to have a better prognosis. Also trisomy 4, 10 and 17 as well as deletion (9p) fare better. The high-risk group includes patients with t(9:22) BCR/ABL (Philadelphia chromosome), t(4:11) MLL-AF4, complex karyotypes, low hypodiploidy or near triploidy. If conventional cytogenetics do not pick up any abnormality, there are multiple molecular/FISH probes and markers for the more common cytogenetic abnormalities. This is helpful when the abnormalities are cryptic. Also these can be useful for determining if there are residual blasts present when morphology or flow cytometry are negative, such as in post-chemotherapy marrow examinations or in patients in remission. Great strides have been made in pediatric B-cell ALL with cure rates of up to 85%. In adults it is reported that 50% of patients can achieve a 50% long-term remission with intensive chemotherapy and allogeneic hematopoietic progenitor cell transplant (HPCT) in eligible patients.

B-Lymphoblastic Leukemia, Pediatric

Mihaela Onciu

Patient An 18-year-old white male, who presented to the emergency room with sore throat, cough, and fever.

Clinical History He had had a 4-week history of low-grade fever, cough and sore throat that were not responding to antibacterial therapy. He was pale and tired. Evaluation showed pancytopenia (WBC $1.5 \times 10^3/\mu L$, hematocrit 14.9%, platelets $53 \times 10^3/\mu L$). After transfusion of packed red cells, the patient was admitted for further evaluation.

Family History Multiple cancers on both the maternal and paternal sides of the family.

Medications None.

Physical Examination Notable for low-grade fever, pallor, and diffuse peripheral lymphadenopathy and hepatosplenomegaly.

Initial Work-Up

CBC		WBC Differential	%	# ($\times 10^3/\mu L$)
WBC ($\times 10^3/\mu L$)	1.7	Neutrophils	30	0.5
RBC ($\times 10^6/\mu L$)	2.36	Bands	3	0.1
HGB (g/dL)	8.1	Lymphocytes	52	0.9
HCT (%)	22.4	Monocytes	1	0.0
MCV (fL)	95	Eosinophils	2	0.0
MCH (pg)	34.1	Basophils	1	0.0
MCHC (g/dL)	35.9	Metamyelocytes	1	0.0
PLT ($\times 10^3/\mu L$)	35	Blasts	10	0.2
RDW-CV (%)	19.2	Nucleated red cells	1/100WBC	
MPV (fL)	8.3			

LDH 296 U/L (normal 94-260); chest X-ray: no active disease, no mediastinal mass.

Section B: Acute Leukemias
B-Lymphoblastic Leukemia, Pediatric

Differential Diagnosis Diagnostic considerations included acute leukemia (lymphoblastic, myeloid or mixed-lineage), leukemic phase of non-Hodgkin lymphoma (hepatosplenic lymphoma, small cell variant of anaplastic large cell lymphoma), myelodysplastic syndrome, and viral infection with secondary myelosuppression.

Additional Work-Up Bone marrow biopsy showed a hypercellular (100%) marrow, with most of the cellularity consisting of sheets of blastic cells, with scanty cytoplasm, often indented nuclear outlines, finely dispersed nuclear chromatin and very small or absent nucleoli. Normal hematopoietic elements were markedly decreased in number (**Figures 1** and **2**).

The bone marrow aspirate smears numerous blasts that were predominantly small to intermediate in size, with scant cytoplasm, indented nuclear outlines, homogeneously condensed nuclear chromatin, and absent or inconspicuous nucleoli. Normal hematopoietic elements were markedly decreased in number and morphologically unremarkable (**Figure 3**).

Flow cytometric analysis performed on the marrow aspirate showed a population of cells with low side-scatter and dim CD45 expression, with the following immunophenotype: CD10+, CD19+, surface and cytoplasmic CD22+, CD20–, CD24+, CD34+, cytoplasmic CD79a+, Tdt+, surface Igμ–/Igκ–/Igλ–, cytoplasmic Igμ–, also expressing the myeloid-associated antigens CD13 (dim) and CD33 (dim), while negative for myeloperoxidase. Flow cytometric cell cycle analysis showed a normal diploid DNA content, with a DNA index of 1.00 and an S-phase of 6.54%.

Cytogenetics (Bone Marrow Aspirate) Normal diploid male karyotype, 46, XY [20]. Fluorescence in situ hybridization was negative for *MLL* gene rearrangements.

Molecular Analysis (Bone Marrow Aspirate) RT-PCR was negative for CML and ALL type *BCR/ABL*, *E2A/PBX*, *MLL/AF-4* and *TEL/AML-1* fusion transcripts.

Final Diagnosis B-lymphoblastic leukemia (WHO classification 2008).

Management Approach The current management of acute lymphoblastic leukemia of both B-cell

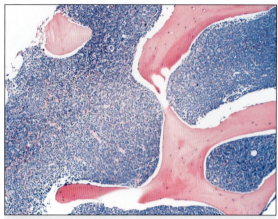

Figure 1 Bone marrow biopsy (H&E, ×100) showing a hypercellular marrow with most of the cellularity replaced by sheets of leukemic cells.

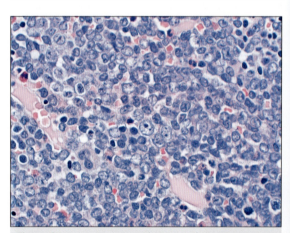

Figure 2 Bone marrow biopsy (H&E, ×600) showing replacement of the cellularity by leukemic blastic cells with scanty cytoplasm, indented nuclear outlines, finely dispersed nuclear chromatin and very small nucleoli.

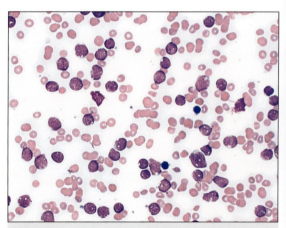

Figure 3 Bone marrow aspirate (Wright-Giemsa, ×600) showing blasts that are predominantly small, with scanty cytoplasm, indented nuclear outlines, homogeneously condensed nuclear chromatin. Nucleoli are absent.

and T-cell lineage involves intensive multiagent chemotherapy. The intensity of chemotherapy is risk-adapted. The level of risk (for relapse) is dictated by presenting features (patient age, leukocyte counts), leukemia-associated parameters (lineage of acute leukemia, genetic lesions present in the leukemic blasts) and initial response to remission induction chemotherapy. Chemotherapy only is employed in patients of low and intermediate risk, while in patients of high-risk, allogeneic hematopoietic progenitor cell transplantation (HPCT) is also considered. The latter modality is also considered in patients with relapsed acute lymphoblastic leukemia. This patient was treated with combination chemotherapy. It included remission induction with methotrexate, prednisone, daunorubicin, and asparaginase, followed by cyclophosphamide, 6-mercaptopurine and cytarabine. Consolidation therapy included methotrexate, hydrocortisone, cytarabine and 6-mercaptopurine, and was followed by maintenance therapy with mercaptopurine, methotrexate, dexamethasone and vincristine. He achieved remission and remains free of disease after 2 years of follow-up.

General Discussion Precursor B-lymphoblastic leukemia is a B-lineage neoplasm derived from bone marrow-based B-lymphoid progenitors. The patients typically present with extensive bone marrow replacement by leukemic cells, associated with peripheral blood pancytopenia or variable degrees of leukocytosis associated with neutropenia, anemia and/or thrombocytopenia. Often there is extensive infiltration of lymph nodes, liver and spleen, and many patients may also present with involvement of the central nervous system (with blasts detected in the cerebrospinal fluid). The diagnosis is based on the identification of blasts in peripheral blood and/or bone marrow and on the demonstration of a precursor B immunophenotype on these cells. The latter includes the expression of B-lineage-specific antigens (CD19, CD20, CD22, CD24, CD79a), CD10, TdT and CD34, and absence of surface immunoglobulin expression (although the leukemic cells may express cytoplasmic Igμ chains). These blasts often show aberrant lineage-inappropriate expression of 1 or several myeloid-lineage antigens (most often CD13 and CD33). Precursor B-ALL encompasses several genetic subtypes with distinct clinical, biological and pharmacological features, which are therefore used in the risk stratification of these patients, especially in pediatric centers. Genetic abnormalities with good prognostic significance (low risk) include hyperdiploidy (>50 chromosomes), t(12;21) (p13;q22) and TEL-AML1 (ETV6-RUNX1). Genetic abnormalities with poor prognostic significance (often high risk) include Philadelphia chromosome or t(9;22) (q34;q11.2), *BCR-ABL,* translocations involving chromosome 11q23 with *MLL* gene rearrangements, and hypodiploidy (<46 chromosomes). The t(1;19) (q23;p13.3); *E2A-PBX1(TCF3-PBX1)* is currently associated with standard risk in the pediatric population. The presence of these genetic lesions along with immunophenotypic aberrancies seen by flow cytometry and specific immunoglobulin and T-cell receptor gene rearrangements may be used to monitor minimal ("sub-microscopic") residual disease in these patients during therapy.

T-Lymphoblastic Leukemia, Pediatric

Mihaela Onciu

Patient A 6-year-old white female brought to the emergency room with fevers, petechiae and ecchymoses.

Clinical History Evaluation in the emergency room showed leukocytosis with anemia and thrombocytopenia. The patient was admitted for further evaluation.

Family History Noncontributory.

Medications None.

Physical Examination Notable for low-grade fever, pallor, multiple petechiae and ecchymoses on extremities, diffuse peripheral lymphadenopathy, and splenomegaly.

Initial Work-Up

CBC		WBC Differential	%	# (×10³/μL)
WBC (×10³/μL)	63.8	Neutrophils	2	1.3
RBC (×10⁶/μL)	3.41	Bands	0	
HGB (g/dL)	10.0	Lymphocytes	1	0.6
HCT (%)	27.7	Monocytes	1	0.6
MCV (fL)	81.3	Eosinophils	1	0.6
MCH (pg)	29.2	Basophils	0	
MCHC (g/dL)	35.9	Myelocytes	1	0.6
PLT (×10³/μL)	60	Blasts	94	60.0
RDW-CV (%)	15.2	Nucleated red cells	0	
MPV (fL)	7.4			

LDH 1,482 U/L (normal 165-310); chest CT examination: anterior mediastinal mass, enlarged thymus, multiple enlarged lymph nodes in the middle mediastinum, right lung hilum and subcarinal area, with mild airway compression.

Differential Diagnosis Diagnostic considerations included acute lymphoblastic leukemia, acute myeloid leukemia, and biphenotypic or mixed lineage leukemia.

Additional Work-Up Bone marrow biopsy showed a hypercellular (100%) marrow, with most of the cellularity replaced by sheets of blastic cells, with scanty cytoplasm, smooth nuclear outlines, finely dispersed nuclear chromatin and very small or absent nucleoli. Normal hematopoietic elements were markedly decreased in number (**Figures 1** and **2**). Bone marrow aspirate smears contained hypercellular marrow particles. Most of the cellularity (97%) consisted of leukemic blasts that were predominantly intermediate to large, with scant to moderate cytoplasm, variably condensed nuclear chromatin and frequent prominent nucleoli (**Figure 3**). Many of the blasts had small cytoplasmic vacuoles. Normal hematopoietic

Section B: Acute Leukemias
T-Lymphoblastic Leukemia, Pediatric

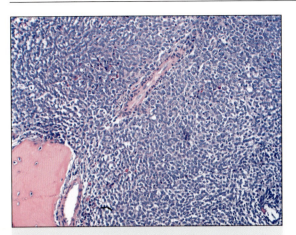

Figure 1 Bone marrow biopsy (H&E, ×200) showing hypercellular marrow with near complete replacement of the cellularity by sheets of blastic cells.

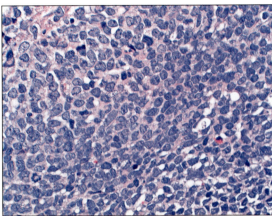

Figure 2 Bone marrow biopsy (H&E, ×600) showing blastic cells with scanty cytoplasm, smooth nuclear outlines, finely dispersed nuclear chromatin and small nucleoli.

elements were markedly decreased in number and morphologically unremarkable, with no evidence of dysplasia. A cytochemical stain for myeloperoxidase was negative in the blasts, with adequate internal positive controls. Flow cytometric analysis of the bone marrow aspirate showed a population of cells with low side-scatter and dim CD45 expression, with the following immunophenotype: CD1a–, CD2–, surfaceCD3–, cytCD3+ (moderate), CD4+, CD5+ (dim), CD7+, CD8–, CD10–, CD56+, CD11b+, CD13+, CD33+, CD34+, CD117+, Tdt–, myeloperoxidase–. Flow cytometric cell cycle analysis showed a normal diploid DNA content, with a DNA index of 1.00 and an S-phase of 0.1%.

Cytogenetics (Bone Marrow Aspirate) Abnormal, low hyperdiploid male karyotype, 47, X, –X, ins(12;9)(p12;q13q34), +16, +19[9]/ 48, idem, +del(X)(q24)[9]. Molecular analysis was not performed.

Final Diagnosis T-lymphoblastic leukemia (WHO classification 2008) or precursor T acute lymphoblastic leukemia (WHO classification 2001).

Management Approach The current management of acute lymphoblastic leukemia (ALL) of both B-cell and T-cell lineage involves intensive multiagent chemotherapy. The intensity of chemotherapy is risk-adapted. The level of risk (for relapse) is dictated by presenting features (patient age, leukocyte counts), leukemia-associated parameters (lineage of acute leukemia, genetic lesions present in the leukemic blasts) and initial response to remission induction

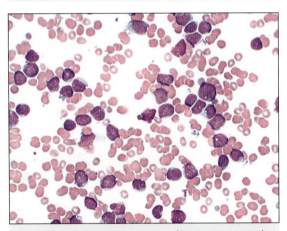

Figure 3 Bone marrow aspirate smear (Wright-Giemsa, ×600) showing intermediate to large blasts, with scant to moderate amounts of cytoplasm, variably condensed nuclear chromatin and occasional prominent nucleoli.

chemotherapy. While well-defined genetic subgroups are used in the risk stratification of B-lineage ALLs, such groups are not in clinical use for T-ALLs at the current time. However, a recently described subgroup of pediatric T-ALL, designated early T-ALL (similar in immunophenotype to this case), is considered a high-risk subtype of leukemia and treated accordingly in some pediatric oncology centers. Chemotherapy only is employed in patients of low and intermediate risk, while in patients of high risk allogeneic hematopoietic progenitor cell transplantation (HPCT) is also considered upfront. The latter modality is also employed in patients with relapsed acute lymphoblastic leukemia. This patient received induction chemotherapy with methotrexate, prednisone, daunorubicin, and asparaginase, followed by cyclophosphamide, 6-mercaptopurine and cytarabine. Consolidation therapy included methotrexate, hydrocortisone, cytarabine and 6-mercaptopurine, and was followed by continuation therapy with 6-mercaptopurine, methotrexate, dexamethasone and vincristine. She achieved remission and remains free of disease after 4 years of follow-up.

General Discussion Precursor T-lymphoblastic leukemia is a T-lineage lymphoid neoplasm derived from thymus-based T-lymphoid progenitors. The patients often present with an anterior mediastinal mass, lymphadenopathy and hepatosplenomegaly. The mediastinal mass may be associated with compression of major airways and other mediastinal structures, resulting in respiratory compromise and superior vena cava syndrome. These findings may or may not be associated with bone marrow infiltration and peripheral blood involvement. The degree of bone marrow infiltration by leukemia is often more extensive than it would be predicted by the peripheral blood cytopenias (in some cases the peripheral blood counts may be normal in the context of extensive bone marrow involvement). By convention, cases with <25% bone marrow replacement by leukemic blasts are staged and treated as non-Hodgkin lymphomas (T-lymphoblastic lymphomas) with bone marrow involvement; cases with more extensive bone marrow involvement are considered T-lymphoblastic leukemias. Patients may also present with involvement of the central nervous system (with blasts detected in the cerebrospinal fluid). The diagnosis is based on the identification of blasts in peripheral blood and/or bone marrow and/or extramedullary tissue biopsies, and on the demonstration of a precursor T immunophenotype on these cells. The latter includes the expression of T-lineage-specific antigens: CD2, cytoplasmic ± surface CD3, CD4, CD5, CD7, CD8, CD10, Tdt, HLA-DR and CD34, and often presence of CD1a (normally expressed in thymocytes present in the thymic cortex). Precursor T-ALLs may be sub-classified according to their resemblance to normal stages of thymocyte maturation into:
- early T/pro-T (CD1a–, cyCD3+, CD2+, CD5– or dim+, CD7+CD8–),
- cortical thymic (CD1a+, CD4+ and/or CD8+, cytoplasmic ± surfaceCD3+, CD2+, CD5+, CD7+), and
- mature/post-thymic (CD1a–, CD4+ or CD8+, cytoplasmic and surfaceCD3+, CD5+, CD7+, often negative for Tdt, CD34, HLA-DR).

Of note, early T/pro-T ALL cases often show aberrant expression of multiple myeloid antigens, including CD11b, CD13, CD33, and most remarkably CD117 (as seen in this case). This immunophenotype, shown to portent a particularly poor prognosis in pediatric patients, raises the differential diagnosis with mixed lineage acute leukemias (of myeloid/T-lymphoid lineage). Importantly, early T-ALLs lack expression of myeloperoxidase. As defined in the most recent WHO classification (2008), a diagnosis of mixed-lineage (T/myeloid) leukemia requires coexpression by the leukemic cells of cytoplasmic CD3 and myeloperoxidase, regardless of the markers expressed on the surface of these cells. The immunophenotypic aberrancies seen by flow cytometry, and specific T-cell receptor gene rearrangements and lineage-inappropriate immunoglobulin gene rearrangements detected at diagnosis may be used to monitor minimal ("sub-microscopic") residual disease in these patients during therapy. Of note, as opposed to patients with B-ALL, in patients with T-ALL monitoring of blood samples has been shown to be of equal value to bone marrow samples for this purpose.

T-Lymphoblastic Leukemia

Sandra Hollensead, Roger H Herzig

Patient A 37-year-old male, who presented with a 2-month history of decreased appetite, fatigue, listlessness, and swelling of the hands and feet.

Clinical History The patient related a single febrile illness and cold sweats, but no night sweats. He had occupational exposure to pesticides and hydrocarbons working in lawn/turf management. He rarely used alcohol, but had smoked for 27 years.

Family History Negative for leukemia, lymphoma, and myeloma. His father died of colon cancer.

Physical Examination Notable only for a red, nonpruritic rash on the hands and trunk and a 0.5 cm slightly tender lymph node in the left axilla.

Initial Work-Up	
CBC	
WBC (×10³/μL)	48.0
RBC (×10⁶/μL)	4.32
HGB (g/dL)	13.5
HCT (%)	38.6
MCV (fL)	89.4
MCH (pg)	31.3
MCHC (g/dL)	35.0
PLT (×10³/μL)	102
RDW-CV (%)	14.3
MPV (fL)	10.3

WBC Differential	%	# (×10³/μL)
Neutrophils	18	8.6
Lymphocytes	45	21.6
Monocytes	6	2.9
Eosinophils	26	12.5
Blasts	5	2.4

On peripheral blood smear review, blasts were small, with finely dispersed nuclear chromatin without prominent nucleoli, and convoluted nuclear membranes (**Figure 1**).

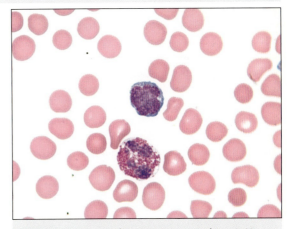

Figure 1 Blood smear (Wright-Giemsa, ×1000) lymphoblast.

Differential Diagnosis Diagnostic considerations included acute lymphoblastic leukemia (ALL), acute myeloid leukemia (AML), leukemic phase of lymphoma, and reactive lymphocytosis.

Additional Work-Up Immunophenotyping by flow cytometry of peripheral blood showed blasts positive for expression of CD45, 2, 3, dual 4/8, 5, 7, dim 25, 43, 52, and TCR α/β, and negative for CD1, 10, 11c, 13, 14, 19, 20, 33, 34, 56, 117, HLA-DR, and TCR γ/δ, TdT, and surface κ and λ light chains. β chain T-cell clonal distribution confirmed monoclonality. Bone marrow biopsy revealed cellularity to be approximately

60%, and the aspirate smear was significant for 20% lymphoblasts, which appeared identical to those seen in the peripheral blood (**Figure 2**). By immunohistochemical staining, the blasts in the marrow were positive for CD3, CD45, and MIB-1 and negative for CD20, CD30, CD15, CD33, and CD34 by immunohistochemistry, and negative for t(8;13) and the *BCR/ABL* fusion gene by FISH. Cerebrospinal fluid was negative for blasts. Lymph node was not biopsied. Immunophenotyping and morphology suggested a more mature T-lymphocyte phenotype. Dual CD4/8 expression; however, is consistent with immaturity, as is the open, lacy appearance of the nuclear chromatin of the blasts. These findings in conjunction with an aggressive clinical course were in keeping with ALL, rather than peripheral T-cell lymphoma in leukemic phase.

Final Diagnosis T- lymphoblastic leukemia.

Management Approach Systemic multiagent chemotherapy and intrathecal prophylactic chemotherapy are usually given. For younger patients, improved outcomes are obtained if asparaginase is included in the chemotherapy regimen. This patient was given 2 cycles of hyper CVAD, but failed to achieve remission. A 3-month remission was obtained with high-dose cytarabine and idarubicin. On relapse, CBC showed 32% lymphoblasts; cytogenetic analysis of the blasts revealed multiple chromosomal abnormalities, but no translocation of the long arm of chromosome 5 (PDGFRB). In relapse, the patient underwent transplant from a matched volunteer. His course was complicated by acute graft-vs-host disease (GVH), primarily of the skin (**Figure 3**). Over a year later, he remains in remission with chronic GVH.

General Discussion T-ALL is classified as acute leukemia when blood and bone marrow are involved, or as T-cell lymphoblastic lymphoma (T-LBL) when thymus, lymph nodes, or extranodal sites are involved, but not blood or bone marrow. However the clinical findings may overlap, thus the WHO designation of T-lymphoblastic leukemia/lymphoma (T-ALL/LBL). Patients with T-ALL often have relative sparing of the bone marrow compared to B-ALL, despite a large burden of tissue disease. This case illustrates the difficulty of detecting lymphoblasts in the peripheral smear when nucleoli are indistinct, and blasts are small,

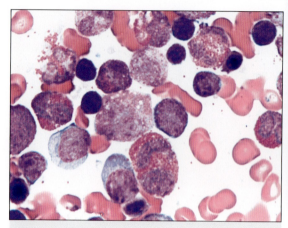

Figure 2 Bone marrow aspirate smear (Wright-Giemsa, ×1000) lymphoblasts and eosinophils.

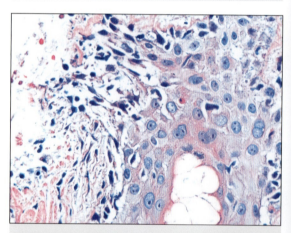

Figure 3 Hair follicle (H&E, ×400) lymphocytic infiltrate, vacuolar interface alteration, and an apoptotic cell (acute GVH disease).

causing confusion with normal or reactive lymphocytes. The recognition may be further confounded by the lack of flagging of the population by the automated cell counting hematology instrument, as was present in this case. In addition, lack of CD34 and TdT expression by the blasts, may lead to the diagnosis of mature T-cell lymphomas in leukemic phase. This patient presented with peripheral eosinophilia. The hematologic neoplasms with eosinophilia and abnormalities of PDGFR A or B, or FGFR1 are described in the 2008 WHO classification. Aberrant tyrosine kinase activity resulting from the fusion gene may make the disease treatable by tyrosine kinase inhibitors such as imatinib.

Acute Ph+ Lymphoblastic Leukemia

Raymond E Felgar

Patient A 36-year-old male presented with lower leg edema and pain. Laboratory work-up revealed leukocytosis, anemia and thrombocytopenia.

Clinical History The patient has a history of pulmonary blebs and spontaneous pneumothorax.

Family History Noncontributory.

Medications None.

Physical Examination No lymphadenopathy, splenomegaly or hepatomegaly. Leg edema noted, thought to be attributable to a deep vein thrombosis.

Initial Work-Up		
CBC		
WBC (×10³/μL)	93.0	
RBC (×10⁶/μL)	3.2	
HGB (g/dL)	9.6	
HCT (%)	29.5	
MCV (fL)	91.6	
MCH (pg)	29.7	
MCHC (g/dL)	32.5	
PLT (×10³/μL)	74.0	
RDW-CV (%)	15.6	
WBC Differential	**%**	**# (×10³/μL)**
Neutrophils	8	7.66
Bands	10	9.3
Lymphocytes	8	
Monocytes	4	
Blasts	64	59.7
Myelocytes	2	1.9
Metamyelocytes	4	3.7

Peripheral blood smear revealed many blasts (**Figure 1**).

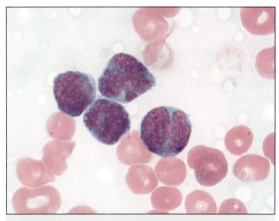

Figure 1 Blood smear (Wright-Giemsa, ×1000) showing blasts.

Differential Diagnosis Excluding the peripheral blood differential findings, the initial diagnostic differential was fairly broad but included infection, as well as leukemia. However, given the percentage and absolute number of circulating blasts, most other diagnoses are excluded, except for an acute leukemia (either lymphoblastic or myeloid type).

Additional Work-Up Bone marrow biopsy was hypercellular and completely infiltrated by blasts (**Figure 2**). A differential performed on the bone marrow aspirate smear revealed 82% blasts (**Figure 3**). Blasts had minimal, basophilic cytoplasm and no Auer rods were seen.

Flow cytometric evaluation of bone marrow aspirate showed 86% blasts with positive staining for CD34, CD19, CD22, CD10, HLA-DR, and terminal deoxynucleotidyl transferase (TdT). A subset of blasts weakly coexpressed CD20. Blasts showed no significant staining for CD13, CD33, CD117, myeloperoxidase, cytoplasmic or surface CD3, or for κ or λ immunoglobulin light chains.

Classical cytogenetic studies demonstrated a mosaic karyotype, with 2 metaphases showing a normal karyotype, 46,XY; 4 metaphases with 46,XY,t(9;22)(q34;q11.2); and 14 metaphases with 46,XY,t(9;22)(q34;q11.2), der (9)t(1;9)(q12;p13) (**Figure 4**).

FISH studies confirmed the presence of a *BCR/ABL1* fusion signal in 172 of 216 (80%) analyzed interphase nuclei (**Figure 5**).

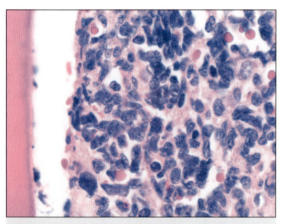

Figure 2 Bone marrow biopsy (H&E, ×400) showing preponderance of blasts.

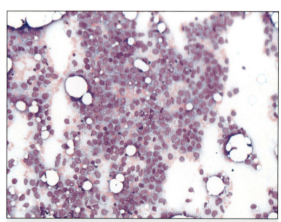

Figure 3 Bone marrow aspirate smear (Wright-Giemsa, ×1000) showing numerous blasts.

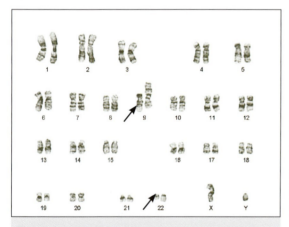

Figure 4 Karyotype showing reciprocal translocation involving chromosomes 9 and 22.

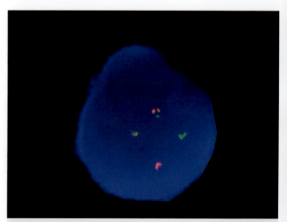

Figure 5 Fluorescent in situ hybridization (FISH) with nucleus showing fusion of red signal (chromosome 9q34, *ABL* gene) and green signal (chromosome 22q11.2, BCR locus) indicating the presence of a *BCR/ABL* fusion.

Final Diagnosis Precursor B-cell lymphoblastic leukemia with t(9;22)(q34;q11.2).

Management Approach Therapy for precursor B-cell lymphoblastic leukemia (B-ALL) differs somewhat from acute myeloid leukemia therapy. Although both employ an intense "induction phase" to induce remission, followed by a "consolidation phase" to remove clinically undetectable residual disease, B-ALL therapy has a third "maintenance phase" of therapy consisting of low-dose chemotherapy given over a 2-year to 3-year follow-up period that is designed to target slowly proliferating neoplastic cells once they re-enter an active cell cycle. There are several commonly used treatment protocols including the Larson protocol employed in this case. Use of the Larson protocol initially appeared to achieve successful induction, with suppression of blasts on a 30-day follow-up marrow. However, approximately 5 months later, peripheral blood showed 38% circulating blasts which were confirmed to have a B-precursor phenotype by flow cytometry, similar to the diagnostic blast population. Cerebrospinal fluid examinations also appeared to show central nervous system involvement by leukemia at that time. Re-induction chemotherapy was administered, along with tyrosine kinase inhibitors imatinib and the newer generation tyrosine kinase inhibitor, dasatinib, with a long-term plan to perform allogeneic hematopoietic progenitor cell transplantation. However, the patient developed pneumonia requiring hospitalization and intubation and subsequently died approximately 1 year following initial diagnosis.

General Discussion Precursor B-cell lymphoblastic leukemia with t(9;22)(q34;q11.2); BCR-ABL1 is currently recognized by the 2008 WHO classification as a subtype of B-lymphoblastic leukemia/lymphoma with recurrent cytogenetic abnormalities and is associated with very poor prognosis, as this case illustrates. Cases are also relatively more common in adults [25% of adult acute lymphoblastic leukemia (ALL) vs 2%-4% of childhood ALL]; this may, in part, account for the relatively poorer outcomes of adult cases of ALL survival in comparison to pediatric cases, but is probably not the sole factor accounting for this. There are no distinct morphologic or cytochemistry features that allow for distinction from other subtypes of ALL and therefore cytogenetic, molecular, and/or FISH studies are key to demonstrating the presence of a *BCR/ABL1* translocation or fusion RNA product. Most cases have a precursor B-cell phenotype with expression of CD19, CD10, and TdT, with variable staining for CD20 and CD22. Although more frequent coexpression of myeloid markers (namely CD13 and CD33) may be seen, this finding is not specific. Very rare cases may also have a precursor T-cell phenotype. The characteristic t(9;22) translocation results in a fusion gene product of the tyrosine kinase ABL1 on 9q34 with the BCR locus on 22q11. The resultant fusion product has tyrosine kinase activity that can be targeted by imatinib and newer generation tyrosine kinase inhibitors that are more typically used to treat chronic myelogenous leukemia. There is clinical data to support that some patients may benefit from this therapy in addition to standard chemotherapy protocols, with improved early event-free survival. The *BCR/ABL* fusion gene product produces a 190 kd (p190) fusion protein in most pediatric cases of B-ALL, but in adult cases, approximately 50% can produce the 210 kd (p210) product that is more often associated with CML.

Section B: Acute Leukemias

Acute Leukemia of Ambiguous Lineage

Powers Peterson

Patient A 16-year-old Caucasian female with recent onset of fever.

Clinical History The patient reported having experienced progressive fatigue over the past several weeks with recent onset of fevers.

Family History Noncontributory.

Medications Over-the-counter analgesics as needed for headaches and fever.

Physical Examination Temperature 102.9°F; BP 100/70 mmHg; heart rate 82/min, respiratory rate 16/min. Her chest was clear to auscultation and percussion. Her skin exam showed petechial hemorrhages on bilateral lower extremities.

Initial Work-Up		
CBC		
WBC (×10³/μL)	192.0	
RBC (×10⁶/μL)	3.2	
HGB (g/dL)	2.7	
HCT (%)	8.3	
MCV (fL)	82	
MCH (pg)	27	
MCHC (g/dL)	32.5	
PLT (×10³/μL)	14	
RDW-CV (%)	11.5	
MPV (fL)	8.6	
WBC Differential	**%**	**# (×10³/μL)**
Neutrophils	3	5.8
Lymphocytes	4	7.7
Blasts	91	174.7
Myelocytes	2	3.8

Peripheral blood smear revealed predominantly immature cells (blasts), some with cytoplasmic granules but no Auer rods were seen (**Figure 1**).

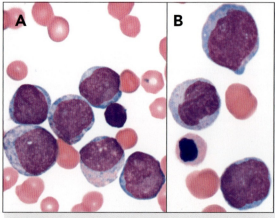

Figure 1 Blood smear (Wright, ×1000) **A** showing several blasts with fine chromatin and occasional nucleoli. A lymphocyte and a probable myelocyte are also present. **B** shows 2 blasts, a monocyte, and a nucleated red cell. One blast has moderate amount of cytoplasm while the other has a little.

Differential Diagnosis Diagnostic considerations included acute myeloid leukemia, acute lymphoid leukemia, and acute leukemia of biphenotypic/bilineal/ambiguous lineage.

Additional Work-Up
- PT 12.2 sec (normal 10.7-13.4)
- INR 1.2 (normal 0.9-1.2)
- PTT 28.4 sec (normal 23-33)

Bone Marrow Aspirate and Clot Section
Predominantly immature cells (blasts) with monocytic features: folded/grooved nuclei, some with nucleoli, abundant cytoplasm and some containing cytoplasmic granules and occasional ones with cytoplasmic vacuoles; no Auer rods were seen (**Figure 2**). Immunophenotypic analysis by flow cytometry performed on blood and bone marrow aspirate generated the following results:

Myeloid CD33 (98.0%), CD117 (66.2%), CD15 (93.3%), CD13 (31.7%), CD14–, CD33 (98.0%), cytoplasmic MPO (53.9%), CD13 (31.7%), CD34 23.2%, CD64 (47.7%), CD11c (35.9%).

B-Cell Cytoplasmic CD22 (98.2%, strong), surface CD22 (10.5%, dim), TdT (54.4%), CD19 (36.5%, strong), cytoplasmic CD79a (34.2%, moderate-strong); CD10–.

T-Cell CD7 (9.3%); <1% of cells expressed CD2, CD3, CD5, CD4, CD8. The population that expressed CD33 co-expressed cytoplasmic CD22.

Cytogenetics (Bone Marrow Aspirate) 46 XX

FISH Negative for all of the following:
BCR/ABL (9q34;22q11.2)
deletion EGR-1 (5q31)
deletion D5S23,D5S721 (5p15.2)
ETV6/RUNX1 (TEL, 12p13; AML, 21q22)
MLL rearrangement (11q23)
RUNX1T1/RUNX1 (ETO, 8q22; AML1, 21q22)
rearrangement 16q22
inversion 16
translocation (16;16)
deletion 9p21
monosomy 7
deletion 7q31

Final Diagnosis Acute leukemia of ambiguous lineage—mixed phenotype acute leukemia, B/myeloid (NOS).

Management Approach Acute leukemias of ambiguous lineage account for <4%-5% of all acute leukemias and generally have a poor prognosis. General management approach includes initial chemotherapy for acute myeloid leukemia; if unsuccessful, then therapy for B-lymphoid leukemia. Evaluation for stem cell transplant is also routinely done. Because of hyperleukocytosis and the mixed myeloid/B-lymphoid phenotype of the leukemia, this patient's induction therapy regimen consisted of cytarabine, daunorubicin and 6-thioguanine. She went into remission and then received consolidation chemotherapy for several months. She is now awaiting hematopoietic progenitor cell transplant (HPCT).

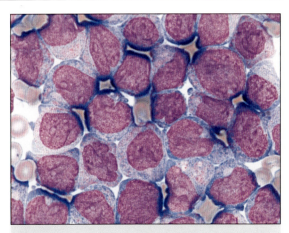

Figure 2 Bone marrow aspirate smear (Wright-Giemsa, ×1000) showing numerous blasts with large, often folded or reniform nuclei and prominent nucleoli. The cytoplasm of many blasts contains granules, but no Auer rods. A few blasts also have cytoplasmic vacuoles.

General Discussion One of the major changes in the 2008 WHO revision of the classification of hematologic malignancies was in the diagnosis of acute leukemias that were neither clearly lymphoid nor myeloid. Previous terminology included the terms biphenotypic, mixed lineage, or ambiguous lineage to describe these diseases. The 2008 classification terminology is acute leukemias of ambiguous lineage; that diagnosis is based on immunophenotyping. Criteria for assigning a single blast cell population to >1 lineage are now clearly stated. To be called myeloid, the blasts should express myeloperoxidase or should express 2 of the monocytic markers NSE, CD11c, CD14, CD64, lysozyme. To be called B-lymphoid, the blasts should express strong CD19 with either strong CD79a, strong cytoplasmic CD22, or strong CD10. Alternatively, if CD19 is weak, then 2 of the following should be strongly expressed: CD79a, cytoplasmic CD22, CD10. To be called T-lymphoid, the blasts should express cytoplasmic CD3 (epsilon chain). Surface CD3 is rare in mixed phenotype leukemias. This patient has a B/myeloid acute leukemia because the blasts express both B-lymphoid and myeloid markers. The evidence for B-lineage is strong CD19 with strong CD79a and moderate-strong cytoplasmic CD2. The evidence for myeloid lineage is the myeloperoxidase.

T-Lymphoblastic Crisis of Chronic Myelogenous Leukemia

James D Cotelingam, Diana M Veillon, Mary Lowery-Nordberg

Patient A 30-year-old white male presented with a 2-week history of abdominal pain, chest pain upon inspiration, shortness of breath, fever, night sweats, and a 10-lb weight loss.

Clinical History The patient had been diagnosed with chronic myelogenous leukemia (CML) 6 months prior (**Figure 1**). He was initially treated with imatinib (400 mg/day), but dosage was increased to 800 mg/day when he failed to respond. He subsequently presented with an elevated white blood cell count (94 × 10^3/μL) with circulating blast forms.

Family History Grandfather with leukemia, grandmother with disseminated cancer (type unknown).

Medications Allopurinol, guaifenisen, hydroxyurea, oxycodone, imatinib, intravenous fluids (normal saline).

Physical Examination He was tachycardic (pulse 119) with a right ventricular heave and febrile at 101.2°F. BP was 118/54, and respiratory rate 18. A right sided retinal hemorrhage was present. A small left supraclavicular lymph node was palpable. The liver was enlarged: liver 2 cm and the spleen 8 cm below the costal margin.

Initial Work-Up

CBC		WBC Differential	%	# (×10^3/μL)
WBC (×10^3/μL)	76.8	Neutrophils	18	13.8
RBC (×10^6/μL)	2.71	Bands	2	1.5
HGB (g/dL)	8.6	Lymphocytes	20	15.4
HCT (%)	24.9	Monocytes	3	2.3
MCV (fL)	91.8	Eosinophils	2	1.5
MCH (pg)	31.9	Basophils	3	2.3
MCHC (g/dL)	34.8	Metamyelocytes	1	0.8
PLT (×10^3/μL)	13	Promyelocytes	9	6.9
RDW-CV (%)	14.3	Blasts	42	32.3
MPV (fL)	10.3			
PT (sec)	20.2 (normal 11.3-15.2)			
INR	1.73 (normal 0.8-1.2)			
PTT (sec)	45.3 (normal 24.7-35.5)			

Differential Diagnosis Blast crisis of CML, type unspecified (myeloid vs lymphoid).

Section B: Acute Leukemias
T-Lymphoblastic Crisis of Chronic Myelogenous Leukemia

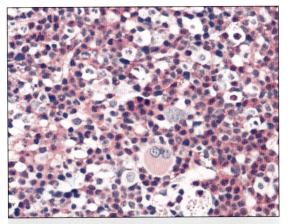

Figure 1 Bone marrow biopsy at the initial diagnosis of CML (H&E, ×400) showing a hypercellular, myeloid predominant bone marrow with <5% blast forms.

Additional Work-Up Bone marrow aspirate and biopsy (**Figure 2**) revealed a marrow cellularity of 100%. Blast forms comprised >70% of the marrow cellularity and were immunoreactive for CD3, CD34 and TdT (**Figure 3**). All other hematopoietic elements were markedly decreased. Moderate reticulin fibrosis was present. Stainable iron was absent. Immunophenotyping by flow cytometry revealed a predominance of blast forms that expressed CD34 (partial), CD2, CD3 (partial), CD5 (partial), CD7, CD38, CD71, and CD79a, but did not express myeloid antigens. Cytogenetic studies (**Figure 4**) revealed an abnormal male karyotype with a 9;22 translocation: 46,XY,t(9;22)(q34;q11.2). No additional chromosomal aberrations were noted. Molecular genetic studies by FISH were positive for BCR-ABL1 (**Figure 5**).

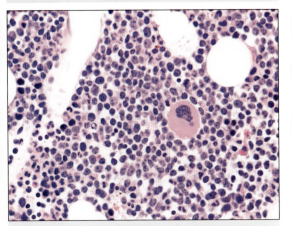

Figure 2 Bone marrow biopsy at current presentation (H&E, ×400) showing a hypercellular marrow with a predominance of blast forms.

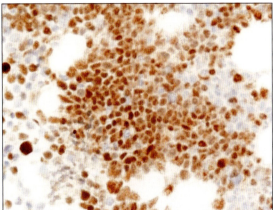

Figure 3 Bone marrow biopsy (TdT, ×400) showing hypercellular marrow with a predominance of blast forms immunoreactive for TdT.

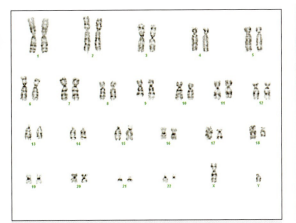

Figure 4 Bone marrow karyotype: showing classic 9;22 translocation 46,XY,t(9;22)(q34;q11.2).

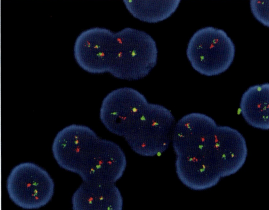

Figure 5 Bone marrow FISH analysis using a dual-color, dual-fusion probe (Abbott, Inc.) for BCR/9q34 (red) and ABL1/22q11.2 (green). Fusion signals are depicted in yellow.

Section B: Acute Leukemias
T-Lymphoblastic Crisis of Chronic Myelogenous Leukemia

Final Diagnosis T-lymphoblastic crisis of CML.

Management Approach The chronic phase of CML is treated with tyrosine kinase inhibitors such as imatinib. Myeloid blast crisis may also respond to imatinib, alone or in combination with other chemotherapies. Patients who develop a lymphoid blast crisis of CML may respond to chemotherapy used for acute lymphoblastic leukemia. In many cases, the initial treatment is followed by an allogeneic hematopoietic progenitor cell transplant for eligible patients. Ideally, transplantation occurs during the chronic phase of the disease. Transplantation while the patient is in blast crisis characteristically has a poor prognosis. For this patient, the treatment with intravenous fluid (normal saline), hydroxyurea, allopurinol, and imatinib was continued. He also underwent leukapheresis without complications. He had evidence of disseminated intravascular coagulation and was treated with appropriate transfusion therapy including fresh frozen plasma and platelets. He was subsequently transferred to another facility for evaluation for allogeneic hematopoietic progenitor cell transplantation (HPCT).

General Discussion Chronic myelogenous leukemia is a myeloproliferative neoplasm that originates in an abnormal bone marrow stem cell. It is characteristically associated with the Philadelphia (Ph) chromosome resulting from a reciprocal t(9;22). CML typically has 3 phases in its natural history: chronic phase, accelerated phase, and a blast phase (or blast crisis). Progression of CML to accelerated phase or blast crisis is usually associated with clonal evolution and the development of additional cytogenetic abnormalities. The blast phase of CML is diagnosed when blasts comprise at least 20% of peripheral blood leukocytes or 20% of the bone marrow cellularity. Alternatively, the blast phase of CML may be diagnosed when the blast proliferation is extramedullary. Such blastic proliferations are also known as chloroma, granulocytic sarcoma, or extramedullary myeloid tumors. They more commonly present in lymph nodes, spleen, bone, central nervous system, and skin. Enumeration of blast forms and identification of blast lineage is essential for diagnosis, classification, and treatment. In about 70% of patients the blast crisis of CML is characterized by blasts of myeloid lineage. However, blasts may also exhibit evidence of monocytic, megakaryocytic, or erythroid differentiation. In 20%-30% of cases, blast crisis is of lymphoid lineage and is usually of precursor B-cell origin. Lymphoblastic crisis of CML is rarely of T-phenotype. T-lymphoblastic crisis of CML is reported in <50 cases in the literature. It is characteristically associated with a poor prognosis. Blastic proliferation may occur within the marrow or in an extramedullary site. In a significant number of case reports, the T-lymphoblastic crisis is predominantly extramedullary. It has been suggested that the use of imatinib may be associated with a mild increase in the incidence of sudden blast crisis as well as an increase in the frequency of lymphoid blast crisis.

Chronic Myelogenous Leukemia

Ari B Molofsky, Jingwei Yu, Imran Siddiqi

Patient A 52-year-old woman with abdominal fullness, early satiety, and mild fatigue.

Clinical History The patient had a large intra-abdominal teratoma removed 3 years prior. Otherwise the history was unremarkable.

Family History Mother with chronic myelogenous leukemia (CML), sister with Crohn disease.

Medications None.

Physical Examination Afebrile, splenomegaly to 7 cm below costophrenic angle.

Initial Work-Up

CBC

WBC (×10³/µL)	249.0
RBC (×10⁶/µL)	2.9
HGB (g/dL)	8.8
HCT (%)	25.2
MCV (fL)	87
MCH (pg)	30.3
MCHC (g/dL)	34.9
PLT (×10³/µL)	913

WBC Differential	%	# (×10³/µL)
Neutrophils/bands	30	74.7
Bands	0	
Lymphocytes	2	5.0
Monocytes	1	2.5
Eosinophils	7	17.4
Basophils	10	24.9
Myelo/Metamyelocytes	46	114.5
Blasts	4	10.0

Peripheral blood smear revealed a significant leukocytosis comprised of mature and immature granulocytes and a few circulating blasts (**Figure 1**). Basophilia and eosinophilia were prominent. Thrombocytosis was marked.

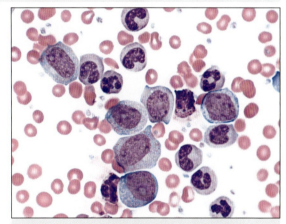

Figure 1 Blood smear (Wright-Giemsa, ×1000) showing leukocytosis with a prominent population of circulating myelocytes ("myelocyte bulge"), increased basophils, and occasional blasts.

Differential Diagnosis Diagnostic considerations include leukemoid reaction (reactive neutrophilia with left shift), chronic myelogenous leukemia BCR-ABL1 positive (CML), atypical chronic myelogenous leukemia BCR-ABL1 negative (aCML), polycythemia vera (PV), primary myelofibrosis (PMF), and chronic neutrophilic leukemia (CNL).

Additional Work-Up The bone marrow biopsy was hypercellular (>90%), composed predominantly of maturing granulocytic elements (**Figure 2**). Megakaryocytes were increased, including several clusters of small, hypolobated forms (**Figure 3**). No

Section C: Chronic Myeloproliferative Neoplasms and Myelodysplastic Syndromes
Chronic Myelogenous Leukemia

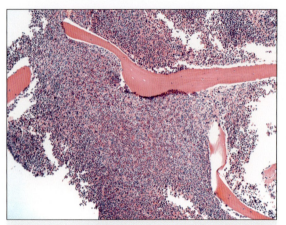

Figure 2 Bone marrow biopsy (H&E, ×100) showing markedly hypercellular marrow.

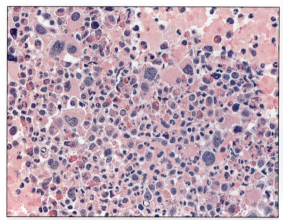

Figure 3 Bone marrow biopsy (H&E, ×400) showing granulocytic hyperplasia with increased, hypolobated megakaryocytes.

sheets or clusters of blasts were appreciated. In the bone marrow aspirate smear, there was marked granulocyte predominance, with a myeloid/erythroid ratio of 40:1. A relative myelocyte "bulge" was appreciated. Blasts were not increased, accounting for <5% of cells. No significant myeloid or erythroid dysplasia was noted. Abundant megakaryocytes were present, including hypolobated micromegakaryocytes. Occasional sea blue histiocytes were also seen. Quantitative PCR on peripheral blood was positive for BCR-ABL1 p210 (b3a2) translocation, with an elevated BCR-ABL1/ABL1 ratio of 22.098. Classical cytogenetics showed a Philadelphia chromosome in all metaphases examined, with a karyotype of 46, XX, t(9;22) (q34;q11.2) (**Figure 4**). Interphase dual-color, dual-fusion FISH analysis for BCR and ABL1 revealed 2 yellow signals, indicative of the reciprocal t(9;22) BCR-ABL1 translocation. One normal chromosome 9 and chromosome 22 signal can also be appreciated (**Figure 5**). No additional chromosomal abnormalities and abnormal FISH signal patterns were detected.

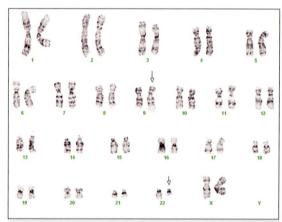

Figure 4 Bone marrow karyotype (G-banding) demonstrating t(9;22) translocation (arrows).

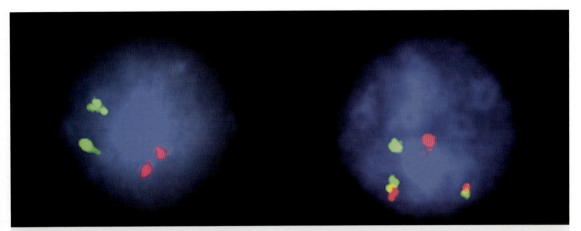

Figure 5 Bone marrow (Interphase dual-color, dual-fusion FISH analysis for BCR and ABL1). The left panel shows a normal cell, with 4 separate signals, 2 for chromosome 9 (red) and 2 for chromosome 22 (green). The right panel shows an abnormal cell with 2 yellow fusion signals, indicating t(9;22) BCR-ABL1 translocation. One normal chromosome 9 and one normal chromosome 22 signal can also be appreciated.

Final Diagnosis Chronic myelogenous leukemia, BCR-ABL1 positive, chronic phase.

Management Approach Treatment of chronic myelogenous leukemia (CML) has been revolutionized over the past decade with the advent of tyrosine kinase inhibitors (TKIs) that block the ATP binding pocket of the ABL1 kinase, inhibiting constitutive activation of the fusion BCR-ABL1. Imatinib is the first-line TKI therapy for CML, yielding 5-year progression free survival between 80%-95%. Unfortunately, primary and secondary treatment failures do occur, often secondary to acquired mutations in the BCR-ABL1 ATP binding pocket. Second generation TKIs are available, including dasatinib and nilotinib, which are effective in most, but not all, treatment failures. Finally, allogeneic progenitor cell transplant can be considered in younger patients or patients with CML in accelerated or blast phase, in which monotherapy with TKIs is less effective. In this case, the patient was begun on imatinib.

General Discussion CML is a chronic myeloproliferative neoplasm (MPN) that results in a proliferation of neutrophils and immature granulocytes in the blood and bone marrow. It is by definition associated with the BCR-ABL1 t(9;22)(q34;q11.2) translocation, present in a hematopoietic stem-like precursor, and resulting in the Philadelphia chromosome (derivative chromosome 22). The translocation can be identified by chromosome analysis, BCR-ABL1 FISH or BCR-ABL1 PCR. Three possible common breakpoints occur in BCR, resulting in BCR-ABL1 fusion proteins of different molecular weights: p190, p210, and p230. The p210 transcript is most common in CML, whereas the p190 transcript is more often associated with BCR-ABL1 positive de novo ALL. Although FISH analysis detects each of these fusions, PCR must be specifically designed to detect each separate product. Quantitative PCR has become standard of care for tracking CML disease response to TKI therapy, with a complete molecular response (>3 log reduction in BCR-ABL1/ABL1 product) associated with the best clinical outcomes. Increased BCR-ABL1 PCR ratios of more than tenfold can indicate treatment failure and disease progression. The natural history of CML begins with a chronic phase (CP) that is often asymptomatic and typically marked by blood neutrophilia with increased immature granulocytes, which will progress over several years to an accelerated phase (AP) and eventual blast phase (BP), resembling acute leukemia. Flow immunophenotyping is integral to assess the immunophenotype of blasts in BP, as approximately 70% of CML progress to a myeloid blast phase and 30% to a lymphoid blast phase. CML can present at any age, but is more common in the elderly. Prior to the advent of TKI therapy, the average survival was 3 years-5 years. With the advent of TKI therapy, CML has been transformed into an often manageable, if not curable, disease.

Atypical Chronic Myelogenous Leukemia, BCR-ABL1 Negative

Yang O Huh

Patient A 74-year-old male presented with fatigue.

Clinical History He had presented to his primary care doctor with increasing fatigue, worsening exercise tolerance and 25-pound weight loss over a period of 9 months. A CBC performed at primary doctor's office revealed a white blood cell (WBC) count of $210 \times 10^3/\mu L$ and hemoglobin of 5.5 g/dL. He was seen by a hematologist and a bone marrow study revealed morphology suggesting chronic myelogenous leukemia. Cytogenetic study; however, revealed trisomy 8, and no evidence of Philadelphia chromosome. The patient was started on hydroxyurea, and received transfusion of 6 units of packed red cells.

Family History Noncontributory.

Medications Hydroxyurea, allopurinol.

Physical Examination Notable for marked splenomegaly and mild hepatomegaly. He had no palpable adenopathy. He had no petechiae or ecchymoses.

Initial Work-Up

CBC		WBC Differential	%	# ($\times 10^3/\mu L$)
WBC ($\times 10^3/\mu L$)	37.4	Neutrophils	85	31.8
RBC ($\times 10^6/\mu L$)	2.98	Bands	0	
HGB (g/dL)	9.1	Lymphocytes	3	1.1
HCT (%)	27.1	Monocytes	6	2.2
MCV (fL)	91	Eosinophils	0	
MCH (pg)	30.5	Basophils	1	0.4
MCHC (g/dL)	3.5	Metamyelocytes	5	1.9
PLT ($\times 10^3/\mu L$)	76			
RDW-CV (%)	23.7			
MPV (fL)	10			

Peripheral blood smear revealed neutrophilia with some dysplastic neutrophils (**Figure 1**).

Section C: Chronic Myeloproliferative Neoplasms and Myelodysplastic Syndromes
Atypical Chronic Myelogenous Leukemia, BCR-ABL1 Negative

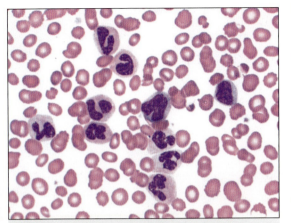

Figure 1 Blood smear (Wright-Giemsa, ×500) showing increased neutrophils, some with dysplastic changes including abnormal nuclear segmentation and chromatin clumping.

Differential Diagnosis Diagnostic considerations included myeloproliferative neoplasms (MPN) including chronic myelogenous leukemia (CML) and myelodysplastic/myeloproliferative neoplasms (MDS/MPN) including chronic myelomonocytic leukemia (CMML).

Additional Work-Up Bone marrow biopsy revealed hypercellular (>90%) marrow with granulocytic hyperplasia, decreased erythroid precursors, and adequate number of megakaryocytes (**Figure 2**). There was mild increase in reticulin fibers without collagen fibrosis. Bone marrow aspirate smears showed increased granulocytes with significant dysplastic features including marked hypogranularity and occasional abnormal segmentation (**Figure 3**).

Erythroid precursors were decreased and showed dyspoietic changes with nuclear irregularities. Some megakaryocytes were also dysplastic. A 500-cell differential count results: blasts 1%, myelocytes 22%, metamyelocytes 22%, neutrophils +bands 33%, eosinophils 1%, basophils 1%, lymphocytes 5%, monocytes 6%, normoblasts 9%, M:E ratio 9:1. Flow cytometric analysis of bone marrow aspirate demonstrated immunophenotypic aberrancies suggesting dysplastic maturation of granulocytes including markedly reduced side scatter, aberrantly increased expression of CD56, and altered expression of CD13 and CD16.

Cytogenetics 47,XY,+8[12]/46,XY[8] and negative result for *BCR/ABL1* by FISH.

Molecular Analysis No *BCR-ABL1* fusion transcript by real-time PCR analysis, positive for *N-RAS* mutation at codon 12, no mutation for *JAK2* at codon 617, and no mutation at codon 515 of *MPL*.

Final Diagnosis Atypical chronic myelogenous leukemia, *BCR-ABL1* negative.

Management Approach Patients with atypical chronic myelogenous leukemia (aCML) have poor prognosis, especially when they have markedly elevated WBC count and anemia, as seen in this patient. Age >65 years, female gender, WBC >50 × 10^3/μL, thrombocytopenia and anemia have been reported to be adverse prognostic factors. In approximately 30% of patients, atypical chronic myeloid leuekmia evolves rapidly to acute myeloid leukemia, and the remainder die of marrow

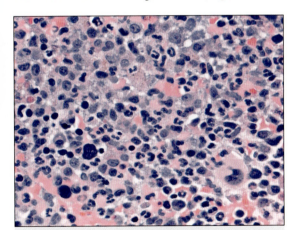

Figure 2 Bone marrow biopsy (H&E, ×400) showing hypercellularity with granulocytic predominance and dysplastic megakaryocytes.

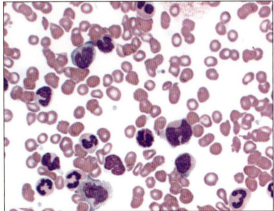

Figure 3 Bone marrow aspirate smear (Wright-Giemsa, ×500) showing dysplastic granulocytes similar to those in the peripheral blood.

failure. Without proven effective therapy, patients with aCML are often treated with hydroxyurea when WBC count is high, as in this patient, and less frequently with intensive induction chemotherapy regimens used for acute myeloid leukemia. In young patients, aggressive therapy including hematopoietic progenitor cell transplantation should be considered. This patient was continued on hydroxyurea and died of bone marrow failure 6 months after initial diagnosis.

General Discussion aCML, *BCR-ABL1* negative is a rare disease in the MDS/MPN category by WHO classification (2008), with estimated incidence of only 1 cases to 2 cases for every 100 cases of *BCR-ABL1*-positive CML. It is characterized by leukocytosis resulting from increased neutrophils and their precursors with prominent dysgranulopoiesis.

Dysplastic granulocytes often show acquired Pelger-Huet anomaly, hypogranularity, and abnormal chromatin clumping. Monocytes are not increased and should be <10% of leukocytes. Dyserythropoiesis with moderate to severe anemia and dysmegakaryopoiesis with thrombocytopenia are common. Blasts are usually <5% and should be <20% of leukocytes in the blood and in the bone marrow.

The neoplastic cells do not have the Philadelphia chromosome or a *BCR-ABL1* fusion gene. Cases with rearrangement of *PDGFRA* or *PDGFRB* genes are also excluded. However, karyotypic abnormalities are frequent up to 80% of patients with a CML, *BCR-ABL1* negative. The most common abnormalities are +8 and del(20q). Mutations of *NRAS* or *KRAS* have been reported in approximately 30% of cases.

Chronic Neutrophilic Leukemia

James D Cotelingam, Menchu G Ong, Mary Lowery Nordberg

Patient A 71-year-old male with a chief complaint of 30-lb weight loss over a 4-month period.

Clinical History At his annual check-up he had a markedly elevated white blood cell count ($300 \times 10^3/\mu L$) with neutrophil predominance. Later, he developed anemia and thrombocytopenia that required red cell and platelet transfusions, and he was referred by his oncologist to our institution for follow-up care and treatment. Past medical history was significant for hypertension and gout. On admission, he received intravenous fluids, allopurinol and hydroxyurea. His WBC count dropped to $68 \times 10^3/\mu L$. A week later, his symptoms improved (better appetite, subjective decrease in splenomegaly); however, his thrombocytopenia worsened.

Family History Positive for diabetes.

Medications Hydroxyurea, lisinopril, colchicine.

Physical Examination Afebrile male, not in acute distress but with a blood pressure of 192/94. Hepatosplenomegaly was present. There was no lymphadenopathy.

Initial Work-Up

CBC		WBC Differential	%	# ($\times 10^3/\mu L$)
WBC ($\times 10^3/\mu L$)	207.0	Neutrophils	84	173.9
RBC ($\times 10^6/\mu L$)	2.3	Bands	3	6.2
HGB (g/dL)	8.8	Lymphocytes	6	12.4
HCT (%)	28.3	Monocytes	5	10.4
MCV (fL)	123.0	Eosinophils	0	
MCH (pg)	38.3	Basophils	0	
MCHC (g/dL)	31.2	Metamyelocytes	1	2.1
PLT ($\times 10^3 u/L$)	70	Myelocyte	1	2.1
RDW-CV (%)	13.7			
MPV (fL)	10.2			

Peripheral blood smear revealed marked neutrophilia, occasional hypersegmented neutrophils, occasional bands, and rare metamyelocytes and myelocytes (**Figure 1**).

Section C: Chronic Myeloproliferative Neoplasms and Myelodysplastic Syndromes
Chronic Neutrophilic Leukemia

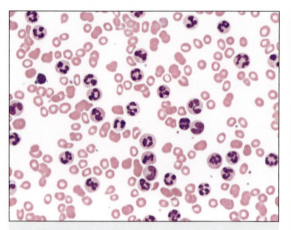

Figure 1 Blood smear (Wright-Giemsa, ×400) showing neutrophilia with a few bands.

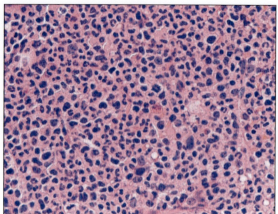

Figure 2 Bone marrow biopsy (H&E, ×400) showing a hypercellular, myeloid predominant marrow with marked expansion of the neutrophilic compartment.

Differential Diagnosis leukemoid reaction, chronic neutrophilic leukemia (CNL) and chronic myelogenous leukemia (CML).

Additional Work-Up

Bone marrow biopsy: Marrow cellularity was 100%. The M:E ratio was >10:1. Myeloid maturation was left shifted, with marked expansion of the neutrophilic compartment (**Figure 2**). CD34+ blasts were not increased. Megakaryocytes were adequate and maturing. Erythropoiesis was normoblastic. Plasma cells were not increased. Lymphocytes were mildly increased, with more T than B cells. Reticulin was moderately increased. No metastatic carcinoma or granuloma was identified. Stainable iron was absent and no ring sideroblasts were found.
- FISH analysis for PDGFR-β, t(9;22) *BCR/ABL*, PDGFR-α/FIP1L1/CHIC2 were negative
- PCR for *JAK2 V617F* was positive
- Karyotype was 46XY
- Serum B_{12}: >1,200 pg/mL (normal 208-964)
- Serum uric acid: 12.9 mg/dL (normal 3.5-7.2)
- LDH: 595 U/L (normal 125-243)

Final Diagnosis Chronic neutrophilic leukemia.

Management Approach Due to the rarity of the condition, the optimal treatment strategy remains controversial. Chemotherapeutic agents including hydroxyurea, busulfan and thioguanine have been administered to control leukocytosis and splenomegaly. Alpha interferon has also been tried for patients unresponsive to hydroxyurea. However, the only therapy that is expected to be curative is allogeneic progenitor cell transplant performed when the disease is stable. This patient received a higher dose of hydroxyurea (2,000 mg) with allopurinol and intravenous fluids to prevent tumor lysis syndrome. His WBC count decreased to $68 \times 10^3/\mu L$. He was subsequently discharged with instruction to follow-up with his primary oncologist.

General Discussion CNL is a rare myeloproliferative neoplasm and only 150 cases have been reported. This is primarily a disease of the elderly but cases of CNL in adolescents and young adults have also been described. There is no sex predilection. The differential diagnosis included a leukemoid reaction, chronic neutrophilic leukemia (CNL) and chronic myelogenous leukemia (CML). All 3 entities present with an elevated WBC count. In both CML and CNL, splenomegaly is present. In the chronic phase of CML, the neutrophils in the peripheral blood are in different stages of maturation, while in CNL, segmented neutrophils and bands constitute the majority of white blood cells. In a leukemoid reaction, splenomegaly and a sustained neutrophilia are not expected findings. Patients may present with weight loss, abdominal discomfort, fatigue, and anorexia. Splenomegaly is consistently seen. Hepatomegaly may also be observed. Easy bruising and epistaxis from severe thrombocytopenia and gouty arthritis have been reported. There is peripheral blood leukocytosis with segmented neutrophils and bands comprising >80% of white blood cells. The bone marrow is hypercellular and myeloid predominant. There is an increased LAP score, serum B_{12} and uric acid. The majority of reported cytogenetics has been normal. In a minority of patients, clonal karyotypic abnormalities may include trisomy 21, del(12p), monosomy 7, del(20q), trisomy 8, trisomy 9, and del (11q14). The Philadelphia chromosome and the *BCR/ABL* fusion gene are absent in CNL. Part of the work-up of Philadelphia chromosome-negative chronic myeloproferative disorders include testing for PDGFRA and PDGFRB fusion genes. In eosinophilia-associated chronic myeloproliferative disorders, the detection of the *FIP1L1-PDGFRA* fusion gene and overexpression of PDGFRA and PDGFRB led to targeted therapy with tyrosine kinase inhibitors. Very rare instances of CNL having JAK2 V617-F mutation have been described and this mutation appears to be associated with a better survival. However, one case reports that progressive disease developed despite an HLA-matched unrelated bone marrow transplant. Additional data is required to assess the relationship of JAK2 mutation and the clinical course of CNL.

Polycythemia Vera

Josef T Prchal, Sujata Narayanan, Mohamad Salama

Patient A 57-year-old Caucasian female presented to the emergency department with blurred vision in her right eye and weakness in the left hand.

Clinical History Clinically the patient was suspected to have had a transient ischemic attack (TIA). However, the CT scan and MRI studies did not show any evidence of TIA. Her past medical history included portal and splenic vein thrombosis and splenectomy.

Family History No family history of bleeding or clotting disorders and malignancy.

Medications Insulin, metformin, warfarin, ferrous sulfate, sumatriptan.

Physical Examination Unremarkable with a well-healed midline abdominal scar.

Initial Work-Up		
CBC		
WBC (×10³/μL)	12.3	
RBC (×10⁶/μL)	7.9	
HGB (g/dL)	15.3	
HCT (%)	51.5	
MCV (fL)	65.4	
MCH (pg)	19.5	
MCHC (g/dL)	29.8	
PLT (×10³/μL)	549	
RDW-CV(%)	24.2	
MPV (fL)	10.1	
WBC Differential	%	# (×10³/μL)
Neutrophils	78.9	9.7
Lymphocytes	14.4	1.7
Monocytes	3.1	0.4
Eosinophils	2.9	0.4
Basophils	0.6	0.1

Serum iron 30 μg/dL, TIBC 550 μg/dL, ferritin 15 ng/mL.

Differential Diagnosis Diagnostic considerations included essential thrombocythemia, primary myelofibrosis, chronic myelogenous leukemia and polycythemia vera (PV) masked by iron deficiency anemia.

Additional Work-Up Bone marrow examination revealed hypercellular marrow (**Figure 1**) with trilineage hyperplasia (**Figure 2**) and minimal reticulin fibrosis (**Figure 3**). *JAK2* V617F mutation was positive with 38.5% mutant allele burden in granulocytes. Testing for *BCR/ABL* and cMPL mutation was negative. Erythropoietin-independent erythroid colony formation was evident by endogenous erythroid colony (EEC) assay.

Final Diagnosis Polycythemia vera masked by coexistent iron deficiency.

Management Approach Phlebotomy is the recommended treatment for PV; however, its usefulness has been questioned recently. Leukocytosis has been established as a predictive factor for thrombotic events in PV patients. Although myelosuppressive therapy is useful in preventing thrombotic complications, it has high leukemogenic potential. Interferon α has been shown to be effective in correcting abnormal blood counts in all 3 lineages and correcting all symptoms in PV patients, thus eliminating the need for phlebotomy

Section C: Chronic Myeloproliferative Neoplasms and Myelodysplastic Syndromes
Polycythemia Vera

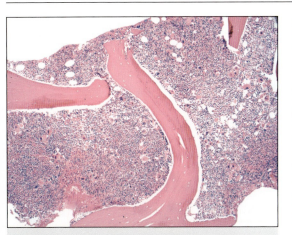

Figure 1 Bone marrow biopsy (H&E, ×100) showing hyperplastic marrow.

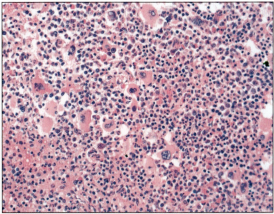

Figure 2 Bone marrow biopsy (H&E, ×400) showing hypercellular marrow with trilineage hyperplasia and loose clustering of megakaryocytes.

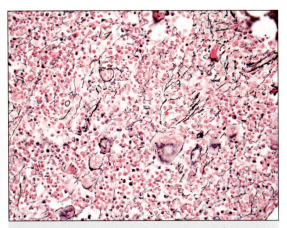

Figure 3 Bone marrow biopsy (reticulin stain, ×400) showing mild reticulin fibrosis.

1) HGB >18.5 g/dL (men) >16.5 g/dL (women) or HGB or HCT >99th percentile of reference range for age, sex or altitude of residence or HGB >17 g/dL (men), or >15 g/dL (women) if associated with a sustained increase of ≥2 g/dL from baseline that cannot be attributed to correction of iron deficiency or elevated red cell mass >25% above mean normal predicted value, 2) presence of *JAK2* V617F or similar mutation.

Minor criteria include: (1) bone marrow trilineage proliferation, (2) subnormal serum erythropoietin level, and (3) endogenous erythroid colony (EEC) growth. *JAK2* V617F mutation is evident in >95% of patients and up to 5% of cases have heterogeneous mutations of exon 12 of *JAK2* gene. Thus, *JAK2* V617F mutation is an excellent PV screen test. PV patients usually have low serum erythropoietin concentrations with specificity of 92%-99 %. High levels of erythropoietin are suggestive of other causes of polycythemia. The demonstration of EEC in cultures in vitro has a 100% sensitivity and specificity in diagnosing patients who have not received any prior chemotherapy. The incidence of PV is ~1.9 per 100,000 per year. Median survival of untreated PV after diagnosis is around 6 months-18 months, but exceeds 10 years for treated patients. According to the Polycythemia Vera Study Group, the most common causes of death included thrombosis (29%), hematologic malignancies (23%), nonhematologic malignancies (16%), hemorrhage (7%) and myeloid metaplasia with myelofibrosis (3%). However, the increased risk of other malignancies is likely caused by chemotherapeutic agents that have been shown to increase risk of leukemic transformation and myelodysplastic syndrome. The leukemogenic risk of hydroxyurea; however, remains controversial.

and decreasing thrombotic complications. This patient was started on hydroxyurea and responded adequately. She was also placed on lifelong anticoagulation with Coumadin. She is followed at regular intervals as an outpatient and has not had any recurrence of any thrombotic events.

General Discussion PV patients usually present with pruritus, erythromelalgia, thrombosis, transient ischemic attacks, splenomegaly and laboratory findings of increased red cell mass, elevated hemoglobin and hematocrit, thrombocytosis and leukocytosis that is secondary to abnormal clonal proliferation of myeloid cells. The 2008 revised WHO criteria for the diagnosis of PV requires meeting either both major criteria and 1 minor criterion or the first major criterion and 2 minor criteria. Major criteria include:

Essential Thrombocythemia

Linda Sandhaus

Patient A 9-year-old African-American girl, who was brought to the emergency department with a chief complaint of neck pain.

Clinical History The patient reported having mild neck pain for the past several days, but the severity had increased over the past several hours.

Family History Unremarkable (there was no family history of blood disorders).

Medications None.

Physical Examination There was tenderness of the right neck with some difficulty in turning the head. There was no lymphadenopathy or organomegaly.

Initial Work-Up		
CBC		
WBC (×10³/μL)	5.9	
RBC (×10⁶/μL)	4.64	
HGB (g/dL)	11.9	
HCT (%)	36.4	
MCV (fL)	78	
MCHC (g/dL)	32.7	
PLT (×10³/μL)	1,480	
RDW-CV (%)	14.3	
WBC Differential	**%**	**# (×10³/μL)**
Neutrophils	68	4.0
Bands	0	
Lymphocytes	24	1.4
Monocytes	7	0.4
Eosinophils	1	0.1
Basophils	0	

Group A Streptococcus screen was positive.

Differential Diagnosis The patient was treated with amoxicillin for the presumed streptococcal infection. The thrombocytosis was interpreted as "probably reactive." A follow-up appointment was scheduled for the pediatric hematology/oncology clinic.

Additional Work-Up The marked thrombocytosis was still present when the patient was seen in the hematology/oncology clinic 3 weeks later (**Figure 1**). A bone marrow aspiration and biopsy were performed. The abnormal findings were limited to the megakaryocytes, which were extremely variable in their nucleation with hypo- and hyperlobated forms and hyperchromasia. As is often the case, the morphologic atypia of the megakaryocytes was most apparent in the biopsy sections, where clustering of megakaryocytes was also a key feature (**Figure 2**). The myeloblast count was not increased and the overall bone marrow cellularity was normal for the patient's age, with the exception of the markedly increased numbers of megakaryocytes.

Cytogenetic analysis for Philadelphia chromosome and FISH for *BCR-ABL* translocation were negative. JAK2 mutation status was negative. An elevated K+ level of 5.2 mEq/L was also noted.

Final Diagnosis Essential thrombocythemia.

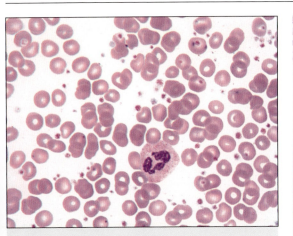

Figure 1 Blood smear (Wright-Giemsa, ×1000) showing marked thrombocytosis.

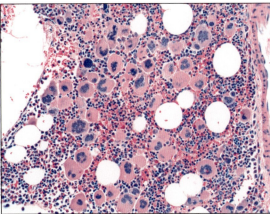

Figure 2 Bone marrow biopsy (H&E, ×400) showing increased number of atypical megakaryocytes in clusters.

Management Approach Most patients with essential thrombocythemia (ET) are asymptomatic at presentation and are diagnosed after an elevated platelet count is found incidentally on a CBC obtained for another clinical indication. Thrombotic and hemorrhagic complications can occur in children, but appear to be less frequent than in adults. ET is an indolent disorder and children appear to have a more benign course than adults. Young asymptomatic patients with platelet counts <1,500 × 10^3/µL are considered at low risk for thrombosis and hemorrhagic events. The goal for treatment of ET is to prevent bleeding and thrombosis without increasing these risks. When treatment is indicated, the combination of hydroxyurea and aspirin appears to provide the best protection. Transformation to acute myelogenous leukemia is extremely rare. Treatment for this child also began with daily aspirin and hydroxyurea.

General Discussion Most thrombocytoses in the pediatric age group are benign and reactive. Causes of reactive thrombocytosis include infection, iron deficiency anemia, hemolytic anemia, acute blood loss, connective tissue diseases, inflammatory bowel disease, malignancies, and splenectomy. Underlying causes of a reactive thrombocytosis should always be excluded before a diagnosis of myelproliferative disorder is considered. This patient's thrombocytosis was initially thought to be reactive, probably secondary to a bacterial infection. Reactive thrombocytosis is mediated by cytokines, and is usually transient. The platelet count in reactive thrombocytosis may exceed 1,000 × 10^3/µL; however, thrombotic or hemorrhagic complications are rare. Platelet morphology is usually normal and may include the presence of many large and even giant platelets. The persistence and magnitude of the thrombocytosis raised the suspicion of a myelproliferative process in this patient. The platelet morphology was normal, and basophilia, which is often present in chronic myeloproliferative disorders (CMPDs), was not apparent in the peripheral blood. The WHO criteria for essential thrombocythemia (ET) include sustained thrombocytosis in excess of 450 × 10^3/µL, increased atypical megakaryocytes, exclusion of other chronic myeloproliferative disorders, and demonstration of a clonal marker or exclusion of reactive thrombocytosis. The platelets usually demonstrate anisocytosis, but more significant morphologic abnormalities, while helpful if present, are not characteristic or necessary for diagnosis. *JAK2 V617F* mutation occurs in about 40%-50% of cases of ET, although the incidence appears to be lower in pediatric cases. Therefore, absence of JAK2 mutation does not exclude the diagnosis of ET. On the other hand, the diagnosis of ET should not be made if the Philadelphia chromosome or molecular evidence of BCR-ABL translocation is detected. ET is rare in children, occurring more commonly in adults with a peak incidence in the 6th decade and a secondary peak in the 3rd decade, especially in women. The presence of erythroid hyperplasia, granulocytic hyperplasia or significant fibrosis in the marrow should raise consideration of another CMPD. The most common chronic myeloproliferative disorder in the pediatric age group is chronic myelogenous leukemia, which was excluded in this case by the absence of a *BCR-ABL* translocation and peripheral blood smear and bone marrow morphology that were inconsistent with CML. Primary familial thrombocytosis has been reported, but was not a consideration in this case. It is worth mentioning that thrombocytosis may cause pseudohyperkalemia, because potassium is released from the platelets during blood clotting in serum tubes. Therefore, pseudohyperkalemia is a pre-analytical laboratory artifact.

Primary Myelofibrosis

Josef T Prchal, Sujata Narayanan, Mohamad Salama

Patient A 76-year-old Caucasian male, who presented with fatigue, and abdominal fullness.

Clinical History The patient also reported having night sweats and weight loss for the past couple of years. He had a history of mild coronary artery disease and an unremarkable social history, and reported exposure to Agent Orange.

Family History There was no family history of hematologic disorders or other cancers.

Medications Aspirin, clopidogrel, metoprolol, lisinopril, atorvastatin and acetaminophen/oxycodone.

Physical Examination Remarkable for an enlarged spleen 12 cm below costal margin. There was no hepatomegaly or peripheral lymphadenopathy.

Initial Work-Up		
CBC		
WBC (×10³/μL)	16.3	
RBC (×10⁶/μL)	5.37	
HGB (g/dL)	14.9	
HCT (%)	44.4	
MCV (fL)	82.9	
MCH (pg)	28.1	
MCHC (g/dL)	33.9	
PLT (×10³/μL)	302	
RDW-CV (%)	18.5	
MPV (fL)	11.7	
WBC Differential	**%**	**# (×10³/μL)**
Neutrophils	70	11.4
Bands	8	1.3
Lymphocytes	11	1.8
Monocytes	6	1.0
Eosinophils	1	0.2
Basophils	2	0.4
Myelocytes	2	0.4

Peripheral blood smear revealed leukoerythroblastic picture, anisopoikilocytosis, polychromasia and teardrops (**Figure 1**). Serum LDH was increased at 1,485 U/L and uric acid of 9.2 mg/dL.

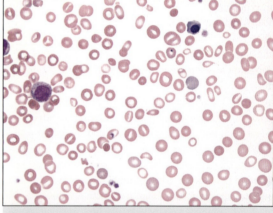

Figure 1 Blood smear (Wright-Giemsa, ×1000) showing anisopoikilocytosis, polychromasia, occasional teardrop cells, a myelocyte and a nucleated red blood cell.

Differential Diagnosis Diagnostic considerations included myeloproliferative neoplasms (MPNs), including chronic myelogenous leukemia, primary myelofibrosis (PMF) and late-onset Gaucher disease.

Additional Work-Up Bone marrow aspiration was dry tap and core biopsy showed hypercellular marrow with prominent osteosclerosis and clustered/abnormally localized megakaryocytes (**Figures 2** and **3**). Megakaryocytes showed atypical hyperchromatic nuclei of variable size and shape (**Figure 3**). There was

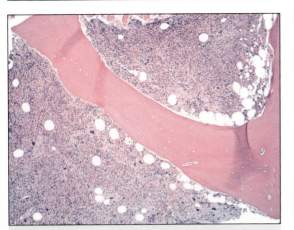

Figure 2 Bone marrow biopsy (H&E, ×100) showing a hypercellular marrow with moderate to severe osteosclerosis.

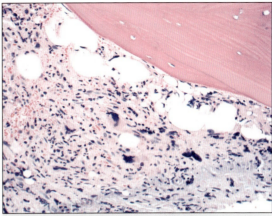

Figure 3 Bone marrow biopsy (H&E, ×500) showing atypical megakaryocytes with hyeprchromatic nuclei of variable sizes and shapes in a fibrotic stroma.

reduced sideroblastic iron and evidence of increased (3+) reticulin fibrosis (**Figure 4**). Karyotype was normal. *JAK2* V617F was positive with 23% mutant allele burden in granulocytes. BCR/ABL and cMPL mutation testing were negative. Peripheral blood CD34+ blast proportion represented 0.2%

Final Diagnosis Primary myelofibrosis, *JAK2* V617F positive.

Management Approach The treatment of PMF is based on the patient's presentation and the presence of constitutional symptoms (splenomegaly with abdominal fullness, anemia etc). In the absence of any of these symptoms, most patients could be followed clinically without interventions. Patients with a higher IPSS score indicating a poor prognosis should be considered for allogeneic hematopoietic stem cell transplantation. Androgens, danazol, erythropoietin, darbepoietin, thalidomide with prednisone, and blood transfusions have shown to improve anemia. Patients symptomatic from splenomegaly can benefit from hydroxyurea and splenectomy. These remain palliative measures and do not offer cure. Alkylating agents like melphalan and busalfan have been used but have high leukemogenic potential. This patient was observed for several months without therapy. At the point where his hemoglobin dropped below 10 g/dL, he was started on thalidomide and prednisone. His hemoglobin remained stable and he continues on therapy a year later.

General Discussion PMF is a myeloproliferative neoplasm that involves abnormal proliferation of the clonal hematopoietic stem cell leading to ineffective erythropoiesis and dysplastic megakaryocytic

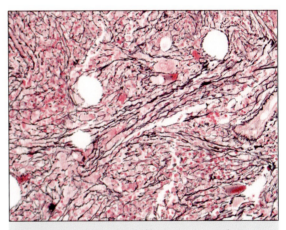

Figure 4 Bone marrow biopsy (Reticulin stain, ×400) showing increased reticulin fibrosis.

hyperplasia. There is bone marrow fibrosis secondary to nonclonal expansion of fibroblasts from increased growth factors, which contributes to the ineffective erythropoiesis and anemia. Extramedullary hematopoiesis occurs in spleen or in other organs. Patients present with severe anemia, splenomegaly and constitutional symptoms. Peripheral smear typically shows anisocytosis, poikilocytosis, teardrop cells (dacrocytes), nucleated red cells and often immature myeloid precursor cells (leukoerythroblastic picture). Additional findings may include elevated levels of alkaline phosphatase, lactate dehydrogenase, uric acid, leukocyte alkaline phosphatase, and vitamin B_{12}. Bone marrow aspirate frequently produces a dry tap. The core biopsy shows fibrosis, osteosclerosis, and granulocytic/megakaryocytic hyperplasia with dysmegakaryopoiesis. Incidence of PMF is 1.5 per

100,000 per year, with median age of diagnosis at 67 years. The 3-year survival rate is estimated at 52%. More than 90% of the chromosomal abnormalities in PMF are represented by 20q–, 13q–, 5–,+8, +9, 12p–, and abnormalities of chromosomes 1 and 7. *JAK2* mutations have been found in 50% of patients with PMF and lead to activation of the JAK/STAT pathway causing increased cellular proliferation. Acquired mutations in *MPL*, the thrombopoietin receptor, are found in an additional 5% of patients (*MPLW515L/K*). Leukemic transformation in PMF occurs in approximately 4% of the patients and is mostly myeloid in nature. More than 3% circulating blasts and platelets <100 × 10^3/μL at the time of diagnosis are the 2 independent risk factors associated with leukemic transformation. Revised WHO criteria for diagnosis of PMF requires meeting all 3 major criteria and 2 minor criteria. Major criteria include 1) presence of megakaryocyte proliferation and atypia, usually accompanied by either reticulin and/or collagen fibrosis, or, in the absence of significant reticulin fibrosis, the megakaryocyte changes must be accompanied by an increzased bone marrow cellularity characterized by granulocytic proliferation and often decreased erythropoiesis (ie, prefibrotic cellular-phase disease), 2) not meeting WHO criteria for polycythemia vera, chronic myelogenous leukemia, myelodysplastic syndrome, or other myeloid neoplasms, and 3) demonstration of *JAK2 V617F* or other clonal marker (eg, *MPLW*515L), or in the absence of a clonal marker, no evidence of bone marrow fibrosis due to underlying inflammatory or other neoplastic diseases. Minor criteria include 1) leukoerythroblastosis, 2) increase in serum lactate dehydrogenase level, 3) anemia, and 4) palpable splenomegaly.

Systemic Mastocytosis with Associated Clonal Hematologic Non-Mast Cell-Lineage Disease

Yang O Huh

Patient A 75-year-old woman presented with complaints of increasing fatigue and weakness over the course of several months.

Clinical History The patient was diagnosed anemic 2 years prior to the current presentation, and she was treated with darbepoetin α with good initial response. A bone marrow biopsy was performed at that time, which showed myelodysplastic syndrome with del(20q) by cytogenetics. She started requiring red blood cell transfusions every other week. Splenomegaly was noted several months later. Splenomegaly rapidly increased, requiring splenectomy 8 months after the original presentation. Pathologic evaluation of the spleen showed mastocytosis. Bone marrow biopsy performed after splenectomy showed mastocytosis and myelodysplasia. 8 months later, she experienced progressive fatigue and started to notice enlarged lymph nodes in the axillae. She was referred to a tertiary care institution for further work-up and management.

Family History Noncontributory.

Medications None.

Physical Examination She had bilateral enlarged axillary lymph nodes. She had no other palpable lymph nodes. Her abdominal exam was remarkable only for the well-healed surgical scar. She had no petechiae or ecchymoses.

Initial Work-Up

CBC		WBC Differential	%	# (×10³/μL)
WBC (×10³/L)	11.4	Neutrophils	35	4.0
RBC (×10⁶/μL)	3.53	Bands	0	
HGB (g/dL)	10.3	Lymphocytes	17	1.9
HCT (%)	32	Monocytes	45	5.1
MCV (fL)	91	Eosinophils	2	0.2
MCH (pg)	29.2	Basophils	1	0.1
MCHC (g/dL)	32.2			
PLT (×10³/μL)	239			
RDW-CV (%)	68.6			
MPV (fL)	11.0			

Differential Diagnosis Diagnostic considerations included myelodysplastic/myeloproliferative neoplasm (MDS/MPN) (chronic myelomonocytic leukemia) and myeloproliferative neoplasm (MPN) (systemic mastocytosis).

Additional Work-Up Bone marrow biopsy revealed a hypercellular (100%) marrow with an extensive infiltration of oval to spindle mast cells, focally forming dense aggregates and sheets (**Figure 1**), replacing about 60% of medullary space. These cells stained

Section C: Chronic Myeloproliferative Neoplasms and Myelodysplastic Syndromes
Systemic Mastocytosis with Associated Clonal Hematologic Non-Mast Cell-Lineage Disease

intensely positive for tryptase (**Figure 2**) and CD117 (**Figure 3**), and weakly positive for CD25 and for CD2 in a small subset. Aspirate smear and touch preparations showed numerous atypical mast cells, averaging 12%, including some spindle cells and oval cells with uneven distribution of granules (**Figure 4**). Increased monocytes that were strongly positive for esterase stain were also present. The 500-cell differential count of bone marrow aspirate smear: promyelocytes 1%, myelocytes 16%, metamyelocytes 11%, neutrophils+bands 21%, eosinophils 1%, lymphocytes 10%, plasma cells 2%, monocytes 8%, normoblasts 18%, mast cells 12%, M:E ratio 2.8:1. Erythrocytes, granulocytes and megakaryocytes were dysplastic. No excess blasts were identified. Flow cytometric analysis of bone marrow aspirate specimen demonstrated a mast cell population that expressed CD117, CD25, and dim CD2. Mutation was detected in codon 816 in exon 17 of the *KIT* gene by PCR-based DNA sequencing analysis (D816V). Serum tryptase was markedly elevated to 697.0 ng/mL (normal <11.5 ng/mL).

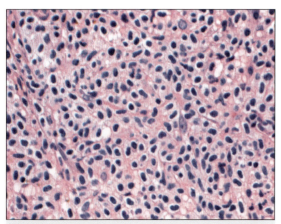

Figure 1 Bone marrow biopsy (H&E, ×400) showing sheets of oval mast cells tightly in aggregate.

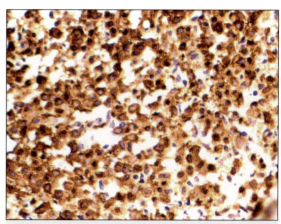

Figure 2 Bone marrow biopsy (tryptase stain, ×400) showing strong reactivity of oval cells.

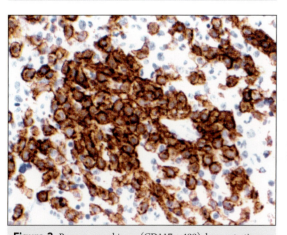

Figure 3 Bone marrow biopsy (CD117, ×400) demonstrating strong positivity of oval cells.

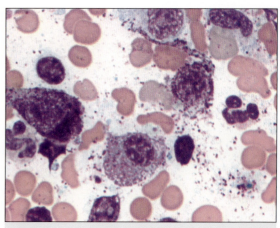

Figure 4 Bone marrow aspirate smear (Wright-Giemsa, ×1,000) showing atypical spindle or oval shaped mast cells with uneven distribution of cytoplasmic granules.

Final Diagnosis Systemic mastocytosis with associated clonal hematologic non-mast cell-lineage disease (SM-AHNMD) by the WHO criteria.

Management Approach There is currently no cure for systemic mastocytosis (SM). The prognosis of SM depends on the type of disease. Patients with high-grade (aggressive) disease may survive only a few months, whereas those with indolent SM usually have a normal life expectancy. Aggressive SM should be treated. If there is an associated hematologic malignancy, therapy should cover the non-mast cell lineage disease as well. Treatment options that have been attempted in some cases, with limited success in prolongation of survival, include chemotherapy (cladribine, imatinib), biological therapy (interferon-α) irradiation, hematopoietic progenitor cell transplant, and splenectomy. Agents used for symptomatic relief include nonsteroidal anti-inflammatory agents, glucocorticoids, ketotifen, and disodium cromoglycate. For this patient, who had extensive SM involving 60% of medullary space and 12% mast cells in aspirate smear, cladribine was used to treat the mast cell disease, as well as cytarabine for the associated chronic myelomoncytic leukemia (CMML). The patient responded to therapy but developed neutropenia and pneumonia.

General Discussion Systemic mastocytosis is characterized by involvement of at least one extracutaneous organ by a clonal neoplastic proliferation of mast cells. The diagnosis of SM can be made when the major criterion and one minor criterion or at least 3 minor criteria are present. The major diagnostic criterion by the WHO classification is a multifocal compact infiltrate of mast cells in bone marrow and/or other extracutaneous organs. The minor criteria include atypical morphology of mast cells, detection of point mutation of *KIT* at codon 816, aberrant immunophenotype with CD2 and/or CD25 expression, and persistent elevation of serum tryptase exceeding 20 ng/mL. SM may coexist with hematopoietic neoplasms, such as acute myeloid leukemia, myelodysplastic syndrome (MDS), myeloproliferative neoplasm (MPN), MDS/MPN, or less commonly lymphoproliferative disease, which is recognized as a subtype of SM in the WHO criteria as systemic mastocytosis with associated clonal hematologic non-mast cell lineage disease (SM-AHNMD). Careful evaluation of peripheral blood and bone marrow is crucial in identifying coexisting hematologic neoplasms. In this case, CMML was evident with absolute monocytosis in the blood, which was further supported by monocytosis and trilineage dysplasia in the bone marrow. CMML is the most common hematologic neoplasm associated with SM.

Congenital Polycythemia

Josef T Prchal, Sujata Narayanan

Patient A 17-year-old Caucasian female, who was referred to our institution for management of previously diagnosed polycythemia vera.

Clinical History The patient was diagnosed with polycythemia vera at the age of 5 years. Her laboratory studies, especially her hemoglobin and hematocrit prior to age 5, were not available. By records, it was known that she had increased red cell volume and a normal hemoglobin oxygen dissociation curve (normal p50). The patient had regular follow-up with a pediatric hematologist/oncologist, and her bone marrow aspiration and biopsy, which revealed erythroid hyperplasia, were interpreted as being consistent with polycythemia vera. She was being treated with phlebotomies every 2 months-3 months. A year before her current presentation, she was started on hydroxyurea because of neurological symptoms thought to be secondary to complications of polycythemia. She was then referred to our clinic for further evaluation. She had normal leukocyte and platelet counts and on exam there was no evidence of splenomegaly. She did not have any previous history of thrombotic complications, erythromelalgia, or aquagenic pruritus. The investigations for possible congenital polycythemia were then initiated.

Family History The patient was adopted and no family history was available.

Medications Hydroxyurea, fluoxetine, lisdexamfetamine.

Physical Examination She appeared well and her vital signs were normal. Her head and neck exam was remarkable for facial erythema. Her skin was otherwise without erythema or rashes. Her spleen was not palpable. Her exam was otherwise unremarkable.

Initial Work-Up on Presentation for Further Evaluation at age 17

CBC		WBC Differential	%	# (×10³/μL)
WBC (×10³/μL)	5.4	Neutrophils	50.5	2.7
RBC (×10⁶/μL)	5.83	Bands	0	
HGB (g/dL)	14.9	Lymphocytes	39.9	2.2
HCT (%)	46.8	Monocytes	5.6	0.3
MCV (fL)	80.2	Eosinophils	3.1	0.2
MCH (pg)	25.6	Basophils	0.8	0.0
MCHC (g/dL)	31.9			
PLT (×10³/μL)	224			
RDW-CV (%)	16.3			
MPV (fL)	8.1			

Peripheral blood smear revealed no morphologic abnormalities.

Differential Diagnosis Polycythemia vera vs congenital polycythemia.

Additional Work-Up
- Arterial and venous blood gases showed normal arterial oxygen saturation and venous blood gases were used for estimation of p50 (1), and the calculated p50 was 27.2 (normal 24-31)
- Erythropoietin level: 34.5 (normal 3-27)
- *JAK2* V671F mutation: negative
- Peripheral blood mononuclear cells were used for measurement of the response of erythroid progenitors to erythropoietin. The erythroid progenitor hypersensitivity to erythropoietin, but not independence from erythropoietin was found
- Sequencing of von Hippel-Lindau gene: no mutation found
- Sequencing of proline hydroxylase type 2 gene: no mutation found

Sequencing of HIF-2 α gene showed a nonsynonymous mutation at exon 12 of the EPAS1/HIF2 α gene changing the amino acid at codon 537 from glycine to arginine.

Final Diagnosis Congenital polycythemia secondary to augmented hypoxic response resulting in increased erythropoietin levels and yet unexplained increased sensitivity of erythroid progenitors to erythropoietin.

Management Approach The management of congenital polycythemia is unknown. In those patients with increased hemoglobin affinity to oxygen, which leads to decreased delivery of oxygen to tissues, phlebotomies are not recommended, as these may further decrease the hemoglobin oxygen carrying capacity and thus decreased tissue oxygen delivery. Sufficient clinical data about value of therapeutic phlebotomies has been generated from another disorder of augmented hypoxic response, ie, Chuvash polycythemia. In this population, the phlebotomized and nonphlebotomized patients had the same risk of cerebrovascular thrombosis. This patient is being followed by hematology but with no specific intervention being taken at present. Her hemoglobin remains stable in the normal range.

General Discussion Congenital polycythemia is suspected when disease onset is at an early age or there is a positive family history of polycythemia. The first described congenital polycythemias were due to globin mutations leading to increased hemoglobin oxygen affinity and thus decreased oxygen delivery to tissues. A much more rare cause is congenital deficiency of 2,3-diphosphoglycerate (DPG) deficiency, both of these entities are characterized by decreased p50; ie, increased hemoglobin oxygen affinity). Hypoxia is a potent stimulator of erythropoiesis via the oxygen sensor signaling pathways. It results in increased production of hypoxia inducible factors (HIF1 and HIF2; composed of 2 subunits HIFα and HIFβ), which are transcription factors responsible for the production of erythropoietin. They also augment iron supplies to the cells, by augmentation of transferrin gene transcription and decreased transcription of hepcidin. There are many other genes that are regulated by HIF transcription factors. It is estimated that in endothelial cells, 3% of all genes are HIF regulated. The α subunits of HIF1 and HIF2 are rapidly destroyed in the presence of oxygen. This is initiated by proline hydroxylase domain-containing enzymes. The prolyl hydroxylated α subunits of HIF1 and HIF2 can then interact with the von Hippel-Lindau tumor suppressor protein, which leads to ubiquitination of the complex, which is rapidly degraded in the proteosome. However, under the absence of oxygen (hypoxia), the degradation of HIF-α is abrogated, HIF1 and HIF2 levels increase, which leads to augmentation of transcription of erythropoietin and many other genes. The effect of erythropoietin on cells is transmitted by a specific erythropoietin receptor, and certain mutations (gain-of-function mutations) of this receptor, that delete its negative regulatory domain, have been associated with some cases of congenital and familial polycythemia.

The classification of congenital polycythemia is as follows:

Decreased p50 (partial pressure of oxygen at which 50% of hemoglobin is saturated with oxygen)
- High-oxygen-affinity hemoglobinopathy
- 2,3-Bisphosphoglycerate deficiency
- Methemoglobinemia
- Normal p50

VHL mutations including Chuvash polycythemia:
- PHD2 mutations
- HIF2-α mutations (increased sensitivity of erythroid progenitors to erythropoietin by yet unknown mechanism)
- EPOR mutations (autosomal dominant) gain of function, leading to increased erythropoietin signaling, leading to compensatory decrease in EPO level and increases sensitivity of erythroid progenitors to erythropoietin

Myeloproliferative Neoplasm, Unclassifiable

John Anastasi

Patient A 73-year-old female, who presented for evaluation prior to cataract surgery.

Clinical History The patient has a history of coronary artery disease, hypertension and adult onset diabetes. She has no history of thrombosis, bleeding or hematologic disease.

Family History Sister with breast cancer; nephew with leukemia.

Medication None.

Physical Examination Unremarkable.

Initial Work-Up

CBC		
WBC (×10³/μL)	9.0	
RBC (×10⁶/μL)	3.63	
HGB (g/dL)	10.9	
HCT (%)	33.5	
MCV (fL)	80.3	
MCH (pg)	30.0	
MCHC (g/dL)	32.5	
PLT (×10³/μL)	591	
RDW-CV (%)	17.8	
WBC Differential	**%**	**# (×10³/μL)**
Neutrophils	54	4.9
Bands	4	0.4
Lymphocytes	32	2.9
Monocytes	6	0.5
Eosinophils	2	0.2
Basophils	2	0.2

Peripheral blood smear revealed slightly microcytic red cells and occasional elliptocytes, but there were no teardrop cells, left shift, or leukoerythroblastosis (**Figure 1**).

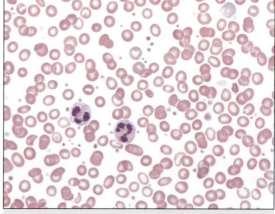

Figure 1 Peripheral blood smear (Wright-Giemsa, ×500) showing mild anisocytosis, microcytic hypochromic red cells, and thrombocytosis.

Differential Diagnosis Reactive thrombocytosis vs essential thrombocytosis, vs primary myelofibrosis, vs other myeloproliferative neoplasm (MPN).

Additional Work-Up The patient was found to have iron deficiency, for which she was treated with oral iron. A *JAK2* V617F mutation was detected. A bone marrow biopsy was undertaken to clarify the nature of the suspected myeloproliferative neoplasm. The marrow was normocellular (**Figure 2**). Megakaryocytes were slightly elevated without clustering (**Figure 3**). Some were normal, others were large with abundant cytoplasm or small with nuclear atypia and karyorrhexis (**Figure 4**). Background hematopoiesis was a mix of myeloid and erythroid cells with a normal ratio of 2.5:1. There were trace iron stores and no significant increase in reticulin fibrosis (**Figures 5** and **6**). Cytogenetic analysis: normal female karyotype. Additional molecular studies: *BCR-ABL1*-negative.

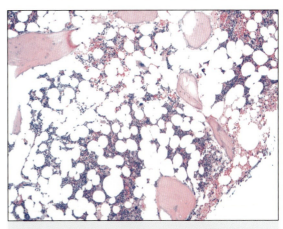

Figure 2 Bone marrow biopsy (H&E, ×100) showing nonmolecular storage.

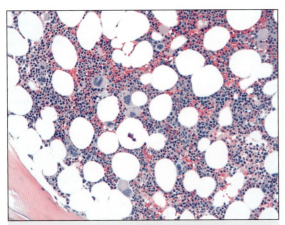

Figure 3 Bone marrow biopsy (H&E, ×200) showing slighly increasing granulocytes without clustering. Background hematopoiesis is myelod and erythroid (normal rates).

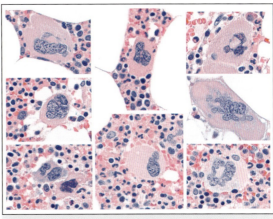

Figure 4 Bone marrow biopsy (H&E, ×500) composite of megakaryocytes. Left column, variable megakaryocytes like in PMF; middle column, normal megakaryocytes; right column, large forms with abundant cytoplasm and nuclear lobulation like in ET.

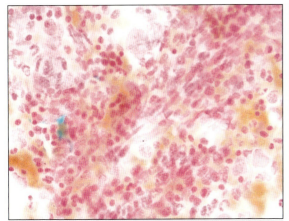

Figure 5 Bone marrow aspirate smear (Prussian blue, ×400) shows trace iron stores (blue).

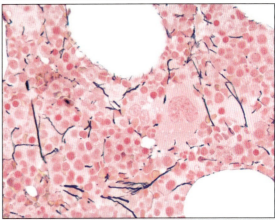

Figure 6 Bone marrow biopsy (reticulin silver stain, ×500) shows minimal reticulin fibrosis.

Section C: Chronic Myeloproliferative Neoplasms and Myelodysplastic Syndromes
Myeloproliferative Neoplasm, Unclassifiable

Final Diagnosis Myeloproliferative neoplasm, unclassifiable, *JAK2* V617F-positive.

Management Approach There is no standard treatment for an early phase of an MPN as in this case. Patients over 60 years of age with previous thrombotic events are at risk for further thromboses Patients with platelet counts over 1.5 million/μL are treated with hydroxyurea or anagrelide to reduce the counts. JAK2 inhibitors are being evaluated in trials, but are not generally available. In this case the patient was treated conservatively (observation) and had no complications for 1 year.

General Discussion The *BCR-ABL1* negative MPN include polycythemia vera (PV), essential thrombocythemia (ET), and primary myelofibrosis (PMF). Although the diagnosis and separation of one from another can be straightforward, the clinical, pathologic and genetic findings overlap, so a clear diagnosis cannot sometimes be made. In 3 situations it may be best to consider the process "unclassifiable."

These include (a) when disease is early and diagnostic features needed to distinguish one from another are not yet apparent; (b) when the disease presents in an advanced stage such that distinguishing characteristics are overshadowed by end-stage fibrosis; or (c) when the initial presentation is complicated by co-morbidities that obscure the diagnosis.

In the case presented, the MPN is in an early phase so that distinguishing characteristics are not apparent. The lack of polycythemia (particularly after correction of the low iron) would rule out PV, and the lack of a leukoerythroblastic picture, fibrosis and sinusoidal hematopoiesis all rule out the fibrotic stage of PMF. However, none of the findings are helpful in distinguishing ET from what has been termed the "prefibrotic stage of PMF." The bone marrow did not show all of the features typical of ET or those of prefibrotic PMF. The *JAK2* mutation was little help as it can be seen in either process. In this case we favored the designation of MPN "unclassifiable."

Refractory Anemia with Ring Sideroblasts

Cheryl Hanau, Bhavna Khandpur, Steve Hou

Patient A 76-year-old woman presented with progressive weakness for the past 1 year.

Clinical History Significant for gastroesophageal reflux disease (GERD).

Family History Noncontributory.

Medications Diazepam, ibuprofen.

Physical examination Unremarkable.

Initial Work-Up		
CBC		
WBC (×10³/μL)	5.0	
RBC (×10⁶/μL)	2.17	
HGB (g/dL)	7.0	
HCT (%)	21.3	
MCV (fL)	98	
MCH (pg)	32.3	
MCHC (g/dL)	32.9	
PLT (×10³/μL)	114	
RDW-CV (%)	21.3	
MPV (fL)	10.1	
WBC Differential	**%**	**# (×10³/μL)**
Neutrophils	58	2.9
Bands	4	0.2
Lymphocytes	32	1.6
Monocytes	4	0.2
Eosinophils	2	0.1
Basophils	0	

Blood smear review revealed anisopoikilocytosis, microcytic red cells, macrocytic red cells, and a few teardrop cells. Occasional nucleated red cells were also present (**Figure 1**).

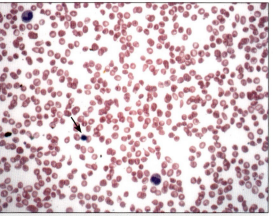

Figure 1 Blood smear (Wright-Giemsa, ×100) showing anisopoikilocytosis, macrocytic red cells, microcytic red cells, elliptocytes and a few teardrop cells. A nucleated red cell is also seen (arrow).

Differential Diagnosis Diagnostic considerations based on findings of bicytopenia and MCV near upper end of normal included megaloblastic (vitamin B_{12} and folate deficiency) and nonmegaloblastic causes. The latter category included conditions such as acute blood loss, hemolysis, bone marrow infiltration, high levels of erythropoietin associated with bone marrow failure, excessive alcohol intake, liver disease, hypothyroidism, myelodysplastic syndrome, and secondary myelodysplasia.

Section C: Chronic Myeloproliferative Neoplasms and Myelodysplastic Syndromes
Refractory Anemia with Ring Sideroblasts

Additional Work-Up

Serum chemistries:
- Folate 17 ng/mL (normal 4-20)
- Red cell folate 200 ng/mL (normal 166-640)
- Vitamin B_{12} 400 mg/mL (normal 200-900)
- Total protein 6.0 g/dL (normal 6.0-7.8) with albumin 3.4 g/dL (normal 3.2-4.5)
- AST 28 U/L (normal 8-33), ALT 20 U/L (normal 4-36)
- Bone marrow biopsy was hypercellular (50%-60 %) and showed marked erythroid hyperplasia (**Figure 2**). The granulocytic and megakaryocytic series were proportionately normal without abnormal localization of immature precursors. Stainable iron was markedly increased
- The aspirate smears revealed morphologically unremarkable megakaryocytes. The erythroid series showed full differentiation with megaloblastoid changes, and bi- and multinucleated erythroid precursors (**Figure 3**). The granulocytic series showed full differentiation with no increase in blasts. Iron stain revealed 30%-40% ringed sideroblasts (**Figure 4**). The M:E ratio was estimated at 2.2:1
- Flow cytometry performed on the aspirate did not reveal any immunophenotypic abnormalities
- Marrow cytogenetics: 46, XX, del(7)(q22q34)

Final Diagnosis Refractory anemia with ring sideroblasts.

Management Approach The patient's IPSS (International Prognostic Scoring System), age and performance status are used in planning therapeutic because they provide a risk-based clinical evaluation. The options for MDS include supportive care, low-intensity therapy, high-intensity therapy, and/or clinical trial. Patients with IPSS (low/intermediate 1) are categorized on the basis of serum erythropoietin (sEpo). Those with levels <500 mU/mL should be treated with recombinant human erythropoietin (Epo) with or without granulocyte colony stimulating factor (G-CSF). Nonresponders should be treated with hypomethylating agents or by lenalidomide therapy. This patient was treated with supportive care.

General Discussion Refractory anemia with ringed sideroblasts (RARS) is a myelodysplastic syndrome (MDS) characterized by anemia, morphologic dysplasia in the erythroid lineage and ring sideroblasts comprising ≥15% of bone marrow erythroid precursors. On an iron-stained aspirate smear, 15% or more of

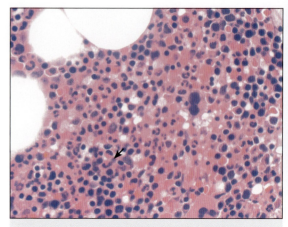

Figure 2 Bone marrow biopsy (H&E, ×400) showing hypercellular marrow with erythroid hyperplasia (arrows).

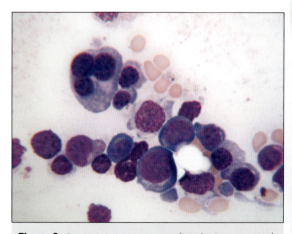

Figure 3 Bone marrow aspirate smear (Wright-Giemsa, ×1000) showing marked erythroid proliferation and dysplastc features in erythroid series, multinucleated erythroid precursor and megaloblastic changes.

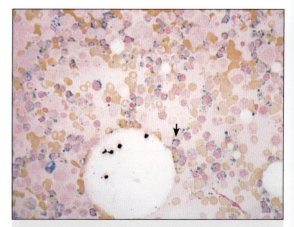

Figure 4 Bone marrow aspirate smear (Prussian blue, ×400) showing numerous ring sideroblasts, as defined by 5 or more iron granules encircling ⅓ or more of the nucleus (arrow).

the red cell precursors are ring sideroblasts, which are defined by 5 or more granules encircling ⅓ of the nucleus. There is no significant dysplasia in the nonerythroid lineages. Myeloblasts comprise <5% of the nucleated bone marrow (BM) cells and are not present in the peripheral blood (PB). Ring sideroblasts (RS) represent erythroid precursors with abnormal accumulation within the mitochondria including some deposited as mitochrondrial ferritin. A primary defect of the mitochondrial iron metabolism is suspected, the defect being caused by somatic mutations or deletions in nuclear or mitochondrial DNA. Primary defects or acquired mutations in heme synthesis have not been demonstrated. Ring sideroblasts may be observed in other types of MDS. When RS are 15% or more of the erythroid precursors but there are 10% or more dysplastic cells in any nonerythroid lineage and blasts are <1% in the PB and <5% in BM with no Auer rods or monocytosis, the case is classified as refractory cytopenia with multilineage dysplasia (RCMD). Aberrant immunophenotypic features of erythroid precursors may be found in RARS by flow cytometric analysis. Clonal chromosomal abnormalities are seen in 5%-20% of cases of RARS and when present typically involve a single chromosome.

Refractory Anemia with Ring Sideroblasts Associated with Marked Thrombocytosis

Yang O Huh

Patient A 68-year-old woman presented with complaints of fatigue and dyspnea on exertion for several months.

Clinical History The patient had a history of low white blood cell count for >10 years, but no specific diagnosis had been made. 10 years following the initial diagnosis of leukopenia, she was noted to have anemia, and a bone marrow biopsy revealed refractory cytopenia with multilineage dysplasia and increased ring sideroblasts. Platelet count at the time was $310 \times 10^3/\mu L$. 3 months later, her platelet count rose to $1,597 \times 10^3/\mu L$ and her hemoglobin was 8.4 g/dL. She was transfusion dependent.

Family History Noncontributory.

Medications None.

Physical Examination Unremarkable. No lymphadenopathy or hepatosplenomegaly.

Initial Work-Up		
CBC		
WBC ($\times 10^3/\mu L$)	4.2	
RBC ($\times 10^6/\mu L$)	3.01	
HGB (g/dL)	8.4	
HCT (%)	27.7	
MCV (fL)	92	
MCH (pg)	27.9	
MCHC (g/dL)	30.3	
PLT ($\times 10^3/\mu L$)	1,597	
RDW-CV (%)	27.1	
MPV (fL)	10.1	
WBC Differential	**%**	**# ($\times 10^3/\mu L$)**
Neutrophils	63	2.6
Bands	0	
Lymphocytes	29	1.2
Monocytes	1	
Eosinophils	3	0.1
Basophils	3	0.1
Metamyelocytes	1	

Peripheral blood smear revealed markedly increased platelets with anisocytosis and occasional giant platelets (**Figure 1**).

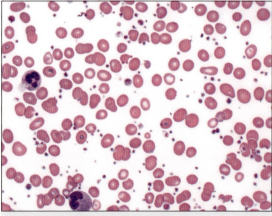

Figure 1 Blood smear (Wright-Giemsa, ×500) showing marked thrombocytosis with occasional giant platelets. Red blood cells showed moderate anisopoikilocytosis with some dacrocytes, ovalocytes, and mild polychromasia. Neutrophils were adequate and mildly dyspoietic with rare cells showing abnormal nuclear segmentations.

Differential Diagnosis Diagnostic considerations included myelodysplastic syndrome (MDS), myeloproliferative neoplasm (MPN), and myelodysplastic/myeloproliferative neoplasm, unclassifiable.

Additional Work-Up Bone marrow biopsy was hypercellular with erythroid predominance, marked atypical megakaryocytic hyperplasia, and mild reticulin fibrosis (**Figure 2**). Aspirate smears showed dysplastic

Section C: Chronic Myeloproliferative Neoplasms and Myelodysplastic Syndromes
Refractory Anemia with Ring Sideroblasts Associated with Marked Thrombocytosis

erythroid hyperplasia and markedly increased dysplastic megakaryocytes. Megakaryocytes were enlarged with abundant amount of cytoplasm and deeply lobulated nuclei. Also identified are atypical forms with multiple separated nuclear lobes (**Figure 3**). Granulocytes were decreased with mild dysplastic features. Blasts were patchy and at 4%. Iron stain of aspirate smear showed markedly increased number of ring sideroblasts, up to 86% of the all erythroid precursors (**Figure 4**). Cytogenetic analysis revealed a normal diploid karyotype. No mutation at codon 617 of JAK2 was identified.

Final Diagnosis Refractory anemia with ring sideroblasts (RARS) associated with marked thrombocytosis (RARS-T) (2008 WHO classification).

Management Approach The current literature does not provide enough information regarding the outcome of patients with RARS-T. Compared to patients with essential thrombocythemia (ET), patients with RARS-T have a worse outcome, more similar to that of patients with RARS. The available evidence is insufficient for recommending any specific treatment. For this patient, who was evaluated by us for a second opinion, recommendations to the referring physician included trial of a combination of filgrastim and erythropoietin, and low-dose anagrelide. The patient was treated with a combination of low dose vidaza, filgrastim, and erythropoietin. She responded well to treatment and became transfusion-independent. At a follow-up visit 4 months after initiation of treatment, her hemoglobin was 10 g/dL and platelet count was $189 \times 10^3/\mu L$.

General Discussion Refractory anemia with ring sideroblasts associated with marked thrombocytosis (RARS-T) has clinical and morphologic features of both MDS and MPN. Patients with RARS-T typically present with severe anemia and marked thrombocytosis. Bone marrow shows atypical erythroid proliferation and prominent ringed sideroblasts, at least 15% of the erythroid precursors on iron stain. In addition, abnormal megakaryocytes resembling those seen in essential thrombocythemia should be present. The cut-off for platelet has been lowered to $450 \times 10^3/\mu L$ from $600 \times 10^3/\mu L$ in the 2008 WHO classification to be consistent with the criteria for ET. In support of a myeloproliferative component of this neoplasm, the majority of cases (about 60%) with RARS-T carry the JAK2 mutation, but JAK2 mutation is not a diagnostic criterion. Less commonly, the MPL W515K/L mutation has been reported. Cases with isolated del(5q), t(3;3)(q21;q26) or inv(3)(q21q26) are excluded from this category. RARS-T is a provisional entity under the category of myelodysplastic/myeloproliferative neoplasm in the 2008 WHO classification.

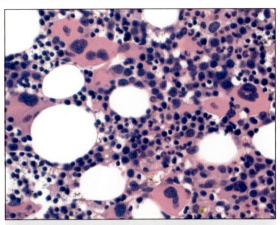

Figure 2 Bone marrow biopsy (H&E, ×400) showing hypercellularity with erythroid hyperplasia and dysplastic megakaryocytic proliferation.

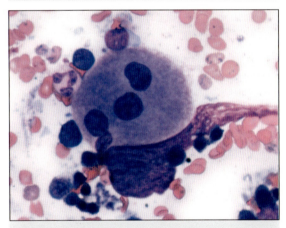

Figure 3 Bone marrow aspirate smear (Wright-Giemsa, ×1000) showing a dysplastic megakaryocyte with abnormal nuclear lobation.

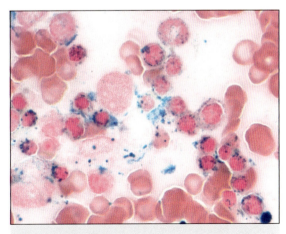

Figure 4 Bone marrow aspirate smear (Prussian blue, ×1000) showing numerous ring sideroblasts.

Refractory Cytopenia with Multilineage Dysplasia

Cheryl Hanau, Bhavna Khandpur, Steve Hou

Patient A 58-year-old female presented with progressive fatigue.

Clinical History The patient stated that she had had low blood counts for the past 5 years and has had 2 prior nondiagnostic bone marrow procedures.

Family History Her mother has coronary artery disease and brother has colon cancer.

Medication History Sustained-release oxycodone, Clonazepam, acetaminophen/oxycodone.

Clinical Examination Notable for left supraclavicular lymphadenopathy.

Initial Work-Up

CBC		WBC Differential	%	# (×10³/μL)
WBC (×10³/μL)	2.0	Neutrophils	68.4	1.4
RBC (×10⁶/μL)	3.70	Lymphocytes	23.0	0.5
HGB (g/dL)	9.5	Monoocytes	7.1	0.1
HCT (%)	28.7	Eosinophils	1.5	0.0
MCV (fL)	78	Basophils	0	
MCH (pg)	25.7	Nucleated red cells	12/100 WBC	
MCHC (g/dL)	33.1			
PLT (×10³/μL)	151			
RDW-CV (%)	15.4			
MPV (fL)	10			

Peripheral blood smear revealed anisopoikilocytosis, microcytic red cells, macrocytic red cells, polychromasia, few target cells, occasional teardrop cells, and nucleated red cells with bi- and trinucleation (**Figures 1** and **2**). Pseudo-Pelger-Huët cells were also present (**Figure 3**).

Differential Diagnosis The conditions associated with bicytopenia, circulating nucleated red cells, and dysplastic features in erythroid and granulocytic lineages include metastatic involvement of marrow, myelodsysplastic process (primary and secondary), myelofibrosis, acute leukemia (aleukemic phase), viral infection, immunodeficiency process, nutritional deficiency (vitamin B_{12}/folate), and exposure to heavy metals or other toxins. Clinical history and presentation along with the peripheral blood findings led us to consider myelodysplastic syndrome (MDS) as the most likely diagnosis.

Additional Work-Up Bone marrow biopsy was hypercellular (60%) with mild erythroid hyperplasia. Megakaryocytes were present in adequate number and many were dysplastic (**Figure 4**). Stainable iron was present. Bone

Section C: Chronic Myeloproliferative Neoplasms and Myelodysplastic Syndromes
Refractory Cytopenia with Multilineage Dysplasia

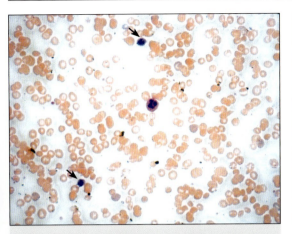

Figure 1 Blood smear (Wright-Giemsa, ×400) showing anisocytosis, microcytic red cells, macrocytic red cells, hypochromasia, and nucleated red cells with dysplastic changes (arrows).

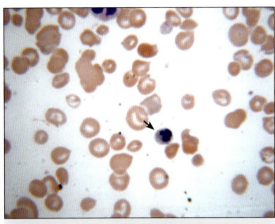

Figure 2 Blood smear (Wright-Giemsa, ×1000) showing anisocytosis, microcytic red cells, macrocytic red cells, polychromasia, and a dysplastic nucleated red cell (arrow).

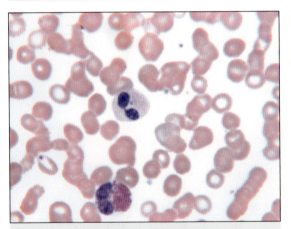

Figure 3 Blood smear (Wright Giemsa, ×1000) showing a pseudo-Pelger-Huët cell.

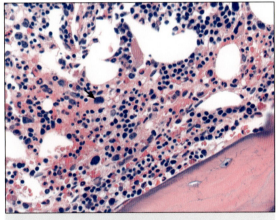

Figure 4 Bone marrow biopsy (H&E, ×400) showing hypercellular marrow with micromegakaryocytes (arrows).

marrow aspirate was diluted with blood and therefore the differential count was performed on biopsy touch imprint. Blasts comprised 2% of bone marrow cellular elements. The myeloid to erythroid ratio (M:E ratio) was estimated at 0.8:1. Dysplastic features were also noted in the erythroid series. Myeloid series showed maturation without abnormal localization of precursors. Flow cytometry performed on bone marrow aspirate demonstrated an abnormal pattern of expression of the myeloid markers CD13/CD16 and HLA-DR and CD11b. Cytogenetic analysis showed a normal female karyotype (46, XX).

Final Diagnosis Refractory cytopenia with multilineage dysplasia (myelodysplastic syndrome).

Management Approach The patient's International Prognostic Scoring System (IPSS), age and performance status are used in planning therapeutic options because they provide a risk-based clinical evaluation. The options for MDS include supportive care, chemotherapy or immune suppressive therapy. Supportive care includes blood transfusions, platelet transfusions, and myeloid growth factors such as filgrastim (G-CSF), sargramostim (GM-CSF), and/or erythroid growth factors—erythropoietin (EPO) or darbepoietin. Chemotherapy may be a treatment option for patients with high IPSS risk score who are in good overall health but do not have a suitable donor for hematopoietic progenitor cell transplant (HPCT). The only known treatment that can bring about a long-term remission from MDS is HPCT. Induction chemotherapy may be used to bring MDS into remission before a patient receives HPCT. In recent years, 3 medicines have been approved by the FDA specifically to treat MDS. These are azacitidine, decitabine and lenalidomide. Azacitidine and decitabine are approved to treat all types of MDS, and lenalidomide is approved to treat only the 5q– syndrome type of MDS. These therapies may be used "upfront" or for patients with low risk disease who fail supportive care strategies discussed above. This patient was treated with supportive care.

General Discussion Refractory anemia with multilineage dysplasia (RCMD) is a type of myelodysplastic syndrome (MDS) that is characterized by the presence of one or more cytopenias and dysplastic changes in 2 or more of the myeloid lineages. Blasts account for <1% of peripheral blood (PB) cells and <5% of bone marrow (BM) nucleated cells. Auer rods are not present and absolute monocyte count in the blood is $<1 \times 10^3/\mu L$. The recommended levels for defining cytopenias are Hb <10 g/dL, absolute neutrophil count is $< 1.8 \times 10^3/\mu L$ and platelet count $< 100 \times 10^3/\mu L$. However, values in excess of these thresholds do not exclude a diagnosis of MDS if definitive morphologic or cytogenetic findings are consistent with a diagnosis. The threshold for dysplasia is >10% of the cells in each of the affected cell lines. Dysplasia may be defined as the presence of one or more of the following features in individual cell lines. Erythroid precursors may show abnormal nuclear morphology megaloblastoid or megaloblastic changes, irregular shape, internuclear chromatin bridging, multilobation, nuclear budding, and/or cytoplasmic vacuoles. Granulocytes may reveal hypogranulatiogranulation, hyposegmentation, (pseudo-Pelger-Huët cells), hypersegmentation, structurally abnormal segmentation, hyperchromatic nuclei and Döhle bodies. Megakaryocytes may be small (micromegakaryocytes), hypolobated (mono or bi), hyperlobated and may show separation of nuclear lobes. Many of these dysplastic features are seen in the bone marrow. Peripheral blood may or may not reveal any of the dysplastic features. When present, blood findings typically include macrocytic red cells (round or oval), pseudo-Pelger-Huët cells, and Döhle bodies.

There is a generally good correlation between the percentage of blasts by morphologic examination of and percentage of CD34 + cells determined by flow cytometry (FC). Erythroid abnormalities, as determined by the pattern of expression of CD71 and CD105 in glycophorin A (GPA)-positive nucleated cells, reportedly can predict morphologic dysplasia with 98% sensitivity. Aberrant maturation patterns in granulopoiesis could predict morphological dysplasia and abnormal cytogenetics in approximately 90% of cases. However, flow cytometry is limited in cases with borderline dysplasia by morphology and no cytogenetic abnormalities. Clonal cytogenetic abnormalities are observed in around 50% of MDS cases. The importance of cytogenetic studies as a prognostic indicator in MDS has been recognized and codified by the International Myelodysplastic Syndrome Working Group. Three major risk categories have been defined: (a) good risk: normal karyotype, isolated del (5q), isolated del (20q) and –Y, (b) poor risk: complex abnormalities, ie, ≥3 abnormalities or abnormalities of chromosome 7; and (c) intermediate risk: all other abnormalities.

Refractory Anemia with Excess Blasts-2

Raymond E Felgar, James T Edinger, Louis Pietragallo

Patient An 84-year-old woman with petechiae on her legs and ecchymoses at recent venipuncture sites on the arms.

Clinical History The patient had fatigue but no other symptoms.

Family History Noncontributory.

Medications Raloxifene, calcium, vitamin E.

Physical Examination Notable only for generalized pallor, ecchymoses and petechiae.

Initial Work-Up

CBC

WBC (×10³/µL)	1.4
RBC (×10⁶/µL)	2.02
HGB (g/dL)	8.0
HCT (%)	23.7
MCV (fL)	117.1
MCH (pg)	39.4
MCHC (g/dL)	33.7
PLT (×10³/µL)	73
RDW-CV (%)	16.5

WBC Differential	%	# (×10³/µL)
Neutrophils	20	.3
Bands	2	
Lymphocytes	60	.8
Monocytes	12	.2
Eosinophils	2	
Basophils	1	
Metamyelocytes	1	
Blasts	2	

Peripheral blood smear revealed mild anisocytosis, toxic granulation, and decreased platelets with occasional large forms, along with rare circulating blasts (**Figure 1**).

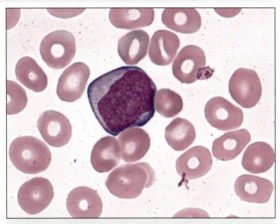

Figure 1 Blood smear (Wright-Giemsa, ×1000) showing a representative blast.

Differential Diagnosis Diagnostic considerations included megaloblastic anemia, myelodysplastic syndrome, and acute leukemia.

Additional Work-Up
- Serum vitamin B_{12}: 166 pg/mL (normal 200-1,100)
- Serum folate, LDH, AST, ALT, reticulocyte count, and total bilirubin were all normal

Bone marrow examination revealed increased blasts on aspirate (14.5%), with no Auer rods. Some intermediate myeloid cells appeared to be hypogranular.

Section C: Chronic Myeloproliferative Neoplasms and Myelodysplastic Syndromes
Refractory Anemia with Excess Blasts-2

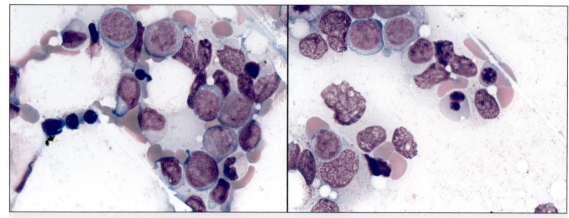

Figure 2 Bone marrow aspirate smear (Wright-Giemsa, ×500) demonstrating numerous blasts with fine chromatin, prominent nucleoli, increased nuclear cytoplasmic ratio, and basophilic cytoplasm. Dyserythropoietic forms were also seen.

Erythroid maturation was slightly megaloblastoid, with dyserythropoietic forms (**Figure 2**). Marrow biopsy was variably cellular (5%-40%), with numerous blasts, both singly and in clusters, and markedly decreased megakaryocytes (**Figure 3**). CD117 and CD34 stains showed many interstitial blasts (**Figure 4**).

Flow cytometric studies on marrow demonstrated increased myeloblasts with the following immunophenotype: CD45 (dim+), CD34+, CD117+, CD33+, CD13+, HLA-DR+, CD36 (partial+), myeloperoxidase (partial+), with negative staining for CD64, CD19, CD56, CD7, CD11b, CD15, and CD3.

Cytogenetic studies showed a normal female karyotype, 46,XX.

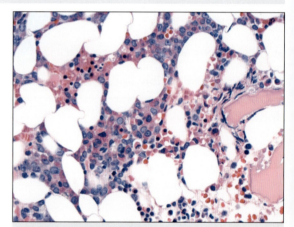

Figure 3 Bone marrow biopsy (H&E, ×400) demonstrating numerous blasts with fine chromatin, increased nuclear cytoplasmic ratio, and conspicuous nucleoli both singly and in clusters.

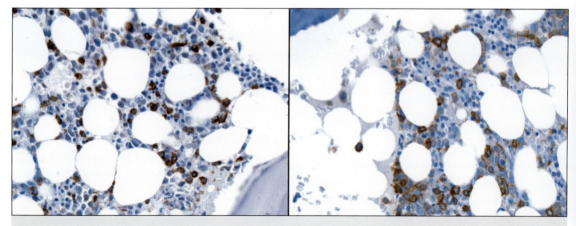

Figure 4 Bone marrow biopsy (CD34 and CD117 stains with hematoxylin nuclear counterstain) highlighting increased blasts and immature precursors with occasional clusters located away from the bony trabeculae. This feature is sometimes referred to as "ALIP" (abnormal localization of immature precursors).

Final Diagnosis Refractory anemia with excess blasts, type 2 (RAEB-2).

Management Approach Therapy for refractory anemia with excess blasts (RAEB) can involve hypomethylating agents (azacitidine and decitabine), other chemotherapeutic agents, and supportive measures (ie, growth factors, erythropoietin, and transfusion). Allogeneic hematopoietic progenitor cell transplantation (HPCT) is the only potentially curative therapy, but many patients do not qualify due to other comorbidities. Initially, B_{12} injections were given with no improvement of her anemia. Marrow examination was then performed to establish a diagnosis. Given the guarded prognosis, the patient was offered chemotherapy with hypomethylating agents. Due to the possible risks, the patient declined chemotherapy and chose supportive care with granulocyte-colony stimulating factor and erythropoietin. She was generally asymptomatic, requiring only minimal transfusion.

General Discussion RAEB is a myelodysplastic syndrome (MDS) with 5%-19% myeloblasts in bone marrow and/or 2%-19% blasts in blood. Due to differences in survival and risk of progression to acute leukemia, RAEB has been divided into RAEB-1 (5%-9% blasts in bone marrow and/or 2%-4% blasts in blood) and RAEB-2 (10%-19% blasts in bone marrow and/or 5%-19% blasts in blood). The presence of Auer rods indicates a diagnosis of RAEB-2, regardless of blast count. RAEB accounts for almost 40% of MDS cases, with most patients over 50 years of age. Signs and symptoms are often related to cytopenias and bone marrow failure. Blood examination often shows dyspoiesis of multiple cell lines, including anisopoikilocytosis, large or hypogranular platelets, and abnormalities of neutrophil granularity or nuclear segmentation. Blasts are often identified. Bone marrow is usually hypercellular, but may be hypocellular, normocellular or fibrotic. Dyspoietic changes must be seen in $\geq$10% of cells within a given lineage to consider it dysplastic. Erythropoiesis is often increased with nuclear budding or lobulation. Granulopoiesis is generally increased with abnormalities of granularity and nuclear segmentation. Megakaryocytes may be increased, with normal-sized and small forms (micromegakaryocytes), as well as multinucleated forms with widely-spaced nuclei. Blasts may be seen in abnormal, interstitial clusters, often referred to as abnormal localization of immature precursors (ALIP), which can be highlighted by CD34 or CD117 stains. CD61 or CD41 stains may emphasize abnormal megakaryocytes. Blasts in RAEB are usually positive for CD34, CD117, CD38, HLA-DR, CD13, and CD33. Aberrant expression of CD7 (a T/NK lineage marker) may correlate with a poor prognosis. Many cases of RAEB will have normal cytogenetic studies, but 30%-50% will have clonal abnormalities including +8, −5, −7, del(5q), del(7q), del(20q), and complex karyotypes. RAEB has a poor prognosis with progression to marrow failure and/or leukemia; 25% of RAEB-1 and 33% of RAEB-2 cases progress to acute myeloid leukemia (AML). The median survival for RAEB-1 and RAEB-2 is 16 and 9 months, respectively. RAEB-2 patients with 5%-19% circulating blasts have a median survival of 3 months, similar to that of MDS-related AML. Cases classified as RAEB-2 based on the presence of Auer rods have a median survival of 12 months, similar to patients with 2%-4% circulating blasts.

Myelodysplastic Syndrome with Isolated del(5q)

Raymond E Felgar, Amanda L Wilson, Sara A Monaghan

Patient An 84-year-old Caucasian man with pancytopenia.

Clinical History The patient has a history of diverticulitis, atrial fibrillation, hypertension and type II diabetes. He had had prior removal of tubular adenomas.

Family History Noncontributory.

Medications Repaglinide, diltiazem, digoxin, lovastatin, and ranitidine.

Physical Examination Unremarkable; no hepatosplenomegaly.

Initial Work-Up

CBC		WBC Differential	%	# (×10³/μL)
WBC (×10³/μL)	1.9	Neutrophils	40	0.8
RBC (×10⁶/μL)	2.3	Bands	5	0.1
HGB (g/dL)	8.3	Lymphocytes	36	0.7
HCT (%)	23.3	Monocytes	10	0.2
MCV (fL)	101.7	Eosinophils	7	0.1
MCH (pg)	36.0	Basophils	2	
MCHC (g/dL)	35.4			
PLT (×10³/μL)	135			
RDW-CV (%)	17.0			
MPV (fL)	10.5			

Peripheral blood smear revealed mild macrocytosis, moderate anisocytosis, occasional ovalocytes, and mild polychromasia. Also noted was neutropenia without overt dysplasia and mild thrombocytopenia.

Differential Diagnosis The differential diagnosis for pancytopenia is broad, and includes both clonal and nonclonal processes. Nutritional deficiencies (especially vitamin B_{12} and folate), heavy-metal toxicity, elemental deficiencies, and many therapeutic agents must be considered. Other considerations include parvovirus B19 infection, autoimmune disorders, and paraneoplastic disorders. Replacement of the bone marrow by malignancies, such as hairy cell leukemia, can result in pancytopenia. Primary production abnormalities, such as congenital hematologic disorders, paroxysmal nocturnal hemoglobinuria, myelodysplastic syndromes, and acute leukemias are also in the differential.

Additional Work-Up

Bone marrow biopsy and aspirate showed a relatively normocellular marrow for age (30% cellular) with an unremarkable myeloid to erythroid ratio and 2.8% blasts. Erythroid and granulocytic precursors demonstrated complete maturation, with rare dyspoietic forms (<10% of cells in each lineage). Megakaryocytes were increased in number, with occasional small clusters

Section C: Chronic Myeloproliferative Neoplasms and Myelodysplastic Syndromes
Myelodysplastic Syndrome with Isolated del(5q)

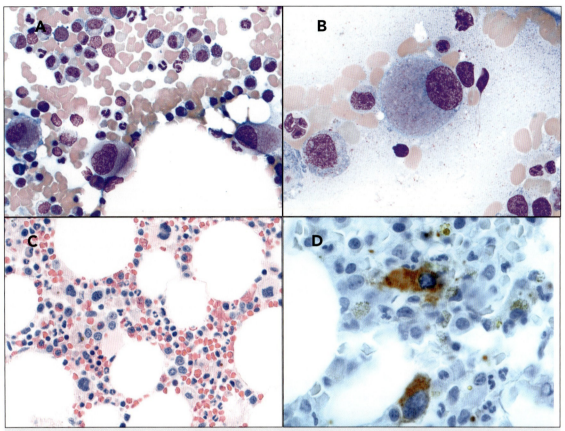

Figure 1 **A** Bone marrow aspirate smear (Wright-Giemsa, ×200) showing normal erythroid and granulocytic maturation and dysplastic megakaryocytes, **B** bone marrow aspirate smear (Wright-Giemsa, ×1000) highlighting dysplastic megakaryocytes, **C** bone marrow biopsy (H&E, ×200) showing normal erythroid and granulocytic maturation and dysplastic megakaryocytes, and **D** bone marrow biopsy (CD61 immunostain with hematoxylin counterstain, ×1000) highlighting atypical megakaryocytic cells.

on the biopsy and many small and monolobated nuclear forms (**Figures 1A-1C**). The presence of numerous mononuclear megakaryocytes in this case was highly suggestive of myelodysplasia with del(5q), also known as "5q– syndrome." No ring sideroblasts were seen on aspirate iron stain, with otherwise adequate iron stores. A CD61 immunohistochemical stain highlights the atypical megakaryocytes (**Figure 1D**). Flow cytometric studies on the bone marrow showed granulocytes, lymphocytes, and monocytes, with no identified abnormality of granulocyte maturation, based on the expression pattern of CD11b, CD13, and CD16. Myeloblasts accounted for <5% of total cells. No abnormal lymphoid population was identified. Bone marrow cytogenetic studies showed an abnormal clone with an interstitial deletion of the long arm of one chromosome 5, resulting in monosomy of the 5q22q35 region (**Figure 2**).

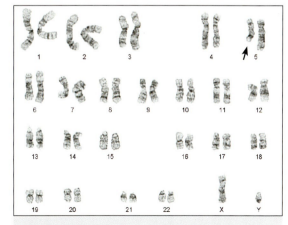

Figure 2 Bone marrow (karyotype); note the one chromosome 5 (arrow) with shortening of the long arm.

Final Diagnosis Myelodysplastic syndrome with isolated del(5q).

Management Approach The prognosis for myelodysplastic syndrome with deletion 5q is generally favorable, with a median survival of 145 months. Since the majority of patients with this disease are women, with a median age of 67 years, and with a low risk of transformation to acute myeloid leukemia (AML), therapy tends to be largely supportive. However, because of progressive, associated anemia, almost all patients eventually become transfusion-dependent, with an associated risk of iron overload, which may require chelation therapy. Neither recombinant erythropoietin (EPO) nor granulocyte colony stimulating factor (G-CSF) has proven to be efficacious. Hematopoietic progenitor cell transplant has not been shown to improve overall survival. In 2005, the US Food and Drug Administration (FDA) approved the oral immunomodulatory, antiangiogenic, and antineoplastic agent lenalidomide for this syndrome. Specifically, it was approved for use in patients with transfusion-dependent anemia who have myelodysplastic syndrome with del(5q) with or without additional cytogenetic abnormalities, and who have an international prognostic scoring system (IPSS) score of low or intermediate-1 risk. Patients with additional cytogenetic abnormalities are eligible only if cytopenias involve a single lineage and the bone marrow blast count is below 5%. This patient's anemia was managed with a combination of outpatient red cell transfusions and lenalidomide.

General Discussion Myelodysplastic syndrome with isolated del(5q) is generally characterized by macrocytic or normocytic anemia, normal or increased platelet count, <5% blasts in the blood and bone marrow, absence of Auer rods, hypolobated micromegakaryocytes, and del(5q) as the sole cytogenetic abnormality. Bone marrow is usually hypercellular with erythroid hyperplasia and normal or increased number of megakaryocytes. A variable degree of dyserythropoisis may also be present. Serum erythropoietin levels are frequently elevated with a downregulated stem cell response to EPO. This likely explains the ineffectiveness of exogenously administered EPO as anemia therapy.

Myelodysplastic Syndrome, Unclassifiable

Emmanuel Besa, Ajay Kandra

Patient An 87-year-old woman with a history of chronic thrombocytopenia.

Clinical History Her platelet counts have ranged from 45 ×10³/μL-75 ×10³/μL for many years. There was no history of occupational exposure to radiation or chemicals and she denied smoking and alcohol use. Despite her low platelet counts, she did not experience abnormal bleeding of any kind.

Family History Noncontributory.

Medications Multivitamins.

Physical Examination No lymphadenopathy or hepatosplenomegaly.

Initial Work-Up

CBC	
WBC (×10³/μL)	5.2
RBC (×10⁶/μL)	4.3
HGB (g/dL)	13.1
HCT (%)	41.3
MCV (fL)	96
MCH (pg)	30.4
MCHC (g/dL)	31.7
PLT (×10³/μL)	55
RDW-CV (%)	13.9

WBC Differential	%	# (×10³/μL)
Neutrophils	60.1	3.1
Eosinophils	5.0	0.3
Lymphocytes	30.8	1.6
Monocytes	4.0	0.2
Basophils	0.1	0.0

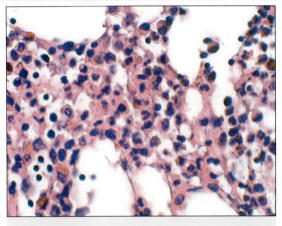

Figure 1 Bone marrow biopsy (H&E, ×400) showing hypercellular marrow.

Differential Diagnosis Conditions typically associated with isolated thrombocytopenia include pseudothrombocytopenia, chronic immune (or idiopathic) thrombocytopenia (ITP), drug-induced thrombocytopenia, liver disease, connective tissue disease, HIV infection, occult lymphoma and myelodysplastic syndrome.

Additional Work-Up In the absence of any indication or evidence for liver disease, connective tissue disorders, alcohol or drug use, the work-up for thrombocytopenia included review of blood smear and bone marrow examination. Peripheral blood smear review revealed decreased number of platelets. All cellular elements appeared morphologically normal. Bone marrow was hypercellular (30%-40%) for her age (**Figure 1**). All hematopoietic elements were present with slight myeloid hyperplasia. Storage iron was increased but no ring sideroblasts were identified. The aspirate smear revealed adequate megakaryocytes with occasional dysplastic forms (**Figure 2**) and dysplastic changes (megaloblastoid and binucleation)

Section C: Chronic Myeloproliferative Neoplasms and Myelodysplastic Syndromes
Myelodysplastic Syndrome, Unclassifiable

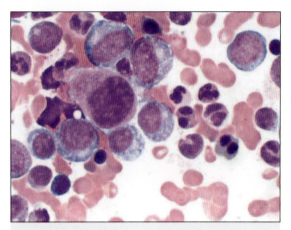

Figure 2 Bone marrow aspirate smear (Wright-Giemsa, ×1000) showing many myeloid cells, a unilobed megakaryocyte and a binucleated red cell.

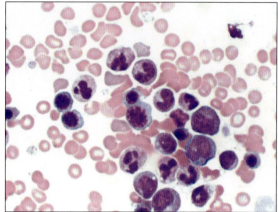

Figure 3 Bone marrow aspirate smear (Wright-Giemsa, ×500) showing myeloid cells and erythroid cells with 1 megaloblastoid erythroid precursor.

in a few (<10%) erythroid precursors (**Figure 3**). There was no increase in blasts and no evidence of any other malignancy. Flow cytometric analysis of bone marrow aspirate revealed no evidence of lymphoid monoclonality, aberrant antigen expression, or an increase in blasts. Cytogenetic analysis of aspirate: 46,XX, del(20)(q11.2)[17 cells]/46,XX[3 cells].

Final Diagnosis Myelodysplastic syndrome (MDS), unclassifiable (MDS-U).

Management Approach Treatment modalities used for patients with MDS include observation, hematopoietic growth factors, blood transfusions, and drug therapy such as azacitadine, decitabine and lenalidomide. Eligible patients are considered for allogeneic progenitor cell transplantation. This patient's international prognostic scoring system (IPSS) score was 0. She therefore had low-risk MDS. She was managed by observation alone. Her blood counts are being monitored every 3 months-6 months to detect progression of thrombocytopenia or development of other cytopenias which could potentially increase her IPSS score and therefore her risk category.

General Discussion Isolated thrombocytopenia is often mistakenly diagnosed as chronic ITP since the condition (ITP) does not require a bone marrow study to establish. A patient diagnosed with ITP who does not have an initial response to steroid therapy, may have a different etiology for thrombocytopenia and should be evaluated by a bone marrow examination including karyotype. The presence of dysplasia in >10% of cells in one or more lineages of the marrow is considered adequate to suggest the diagnosis of MDS. The presence of an abnormal clone by karyotype supports this diagnosis. According to the 2008 WHO classification, the diagnosis of MDS-U subtype can be made when a patient presents with either (a) refractory cytopenia with unilineage dysplasia (RCUD) or refractory cytopenia with multilineage dysplasia (RCMD) but with 1% blasts in the peripheral blood or (b) pancytopenia with unilineage dysplasia, or (c) persistent cytopenia(s) with ≤1% blasts in peripheral blood and <5% blasts in the bone marrow, unequivocal dysplasia in <10% of the cells in one or more myeloid lineages and one or more cytogenetic abnormalities considered as presumptive evidence of MDS. This patient falls into category C. Deletion 20q is a recurrent abnormality observed in myelodysplastic syndromes (MDS) and in other myeloid neoplasms. It is seen in 10% of patients with polycythemia vera and in 4%-5% of MDS patients. The MDS patients with del(20q) have a good prognosis and a low transformation rate to acute leukemia. The deletion may result in the loss of one or several tumor suppressor genes. The diversity of myeloid malignancies with del(20q) could be due to its occurrence in a pluripotent stem cell. The size of 20q deletions was also found to be highly variable in various myeloid disorders. The abnormal translocation along with additional abnormalities in chromosomes 5 or 7, or both, predicts a relatively poor prognosis.

Chronic Myelomonocytic Leukemia

Javed Gill

Patient A 63-year-male, who presented with several months history of progressive fatigue.

Clinical history The patient reported a 20-pound unintentional weight loss over a year.

Family History Noncontributory.

Medications None.

Physical Examination Notable only for spleen tip being palpable below subcostal margin.

Initial Work-Up

CBC		WBC Differential	%	# (×10³/µL)
WBC (×10³/µL)	19.8	Neutrophils	50	9.9
RBC (×10⁶/µL)	4.48	Bands	15	3.0
HGB (g/dL)	9.8	Lymphocytes	14	2.8
HCT (%)	29.9	Monocytes	13	2.6
MCV (fL)	94.8	Eosinophils	0	0
MCH (pg)	25.1	Basophils	0	0
MCHC (g/dL)	30.3	Metamyelocyte	7	1.4
PLT (×10³/µL)	76	Myelocyte	1	0.2
RDW-CV (%)	14.5	Nucleated red cells	occasional	
MPV (fL)	9.5			

Peripheral blood smear examination revealed absolute monocytosis (**Figure 1**), leukoerythroblastosis, and a few neutrophils with marked hypogranulation (**Figure 2**).

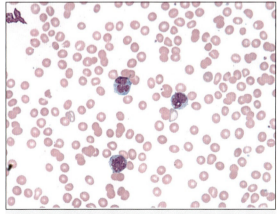

Figure 1 Blood smear (Wright, ×500) showing an increased number of monocytes (3 shown).

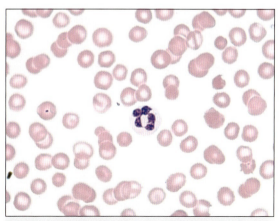

Figure 2 Blood smear (Wright, ×1000) showing a severely hypogranulated neutrophil.

Section C: Chronic Myeloproliferative Neoplasms and Myelodysplastic Syndromes
Chronic Myelomonocytic Leukemia

Differential Diagnosis Diagnostic considerations included acute myeloid leukemia (AML), chronic myelogenous leukemia (CML), atypical chronic myelogenous leukemia (ACML), chronic myelomonocytic leukemia (CMML), and reactive monocytosis.

Additional Work-Up A bone marrow examination revealed 100% cellularity, increased blasts at 7% (**Figure 3**), monocytosis, and myeloid and erythroid dysplasia (**Figure 4**).

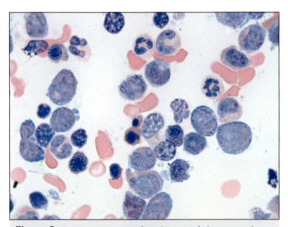

Figure 3 Bone marrow smear (Wright, ×1000) showing nuclear protrusion in an erythroid precursor and increased number of blasts.

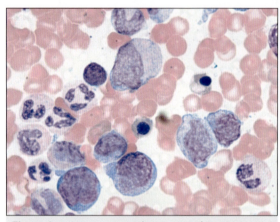

Figure 4 Bone marrow smear (Wright, ×1000) showing myeloid cells, erythroid cells, and a few atypical monocytes.

Flow cytometry performed on bone marrow aspirate revealed 15% monocytes (CD64+ and partial CD14+) and increased CD34+ (7%) and CD117+ (8%) cells.

Final Diagnosis Chronic myelomonocytic leukemia (CMML-1).

Management approach In CMML, life expectancy is highly variable and no consensus on optimal therapy exists. Supportive care remains the hallmark of management. Hypomethylating agents (such as azacytidine) and, in some patients, an allogeneic stem cell transplant may be an option. In the proliferative form of CMML, work-up should include screening for known molecular abnormalities associated with constitutively active tyrosine kinases that may be candidates for targeted therapies. This patient is being closely followed with only supportive care.

General Discussion CMML is a heterogeneous clonal hematopoietic malignancy classified under, "myelodysplastic/myeloproliferative neoplasms (MDS/MPN)" by WHO, with hybrid features. This disorder primarily occurs in older adults. The presenting complaints are usually related to blood cytopenias (fatigue, infections, bleeding), or tissue infiltration (splenomegaly; primarily red pulp infiltration in 30%-50%, hepatomegaly in about 20%, and rare lymph nodes or skin). Other common symptoms are weight loss, fever, and night sweats.

Persistent absolute monocytosis (>1 × $10^3/\mu L$), usually 10% or higher in peripheral blood, dysplasia, and <20% blasts in peripheral blood and bone marrow are the major defining features in CMML. If blasts (promonocytes included) are <5% in the peripheral blood and <10% in the bone marrow, the disorder is classified as CMML-1. And if blasts are 5%-19% in the peripheral blood or 10%-19% in the bone marrow, or Auer rods are present, irrespective of the blast count, it is classified as CMML-2, signaling a poorer prognosis.

To assess the monocytic component, cytochemical stains (α-naphthyl acetate esterase, α-naphthyl butyrate esterase or lysozyme) or immunophenotypic studies (flow cytometry or immunohistochemical stains CD68 and CD163) are very useful. Flow cytometry on peripheral blood and bone marrow demonstrates various phenotypic aberrations in monocytes including decreased expression of monocytic antigens (CD14, HLA-DR, CD13, CD15, CD64 or CD36) and/or aberrant expression of nonmyelomonocytic antigens (CD2 or CD56). An increased percentage or aberrant phenotype of blasts has been associated with early transformation to AML. In the majority of patients at the time of diagnosis, the peripheral blood shows leukocytosis and monocytosis, resembling a myeloproliferative process. It is often accompanied by eosinophilia, anemia, and thrombocytopenia. Granulocytes and monocytes commonly show dysplasia. Red cells are frequently macrocytic, with anisopoikilocytosis. In other patients; however, the WBC count is normal or mildly decreased with variable neutropenia, resembling a myelodysplastic process. The bone marrow is usually hypercellular and in most cases demonstrates significant granulocytic and monocytic proliferation as well as dysplasia. Fibrosis may be present.

Cytogenetic studies show clonal karyotypic abnormalities in about ⅓ of patients, but none is specific. The *JAK2* V617F mutation is present in a minority of cases. By definition, no Philadelphia chromosome or BCR-ABL is demonstrated, excluding CML. The cases of "MDS/MPN" by the 2008 WHO classification, with eosinophilia associated with t(5;12)(q31-33;p12) and ETV6-PDGFRB fusion gene, which were formerly included in the CMML category, are now considered a distinct entity. In these cases there is an aberrant, constitutively activated tyrosine kinase, and these disorders are sensitive to tyrosine kinase inhibitors (such as imatinib).

The prognosis of patients with CMML varies with a median survival of about 2.5 years. Some patients have highly aggressive disease and either transform to AML or succumb to bone marrow failure in a few months, while others have a more indolent clinical course. Overall, the incidence of transformation to AML is about 25%.

Chronic Lymphocytic Leukemia

Kanti R Rai, Tawfiqul A Bhuiya

Patient A 70-year-old male visited his primary care physician for a routine annual check-up.

Clinical History The patient offered no symptoms, and there was no significant past history except for hypercholesterolemia, for which he was being treated.

Family History Father had non-Hodgkin lymphoma for 20 years and died at age 90.

Medications A statin drug for high cholesterol.

Physical Examination Palpably enlarged multiple nodes bilaterally, in the neck, axillae, and inguinal regions. All were discrete, nonmatted, nontender, firm, and were freely movable; none were larger than 2 cm in diameter. Spleen and liver were not palpable.

Initial Work-Up

CBC	
WBC (×10³/μL)	40
RBC (×10⁶/μL)	5
HGB (g/dL)	14
HCT (%)	45
MCV (fL)	92
MCH (pg)	33
MCHC (g/dL)	34
PLT (×10³/μL)	204
RDW-CV (%)	12
MPV (fL)	7

WBC Differential	%	# (×10³/μL)
Neutrophils	20	8
Bands	0	
Lymphocytes	75	30
Monocytes	5	2
Eosinophils	0	
Basophils	0	

Peripheral blood smear revealed increased number of mature-appearing lymphocytes and smudge cells (**Figure 1**).

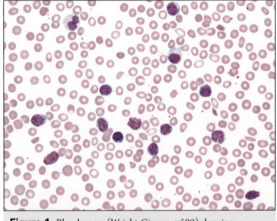

Figure 1 Blood smear (Wright-Giemsa, ×500) showing lymphocytosis and a smudge cell.

Differential Diagnosis Diagnostic considerations included chronic lymphocytic leukemia (CLL), non-Hodgkin lymphoma in leukemic phase, persistent polyclonal B-lymphocytosis, and prolymphocytic leukemia.

Additional Work-Up Flow cytometry of blood lymphocytes revealed a monoclonal population of B lymphocytes that was CD19+, CD20+ (dim), CD5+, CD23+ with κ sIgM (dim) restriction and was negative for CD10, CD103, and CD25. Examination of bone marrow biopsy showed hypercellularity with a heavy lymphocytic interstitial infiltrate (**Figures 2** and **3**). Trilinear hematopoietic elements showed normal maturation but were markedly reduced. Iron stores were adequate and reticulin stain was negative. The aspirate smear revealed preponderance of small and medium-size mature-appearing lymphocytes, which accounted for 80% of the cellular elements (**Figure 4**). By immunohistochemistry, the leukemic cells stained positive with CD20 and CD23 (**Figures 5** and **6**). Immunophenotyping by flow cytometry performed on the marrow aspirate yielded results similar to that of blood lymphocytes.

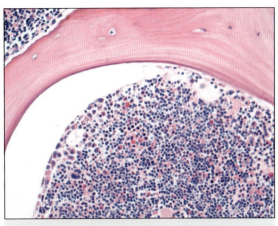

Figure 2 Bone marrow biopsy (H&E stain, ×20) showing infiltrate by small mature lymphocytes.

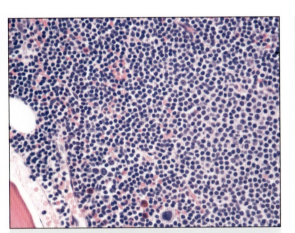

Figure 3 Bone marrow biopsy (H&E stain, ×40) showing diffuse lymphoid infiltrate.

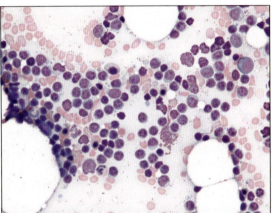

Figure 4 Bone marrow aspirate smear (Wright-Giemsa ×500) showing infiltrate of small mature lymphocytes.

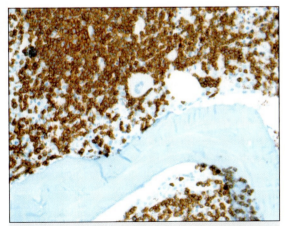

Figure 5 Bone marrow biopsy (CD20, ×40) in which leukemic cells are positive.

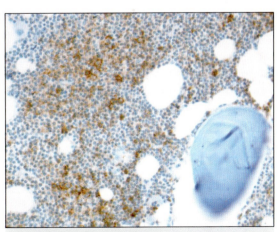

Figure 6 Bone marrow biopsy (CD23, ×40) in which leukemic cells are positive.

Section D: Chronic Lymphoproliferative Disorders
Chronic Lymphocytic Leukemia

Final Diagnosis Chronic lymphocytic leukemia (CLL), clinical stage I.

Management Approach Patients with low-risk disease are usually asymptomatic and managed with a "watch and wait" approach. Those with intermediate-risk or high-risk disease are generally treated with combination chemotherapy and/or monoclonal antibody therapy. A frequently used regimen is an alkylating agent and/or a purine analog with either alemtuzumab, ofatumumab or rituximab. This patient was placed on observation only, with the plan to start with chemo-immunotherapy (rituximab + fludarabine + cyclophosphamide), if the disease showed rapid progression or if the patient developed disease-related symptoms such as weight-loss, night sweats, or fatigue. His follow-up monitoring includes tests for IGVH mutation status, ZAP-70, CD38 and β-2 microglobulin. These are important newly described prognostic markers. If IGVH is mutated, CD38 is negative, ZAP-70 is negative and β-2 microglobulin is low, the prognosis is excellent in early-stage patients, as is the case with this patient.

General Discussion Chronic lymphocytic leukemia (CLL), a B-cell lymphoproliferative disorder, is the most common form of leukemia among the adult populations of the Western hemisphere. It occurs in middle-aged and elderly persons in a male-to-female ratio of approximately 2:1. Clinical presentation is variable. Many patients are asymptomatic at initial diagnosis. Signs and symptoms, if and when present, may include fatigue, weakness, frequent infections, auto-immune hemolytic anemia, lymphadenopathy, splenomegaly, hepatomegaly, extranodal infiltrates, weight loss, fever and/or night sweats. The clinical course is also variable. Some patients run a benign course and live for many years without any complications of the disease while others have an aggressive course and may die within a year or 2. A majority fall in between these extremes with a median survival of a few years. Over time, in a minority of cases the disease may progress to prolymphocytic transformation (CLL/PLL) or to diffuse large B-cell lymphoma, (also known as Richter syndrome). The latest guidelines proposed by the International Workshop on Chronic Lymphocytic Leukemia (IWCLL) for the diagnosis of CLL require (a) peripheral blood B-lymphocyte count of at least 5,000/μL and (b) the B lymphocytes must be monoclonal and have the immunophenotype of CD19+, CD20+ (dim), CD23+ and CD5+ with restriction to either κ or λ immunoglobulin light chains. Examination of bone marrow is not required for diagnosing CLL provided that the 2 above-noted criteria have been met. However, bone marrow findings may be helpful in determining the likely future clinical course of the disease. A nodular or interstitial pattern of lymphocytic infiltration in the bone marrow biopsy specimen is associated with better overall prognosis than a diffuse pattern. Bone marrow examination also helps in judging the response to therapy and determining the reason(s) for cytopenias (anemia, neutropenia and thrombocytopenia) when they occur. Clinical staging systems, which categorize the disease into low-risk, intermediate-risk, and high-risk, can be improved with the utilization of relatively new prognostic markers, such as IGVH mutation status, ZAP-70, CD-38, cytogenetic abnormality as determined by FISH, and β-2 microglobulin. Patients with mutated IGVH genes have significantly longer survival time than those with unmutated IGVH genes. In contrast, patients with ZAP-70 positivity are known to have a relatively aggressive clinical course and shorter life-expectancy than those who are ZAP-70 negative. CD38+ cases have worse prognosis than CD38– cases. Patients with isolated del(13q) have the best overall clinical course and survival time whereas those with del(17p) and del(11q) have a rapid clinical course and relatively short overall survival. Patients with trisomy-12 or normal cytogenetics by FISH probes have the clinical course and survival statistics intermediate between the 2 extremes. The level of β-2 microglobulin has been reported to correlate with the extent of disease and, thus, with the overall prognosis.

Large B-Cell Lymphoma with Underlying Chronic Lymphocytic Leukemia (Richter Transformation)

M James You, Carlos Bueso-Ramos

Patient A 76-year-old man, who presented with right hip pain, night sweats, and anorexia.

Clinical History The patient had a history of chronic lymphocytic leukemia/small lymphocytic lymphoma (CLL/SLL), Rai stage 0, diagnosed 5 months prior to the current presentation. He was followed by observation only. More recently, he developed progressive right hip pain, night sweats and anorexia. The patient also had a past medical history of atrial fibrillation and hypothyroidism. CT of the abdomen and pelvis revealed extensive adenopathy with a large pelvic mass. A PET scan revealed multifocal lymphoma above and below the diaphragm with high standardized uptake value (SUV), suggestive of aggressive disease.

Family History Father with lung cancer and a sister with a reported noncancerous brain tumor.

Medications Niacin, metoprolol, warfarin and levothyroxine.

Physical Examination His exam was remarkable for extensive lymphadenopathy involving neck and inguinal lymph nodes. There was bilateral extremity edema with the right greater than left. There was erythema, warmth, and tenderness over the right lower extremity, which appeared greater than the left lower extremity.

Initial Work-Up

CBC

WBC (×10³/µL)	15.9
RBC (×10⁶/µL)	3.48
HGB (g/dL)	11.0
HCT (%)	32.4
MCV (fL)	93
MCH (pg)	31.6
MCHC (g/dL)	34.0
PLT (×10³/µL)	215
RDW-CV (%)	15.5
MPV (fL)	6.9

WBC Differential	%	# (×10³/µL)
Neutrophils	21	3.3
Bands	3	0.5
Lymphocytes	74	11.8
Monocytes	2	0.3

Peripheral blood smear revealed small and large atypical lymphoid cells (**Figure 1**). Bone marrow biopsy was hypercellular and revealed extensive involvement by large lymphoma cells (**Figure 2**).

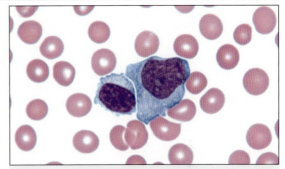

Figure 1 Blood smear (Wright, ×1000) showing small and large atypical lymphoid cells.

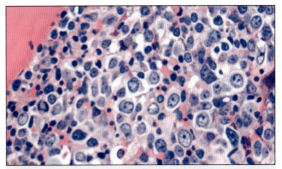

Figure 2 Bone marrow biopsy (H&E, ×400) showing hypercellular marrow with extensive involvement by large lymphoid cells.

Section D: Chronic Lymphoproliferative Disorders
Large B-Cell Lymphoma with Underlying Chronic Lymphocytic Leukemia (Richter Transformation)

Differential Diagnosis Diagnostic considerations included Richter transformation of CLL/SLL and CLL/SLL with concurrent classical Hodgkin lymphoma.

Additional Work-Up Immunohistochemical stains performed on bone marrow sections demonstrated that small B lymphocytes were positive for CD20 and CD5. Large atypical lymphocytes were positive for CD20 (**Figure 3**) and negative for CD5, CD15 and CD30. The majority of the large atypical cells and occasional small lymphocytes were positive for Ki-67 (**Figure 4**).

Flow immunophenotypic analysis on bone marrow aspirate showed aberrant λ light-chain restricted B cells, positive for CD19, CD20, CD5 (partial), CD43 (partial), CD23 (subset) and HLA-DR, and negative for FMC-7, CD34, CD117, CD10, TdT, CD13, CD33, CD7, CD2, CD14, CD64, CD15, CD56 and MPO. Cytogenetic studies showed trisomy 12 and absence of an IGH/CCND1 gene rearrangement. Molecular diagnostic studies showed 22 base pair changes in the IgH variable region.

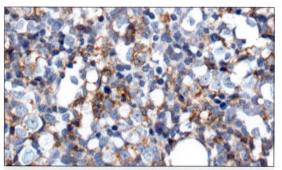

Figure 3 Bone marrow biopsy (CD20, ×400) revealing membrane staining in small and large B cells.

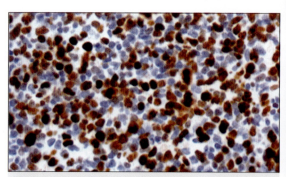

Figure 4 Bone marrow biopsy (Ki-67, ×400) revealing high proliferation index of the large lymphoma cells.

Final Diagnosis Large B-cell lymphoma in a patient with underlying chronic lymphocytic leukemia (Richter transformation).

Management Approach Treatment of Richter transformation of CLL/SLL has generally relied on combination of chemotherapy with or without the addition of rituximab. This patient received aggressive combination chemotherapy with cyclophosphamide, vincristine, doxorubicin and dexamethasone (Hyper-CVAD) and rituximab. He responded well initially. However, the disease was persistent and the patient died approximately 8 months after the treatment.

General Discussion Several types of transformation in chronic lymphocytic leukemia have been described: prolymphocytic transformation, which is relatively low-grade and slowly progressive; diffuse large B-cell lymphoma (Richter syndrome), which is rapidly progressive and accounts for about 5% of all deaths in chronic lymphocytic leukemia; Hodgkin lymphoma and acute leukemia. Transformation to acute leukemia is unusual in untreated CLL/SLL. Richter transformation of CLL/SLL occurs in <10% of patients and may present as extensive lymphadenopathy and/or tumor mass. CLL/SLL may also have a concurrent classical Hodgkin lymphoma with classical Reed-Sternberg cells positive for CD15 and CD30 in a background of reactive small T lymphocytes, histiocytes, plasma cells and eosinophils. The onset of transformation of CLL/SLL is suggested when there is a proliferation of a new population of large lymphoid cells with immature-appearing morphological features, a finer nuclear chromatin pattern, and a prominent nucleolus. This morphological transformation is accompanied by the appearance of complex chromosomal changes that are not present earlier or are in addition to the commonly presenting trisomy 12. A variety of techniques are available to help determine whether the transformation represents a clonal evolution of the original CLL/SLL or an independent disease; these include cytogenetic analysis, immunoglobulin gene rearrangement analysis, and anti-idiotype antibodies. Molecular studies have shown that the development of Richter syndrome in CLL/SLL may represent either the identical clone of cells, present in the preceding CLL/SLL or a different malignant clone. The majority of Hodgkin lymphoma cases occur in unmutated (>98% homology with germline) CLL/SLL. Comprehensive immunophenotyping by flow immunophenotypic analysis and immunoperoxidase studies are essential in supporting the diagnosis of large B-cell lymphoma in a patient with underlying chronic lymphocytic leukemia.

B-Cell Prolymphocytic Leukemia

Alina Dulau Florea, Jerald Gong, Gene Gulati

Patient A 67-year-old Caucasian male, who was admitted to the hospital because of anemia and massive splenomegaly.

Clinical History The patient was in his usual state of health until 3 months before admission, when he presented to his family practitioner with fatigue and early satiety, and was found to have a WBC of $65 \times 10^3/\mu L$ with 85% lymphocytes. He reported unintentional weight loss of >15 lbs over the last 6 months. He had a history of hypertension but no other significant clinical history.

Family History Noncontributory.

Medications Metoprolol, furosemide.

Physical Examination Notable for massive splenomegaly without hepatomegaly. He had no lymphadenopathy.

Initial Work-Up

CBC		
WBC (×10³/μL)	130.2	
RBC (×10⁶/μL)	3.87	
HGB (g/dL)	10.9	
HCT (%)	33.3	
MCV (fL)	89	
MCH (pg)	28.2	
MCHC (g/dL)	32.7	
PLT (×10³/μL)	68	
RDW-CV (%)	14.1	
WBC Differential	**%**	**# (×10³/μL)**
Neutrophils	4	5.2
Lymphocytes	4	5.2
Monocytes	1	1.3
Atypical lymphs	91	118.5

Results of routine coagulation studies (PT and PTT), serum glucose, electrolytes, alkaline phosphatase and renal-function tests were normal. Peripheral blood smear revealed marked lymphocytosis with over 90% atypical lymphoid cells (**Figure 1**).

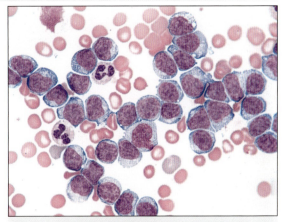

Figure 1 Blood smear (Wright-Giemsa, ×500) showing numerous prolymphocytes. The atypical lymphoid cells are medium-sized, with round nuclei, regular nuclear contours, moderately condensed nuclear chromatin, prominent nucleoli and moderate amount of blue cytoplasm.

Differential Diagnosis Diagnostic considerations based on peripheral blood findings along with clinical presentation included chronic lymphocytic leukemia (CLL), prolymphocytic leukemia (PLL), chronic lymphocytic leukemia in prolymphocytic transformation (CLL/PLL), and leukemic phase of non-Hodgkin lymphoma involving the spleen. Hairy cell leukemia, though usually presents

Section D: Chronic Lymphoproliferative Disorders
B-Cell Prolymphocytic Leukemia

with splenomegaly without lymphadenopathy, was considered unlikely because of extreme leukocytosis. Diffuse large B-cell lymphoma, follicular lymphoma, and mantle cell lymphoma can have splenic involvement, but are usually associated with lymphadenopathy. Diffuse spleen enlargement, absence of lymphadenopathy, and peripheral lymphocytosis with cellular morphology of prolymphocytes narrowed the differential diagnosis to CLL/PLL and PLL.

Additional Work-Up Flow cytometry performed on the peripheral blood showed a κ light-chain restricted, abnormal mature B-lymphoid population comprising 95% of all analyzed cells, with the following immunophenotype: CD19+, CD20+, CD22+, CD79a+, CD38+, bright surface IgM κ+, FMC7+, CD5–, CD23– and TDT–. No blast population was identified. Examination of bone marrow biopsy revealed lymphoid aggregates that comprised approximately 10% of the marrow cellularity and increased interstitial atypical lymphoid cells (**Figure 2**). Morphologically, the majority of atypical lymphoid cells were medium sized, with moderately condensed nuclear chromatin, prominent single nucleoli, and moderate amount of basophilic cytoplasm (**Figure 3**). A differential count performed on the aspirate smear yielded a lymphoid cell count of 60%. Flow cytometry performed on a bone marrow aspirate sample demonstrated a clonal B-cell population with immunophenotype identical to that found in the peripheral blood. FISH analysis on the bone marrow was positive for del(17p).

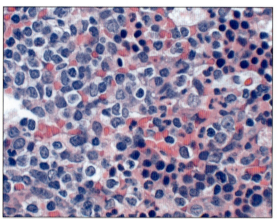

Figure 2 Bone marrow biopsy (H&E, ×400) showing hypercellular marrow with interstitial atypical infiltrate of prolymphocytes.

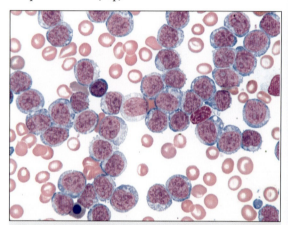

Figure 3 Bone marrow aspirate smear (Wright-Giemsa, ×500) showing infiltrate of prolymphocytes (cells with moderately condensed nuclear chromatin and a prominent nucleolus in each).

Final Diagnosis B-cell prolymphocytic leukemia, de novo.

Management Approach The clinical course is usually aggressive, and the response to therapy is poor, with a median survival ranging from 30 months-50 months. A combination of immunotherapy with rituximab (anti-CD20 antibody) and chemotherapy with cyclophosphamide, doxorubicin, vincristine and prednisone(R-CHOP) is most commonly used. Nucleoside analogs, such as fludarabine and cladribine, and antibody therapies such as alemtuzumab (an anti-CD52 antibody) have also been used with variable degree of success. Splenectomy may improve symptoms. This patient was started on a regimen of R-CHOP. He also received external beam radiation to the spleen. He responded poorly to the therapeutic regimen and died of sepsis 15 days after the start of therapy.

Discussion Prolymphocytic leukemia (PLL) is defined as a B-cell leukemia that is composed of >55% prolymphocytes in the peripheral blood. PLL can arise from a preexisting CLL, in which case this is called prolymphocytic transformatioin of chronic lymphocytic leukemia (CLL/PLL). A de novo form (PLL) may also occur in which there is no prior history of CLL. De novo PLL is an uncommon disorder. It is a disease of the elderly with a slight male predominance. The median age of the affected individuals is about 70 years. Approximately 80% of cases are of B-cell type (B-PLL) with the remainder being T-cell type (T-PLL). Most patients present with B symptoms, massive splenomegaly, marked lymphocytosis (usually over $100 \times 10^3/\mu L$). Anemia, thrombocytopenia and neutropenia are common findings. The diagnosis is based on morphology and immunophenotype of the circulating and bone marrow lymphoid cells along with the history and clinical presentation. B-PLL cells usually express a mature B-cell phenotype, being positive for CD19, CD20, CD22, CD79a, FMC7, with strong surface IgM ± IgD. The most common cytogenetic abnormality is del(17p), found in 50% of the cases, and it is associated with TP53 gene mutations.

Hairy Cell Leukemia

Kanti R Rai, Tawfiqul A Bhuiya

Patient A 48-year-old male, who was found to be pancytopenic by his primary care physician.

Clinical History The patient has a history of gout and gastroesophageal reflux disorder (GERD), and has had appendectomy in childhood. He was found to be pancytopenic (anemic, leukeopenic and thrombocytopenic) during routine follow-up for his gout.

Family History Father died of myocardial infarction at age 80.

Medications Allopurinol, Indomethacin, and exomeprazole.

Physical Examination No acute distress. No palpable lymphadenopathy in cervical, axillary or inguinal regions. Spleen was enlarged upon palpation, reaching 8 cm below the left costal margin. Liver was not palpable. No petechiae, purpura or bruises noted. Vital signs: temperature 95.7°F, pulse 70/min, blood pressure 150/90.

Initial Work-Up		
CBC		
WBC (×10³/μL)	5.0	
RBC (×10⁶/μL)	3.8	
HGB (g/dL)	10.9	
HCT (%)	31	
MCV (fL)	92.1	
MCH (pg)	31.3	
MCHC (g/dL)	34	
PLT (×10³/μL)	100	
RDW-CV (%)	14.5	
MPV (fL)	6.1	
WBC Differential	**%**	**# (×10³/μL)**
Neutrophils	20	1.0
Bands	0	
Lymphocytes	80	4.0
Monocytes	0	
Eosinophils	0	
Basophils	0	

Peripheral blood smear revealed no blasts but several lymphoid cells with the appearance of hairy cells (**Figure 1**).

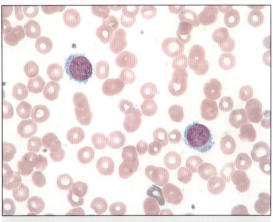

Figure 1 Blood smear (Wright-Giemsa, ×1000) showing 2 hairy cells.

Differential Diagnosis The list of clinical conditions associated with pancytopenia is large and includes benign and malignant entities. From the clinical standpoint, myelodysplastic syndrome (MDS) and drug-induced (allopurinol/indomethacin) cytopenias were considered likely. However, the peripheral blood smear finding of possible hairy cells along with the finding of splenomegaly led us to consider hairy cell leukemia as the most likely potential diagnosis.

Section D: Chronic Lymphoproliferative Disorders
Hairy Cell Leukemia

Additional Work-Up Bone marrow was hypercellular (70%) with all marrow elements present in all stages of maturation and a mild increase in the erythroid series. The M:E ratio was 2:1. Megakaryocytes were increased with normal morphology. There was a mild increase in reticulin fibers. A small number of scattered plasma cells were also present. There was a moderate, interstitial infiltrate of small lymphocytes with hyperchromatic nuclei and apparently large amounts of cytoplasm. Some clusters of lymphocytes had a fried-egg appearance (**Figures 2** and **3**). By immunohistochemical staining, lymphocytes were monoclonal with sIgG/κ restriction and were positive for CD20bright (**Figure 4**), CD19, CD25, CD11c, CD103, DBA-44 (**Figure 5**) and TRAP (**Figure 6**). Lymphocytes were negative for CD5, CD10 and BCL1. Flow cytometry performed on peripheral blood demonstrated a monoclonal B-cell population with the following immunophenotype: CD19+, CD20+, CD22+, CD25+, CD11c+, CD103+, CD5– and CD10–.

Cytogenetics Normal male karyotype.

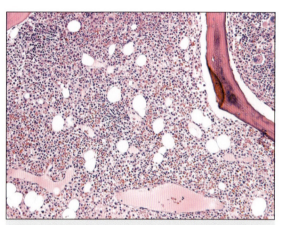

Figure 2 Bone marrow biopsy (H&E, ×40) showing lymphoid infiltrate.

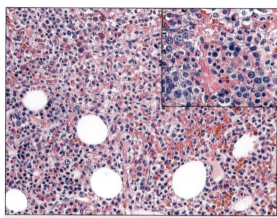

Figure 3 Bone marrow biopsy (H&E, ×60, and inset, ×100) showing monotonous population of lymphoid cells with abundant cytoplasm and clearing around nucleus, or "fried egg" appearance.

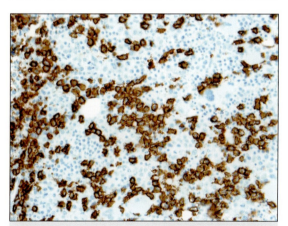

Figure 4 Bone marrow biopsy (CD20, ×100) showing lymphoid cells are positive.

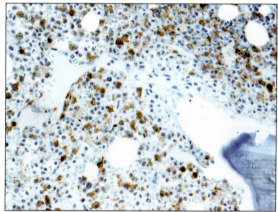

Figure 5 Bone marrow biopsy (DBA44, ×40) showing lymphoid cells are positive.

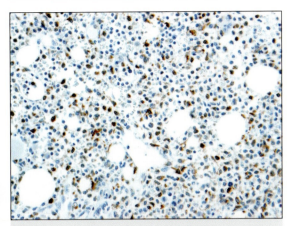

Figure 6 Bone marrow biopsy (tartrate-tesistant acid phosphatase, ×40) showing lymphoid cells are positive.

Final Diagnosis Hairy cell leukemia (HCL).

Management Approach Until the emergence of 2 nucleoside analogues, cladribine and pentostatin, the treatment of hairy cell leukemia consisted of α interferon and splenectomy. All that changed because the complete remissions (CR) and overall remissions are achievable in the range of 80%-90% and 90%-95%, respectively, with either cladribine or pentostatin. Monoclonal antibody therapy with either rituximab (anti-CD20 antibody) or immunotoxin BL22 (anti-CD22 antibody) has also been used with variable degree of success particularly in cases refractory to or relapsing after purine nucleoside analogue therapy. This patient received cladribine and he has been in CR ever since. In most cases CRs last for up to 20 years.

General Discussion HCL is an uncommon B-cell lymphoproliferative disorder generally characterized by pancytopenia, splenomegaly, and circulating hairy cells. Middle-aged males are afflicted more so than females in a ratio of 4:1. Patients may present with weakness, weight loss, abdominal discomfort due to splenomegaly, and/or recurrent infections. Lymphadenopathy, if present, is minimal. Pancytopenia or some other combination of cytopenias are common findings but some cases may have leukocytosis. The number of hairy cells in the blood is variable from a few to many. Hairy cells generally infiltrate bone marrow and spleen but may also infiltrate liver and/or lymph nodes in some cases. In the bone marrow, the "fried-egg appearance" is considered characteristic of hairy cell leukemia. The bone marrow may be non-aspirable in many cases generally due to fibrosis. The spleen often shows red pulp infiltration by hairy cells and "red cell lakes," which are blood-filled spaces lined by hairy cells. Hairy cells often express CD45, CD19, CD20, CD22, CD25, CD11c, CD103, CD79a, CD79b, FMC7, DBA44, and tartrate-resistant acid phosphatase (TRAP). The immunophenotypic features of CD103+, CD25+, CD11c+, and CD20+ when all present, makes the diagnosis unambiguous. Annexin A1 (ANXA1), a relatively new immunohistochemical marker, has been described as highly sensitive and specific for the diagnosis of hairy cell leukemia. Overall prognosis with purine nucleosiode analogue therapy is good.

Section D: Chronic Lymphoproliferative Disorders

Post-Transplant Lymphoproliferative Disorder

Neal Flomenberg, Ubaldo Martinez Outschoorn, Joanne Filicko-O'Hara

Patient A 25-year-old female, who presented with right axillary swelling, fever and weight loss over the month prior to presentation.

Clinical History The patient's past medical history included T-cell acute lymphoblastic leukemia, status post T cell depleted allogeneic matched sibling stem cell transplant 7 years earlier, complicated with polymorphic B-cell post-transplant lymphoproliferative disorder (PTLD) treated with rituximab within the first year post-transplant, grade I graft-vs-host disease of the skin during the immediate post-transplant period, recurrent pneumonias and upper respiratory infections.

Family History Noncontributory. HLA identical brother who was her stem cell donor is alive and well.

Medications None.

Physical Examination Temperature 102.4°F Right axillary lymphadenopathy measuring 5 × 3 cm, tender to palpation, hepatomegaly spanning 16 cm in the midclavicular line, splenomegaly spanning 4 cm below costal margin in the anterior axillary line. She had no other palpable adenopathy.

Initial Work-Up		
CBC		
WBC (×10³/µL)	2.4	
RBC (×10⁶/µL)	4.36	
HGB (g/dL)	11	
HCT (%)	33.8	
MCV (fL)	78	
MCH (pg)	25.2	
MCHC (g/dL)	32.5	
PLT (×10³/µL)	143	
RDW-CV (%)	14.3	
MPV (fL)	11.5	
WBC Differential	**%**	**# (×10³/µL)**
Neutrophils	48	1.2
Bands	24	0.6
Lymphocytes	18	0.4
Monocytes	6	0.1
Eosinophils	4	0.1
Basophils	0	

Differential Diagnosis Diagnostic considerations included neoplastic, infectious and non-infectious inflammatory diseases. The primary concern was that the patient had a lymphoma which in the post-transplant setting is generally classified as post-transplant lymphoproliferative disorder (PTLD). Possible infectious etiologies for her symptoms include bacterial infections such as an abscess, cellulitis, folliculitis, cat scratch disease, tuberculosis, secondary syphilis, viral infections such as EBV infection, CMV disease, hepatitis B virus (HBV) infection, hepatitis C virus infection (HCV), HIV, parasitic diseases such as toxoplasmosis and autoimmune lymphadenopathy related to systemic lupus erythematosus.

Additional Work-Up The patient had blood cultures, infectious disease serologies and PCR tests for EBV, CMV, HIV, HBV, HCV, toxoplasmosis, syphilis, bartonella henselae, and ANA, which were all negative. She had an axillary lymph node excisional biopsy and bone marrow biopsy which showed infiltration by histiocytes and large cells with irregular nuclei and an eosinophilic perinuclear region (**Figure 1**). The large cells stained positive for CD30 (**Figure 2**), anaplastic

Section D: Chronic Lymphoproliferative Disorders
Post-Transplant Lymphoproliferative Disorder

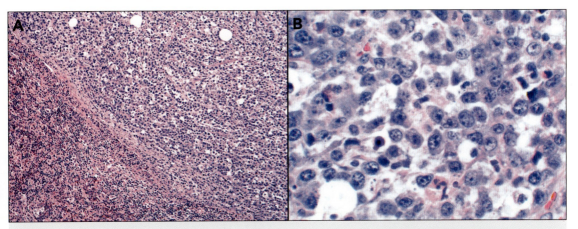

Figure 1 Axillary lymph node biopsy **A** (H&E, ×100), and **B** (×400), showing large atypical pleomorphic cells with irregular nuclei.

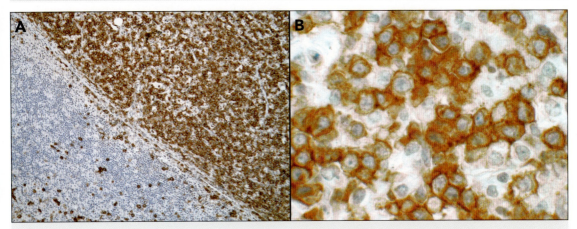

Figure 2 Axillary lymph node biopsy **A** (CD30, ×100), and **B** (×400) showing that large atypical cells are positive.

lymphoma kinase (**Figure 3**), epithelial membrane antigen (EMA), and CD4. EBV, testing by Epstein-Barr encoded RNA (EBER) was also positive. FISH analysis revealed that cells were XY consistent with neoplastic transformation of donor lymphocytes. Skin biopsy due to development of rash and colon biopsy due to diarrhea also revealed involvement by the same population of cells.

Final Diagnosis Post-transplant lymphoproliferative disorder, stage IV, donor-derived anaplastic large cell lymphoma ALK+.

Management Approach PTLD is treated by tapering immune suppression, administering donor lymphocyte infusions, rituximab, or cytotoxic chemotherapy in varying combinations. In B-cell, EBV+ PTLD, tapering immune suppression or administering a donor lymphocyte infusion may allow for a strong anti-EBV response which may be sufficient therapy. Rituximab is also useful in B-cell PTLD, both EBV+ or EBV–. In

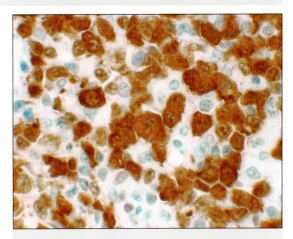

Figure 3 Axillary lymph node biopsy (ALK, ×400) revealing large atypical cells that show nuclear, nucleolar, and cytoplasmic staining.

other respects, treatment of PTLD, particularly, EBV– cases, is based on treating the lymphoma in the same way as in nontransplanted individuals. If a patient is still receiving immunosuppression tapering the immunosuppression, if feasible, may be an appropriate first step in treatment. This patient was treated with CHOP chemotherapy (cyclophosphamide, doxorubicin, vincristine and prednisone). She went into complete remission by the third of 6 cycles of CHOP, but relapsed 4 months later. She is currently undergoing salvage therapy and preparing for second allogeneic hematopoietic progenitor cell transplant, from a haplo-identical donor.

General Discussion Post-transplant lymphoproliferative disorders are lymphoid proliferations that develop in individuals who are immunosuppressed after a solid organ or stem cell allograft. PTLD includes lymphoid neoplastic and nonneoplastic proliferations ranging from infectious mononucleosis-type B-cell polyclonal proliferations to neoplastic lymphoid proliferations. Indolent small B-cell lymphomas or detection of EBV+ cells without lymphoid proliferation are not considered PTLD. Neoplastic lymphoid proliferations are indistinguishable from lymphomas found in immunocompetent adults. Most cases of PTLD are B-cell lymphomas and are EBV+. However, T-cell PTLD constitutes approximately 7%-15% of all PTLD cases and about 40% of T-NK cell PTLD cases are EBV+. It has been suggested that T-cell PTLD EBV+ may be the result of chronic antigenic stimulation rather than being driven by the virus. T-cell PTLD has a worse prognosis than B-cell PTLD and there are no early polyclonal variants of T-cell PTLD. This patient had an anaplastic large cell lymphoma (ALCL) derived from donor T cells. ALCL is an aggressive T-cell lymphoid neoplasm and this patient had the characteristic t(2;5) translocation which leads to the fusion of anaplastic lymphoma kinase (ALK) with nucleophosmin (NPM). This patient had previous B-cell clonal PTLD treated with rituximab. Metachronous PTLD of different subtypes is well described. T-cell PTLD typically occurs much later than other types of PTLD. Although transfer of donor T cells is another treatment option that can be considered for this patient, T-cell PTLD usually does not respond to a decrease in immunosuppression or restoration of T-cell function, in contrast to the B-cell forms of this disorder.

T-Cell Prolymphocytic Leukemia

Mingyi Chen, Auayporn Nademanee, Karen Chang

Patient A 61-year-old male, who presented with complaints of progressive weakness and fatigue.

Clinical History Following an initial diagnosis of T-cell lymphoma, the patient was transferred to our hospital for management.

Family History Noncontributory.

Medications None at presentation.

Physical Examination The patient had prominent splenomegaly and peripheral lymphadenopathy.

Initial Work-Up CT scans revealed marked lymphadenopathy, bilateral pulmonary infiltrates and pleural effusions, splenomegaly, hepatomegaly and diffuse infiltrates of the right iliac and gluteal muscles. CBC showed a marked leukocytosis ($49 \times 10^3/\mu L$) with 80% lymphocytes. At the time of presentation to our hospital, the patient was anemic and thrombocytopenic, and had leukocytosis of $27.6 \times 10^3/\mu L$ with 83% lymphocytes (**Figure 1**). Over the course of the first 4 chemotherapy attempts, the patient's leukocyte count fluctuated between $15 \times 10^3/\mu L$ and $30 \times 10^3/\mu L$, and finally peaked at $87 \times 10^3/\mu L$ with 56% lymphocytes.

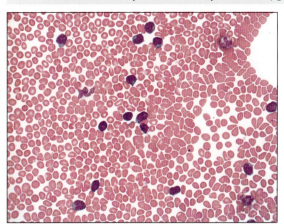

Figure 1 Blood smear (Wright-Giemsa, ×600) showing abnormal prolymphocytes that are medium-sized with single nucleoli and basophilic cytoplasm with occasional blebs or projections. The nuclei are round to oval in shape.

Differential Diagnosis The differential diagnosis of this T-cell lymphoproliferative disorder includes T-cell prolymphocytic leukemia (T-PLL), T-cell large granular lymphocytic leukemia (T-LGL), Sézary syndrome, and adult T-cell leukemia/lymphoma (ATLL).

- T-cell prolymphocytic leukemia is the favored diagnosis because of the cytology. The presence of splenomegaly is also consistent with this diagnosis. The presence of a CD4+ mature T-cell phenotype would also favor T-PLL
- T-LGL should be easy to distinguish from T-PLL. The presence of small irregular nuclei with scant cytoplasm and no cytoplasmic granules strongly favors T-PLL. In addition, a negative granzyme-B immunohistochemistry would strongly favor a diagnosis of T-PLL
- Sézary syndrome/mycosis fungoides should always be considered in the differential diagnosis of circulating T-cell lymphoma cells. The distinguishing features from T-PLL include the clinical setting and the immunophenotype. The skin involvement in Sézary syndrome is distinctive (generalized erythroderma), whereas in T-PLL skin involvement is mostly spotty and occurs in only about 20% of cases. Sézary syndrome cases are usually CD7−
- ATLL is not favored because of the morphology and the immunophenotype, as well as the lack of HTLV-1 serology or hypercalcemia. ATLL cells always express CD25 by flow cytometry

Section D: Chronic Lymphoproliferative Disorders
T-Cell Prolymphocytic Leukemia

Additional Work-Up The bone marrow was diffusely infiltrated by abnormal lymphoid cells (**Figure 2**). By immunohistochemical staining, the neoplastic cells were positive for CD3, and CD4, but not CD8, CD1a, or TdT. Flow cytometry showed CD4 predominance, with a mature phenotype. The lymphoid cells expressed CD2, CD3, CD5, and CD7, and not CD20, CD8, CD16, CD56, or CD57. There was no aberrant antigen loss. T-cell receptor γ chain gene rearrangements were detected by PCR analysis. Pretreatment cytogenetics showed no growth. Cytogenetic study after treatment showed complex cytogenetic abnormalities including isochromosome 8.

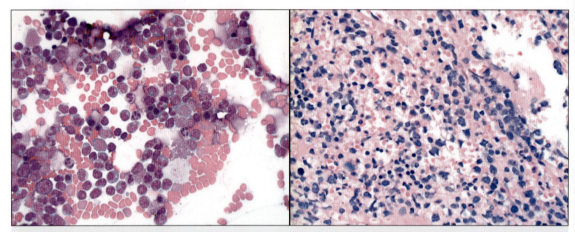

Figure 2 Bone marrow **A** aspirate smear (Wright-Giemsa, ×500) and **B** core biopsy (H&E, ×400) showing infiltration by lymphoid cells that are larger than normal mature lymphocytes and that have single prominent nucleoli with chromatin condensation around the periphery of the nuclei. Marrow involvement is typically diffuse.

Diagnosis T-cell prolymphocytic leukemia.

Management Approach The median survival of a patient with T-cell prolymphocytic leukemia (T-PLL) is <1 year. Most patients with T-PLL require immediate treatment, but the disease does not respond to most available chemotherapeutic drugs or irradiation. Partial remission may be achieved in approximately 30% of patients undergoing combination chemotherapy treatment with alkylating agents including cyclophosphamide, doxorubicin, vincristine and prednisone (CHOP) and the nucleoside purine analogs (2-deoxycoformycin, fludarabine, or leustatin). However, these treatment modalities do not have a significant impact on overall patient survival. Alemtuzumab, a monoclonal anti-CD52 antibody, has been used in treatment of T-PLL, with varying success. Some patients who successfully respond to treatment also undergo stem cell transplantation to consolidate the response. This patient was initially treated by combination chemotherapy with CHOP but without any response. Subsequent single-agent chemotherapy with leustatin (2 cycles), pentostatin (2 doses), and then gemcitabine (1 dose) also did not induce remission. However, he did respond to combination chemotherapy with etoposide, high-dose cytarabine, and ifosfamide, and that prepared him for hematopoietic progenitor cell transplantation with unrelated donor stem cells. He engrafted normally but developed mild graft-vs-host disease of the intestinal tract, which responded to steroid treatment. Four months after the transplant, the disease relapsed, with lymphocytosis of $50 \times 10^3/\mu L$; a bone marrow biopsy revealed recurrent disease. He also developed renal failure and recurrent pleural effusions. Thoracentesis revealed involvement by prolymphocytic leukemia. The clinical course was complicated by respiratory failure, which ultimately led to the patient's death.

General Discussion T-PLL is an aggressive T-cell leukemia characterized by the proliferation of small to medium prolymphocytes with a mature post-thymic phenotype. T-PLL patients typically present with a marked lymphocytosis (>$100 \times 10^3/\mu L$), normocytic anemia, and thrombocytopenia. Physical findings often include generalized lymphadenopathy and hepatosplenomegaly but some cases may also present with skin lesions and/or serous effusions. HTLV-1 serologies are negative. Examination of the peripheral blood film and bone marrow smears are essential for directing the work-up and rendering a diagnosis of T-PLL. Peripheral blood smear often reveals a monotonous population of prolymphocytes. The cells are variable in size, have round nuclei, condensed chromatin usually with a single prominent nucleolus, and a moderate amount of basophilic cytoplasm. Cytoplasmic protrusions or blebs are common. A common small-cell variant of T-PLL represents approximately 25% of all T-PLL cases. A less common variant shows highly irregular nuclear contours. The bone marrow core biopsy of a T-PLL patient will show diffuse, interstitial, and/or focal lymphoid infiltrates along with marrow fibrosis. In lymph nodes, the T-PLL cells may diffusely replace the normal nodal architecture or may concentrate in the paracortical areas, with sparing of the follicles. Prominent high-endothelial venules may be numerous and often infiltrated by neoplastic cells. Cutaneous involvement consists of perivascular or more diffuse dermal infiltrates without epidermotropism. Spleen involvement shows dense red pulp concentration with invasion of the splenic capsule and blood vessels. The neoplastic cells in T-PLL are characteristically post-thymic T cells (TdT–, CD1a–, CD3+), with expression of other pan-T-cell antigens including CD2, CD5, and CD7. The majority of cases are of T-helper phenotype (CD3+, CD4+), with a smaller number of cases expressing T-cytotoxic/suppressor phenotype (CD3+, CD8+). Clonal rearrangement of the TCR is seen in all cases. The neoplastic prolymphocytes express the TCR α/β phenotype. The overexpression of the oncogene TCL1 can be demonstrated by immunohistochemistry and this method is useful for detecting residual T-PLL on bone marrow sections after therapy. Cytogenetic studies have reported a variety of karyotypic abnormalities associated with T-PLL; karyotypes are usually complex and typically involve chromosomes 14 and/or 8.

Section D: Chronic Lymphoproliferative Disorders

T-Cell Large Granular Lymphocytic Leukemia

M James You, Carlos Bueso-Ramos

Patient A 61-year-old man with symptoms of persistent fatigue and dizziness.

Clinical History This patient has a medical history of hypertension, coronary artery disease, reactive airway disease and allergic rhinitis. He went to his primary care physician with symptoms of fatigue and dizziness and was noted to have anemia. A laboratory work-up performed at the physician's office revealed HGB of 8.8g/dL and HCT of 26.3 %. Platelet count was $311 \times 10^3/\mu L$, and WBC count was $7.1 \times 10^3/\mu L$.

Family History Noncontributory.

Medications Simvastatin, metoprolol, cetirizine, aspirin and albuterol inhaler.

Physical Examination Blood pressure was high (159/77). His spleen was palpable. The liver was not palpable and there was no overt lymphadenopathy.

Initial Work-Up		
CBC		
WBC ($\times 10^3/\mu L$)	10.2	
RBC ($\times 10^6/\mu L$)	2.60	
HGB (g/dL)	9.0	
HCT (%)	26.2	
MCV (fL)	101	
MCH (pg)	34.5	
MCHC (g/dL)	34.3	
PLT ($\times 10^3/\mu L$)	324	
RDW-CV (%)	22.5	
MPV (fL)	7.5	
WBC Differential	**%**	**# ($\times 10^3/\mu L$)**
Neutrophils	11	1.1
Bands	1	0.1
Lymphocytes	84	8.6
Monocytes	3	0.3
Eosinophils	1	0.1
Basophils	0	

Peripheral blood smear revealed neutropenia and many lymphocytes containing pink cytoplasmic granules (**Figure 1**).

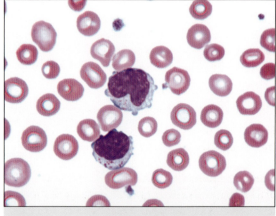

Figure 1 Blood smear (Wright, ×1000) showing lymphocytosis with increased numbers of large granular lymphocytes.

Differential Diagnosis Diagnostic considerations included reactive lymphocytosis and a lymphoproliferative disease.

Additional Work-Up A complete gastrointestinal work-up was negative except for some diverticulosis. Examination of bone marrow biopsy revealed normal cellularity (50%-60%) and an increased number of interstitial and intrasinusoidal lymphocytes (**Figure 2**). Immunohistochemical stains on bone

Section D: Chronic Lymphoproliferative Disorders
T-Cell Large Granular Lymphocytic Leukemia

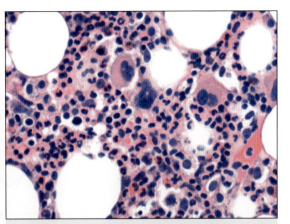

Figure 2 Bone marrow biopsy (H&E, ×400) showing normal cellularity for age (50%-60%) with increased number of interstitial and intrasinusoidal lymphocytes.

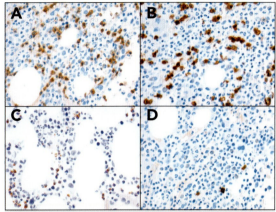

Figure 3 Bone marrow biopsy (immunohistochemical stains, ×400). Lymphoid infiltrates are positive for **A** CD3, **B** CD8, and **C** TIA1. These stains also highlighted the pattern of sinusoidal infiltration that is not uncommon in T-LGL. **D** There are occasional CD20+ B lymphocytes.

marrow specimen demonstrated that the majority of the interstitial lymphocytes were T cells, positive for CD3, CD8 and TIA1 (**Figure 3A**, **3B** and **3C**). Occasional marrow cells were B lymphocytes, positive for CD20 (**Figure 3D**). Flow cytometric analysis of the marrow aspirate showed a distinct population of T cells, positive for CD2, CD3, CD5, CD7, CD8, CD52, CD57 (partial) and TCRαβ, and negative for CD16 and CD56. Molecular diagnostic studies (by PCR) revealed monoclonal T-cell receptor γ chain gene rearrangement. Cytogenetic studies showed a normal male karyotype, 46, XY.

Final Diagnosis T-cell large granular lymphocytic leukemia.

Management Approach The most promising results of treatment of T-cell large granular lymphocytic leukemia (T-LGL) have been reported following the use of low-dose oral methotrexate, cyclosporine, or cyclophosphamide, either as single agents or in combination with prednisone. This patient underwent blood transfusion and received darbepoietin for anemia. In addition, cyclosporine and prednisone were administered. The patient responded with sustained improvement in neutrophil counts, and transfusion independence.

General Discussion T-LGL is typically an indolent clonal T-cell neoplasm. Thus, T-LGL should be distinguished from benign reactive lymphocytosis. Demonstration of clonality is essential to establish T-LGL leukemia. The average age at initial diagnosis is approximately 60 years, and the median survival is >10 years. Systemic symptoms and neutropenia are common. Lymphocytosis composed of lymphocytes with cytoplasmic azurophilic granules is identified in peripheral blood film and bone marrow aspirate smears. In typical cases, there is no evidence of significant trilineage dysplasia. T-LGL involves bone marrow, although morphologic findings may be subtle. The immunophenotype is typically that of CD3+, CD8+ cytotoxic T cells. In situ hybridization study for Epstein-Barr virus is negative.

Adult T-Cell Lymphoma/Leukemia

Beverly P Nelson

Patient A 55-year-old African-American man, who presented with bilateral groin pain and fatigue for 3 days.

Clinical History The patient is a native of the Caribbean, served in the armed services for 25 years, and has hypertension.

Family History His mother died of a T-cell lymphoma. He has a healthy sister (age 48).

Medications Hydrochlorothiazide for hypertension.

Physical Examination Notable for generalized lymphadenopathy and hepatosplenomegaly. Skin was normal without rash or other lesions.

Initial Work-Up

CBC	
WBC (×10³/µL)	34.0
RBC (×10⁶/µL)	3.20
HGB (g/dL)	10.9
HCT (%)	30.9
MCV (fL)	97.0
MCH (pg)	34.3
MCHC (g/dL)	35.4
PLT (×10³/µL)	176
RDW-CV (%)	13.2

WBC Differential	%	# (×10³/µL)
Neutrophils	39	13.3
Bands	0	
Lymphocytes	54	18.4
Monocytes	7	2.4
Eosinophils	0	
Basophils	0	

Serum chemistries: ionized serum Ca 1.47 mmol/L (normal 1.12-1.32), LDH 1,608 U/L (normal 80-170), uric acid 7.1 mg/dL (normal 2.5-8.0), phosphorous 6.2 mg/dL (normal 2.5-5.0). Peripheral blood smear revealed increased numbers of lymphocytes that varied from small to large and included many with irregular nuclear contours (**Figure 1**) and some with visible nucleoli.

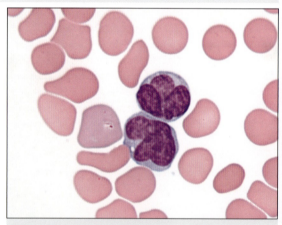

Figure 1 Blood smear (Wright/Giemsa, ×1000) showing 2 ATLL cells with condensed chromatin, and irregular nuclei.

Differential Diagnosis Diagnostic considerations included adult T-cell leukemia/lymphoma, Sézary syndrome, and T-cell prolymphocytic leukemia.

Additional Work-Up PET/CT showed extensive abnormal metabolic activity in the entire skeleton consistent with bone marrow involvement.
- Flow cytometric immunophenotyping of the blood showed a predominant population of T cells that were CD2+, CD3+, CD4+, CD5+, CD25+, α/β+, and negative for the cytotoxic T-cell markers (TIA1, granzyme B)

- Human T-cell leukemia virus (HTLV) 1/2 serology performed on the blood was positive
- Histologic sections of the lymph node biopsy showed complete effacement of the architecture by an abnormal proliferation of T cells associated with many histiocytes containing cytoplasmic debris (**Figure 2**)
- The bone marrow biopsy section showed an abnormal lymphoid infiltrate in clusters (**Figure 3**, arrow) and also as single cells among the normal bone marrow cells. The lymphocytes were large with a moderate amount of cytoplasm, open chromatin pattern, and visible nuclei, and were positive with immunohistochemical stains for CD3 (**Figure 4A**) and FOXP3 (**Figure 4B**)

Final Diagnosis Adult T-cell lymphoma/ leukemia (ATLL).

Management Approach Acute and lymphomatous ATLL are aggressive malignancies with poor prognosis; median survival is about 12 months. Antiretroviral agents with interferon α, ± chemotherapy, have shown promising results (>50% complete response). For this patient, the initial therapy included methyl prednisone to lower the WBC, pamidronate to lower serum calcium, and rasburicase for tumor lysis syndrome prophylaxis. Following ATLL diagnosis, he received zidovudine, a reverse transcriptase inhibitor, and interferon α.

General Discussion Adult T-cell lymphoma/leukemia (ATLL) develops in the setting of HTLV1 infection; a virus transmitted via breast milk and blood. HTLV1 is endemic in regions of Japan, Africa, and in the

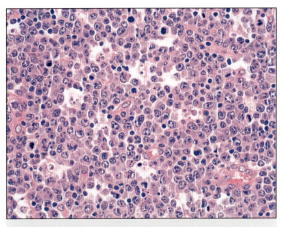

Figure 2 Lymph node (H&E, ×400) showing large lymphoma cells with visible nucleoli and an ample amount of cytoplasm, histiocytes and many mitoses.

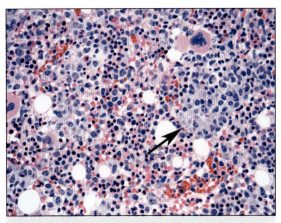

Figure 3 Bone marrow aspirate smear (Wright, ×400) showing extensive replacement of normal marrow elements by blasts.

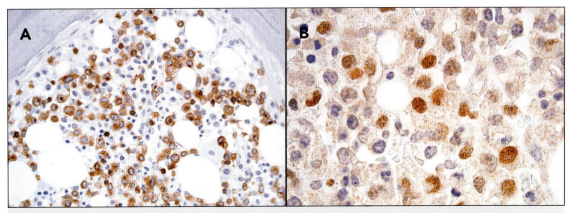

Figure 3 Bone marrow biopsy **A** (CD3, ×400) showing CD3+ lymphoma cells intercalating among the normal cells. **B** (FOXP3, ×1000) showing lymphoma cells that are positive for FOXP3+, a marker of follicular helper T cells.

Section D: Chronic Lymphoproliferative Disorders
Adult T-Cell Lymphoma/Leukemia

Caribbean. Exposure to HTLV1 often occurs during infancy. The latency period between infection and symptomatic disease is long with the median age of ATLL diagnosis in the mid-60s. Less than 5% of those infected develop disease. The clinical forms of ATLL include acute, lymphomatous, chronic, and smoldering. The acute from is the most common and presents with increased lymphocytes, generalized lymphadenopathy, hepatosplemogaly, hypercalcemia, and increased LDH. Eosinophilia is common, and a skin rash is present in 50% of the acute cases. The lymphomatous form presents with lymphadenopathy and a normal lymphocyte count. Onset of the chronic form is insidious; lymphocytosis can persist for months or years without overt disease, and hypercalcemia and significant organomegaly are not typically present. The smoldering form is associated with a skin rash and abnormal lymphocytes in the blood (>5%), but the lymphocyte count is normal, and there is no organomegaly or hypercalcemia. Median survivals for the smoldering, chronic, and acute variants are approximately 62, 42, and 13 months respectively. The smoldering and chronic variants may progress to the acute form. Acute ATLL is an aggressive generalized disease. ATLL cells in the bone marrow may form small clusters or occur as single cells and are frequently FOXP3+. In some cases, the lymphoma cells efface the entire lymph node, and may resembling anaplastic large cell lymphoma (ALCL). ATLL cells are CD30+, EBV±, but are ALK–, granzyme B–, and TIA1– unlike ALCL that is uniformly granzyme B+, and TIA1+, EBV–, and ALK±. The clinical and laboratory features of ATLL, T-cell prolymphocytic leukemia (T-PLL), and Sézary syndrome (SS) overlap, but each disorder has distinctive features. A generalized, erythrodermic skin rash involving the palms of the hands and soles of the feet is present in SS but not in ATLL. The lymphocytes in ATLL often have irregular nuclear contours referred to as "flower cells" but may at times resemble Sézary cells. In the latter cases, hypercalcemia is helpful in distinguishing between the 2 entities since hypercalcemia is not a feature of SS. The phenotypes of ATLL, T-PLL cells and SS cells are also different. ATLL cells are brightly CD25+, but SS cells are CD25–. T-PLL cells may be CD4+/CD8– similar to ATLL, but HTLV serology helps to distinguish ATLL.

Autoimmune Lymphoproliferative Syndrome

Lakshmanan Krishnamurti, Marian Rollins-Raval, Raymond E Felgar

Patient A 4½-month-old male brought to the emergency department because of persistent vomiting.

Clinical History The infant was normal at birth. At approximately 2 months of age, he started developing some "projectile" vomiting 2-3 times a day which consisted of formula without blood or mucus.

Family History There was no history of consanguinity. The older sibling, a 7-year-old male, was asymptomatic. There is a family history of autoimmune disorders.

Medications None.

Physical Examination The patient is a cheerful normal looking infant with massive splenomegaly to the umbilicus). Liver was palpable 3 cm-4 cm. No skeletal abnormalities. Cardiovascular examination was normal. Eyes, ears, and throat showed no abnormalities.

Initial Work-Up

CBC		WBC Differential	%	# (×10³/µL)
WBC (×10³/µL)	5.6	Neutrophils	36	2.74
RBC (×10⁶/µL)	2.29	Lymphocytes	51	3.87
HGB (g/dL)	6.1	Bands	3	0.23
HCT (%)	18.1	Monocytes	6	0.46
MCV (fL)	80	Eosinophils	2	0.15
MCH (pg)	26.7	Basophils	0	
MCHC (g/dL)	333.7	Atypical lymphocytes	0	
PLT (×10³/µL)	121	Nucleated RBC (/100 WBC)	5	
RDW-CV (%)	22.5	Reticulocyte count	5	115

Peripheral blood smear revealed rouleaux, occasional nucleated red cells and a few atypical lymphocytes (**Figure 1**). Since rouleaux formation occurs when the plasma protein concentration is high, it prompted testing for quantitative immunoglobulins, which were found to be high. Nucleated red cells in the circulation suggested marrow regeneration consistent with the diagnosis of hemolytic anemia.

Differential Diagnosis The differential diagnoses for anemia, thrombocytopenia and hepatosplenomegaly include storage disorders such as Gaucher disease, malignant disorders such as leukemia or lymphoma, infectious diseases such as cytomegalovirus, and autoimmune disorders such as systemic lupus erythematosus and autoimmune lymphoproliferative syndrome (ALPS). The ALPS are a group of immune disorders characterized or complicated by lymphoproliferation, autoimmune disease, and lymphoma.

Additional Work-Up The hemoglobin electrophoresis was normal. Evaluation for lipid storage disorders, mucopolysaccharidoses and organic aminoaciduria was negative. There was no evidence of current or past infections with cytomegalovirus, *Rubella*, toxoplasmosis or HIV.

Section D: Chronic Lymphoproliferative Disorders
Autoimmune Lymphoproliferative Syndrome

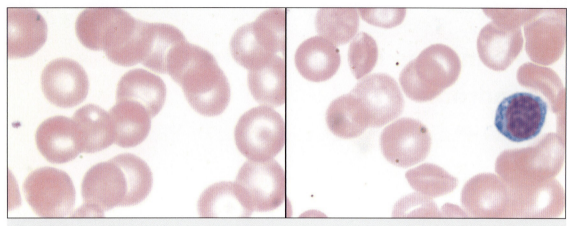

Figure 1 Blood smear (Wright-Giemsa, ×1000) showing rouleaux and an atypical lymphocyte.

Bone marrow was normocellular (100%) and showed trilineage hematopoiesis. The myeloid:erythorid ratio was unremarkable. Erythroid and myeloid maturation was complete and megakaryocytes were present in normal numbers.

Test	Result	Normal
IgA (mg/dL)	98	4-63
IgG (mg/dL)	1,960	55-795
IgM (mg/dL)	93	9-73
Pyruvate kinase, erythrocytes (U/g)	31.1	9.0 to 22.0
RBC fragility, unincubated	Increased	

Flow cytometry (**Figure 2**) performed on peripheral blood demonstrated an increased proportion of CD3+, TCR-α/β+, CD4–, CD8– T lymphocytes, comprising about 4%-9% of total cells. The B lymphocytes were CD19+, CD22+, CD20+, CD5 (partial dim+), CD10 (dim+), FMC7 (predominantly+), CD23 (predominantly+), CD38+ and surface immunoglobulin+. The overall κ:λ ratio was 0.9. Molecular studies established the presence of the FAS(TNFRSF6) mutation in the FAS gene on chromosome 10q24.1.

Final Diagnosis Autoimmune lymphoproliferative syndrome.

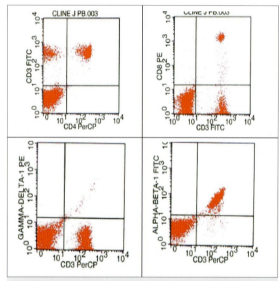

Figure 2 Representative flow cytograms of peripheral blood, with gating on lymphocytes approximately 13% of the lymphocytes appear to be CD3+, CD4–, CD8–, T cells ("double negative T cells"), with only 2% of these being γ-δ T cells and approximately 11% being apparently CD3+, CD4–, CD8–, T-cell receptor αβ+.

Management Approach Clinical management of ALPS generally is directed at autoimmune manifestations such as autoimmune anemia and thrombocytopenia and malignancies. Lymphoproliferation, as manifested by lymphadenopathy and splenomegaly, does not warrant the use of immunosuppressive agents, unless associated with significant obstructive complications or hypersplenism which may require splenectomy. Thrombocytopenic purpura in ALPS may not respond as well to intravenous immunoglobulin and may require the intermittent use of short courses of high-dose corticosteroids. Occasionally autoimmune manifestations may require more intensive therapy, including prolonged corticosteroid treatment and chemotherapeutic agents. Pyrimethamine/sulphadoxine, mycophenolate mofetil, and rituximab have been used in refractory cases. Most patients experience a partial or complete regression of lymphadenopathy and splenomegaly, usually in the second decade of life but autoimmune manifestations may follow a course of remission and exacerbations. This patient was treated initially with oral prednisone. He showed a good response and became transfusion independent. However, on weaning steroids he again became transfusion dependent. He received treatment with anti-CD-20 monoclonal antibody (rituximab), to which he did not respond. He underwent a partial splenectomy and eventually a total splenctomy. His anemia and thrombocytopenia responded to the splenectomy. He had a recurrence of anemia and thrombocytopenia. This was treated with 6 weekly doses of vincristine. He was them placed on mycophenolate mofetil. At 7 years of age, he remained with mild thrombocytopenia, no anemia, extensive lymphadenopathy and no evidence of endocrine disorders.

General Discussion ALPS is a clinical condition with heterogenous phenotype manifest by lymphoproliferative disease, autoimmune cytopenias and susceptibility to malignancy. Defective FAS-induced apoptosis, with resultant dysregulation of lymphocyte homeostasis is the central pathogenetic mechanism. The majority of patients have heterozygous mutations in the FAS (TNFRSF6) gene, but the condition is genetically heterogeneous and mutations in FAS ligand and caspase-8 and caspase-10, all of which are involved in Fas mediated signalling, have also been identified. This results in an accumulation of lymphocytes in organs such as lymph nodes and spleen. Peripheral blood may show reactive changes, but no specific morphologically identifiable abnormalities. Flow cytometric studies generally demonstrate a relative increase in CD3+, CD4–, CD8–, T cells that express T-cell receptors of the α-β type.

Classical Hodgkin Lymphoma with Paraneoplastic Neuromyotonia

Craig Okada, Elie Traer, Jennifer Dunlap

Patient A 24-year-old woman, who presented to the emergency department with progressive difficulty walking.

Clinical History The patient's symptoms began 9 months prior, when she noticed that her legs would become stiff while running. Her symptoms gradually progressed until she began having multiple falls and painful cramps in her legs at night. Six months prior, she was diagnosed with left eye optic neuritis of unknown etiology at an outside hospital and given 3 days of methylprednisolone, with improvement in vision but no improvement in her abnormal gait. She also complained of recent difficulty with swallowing, and had the sensation that food was getting stuck in her esophagus. She denied any fevers, chills, night sweats, or unintentional weight loss. Past medical history was remarkable for reported history of seizures as an infant. However, she was never diagnosed with epilepsy or started on anti-epileptic medication.

Family History Noncontributory.

Medications Meloxicam for pain.

Physical Examination The neurologic exam was notable for a wide-spaced gait, decreased foot proprioception, and positive Romberg test. Her physical exam was otherwise unremarkable. She had no palpable lymph nodes. She had no palpable liver or spleen.

Initial Work-Up

CBC		WBC Differential	%	# ($\times 10^3/\mu L$)
WBC ($\times 10^3/\mu L$)	12.5	Neutrophils	79	9.9
RBC ($\times 10^6/\mu L$)	3.95	Bands	0	0
HGB (g/dL)	11.2	Lymphocytes	11	1.4
HCT (%)	33.9	Monocytes	7	0.9
MCV (fL)	85.7	Eosinophils	2	0.3
MCHC (g/dL)	33.2	Basophils	0	
PLT ($\times 10^3/\mu L$)	480			
RDW-CV (%)	13			

Results of basic metabolic panel, liver panels and serum protein electrophoresis (SPEP) were within normal limits.
She was evaluated initially by neurology and admitted to the hospital for further evaluation. A brain MRI was unremarkable. She had an electromyogram (EMG), which was consistent with neuromyotonia. It was felt that her neuromyotonia might be related to underlying malignancy. A CT scan of her chest, abdomen and pelvis was obtained. The CT was notable for a 7.6 × 5.4 cm cystic mass located in the anterior mediastinum (**Figure 1**). The hematology/oncology service was consulted for further work-up.

Differential Diagnosis The differential diagnosis of neuromyotonia can be broadly categorized into either an autoimmune or a paraneoplastic process. The differential diagnosis of an anterior mediastinal mass includes germ cell tumor, thymoma, lymphoma, thyroid malignancies, parathyroid-related masses and congenital cysts.

Section E: Lymphomas and Their Mimics
Classical Hodgkin Lymphoma with Paraneoplastic Neuromyotonia

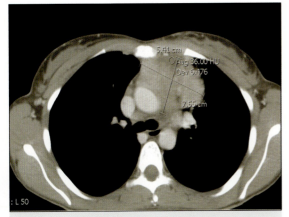

Figure 1 Chest CT with anterior mediastinal mass the dimensions are shown as well as the cystic nature of the lesion (lower density marked by the circle measuring Hounsfield units [HU]).

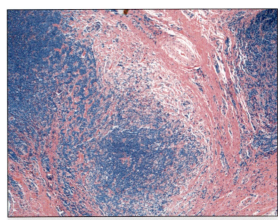

Figure 2 Mediastinal lymph node biopsy (H&E, ×50) showing sclerotic bands of connective tissue surrounding nodules of lymphoid cells.

Additional Work-Up The patient initially had a CT-guided biopsy of her mediastinal mass but there was insignificant tissue to make a diagnosis. She then underwent a mini-thoracotomy and a mediastinal lymph node biopsy was obtained. The biopsy revealed bands of dense sclerotic connective tissue surrounding nodules of lymphoid tissue (**Figure 2**). Within these lymphoid nodules were lacunar Reed-Sternberg cells (**Figures 3** and **4**). These cells were CD30+ (**Figure 5**). Her pretreatment PET scan demonstrated disease in the anterior mediastinum and right supraclavicular/infraclavicular regions. She had a bone marrow biopsy that was negative for involvement with Hodgkin lymphoma.

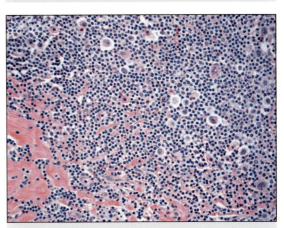

Figure 3 Mediastinal lymph node biopsy (H&E, ×200) showing several lacunar Reed-Sternberg (RS) cells.

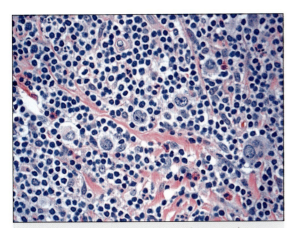

Figure 4 Mediastinal lymph node biopsy (H&E, ×400) showing several lacunar Reed-Sternberg (RS) cells at higher magnification.

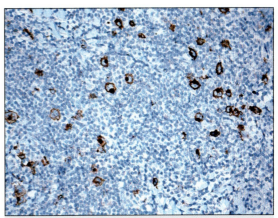

Figure 5 Mediastinal lymph node biopsy (CD30, ×200) highlighting the CD30+ RS cells.

Section E: Lymphomas and Their Mimics
Classical Hodgkin Lymphoma with Paraneoplastic Neuromyotonia

Final Diagnosis Classical Hodgkin lymphoma, nodular sclerosis subtype, with paraneoplastic neuromyotonia.

Management Approach Unfavorable risk factors include large mediastinal adenopathy (mass >1/3 of intrathoracic width or intrathoracic transverse diameter at T5/6 or any mass >10 cm), B symptoms (fevers, night sweats, weight loss of >10%), ESR>50 in the absence of B symptoms, >3 nodal groups, and 2 more extranodal sites. Recommended treatment is doxorubicin, bleomycin, vinblastine and dacarbazine (ABVD), doxorubicin, vinblastine, mechlorethamine, etoposide, vincristine, bleomycin and prednisone (Stanford V) or bleomycin, etoposide, doxorubicin, vincristine, procarbazine and prednisone (BEACOPP). Choice of regimen for Hodgkin lymphoma is based upon stage at presentation and prognostic factors, as well as individual institution guidelines. Most patients are restaged after the 2nd or 3rd cycle of therapy using PET/CT scan, the results of which are used to guide further chemotherapy and/or radiation.

Future fertility was a concern for this patient given her age. Chemotherapy with ABVD has about a 10%-20% infertility rate in Stage I and II Hodgkin lymphoma. The exact rate of infertility with Stanford V is not known but suspected to be less than that of ABVD since the total dose of doxorubicin and bleomycin is less with Stanford V. She opted for a full course of Stanford V chemotherapy (holding the vinca alkaloids after week 4 due to neuropathy) and had complete resolution of her disease by PET scan. Since her original mediastinal disease was >5 cm she was offered involved-field radiation therapy (IFRT) but refused out of concern for late side effects.

General Discussion Hodgkin lymphoma most commonly presents as an enlarging neck mass or mediastinal mass on chest X-ray. The typical B symptoms are fever, night sweats and unintentional weight loss. Less typical associated symptoms are pruritis, pain with drinking alcohol, abdominal swelling or rash. Rarely, Hodgkin lymphoma presents with a paraneoplastic syndrome, as in this case. Neuromyotonia is just one of a subset of paraneoplastic neurologic syndromes believed to result from autoimmune attack of normal neuronal tissue. The paraneoplastic syndromes can affect the CNS, peripheral nerves and muscle activity. A number of antibodies have been associated with different syndromes and may help in diagnosis. Neuromyotonia, also known as Isaac syndrome, is characterized by muscle stiffness caused by continuous muscle fiber activity. Electromyography typically demonstrates spontaneous doublet, triplet or multiplet discharges to individual motor units that occur at irregular intervals. The physiologic consequence of this increased muscle activation is muscle twitching (myokymia), cramps, and delayed muscle relaxation. The etiology of neuromyotonia is thought to be antibodies against voltage-gated potassium channels, and consistent with this model, neuromyotonia reportedly responds well to plasma exchange. The muscular symptoms are managed with anti-epileptic drugs such as phenytoin and carbamazepine. Thymoma, small cell lung cancer and Hodgkin lymphoma are the most commonly associated malignancies. In this case, the patient's neuromyotonia symptoms initially improved with treatment, but then returned a few months after chemotherapy was complete. There is no evidence that her Hodgkin has recurred. In cases where neuromyotonia is not responsive to anti-epileptic drugs, immunosuppressive medications are sometimes effective; however, in this case, immune suppression might increase risk of relapse. She continues to be followed by neurology.

Nodular Lymphocyte-Predominant Hodgkin Lymphoma

Lauren B Smith, Bertram Schnitzer

Patient A 32-year-old African-American man with a 2-year to 3-year history of an enlarging mass in the left inguinal region.

Clinical History The patient was otherwise asymptomatic.

Family History No history of malignancy.

Medications None.

Physical Examination Large, nontender left inguinal mass. No other lymphadenopathy or hepatosplenomegaly.

Initial Work-Up Normal CBC and WBC differential. A core biopsy of the inguinal mass (tan, firm mass with vague nodules)/lymph node, was obtained. It measured 7.5 × 6.0 × 3.5 cm. Microscopically, the lymph node architecture was effaced by large nodules (**Figure 1**) composed of lymphocytes, histiocytes, and occasional large cells (**Figure 2**). The large cells had lobulated nuclei. A compressed rim of normal appearing lymphoid tissue was present at the periphery.

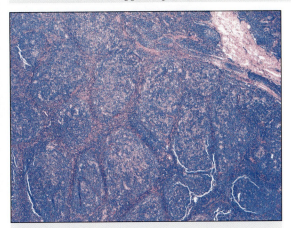

Figure 1 Lymph node biopsy (H&E, ×20) showing large nodules.

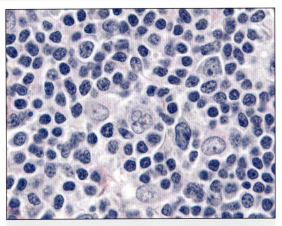

Figure 2 Lymph node biopsy (H&E, ×100) showing large neoplastic (LP) cells.

Differential Diagnosis Diagnostic considerations based on histologic findings included nodular lymphocyte-predominant Hodgkin lymphoma (NLPHL), nodular lymphocyte-rich classical Hodgkin lymphoma (NLRHL), and follicular hyperplasia with progressive transformation of germinal centers (PTGC).

Additional Work-Up By immunohistochemical stains the nodules were composed of a large number of small CD20+ B cells (**Figure 3**). The large atypical cells were strongly positive for CD20 (**Figure 4**) and LCA. CD21 showed an expanded follicular dendritic cell meshwork (**Figure 5**). CD3 and PD-1 showed T-cell rosettes around the LP (lymphocyte predominant) cells (**Figure 6**). CD30 and CD15

Section E: Lymphomas and Their Mimics
Nodular Lymphocyte-Predominant Hodgkin Lymphoma

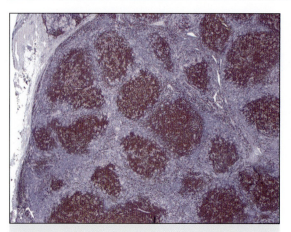

Figure 3 Lymph node biopsy (CD20, ×20) showing large nodules of small B cells.

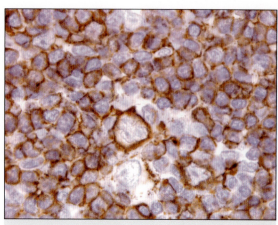

Figure 4 Lymph node biopsy (CD20, ×40) showing positive LP cell and surrounding small B lymphocytes.

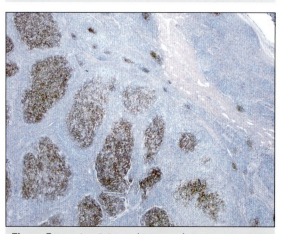

Figure 5 Lymph node biopsy (CD21, ×20) showing expanded follicular dendritic cell meshwork within the nodules.

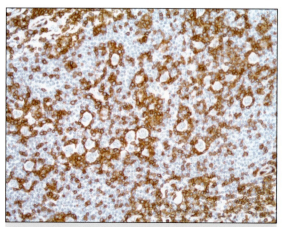

Figure 6 Lymph node biopsy (PD-1, ×20) showing T-cell rosettes around LP cells.

were negative. Flow cytometry showed no evidence of monoclonal B-cell or aberrant T-cell population.

Final Diagnosis Nodular lymphocyte-predominant Hodgkin lymphoma (NLPHL).

Management Approach Distinguishing between classical Hodgkin lymphoma (CHL) and NLPHL is important because the clinical behavior and treatment of these entities can differ. For both CHL and NLPHL, Stage I disease may be irradiated or treated with single agent rituximab. Patients may avoid chemotherapy unless they relapse. For later-stage disease (stages II to IV) combination chemotherapy is warranted possibly followed by involved field radiation. In most cases, the standard therapy is doxorubicin, bleomycin, vinblastine, and dacarbazine (ABVD). At many centers there is a move towards treating these patients with regimens commonly used for non-Hodgkin lymphoma, such as cyclophosphamide, doxorubicin, vincristine and prednisone (CHOP), in combination with rituximab. Two other more aggressive combination regimens are gaining popularity for CHL at some centers: doxorubicin, vinblastine, mechlorethamine, etoposide, vincristine, bleomycin, and prednisone (Stanford 5) or bleomycin, etoposide, doxorubicin, cyclophosphamide, vincristine, procarbazine and prednisone (BEACOPP).

Clinically, NLPHL can have frequent or late relapses, which do not necessarily shorten survival. Treatment-related morbidity/mortality is an important concern in this disease as patients may develop new malignancies after therapy. This patient was treated with local radiation therapy to the inguinal region and was free of disease 2 years later.

General Discussion In the 2008 WHO classification, Hodgkin lymphoma (HL) is divided into 2 disease entities: CHL and NLPHL. NLPHL is uncommon, representing only 5% of the Hodgkin lymphoma cases. Clinically, NLPHL tends to occur in middle-aged male patients and typically involves peripheral lymph nodes, often sparing the spleen, bone marrow and mediastinum. The nodal architecture is completely or partially replaced by nodular or nodular and diffuse infiltrate. Both CHL and NLPHL are characterized by a predominance of nonneoplastic inflammatory cells with small numbers (usually <1%) of malignant cells. These malignant cells are called Reed-Sternberg (RS) and Hodgkin (H) cells in CHL, whereas in NLPHL they are called LP (lymphocyte predominant) cells. LP cells tend to have overlapping nuclear lobes resembling a kernel of exploded corn (thus the name "popcorn" is often used). The neoplastic cells reside in large nodules composed predominantly of small benign B lymphocytes and varying numbers of histiocytes. The cells of the nodules are contained in large, expanded CD21+ follicular dendritic cell meshworks. Diffuse areas may be present along with nodular areas. In contrast to the B cells within the nodules, the small lymphocytes in the diffuse areas are rich in T cells. NLPHL can be distinguished from follicular hyperplasia with PTGC in most cases. The transformed follicles in PTGC are often surrounded by reactive germinal centers, a feature not typically seen in NLPHL. On close examination of PTGC, no LP cells should be present. In rare cases of NLPHL, the nodules may become rich in T cells and lose their nodular architecture, making classification more challenging. In cases with diffuse areas, NLPHL can mimic T-cell/histiocyte rich large B-cell lymphoma (TC/HRLBCL). Differentiating diffuse areas from TC/HRLBCL is important because the latter lymphoma is aggressive and thus requires more aggressive therapy. Immunophenotypically, CHL can be distinguished from NLPHL. H/RS cells are CD30 and typically CD15+. If CD20 is expressed in CHL, it is typically weak and found only in a subset of the H/RS cells. In contrast, the LP cells in NLPHL are characteristically strongly positive for CD20 and LCA (CD45). A number of aberrant somatic mutations (in PAX5, MYC, P1M1, etc) have been found in cases of NLPHL.

Lymphocyte-Rich Classical Hodgkin Lymphoma

Craig Okada, Xu Gang

Patient An 81-year-old Caucasian woman, who presented with right axillary swelling.

Clinical History The patient has a history of a left breast invasive ductal carcinoma that was diagnosed 2 years previously and treated with a simple mastectomy followed by letrozole. She was noted on a routine breast cancer follow-up examination to have an asymptomatic right axillary adenopathy. There was no other palpable superficial adenopathy.

Family History Noncontributory.

Medications Diltazem, omeprazole, aspirin, and letrozole.

Physical Examination She was an elderly but well-appearing woman. She had a well-healed left mastectomy scar and bilateral axillary biopsy scars. Her heart was regular and her lungs clear to examination. She did not have a palpable liver or spleen. She did not have any other palpable adenopathy.

Initial Work-Up

CBC		WBC Differential	%	# (×10³/µL)
WBC (×10³/µL)	4.5	Neutrophils	65.4	3.0
RBC (×10⁶/µL)	4.20	Bands	0	
HGB (g/dL)	11.7	Lymphocytes	29.3	1.3
HCT (%)	35.0	Monocytes	5.3	0.2
MCV (fL)	83.0	Eosinophils	0	
MCH (pg)	27.8	Basophils	0	
MCHC (g/dL)	33.5			
PLT (×10³/µL)	267			
RDW-CV (%)	14.0			

Chemistry panel was normal including an albumin of 4.5. LDH 120 U/L (normal 100-250), β2 microglobulin 2.94 mg/L (normal 0.00-2.70) ESR 9 mm/hour (normal 0-30). A CT scan of her chest, abdomen and pelvis revealed numerous right axillary lymph nodes with the largest measuring 18 mm in the short axis. There were no other sites of adenopathy. A PET scan showed a large area of increased activity in the right axilla corresponding to the enlarged lymph nodes with a maximal standard uptake value (SUV) of 9.8. There was a faint focus of activity in the inferior sternum with the maximal SUV of 5.2.

An excisional right axillary lymph node biopsy was obtained and the histology was initially interpreted as lymphocyte-predominant Hodgkin lymphoma. She was referred to a tertiary care institution for a second opinion. A review of the lymph node biopsy section at the tertiary care institution revealed that there was complete effacement of the normal architecture by a vaguely nodular lymphocyte proliferation consisting of mostly small lymphocytes with scattered large lymphocytes, some demonstrating bilobed nuclei with prominent nucleoli and peri nucleolar halos. Many of the large atypical cells were mononuclear, and rare binucleated forms were seen. Rare eosinophils were identified. There were no fibrous bands separating the nodules (**Figures 1** and **2**).

Section E: Lymphomas and Their Mimics
Lymphocyte-Rich Classical Hodgkin Lymphoma

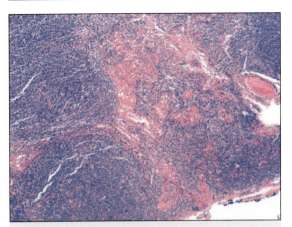

Figure 1 Right axillary lymph node biopsy (H&E, ×50) revealing that the normal lymph node architecture is effaced by a nodular lymphocytic process

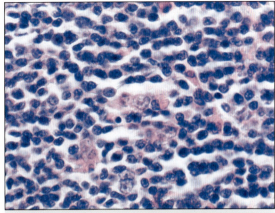

Figure 2 Right axillary lymph node biopsy (H&E, ×400) showing many large mononuclear and occasionally binucleated Reed-Sternberg (RS) cells.

Differential Diagnosis Diagnostic considerations included lymphocyte-rich classical Hodgkin lymphoma and lymphocyte-predominant Hodgkin lymphoma.

Additional Work-Up By immunohistochemical staining, the large atypical cells were CD30+ (**Figure 3**) and dim Pax5+ (**Figure 4**), with variable CD20 expression (mostly negative with few positive cells) and negative for CD15. A CD21 immunostain highlighted the expanded follicular dendritic meshworks throughout the lymph node. CD3 demonstrated numerous T cells, some of which surrounded the large atypical lymphocytes. The absence of LP cells (L&H cells or popcorn cells) and immunophenotypic features were considered most consistent with lymphocyte-rich classical Hodgkin lymphoma. Bone marrow showed focal areas of involvement with Hodgkin lymphoma.

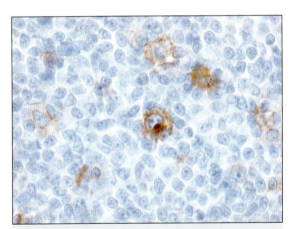

Figure 3 Right axillary lymph node biopsy (H&E, ×50) revealing that the normal lymph node architecture is effaced by a nodular lymphocytic process

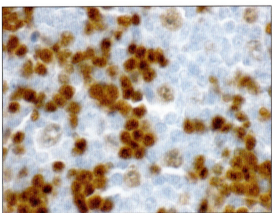

Figure 4 Right axillary lymph node biopsy (H&E, ×400) showing many large mononuclear and occasionally binucleated Reed-Sternberg (RS) cells.

Diagnosis Lymphocyte-rich classical Hodgkin lymphoma.

Management Approach Treatment for Hodgkin lymphoma is based upon stage at presentation and prognostic factors. The adverse risk factors for advanced stage disease include albumin <4 g/dL, hemoglobin <10.5 g/dL, male, age ≥45 years, stage IV disease, leukocytosis (WBC ≥15 × 10^3/μL), and lymphocytopenia (lymphocyte percentage <8% and/or absolute lymphocyte count <0.6 × 10^3/μL). Treatment options usually include combination chemotherapy followed by involved field radiation. A number of combination chemotherapy regimens, including doxorubicin, bleomycin, vinblastine and dacarbazine (ABVD), bleomycin, etoposide, doxorubicin, cyclophosphamide, vincristine, procarbazine, and prednisone (BEACOPP), and vinblastine, doxorubicin, vincristine, bleomycin, nitrogen mustard, etoposide and prednisone (Stanford V) have been used generally with good responses. This patient had stage IVA disease, non-bulky, with adverse risk factors; namely, age and stage. She had a normal left ventricular ejection fraction and pulmonary function study. She was started on doxorubicin, bleomycin, vinblastine and dacarbazine (ABVD) with close monitoring of her cardiac and pulmonary function.

General Discussion Lymphocyte-rich classical Hodgkin lymphoma (LRCHL) accounts for approximately 3%-5% of classical Hodgkin lymphoma (cHL) cases. LRCHL is characterized by infrequent Hodgkin-Reed-Sternberg cells in a background of small mature lymphocytes and rare eosinophils or neutrophils. The growth pattern is typically nodular although there can be a diffuse growth pattern. The Hodgkin cells are mostly binucleated but there is a mononuclear variant. The immunophenotype of the Hodgkin cells in LRCHL is usually the same as in the other subtypes of cHL, namely CD30+ and CD15+. The Hodgkin cells usually lack the expression of pan-B-cell proteins CD19, CD20 and CD79a. PAX-5 expression helps distinguish cHL from unusual T-cell lymphoma. Nodular lymphocyte-predominant Hodgkin lymphoma (NLPHD) is the major morphological mimic of LRCHL. Patients with LRCHL are on average older and present with earlier stages of disease and less mediastinal involvement than patients with other subtypes of cHL. They have fewer adverse prognostic factors and an excellent prognosis with standard treatment used for cHL. This patient presented with asymptomatic adenopathy, which was initially thought to be due to NLPHD. NLPHD might be treated in the same manner as an indolent non-Hodgkin lymphoma, using rituximab in combination with cyclophosphamide, doxorubicin, vincristine and prednisone (R-CHOP), rituximab in combination with ABVD, or other combination chemotherapy regimens. The clarification of her diagnosis resulted in a different treatment recommendation, namely ABVD, without rituximab. The immunophenotype of this case is not quite classical with no detectable expression of CD15. The lack of LP cells (lymphocyte-predominant cells), which are also known as L&H cells (lymphocyte and/or histiocytic Reed-Sternberg cell variants) and the other histologic findings described above; however, best fit with a diagnosis of LRCHL.

Mixed Cellularity Classical Hodgkin Lymphoma

Lauren B Smith, Bertram Schnitzer

Patient A 42-year-old male with a 2-month history of painless enlargement of a left cervical lymph node.

Clinical History The patient reported that 2 weeks of antibiotic therapy did not result in improvement. He also noted a 10-lb weight loss during the previous 2 months.

Family History No history of malignancy.

Medications None.

Physical Examination He appeared well, with normal vital signs. He had an enlarged left cervical lymph node (2 × 2 cm, firm), but no other palpable lymphadenopathy. He had no hepatosplenomegaly.

Initial Work-Up CBC and WBC differential results were within normal limits. A cervical lymph node biopsy was performed. H&E sections revealed large cells with prominent nucleoli, some binucleate, in a mixed inflammatory background including many eosinophils (**Figure 1**).

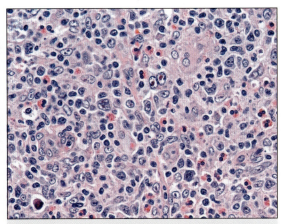

Figure 1 Lymph node biopsy (H&E, ×400) showing large cells, some binucleate, with prominent nucleoli (Reed-Sternberg cells) in a mixed inflammatory background including numerous eosinophils.

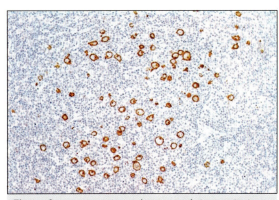

Figure 2 Lymph node biopsy (CD30, ×200) showing that large cells (Reed-Sternberg and Hodgkin cells) are positive.

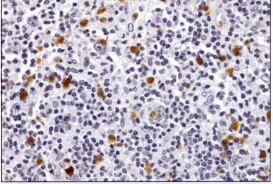

Figure 3 Lymph node biopsy (CD15, ×400) showing large cells (Reed-Sternberg cells) with CD15 expression.

Differential Diagnosis Diagnostic considerations based on histologic findings included classical Hodgkin lymphoma and non-Hodgkin lymphoma. Based on history, metastatic carcinoma was also considered.

Additional Work-Up By immunohistochemical stains, the large cells were positive for CD30 and CD15 (subset), consistent with Reed-Sternberg cells (**Figures 2** and **3**). The background lymphocytes were predominantly CD3+. EBER (in-situ hybridization for Epstein-Barr virus) was positive in many of the large cells (**Figure 4**). Flow cytometry showed no evidence of a monoclonal B-cell population or aberrant T-cell population.

Final Diagnosis Classical Hodgkin lymphoma, mixed cellularity type.

Management Approach Classical Hodgkin lymphoma (CHL) is treated with chemotherapy, often with adjunct radiation therapy. Stage I disease may be treated with local radiation. For later-stage disease (stage II-IV) combination chemotherapy is warranted followed by involved field radiation in some cases. The standard therapy is doxorubicin, bleomycin, vinblastine, and dacarbazine (ABVD). Relapsed disease may be treated with autologous or allogeneic hematopoietic progenitor cell transplant (HPCT). This patient underwent chemotherapy with ABVD and was in remission for 2 years. At relapse, he was treated with an autologous HPCT and is currently in remission.

General Discussion In the 2008 WHO classification, mixed cellularity classical Hodgkin lymphoma (MCCHL) is defined as a type of classical Hodgkin lymphoma (CHL) composed predominantly of a typically diffuse mixed cellular infiltrate composed of benign inflammatory cells with scattered Hodgkin (H) and classical RS cells. The benign background cells consist of variable numbers of small, nonneoplastic lymphocytes, eosinophils, histiocytes, plasma cells, neutrophils, and fibroblasts. Also included in this category are cases that do not fulfill the morphologic criteria for other subtypes of CHL. MCCHL comprises approximately 20%-25% of cases of CHL in industrialized nations. Mixed cellularity (MC) and lymphocyte depleted (LD) are the major subtypes in HIV-infected patients. The median age at diagnosis is 37 years, and approximately 70% of patients are male. Peripheral lymph nodes are usually involved. MCCHL is most often diagnosed in advanced stage (III/IV), and most patients have B symptoms. Unlike nodular sclerosis HL, mediastinal involvement is rare. Prior to the advent of modern therapy, the prognosis of mixed cellularity classical Hodgkin lymphoma (MCCHL) was worse than that of nodular sclerosis subtype and better than that of lymphocyte-depleted subtype. However, with modern therapeutic regimens, these differences are no longer seen. The immunophenotype of H/RS cells is identical to that of other types of CHL. In most cases the H/RS cells express CD15 and CD30. Fascin is expressed in the cytoplasm of almost all cases of CHL. If CD20 is expressed, it usually is present only a subset of H/RS cells. H/RS cells are negative for CD45 but show weak positivity for the B-cell transcription factor PAX5. EBER is expressed by H/RS cells more frequently in MCCHL than in other types of CHL. The differential diagnosis of

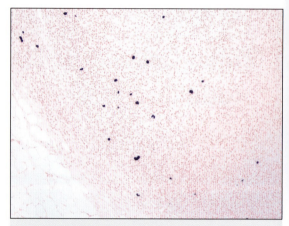

Figure 4 Lymph node biopsy (EBER in situ hybridization, ×100) showing EBV+ Reed-Sternberg cells.

MCCHL includes both benign lymphoid proliferations as well as non-Hodgkin lymphomas. Benign mimickers include immunoblastic proliferations such as those seen in viral infections. The prototypes include infectious mononucleosis and hypersensitivity reactions, most of which are drug-induced. Peripheral T-cell lymphoma (PTCL) can also resemble MCCHL. Both infectious mononucleosis and drug-induced hypersensitivity reactions differ from characteristic cases of MCCHL in that reactive and even hyperplastic follicles are usually present and the atypical immunoblastic proliferation is in the interfollicular areas. Eosinophils are present in drug-induced hypersensitivity reactions. Both benign processes are characterized by a proliferation of immunoblasts, some of which may be binucleated, thus resembling RS cells. The immunoblasts, including the RS-like cells, usually express CD30 but, in contrast to classic RS cells, are CD15 and fascin negative. Unlike the staining of H/RS cells, the immunoblasts in these benign proliferations are predominantly CD20+ B cells, and a smaller population of these cells express T-cell markers. Histologically, MCCHL may closely resemble PTCL, and, therefore, immunophenotyping is necessary to distinguish MCCHL from PTCL. Both MCCHL and PTCL, especially angioimmunoblastic T-cell lymphoma (AITL), are characterized by a polymorphous proliferation of benign inflammatory cells including lymphocytes, eosinophils, histiocytes, plasma cells and H/RS-like cells. Proliferation of high endothelial venules (HEV) is a feature of most PTCL (especially AITL) but not of HL. The H/RS-like cells in PTCL are, with rare exceptions, CD15–. The large cells in PTCL express T-cell markers, although in some cases, especially in AITL, some large cells are CD20+ B cells. These large B cells in AITL are often EBER positive. Finally, a clonal T-cell proliferation demonstrated by PCR on whole tissue sections also supports the diagnosis of PTCL.

Follicular Lymphoma

Beverly P Nelson

Patient A 70-year-old male, who presented with lumps in his neck. The lumps had endured for 1 year prior.

Clinical History The patient reported having these lumps for about a year. His past history is significant for hypertension and prostate carcinoma treated with prostatectomy.

Family History Father deceased at age 78 from colon cancer. Mother died at age 96 of unspecified cause (she had a non-Hodgkin lymphoma that was treated with radiation therapy). Sister (age 65) is healthy.

Medications Atelenol for hypertension.

Physical Examination Notable for enlarged bilateral axillary and inguinal lymph nodes.

Initial Work-Up

CBC

WBC (×10³/μL)	8.1
RBC (×10⁶/μL)	4.54
HGB (g/dL)	13.8
HCT (%)	41.3
MCV (fL)	91
MCH (pg)	30.4
MCHC (g/dL)	33.4
PLT (×10³/μL)	130
RDW-CV (%)	12.1

WBC Differential

	%	# (×10³/μL)
Neutrophils	75.1	6.1
Bands	0	
Lymphocytes	14.6	1.2
Monocytes	5.4	0.4
Eosinophils	4.4	0.4
Basophils	0.5	

CAT scans showed bilateral, axillary and inguinal lymphadenopathy.
Cervical lymph node biopsy: the architecture was effaced by follicular lymphoma (FL) composed of closely spaced, neoplastic follicles with indistinct mantle zones (**Figure 1**). The neoplastic germinal centers (**Figure 2**) contained follicular dendritic cells, centrocytes, and centroblasts that were <15/10 hpf.

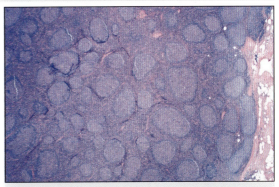

Figure 1 Lymph node (H&E, ×20) in which the malignant follicles are closely spaced, lack well-defined mantle zones, and destroy the architecture of the lymph node.

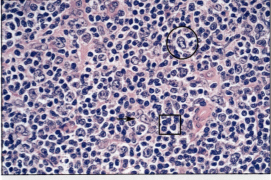

Figure 2 Lymph node (H&E, ×600) showing the malignant germinal center contains mostly centrocytes (square) with occasional centroblasts (circle). Follicular dendritic cells (arrow) should not be confused with centroblasts.

Differential Diagnosis Diagnostic considerations included low-grade non-Hodgkin lymphomas including follicular lymphoma and small lymphocytic lymphoma/chronic lymphocytic leukemia. Hodgkin lymphoma and more aggressive lymphomas such as diffuse large B-cell lymphoma were considered less likely given the clinical presentation.

Additional Work-Up A CD21 immunohistochemical stain of the lymph node highlighted the follicular dendritic meshwork in the neoplastic follicles (**Figure 3**), and a BCL2 stain showed that the germinal centers were BCL2+ (**Figure 4**). Flow cytometric immunophenotyping demonstrated λ surface immunoglobulin light chain restricted B cells that were , CD10+, CD19+, CD20+, CD22+, and negative with the other T-cell associated markers evaluated (CD2, CD3, CD7).

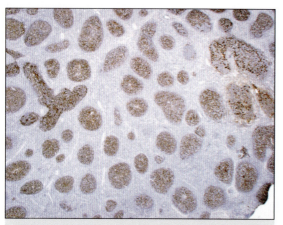

Figure 3 Lymph node (CD21, ×20) showing follicular dendritic cell meshwork is confined to the germinal centers and is helpful to identify follicles that are subtle on H&E stain.

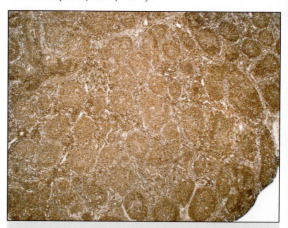

Figure 4 Lymph node (BCL2, ×20) showing the malignant germinal centers are BCL2+.

Final Diagnosis Follicular lymphoma (FL), grade 1-2.

Management Approach Prior to the rituximab era, asymptomatic patients with low-grade FL and low tumor burden were often observed without therapy until symptoms developed, but rituximab is now used alone for asymptomatic patients or in combination with chemotherapy for the symptomatic. This patient received rituximab with cyclophosphamide, vincristine and prednisone (R-CVP) 12 months after diagnosis when hepatomegaly, splenomegaly, and progressive adenopathy developed and repeat lymph node biopsy showed grade 1 fL-2 fL.

General Discussion Follicular lymphoma (FL) is the second most common non-Hodgkin lymphoma (NHL) representing about 25% NHL in the United States and Europe. The usual presenting sign is enlarged superficial lymph nodes. Diagnosis at extranodal sites is rare, but the gastrointestinal tract, especially the duodenum, is the most common extranodal site where FL is initially diagnosed. Lymphoma is usually localized to the duodenum and has excellent prognosis.

Characteristically FL shows a nodular/follicular growth pattern. The nodules are crowded, lack well defined mantle zones, and obliterate the normal tissue. Nodules are subtle in some cases, and may be absent in rare FL with a completely diffuse growth pattern. The neoplastic follicles contain cells typically present in benign follicles: centrocytes, centroblasts, and follicular dendritic cells (FDC). Centrocytes are small lymphocytes with condensed chromatin, angulated/cleaved nuclei, and scant cytoplasm. Centroblasts are large lymphocytes with slightly dispersed chromatin, and visible nucleoli located adjacent to the nuclear membrane. The proportion of centroblasts and centrocytes in each case correlates with clinical behavior and is used to grade each tumor. At least 10 randomly selected neoplastic follicles should be evaluated for grading. Grade-1 FL-grade-2 FL has up to 15 centroblasts per 40× field, and grade-3 FL has >15 centroblasts. Grade-3 FL is subdivided into 3A (centrocytes and centroblasts in the follicle), and 3B (only centroblasts in the follicle). Sheets of centroblasts without FDC meshwork represent diffuse large B-cell lymphoma (DLBCL) and confers less favorable outcome. FL may be diagnosed from H&E-stained tissue sections showing unequivocal neoplastic follicles. Cases with more subtle follicles often require ancillary studies to establish the diagnosis. FL cells are monotypic and are, CD10+, CD19+, CD20+, and CD22+. Neoplastic germinal centers are BCL2+ in up to 90% of grade-1-grade-2 tumors, but only in about 50% of grade-3 tumors. Benign follicles are BCL2–. CD21 show FDC meshwork and is useful to detect follicles that are difficult to appreciate in H&E-stained sections. Molecular analysis for *BCL2* gene rearrangement may be necessary in some cases such as in situ follicular lymphoma characterized by isolated BCL2+ germinal center among benign follicles. This is a rare occurrence with unclear clinical significance. Careful evaluation for FL at other anatomic sites is warranted since in situ FL could represent follicular colonization by FL located elsewhere. But lymphoma is not always found at other anatomic sites, and may not subsequently develop.

Mantle Cell Lymphoma

Tsieh Sun

Patient A 61-year-old man with bilateral neck masses.

Clinical History The patient noticed rapid growth of the neck masses over the past 3 months. He has not had any fever, weight loss or night sweats. He presented to his family physician about 2 months prior, and had been started on antibiotics but with no resolution of the neck masses/adenopathy.

Family history There is no history of malignancy among family members.

Medication None.

Physical Examination He appears comfortable and in no distress. His vital signs are normal. He has bilateral cervical lymphadenopathy. There are also palpable lymph nodes in axillary and femoral areas. He does not have hepatosplenomegaly.

Initial Work-Up

CBC			WBC Differential	%	# (×10³/µL)
WBC (×10³/µL)		7.8	Neutrophils	69.0	5.4
RBC (×10⁶/µL)		5.74	Bands	0	
HGB (g/dL)		17.5	Lymphocytes	17.9	1.4
HCT (%)		51.3	Monocytes	9.3	0.7
MCV (fL)		89.3	Eosinophils	2.1	0.2
MCH (pg)		30.5	Basophils	1.7	0.1
MCHC (g/dL)		34.1			
PLT (×10³/µL)		272			
RDW-CV (%)		13.3			
MPV (fL)		6.6			

Differential Diagnosis Lymphoma vs infectious disease. The clinical setting is most consistent with non-Hodgkin lymphoma. The absence of fever and leukocytosis makes infectious disease less likely.

Additional Work-Up A cervical lymph node biopsy was performed. It showed a nodular pattern with several naked germinal centers surrounded by a greatly expanded paracortical zone composed of small lymphocytes with irregular nuclei and inconspicuous nucleoli (**Figure 1**). Immunohistochemical stains revealed that the tumor cells were immunoreactive with CD20 (**Figure 2**), CD5 and cyclin D1 (**Figure 3**), but were negative for CD3, and CD10. CD23 demonstrated a follicular dendritic cell meshwork in a few nodules. Flow cytometric analysis demonstrated a monoclonal λ B-cell population with coexpression of CD19, CD5, and FMC-7, but low percentages of CD23 and CD10. Cytogenetic karyotype showed t(11;14)(q13;q32).

Section E: Lymphomas and Their Mimics
Mantle Cell Lymphoma

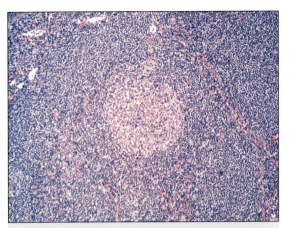

Figure 1 Lymph node biopsy (H&E, ×50) showing a naked germinal center surrounded by a sea of lymphoma cells.

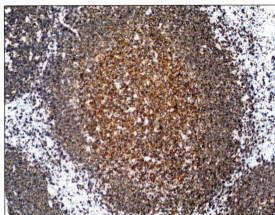

Figure 2 Lymph node biopsy (CD20, ×100) in which the tumor nodule stains positive.

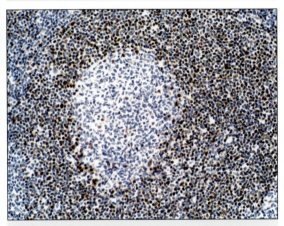

Figure 3 Lymph node biopsy (cyclin D1, ×200) in which the tumor cells in mantle zone stain positive.

Final Diagnosis Mantle cell lymphoma.

Management approach Most of mantle cell lymphoma (MCL) patients have an aggressive clinical course. The median survival time for MCL patients is 3 years-5 years, but some patients may have a comparatively indolent clinical course and may survive for >10 years. The most powerful tool to predict the prognosis is gene expression profiling (GEP), which is able to stratify MCL cases into various subtypes in terms of IgH gene mutation status, proliferation rate, and blastoid morphology. The indolent clinical subtype is usually associated with fewer high-risk chromosomal aberrations. MCL is responsive to multidrug chemotherapy (cyclophosphamide/doxorubicin/vincristine and prednisone, dexamethasone/ high-dose cytarabine/cis-platin, fractionated cyclophosphamide/doxorubicin/vincristine and dexamethasone), but it appears incurable with all of the regimens that have been tried. Rituximab alone or in combination with chemotherapy or chemotherapy followed by allogeneic hematopoietic progenitor cell transplantation (HPCT) seems to hold some hope for long-term remissions. This patient received 3 cycles of rituximab and CHOP that he tolerated well. His cervical lymph nodes were reduced in size following treatment.

General Discussion MCL, a B-cell neoplasm, represents 3%-10% of non-Hodgkin lymphomas. Lymph nodes are the most commonly involved sites but any tissue or organ may be involved, including, blood, marrow, spleen, liver, and gastrointestinal tract. MCL is also responsible for most cases of lymphomatous polyposis of the gastrointestinal tract. It is not uncommon for patients to present with generalized lymphadenopathy, splenomegaly, hepatomegaly, bone marrow and blood involvement. MCL is a small cell lymphoma originating from the mantle zone of the lymphoid follicle. The most characteristic cytology is the centrocyte-like morphology and this was why this tumor was originally designated centrocytic lymphoma. However, the tumor cells can also assume the morphology of small and monocytoid lymphocytes. The cells in the centrocytic variant are identical to the centrocytes in the lymphoid follicles. The small cell variant shows slight or moderate nuclear irregularity or cleft, with clumped chromatin pattern, no nucleoli, and scant cytoplasm. The cells in monocytoid or marginal zone B-cell variant show abundant pale cytoplasm, resembling the tumor cells of marginal zone B-cell lymphoma. In the aggressive form of MCL, the tumor cells may assume a blastoid feature resembling lymphoblasts with immature chromatin pattern and high mitotic rate. Alternatively, the tumor cells may be pleomorphic with large nuclei, prominent nucleoli, and pale cytoplasm. Unlike other small cell lymphomas, MCL does not transform into diffuse large B-cell lymphoma. When large cell morphology is present, it should be classified as MCL, blastoid form or pleomorphic form. There are 3 histologic patterns: diffuse, mantle zone and nodular. The diffuse type is most commonly seen. The mantle zone type is characterized by the presence of large sheets of small lymphocytes around a naked germinal center. However, this pattern can be also seen in nodal marginal zone B-cell lymphoma. The nodular type is either the result of follicular colonization or may arise from the primary lymphoid follicles. However, coexistence of several patterns is frequently encountered. In addition, the difference in histologic pattern does not correlate with any clinical presentation or prognosis. Rather, the cytology of tumor cells can help predict the prognosis: the blastoid or pleomorphic subtype is always seen in patients with aggressive clinical course. Immunophenotyping is important in the differentiation between MCL and other small cell lymphomas. The characteristic feature of MCL is the coexpression of B-cell antigens (CD19 or CD20) with CD5 on the tumor cells. However, this feature is also seen in chronic lymphocytic leukemia/small lymphocytic lymphoma (CLL/SLL). Therefore, CD23 and FMC-7 are used to distinguish them: CD23 is positive in CLL/SLL but not MCL, while FMC-7 is expressed in a high percentage in MCL cases. Nevertheless, CD23+ MCL or CD23– CLL/SLL has been reported from time to time. Immunohistochemistry is reliable in diagnosing MCL, because cyclin D1 is a highly specific marker for MCL. For the mantle zone subtype, the demonstration of the expanded mantle zone by CD20 and CD5 is also highly supportive. The demonstration of the follicular dendritic cell meshwork among the tumor cells by CD21, CD23 or CD35 in MCL also helps to exclude CLL/SLL. The staining of Ki-67 and Survivin (inhibitor of apoptosis) is useful in predicting the prognosis. MCL is characterized by the presence of t(11;14)(q13;q32) that represent the translocation of the proto-oncogene, BCL1 (11q13) juxtaposed to the heavy chain (IgH) gene (14q32). As the IgH enhancer cannot control BCL1, the proto-oncogene becomes deregulated, resulting in over-expression of cyclin D1 (CCND1). Cyclin D1 plays an important role in the control of G1 phase and its elevation results in acceleration of G1/S phase transition and thus tumor cell proliferation. Immunoglobulin genes are rearranged in MCL, but most cases show unmutated variable region genes.

Gastric MALT Lymphoma with Associated *H pylori* Infection

Juan P Palazzo, Adam D Toll

Patient A 72-year-old woman presented with reflux symptoms.

Clinical History The patient reported having reflux and epigastric pain for 5 months. She used antacids without relief.

Family History Noncontributory.

Medications Antacids as needed, low-dose aspirin.

Physical Examination Notable for mild epigastric tenderness to palpation. The liver and spleen were not palpable. She had no palpable lymph nodes.

Initial Work-Up		
CBC		
WBC (×10³/µL)	7.2	
RBC (×10⁶/µL)	3.41	
HGB (g/dL)	11.8	
HCT (%)	32.1	
MCV (fL)	96	
MCH (pg)	35	
MCHC (g/dL)	34.7	
PLT (×10³/µL)	334	
RDW-CV (%)	14.6	
WBC Differential	**%**	**# (×10³/µL)**
Neutrophils	58.8	4.2
Bands	0	
Lymphocytes	29.6	2.1
Monocytes	7.2	0.5
Eosinophils	3.0	0.2
Basophils	1.4	0.1

An esophagogastroduodenoscopy (EGD) with biopsy was performed and showed diffuse gastritis with focal superficial ulceration. Histologic sections showed a prominent lymphocytic infiltrate in the lamina propria and lymphoepithelial lesions with glandular destruction (**Figure 1A**). The lymphocytes were medium-sized with scattered monocytoid forms and inconspicuous nucleoli. Foci of active neutrophilic infiltration into mucosal glands were noted (**Figure 1B**).

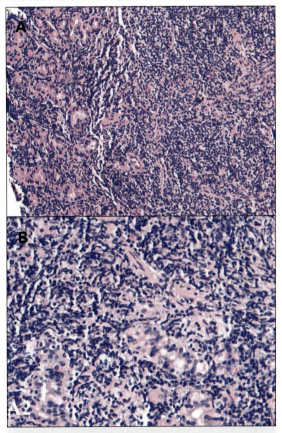

Figure 1 Gastric biopsy **A** (H&E, ×200) and **B** (H&E, ×400) showing a diffuse lymphoid infiltrate in the mucosa with associated lymphoepithelial lesions and glandular destruction.

Section E: Lymphomas and Their Mimics
Gastric MALT Lymphoma with Associated H pylori Infection

Differential Diagnosis Lymphoma vs a reactive or inflammatory condition.

Additional Work-Up A Warthin-Starry stain highlighted numerous curved bacilli morphologically consistent with *Helicobacter pylori* (**Figure 2**). By immunohistochemical stains (IHC) the cells infiltrating mucosal glands were CD3–, CD5–, CD10–, CD20+ (**Figure 3**), BCL1–, BCL2+ (**Figure 4**), and BCL6–. Molecular analysis of the immunoglobulin heavy chain (IgH) gene rearrangement by polymerase chain reaction (PCR) demonstrated a monoclonal B-cell population.

Final Diagnosis Low-grade extranodal marginal zone lymphoma, MALT type, *Helicobacter pylori* +.

Management Approach In cases of *H pylori*-associated gastric MALT lymphomas, attention should be paid to ensure eradication of the infection. Histologic remission can be seen within 6 months of *H pylori* eradication in gastric-confined (stage I) MALT lymphoma. Of note, molecular follow-up may show persistence of the monoclonal B-cell population despite histologic remission, and careful follow-up is warranted in this subset of patients. Treatment regimens typically employ a triple therapy including a proton pump inhibitor in association with various antibiotics. There is no standardized therapy for patients with *H pylori*-negative lymphoma, or those who fail antibiotic therapy. This patient was treated for reflux and *H pylori* infection with omeprazole, amoxicillin, and clarithromycin. Follow-up EGD at 6 months showed minimal chronic gastritis, and no evidence of lymphoma. A Warthin-Starry stain no longer identified *H pylori*, and a urease breath test was negative. PCR analysis failed to identify a monoclonal population.

General Discussion Marginal zone lymphomas are generally tumors of adults with a median age at diagnosis of 60 years. They are believed to be derived from B cells normally present in the extranodal zone and are broadly categorized as nodal, extranodal, and splenic. These lymphomas are comprised of mature B cells, and express pan-B antigens including CD19, CD20, and CD79a. Further, they may also express the marginal zone antigens CD21 and CD35. Reactive T cells expressing CD3 are commonly identified, and play an important role in driving B-cell proliferation early in the disease course. Extranodal marginal zone lymphoma of the mucosa-associated lymphoid tissues (MALT) is relatively common and represent approximately 7%-10% of all non-Hodgkin lymphomas

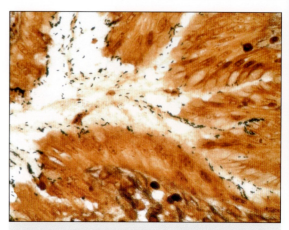

Figure 2 Gastric biopsy (Warthin-Starry stain, ×400) showing numerous curved bacilli consistent with *H pylori*.

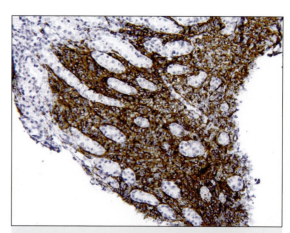

Figure 3 Gastric biopsy (CD20, ×100) showing diffuse staining of lymphoid cells.

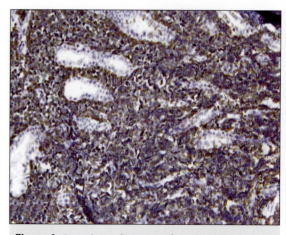

Figure 4 Gastric biopsy (BCL2, ×200) showing diffuse staining of lymphoid cells.

in the United States and Europe. Within this category, primary gastric MALT lymphoma is the most common. Histopathologically, this entity shows a heterogeneous collection of cells, most notably medium-sized monocytoid centrocyte-like marginal zone cells with irregular nuclei. The most important feature; however, is the presence of lymphoepithelial lesions consisting of malignant cells invading and ultimately destroying mucosal glands. MALT lymphomas typically arise in sites where lymphocytes are not commonly found, and have migrated to following an antigenic stimulus. With chronic stimulation, abnormal B-cell clones acquire successive genetic mutations ultimately replacing the normal, reactive B-cell population. Eradication of *H pylori* infection with antibiotic therapy has been shown to lead to regression in a majority (>80%) of early-stage tumors. Multiple translocations affecting the nuclear factor κ B pathway have been identified in MALT lymphomas; the most common implicated in gastric MALT is t(11;18)(q21;q21). The development of this translocation has significant prognostic and therapeutic implications. Identification of the t(11;18) predicts a poor response to *H pylori* eradication, and is commonly seen in disseminated disease. Most patients with gastric MALT; however, have a favorable outcome with >85% 5-year survival. The most common presentation of *H pylori*-associated gastric MALT lymphomas are nonspecific upper gastrointestinal symptoms (epigastric pain, nausea, etc). EGD typically shows gastritis or acute mucosal ulceration. Discrete mass lesions are not typically identified, and their presence should raise suspicion for a diffuse large B-cell lymphoma. Multiple gastric and duodenal biopsies are recommended to establish a diagnosis, as well as determine depth of invasion. PET testing is not warranted as gastric MALT lymphomas typically show low uptake of flurodeoxyglucose (FDG). Southern blotting or polymerase chain reaction (PCR) can aid in demonstrating monoclonality. Molecular findings; however, must be interpreted carefully as *H pylori*-associated gastritis may show monoclonality in the absence of MALT lymphoma.

Burkitt Lymphoma

David S Bosler, Eric D Hsi

Patient A 31-year-old white male with a 2-week history of intermittent abdominal discomfort.

Clinical History The patient reported that the abdominal discomfort started on the right side and then radiated into the rest of the abdomen and down into the right testis. More recently, he had also noticed enlargement of the right testis. CT imaging showed numerous soft tissue density masses ranging from 2 cm - 9 cm in greatest dimension and involving the cecum and terminal ileum, mid transverse colon, splenic flexure and descending colon, as well as enlargement of the pancreatic head and numerous enlarged right peritoneal and periportal lymph nodes. PET scanning showed intense hypermetabolism of the described masses, as well as small hypermetabolic foci in the liver and a left lower rib. Colonoscopy showed distortion of the cecal base by an extrinsic mass, with no mucosa-based lesions.

Family History No history of malignancies except smoking-related lung cancer.

Medications None.

Physical Examination Fit, well-nourished male in no acute distress. Vital signs normal. No palpable lymphadenopathy. A large tender mass is palpated in the right mid-lower abdomen, and the right testis is enlarged and tender. No skin rashes or lesions. Physical exam is otherwise normal.

Initial Work-Up		
CBC		
WBC ($\times 10^3/\mu L$)	8.5	
RBC ($\times 10^6/\mu L$)	4.65	
HGB (g/dL)	13.2	
HCT (%)	38.8	
MCV (fL)	83.4	
MCH (pg)	28.4	
MCHC (g/dL)	34	
PLT ($\times 10^3/\mu L$)	300	
RDW-CV (%)	12.1	
MPV (fL)	10.4	
WBC Differential	**%**	**# ($\times 10^3/\mu L$)**
Neutrophils	71	6.0
Lymphocytes	19	1.6
Monocytes	9	0.8
Eosinophils	2	0.2

*Right lower quadrant mass, needle biopsy: histologic sections showed a dense monotonous lymphoid infiltrate of intermediate-sized cells with relatively round nuclei, granular chromatin and indistinct nucleoli. Numerous mitotic and apoptotic figures were present (**Figure 1**).*

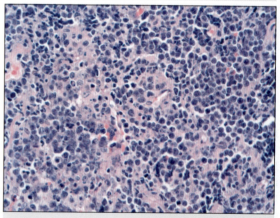

Figure 1 Abdominal mass needle core biopsy (H &E, ×400) showing dense monotonous lymphoid infiltrate of intermediate-size cells and many mitotic and apoptotic figures.

Differential Diagnosis Based on the morphologic features, including the intermediate size of the neoplastic cells, the differential diagnosis included Burkitt lymphoma, lymphoblastic lymphoma, diffuse large B-cell lymphoma and blastoid variant of mantle cell lymphoma.

Additional Work-Up By immunohistochemical stains the neoplastic cells were positive for CD20 (**Figure 2**) and CD10, and negative for BCL2, BCL6, TdT, MUM1, and cyclin D1. Ki-67 stained 100% of the neoplastic cells (**Figure 3**). Immunophenotyping by flow cytometry demonstrated a monotypic B-cell population expressing CD19, CD20, CD10 and surface λ light chains. Fluorescence in situ hybridization (FISH) studies using a dual-color breakapart probe to detect translocations involving the MYC gene (8q24) were positive (**Figure 4**). FISH studies to detect the t(14;18)(q32;q21) IGH/BCL2 fusion were negative.

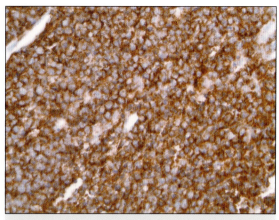

Figure 2 Abdominal mass needle core biopsy (CD20, ×400), in which positivity reflects B-cell lineage.

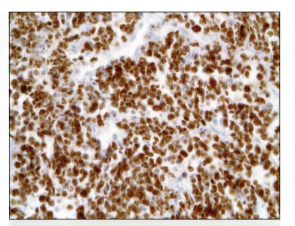

Figure 3 Abdominal mass needle core biopsy (Ki-67, ×400) showing a near 100% proliferative rate.

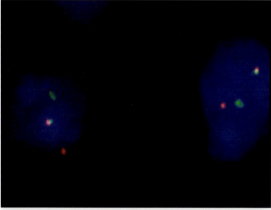

Figure 4 Abdominal mass needle core biopsy (MYC breakapart FISH, ×1000) showing 1 split signal indicating an MYC translocation.

Final Diagnosis Burkitt lymphoma.

Management Approach The patient came to our institution for diagnosis and recommendations for treatment. Standard management approaches were discussed, including R-CODOX-M/IVAC—composed of rituximab (R), cyclophosphamide (C), vincristine (O), doxorubicin (DOX), methotrexate (M), ifosfamide (I), etoposide (V, also known as VP-16), and cytarabine (AC). Intensive chemotherapeutic regimens including intrathecal prophylaxis, such as that described above, are generally part of the therapeutic approach for Burkitt lymphoma. The increased intensity of therapy compared with the standard rituximab, cyclophosphamide, vincristine, prednisone (R-CHOP) that is used in diffuse large B-cell lymphoma reflects the aggressive behavior of this neoplasm. Patients with this disease are at high risk for tumor lysis syndrome and must receive adequate hydration, allopurinol and electrolyte monitoring during the early phases of therapy. This patient was treated with R-CODOX-M/IVAC with a rapid response to therapy and subsequently referred for discussion of allogeneic hematopoietic progenitor cell transplant.

General Discussion The diagnosis of Burkitt lymphoma (BL) is initially suspected based on the morphologic findings. Specifically, the intermediate size of the cells, the monotonous cytologic appearance with relatively round nuclei, granular chromatin and indistinct nucleoli, and the high frequency of mitosis and apoptosis suggest this possibility. Immunohistochemistry findings also support this diagnosis, with coexpression of CD20 and CD10 as well as 100% expression of Ki-67, a marker of proliferation. Lack of TdT staining and expression of surface light chain by flow cytometry help to exclude lymphoblastic lymphoma, and lack of cyclin D1 expression virtually excludes blastoid variant of mantle cell lymphoma. Finally, the presence of an MYC gene translocation by FISH confirms the diagnosis. Although the immunophenotypic and FISH findings described could also be compatible with diffuse large B-cell lymphoma (DLBCL), the 100% Ki-67 staining is unusual for this entity, and the cytologic features (intermediate size, round nuclei, monotony) do not support a diagnosis of DLBCL. DLBCL is more characteristically composed of unequivocally large cells with a greater degree of nuclear irregularity and pleomorphism. Nonetheless, high-grade large B-cell lymphomas can show morphologic, immunophenotypic, and genetic features that overlap with BL. Non-Burkitt high-grade lymphomas can have high mitotic and apoptotic rates that sometimes result in the "starry sky" appearance that, while nonspecific, is classically attributed to BL. MYC translocations, while almost invariant in BL, can occur in approximately 10% of de novo DLBCL. The overlap between these entities has been a source of confusion, and has resulted in the inclusion of "B-cell lymphoma, unclassifiable, with features intermediate between DLBCL and BL" (BCL-U) in the 2008 WHO classification. The WHO authors acknowledge that this is not regarded as a distinct entity, but rather a heterogeneous collection of lymphomas that do not fit purely into either DLBCL or BL. Cases with otherwise classic morphology and immunophenotype for either DLBCL or BL but with incongruent genetics results (ie, presence of MYC translocation in DLBCL or absence of it in BL) should not be put into the intermediate category, but rather assigned according to their morphologic and immunophenotypic features. Some additional characteristics may also help to distinguish between these entities. For example, while MYC translocations can occur in both, they most often occur as a single abnormality in BL and as part of a complex karyotype in diffuse large B-cell lymphoma. Additionally, strong BCL2 expression is not a feature that is associated with BL. Such cases should be evaluated for additional abnormalities such as BCL2 translocation, as cases with translocations of both MYC and BCL2 or MYC with other translocations such as BCL6 are highly aggressive and fall into the BCL-U category. Distinction between these entities is important because, while both are considered aggressive high-grade lymphomas, established intensive chemotherapeutic regimens have a substantial chance of cure in BL, while the optimal therapy and clinical course is less well established for those cases falling into the category of BCL-U.

Diffuse Large B-Cell Lymphoma

Beverly P Nelson

Patient A 61-year-old woman, who presented with multiple painful, tender neck masses.

Clinical History The patient reported having these masses for about 4 months. Her past medical history is significant for hepatitis C, ascites, and cirrhosis.

Family History Noncontributory.

Medications Furosemide, spironolactone.

Physical Examination Notable for ascites and enlarged left-neck lymph nodes.

Initial Work-Up

CBC	
WBC (×10^3/μL)	19.8
RBC (×10^6/μL)	3.29
HGB (g/dL)	11.6
HCT (%)	32.1
MCV (fL)	98
MCH (pg)	35.2
MCHC (g/dL)	35.7
PLT (×10^3/μL)	41
RDW-CV (%)	14.3

WBC Differential	%	# (×10^3/μL)
Neutrophils	99	19.6
Bands	0	
Lymphocytes	1	0.2
Monocytes	0	
Eosinophils	0	
Basophils	0	

A left supraclavicular lymph node biopsy was performed. Histologic sections of the 2 × 1.5 × 0.3 cm lymph node with a tan, fleshy parenchyma showed effacement of the architecture by a lymphoid proliferation with a diffuse growth pattern. The lymphocytes were large with open chromatin and mostly centroblastic morphology characterized by visible nucleoli located adjacent to the nuclear membrane (**Figure 1**).

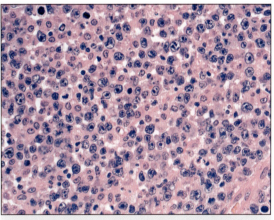

Figure 1 Lymph node (H&E, ×600) showing most lymphoma cells are centroblasts with small nucleoli adjacent to the nuclear membrane.

Differential Diagnosis Diagnostic considerations included a lymphoma vs a reactive condition.

Additional Work-Up By immunohistochemical stains (IHC) the lymphoma cells were CD10–, BCL6-, BCL2+, and MUM-1+ (**Figure 2**). Flow cytometric immunophenotyping of the lymph node showed κ monotypic B cells that were CD5–, CD10–, CD19+, CD20+, CD22+, dim CD25+, and CD52+. Bone marrow biopsy was hypercellular without evidence of lymphoma.

Final Diagnosis Diffuse large B-cell lymphoma, not otherwise specified (NOS).

Management Approach Diffuse large B-cell lymphomas (DLBCL) are rapidly growing but curable with appropriate therapy. Prior to the advent of rituximab, standard treatment for DLBCL was cyclophosphamide, doxorubicin, vincristine, prednisone (CHOP). Rituximab is now routinely used with CHOP (R-CHOP). This patient received 3-cycles of R-CHOP and is completely free of disease 9 months after diagnosis.

General Discussion DLBCL is a heterogeneous group of non-Hodgkin lymphomas (NHL) composed of large lymphocytes with dispersed chromatin and one or more visible nucleoli. The lymphoma cells are CD45+ and positive for B-cell associated markers such as CD19, CD20, CD22, CD79, and PAX 5. Lymphomas included in the DLBCL NOS category should not meet criteria for specific subtypes of DLBCL, such as Burkitt, intravascular large B-cell lymphoma and several others recognized in the WHO 2008 classification. Overall, DLBCL is the most common lymphomas in western countries, representing approximately 30% of NHL, and affect men more commonly than women. Single or multiple masses involving lymph nodes or extranodal sites is the typical clinical presentation. The most common extranodal anatomic sites of presentation are gastrointestinal tract, bone, testis, spleen and Waldeyer ring. The morphology of DLBCL tumor cells is variable. The centroblastic (present in this case) and the immunoblastic variants are the most common. An example of the immunoblastic variant from another patient is illustrated in **Figure 3**. Other less common variants include the anaplastic, cases with a myxoid stroma, spindle cells, and signet ring cells. Survival in DLBCL is linked to genetic subgroups and parameters (age, serum LDH, Ann Arbor stage, performance status, number of extranodal sites with disease) in the International Prognostic Index (IPI). Large-cell lymphoma in the bone marrow is associated with shorter survival (10% survival at 5 years) than no bone marrow involvement or small lymphoma cells (discordant morphology) in the bone marrow (~60% survival at 5 years). 2 reproducible subgroups of DLBCL with different prognosis that is independent of the IPI have been recognized using gene expression profiling (GEP): the germinal center B-cell type (GCB) and the activated B-cell type (ABC). The GCB subgroup has better survival (~60% at 5 years) than the ABC subgroup (~30% at 5 years), but Rituximab may negate the GCB survival advantage. Since GEP is not readily available, IHC algorithms have been proposed as surrogate markers to stratify DLBCL into GCB and ABC subgroups. These IHC algorithms may not be routinely used in the clinical setting, and do not show perfect correlation with the GEP data. An algorithm of 5 antibodies (**Table 1**) shows

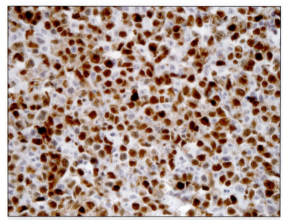

Figure 2 Lymph node (MUM1, ×400) in which at least 80% of the lymphoma cells show nuclear staining.

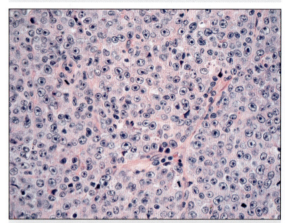

Figure 3 Lymph node from a different case of immunoblastic variant of diffuse large cell lymphoma (H&E, ×600) showing >90% of the lymphoma cells have a single, central, prominent nucleolus.

96% concordance with GEP groups while another using MUM1, CD10, and BCL6 shows 86% concordance.

Table 1. Staining pattern of DLBCL prognostic groups

Germinal center B-cell type (GCB)	Activated B-cell type (ABC)
Must be MUM1– and FOXP1–	MUM1+ or FOXP1+
AND	OR
Positive with one or more of the GCB cell markers: GCET1, CD10, or BCL6	Negative for GCET1, CD10, and BCL6 if MUM1 and FOXP1 are both negative

To be interpreted as positive, GCET1, MUM1, & FOXP1 require ≥80% positive malignant cells, and CD10 & BCL6 require ≥30% positive malignant cells.

Double-Hit High-Grade B-Cell Lymphoma

Pei Lin

Patient A 54-year-old male, who sought medical attention for fatigue, night sweats and weight loss.

Clinical History The patient reported losing 10 lb over a 3-week period. He had noted blood in his stool. He was becoming progressively more fatigued and had been having drenching night sweats for the last 2 weeks-3 weeks. He underwent colonoscopic examination and was found to have a 5 cm ulcerated mass at the illeocecal valve.

Family History Noncontributory.

Medications None.

Physical Examination His vital signs were normal. He had a distended abdomen that was tender to palpation. There was no palpable liver or spleen. He had no palpable lymph nodes.

Initial Work-Up

CBC			Serum Chemistry	
WBC (×10³/μL)	7.0		LDH (IU/L)	1,602 (normal 313-618)
RBC (×10⁶/μL)	3.94		Uric Acid (mg/dL)	8.7 (normal 2.6-7.1)
HGB (g/dL)	8.0		Albumin (g/dL)	2.9 (normal 3.5-4.7)
HCT (%)	25.6		Calcium (mg/dL)	8.3 (normal 8.4-10.2)
MCV (fL)	65		ASP (IU/L)	116 (normal 15-46)
MCH (pg)	20.3		ALP (IU/L)	98 (normal 7-56)
MCHC (g/dL)	31.1		B2M (mg/L)	4.3 (normal 0.6-2.0)
PLT (×10³/μL)	671		Creatinine (mg/dL)	1.6 (normal 0.8-1.5)
RDW-CV (%)	19.6			
MPV (fL)	6.2			

WBC Differential	%	# (×10³/μL)
Neutrophils	90	6.3
Bands	0	
Lymphocytes	3	0.2
Monocytes	6	0.4
Eosinophils	1	0.1
Basophils	0	

CT scan showed right pleural effusion. CT of abdomen and pelvis showed a 10-cm mass in the mid pelvic region.
PET scan showed multiple nodes in the mediastinum, peritoneal, mesenteric lymph nodes as well as mucosal and serosal involvement of the gut from the hemidiaphragm to the lower pelvis with a large conglomerate mass of activity in the pelvis.
A biopsy of the mass at the ileocecal valve was obtained which showed diffuse infiltration of neoplastic lymphoid cells of intermediate size (**Figures 1** and **2**).

Section E: Lymphomas and Their Mimics
Double-Hit High-Grade B-Cell Lymphoma

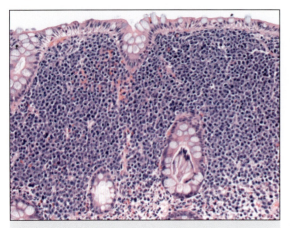

Figure 1 Ileocecal valve mass biopsy (H&E, ×200) showing a diffuse infiltrate of the intermediate sized lymphoid cells in the lamina propria.

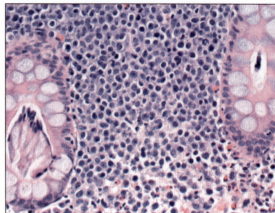

Figure 2 Ileocecal valve mass biopsy (H&E, ×400), high-power view of the diffuse infiltrate of the intermediate-sized lymphoid cells in the lamina propria.

Differential Diagnosis Diagnostic considerations based on histologic findings and clinical presentation included Burkitt lymphoma, diffuse large B-cell lymphoma, "gray zone lymphoma," and mantle cell lymphoma, blastoid variant. Additionally, the CBC findings of microcytic hypochromic anemia with thrombocytosis reflected iron deficiency that was confirmed by iron studies and was thought to be related to the malignant disease involving the gastrointestinal tract and associated blood loss.

Additional Work-Up Immunophenotypic study revealed a high-grade B-cell lymphoma positive for CD20, CD45, BCL2, strong (**Figure 3**) and negative for CD5 and cyclin D1. Ki67 highlighted nearly 100% of cells in the tumor (**Figure 4**). Florescence in situ hybridization performed on sections of the formalin fixed paraffin embedded biopsy tissue found *MYC* rearrangement and *IGH/BCL2* gene fusion in approximately 80% of interphases.

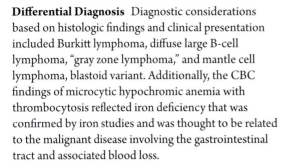

Figure 3 Ileocecal valve mass biopsy (BCL2, ×200) showing the neoplastic cells are strongly positive.

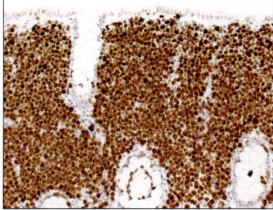

Figure 4 Ileocecal valve mass biopsy (Ki-67 or MIB1, ×200) highlighting 100% of neoplastic cells.

Final Diagnosis High-grade B-cell lymphoma with both *MYC* and *IGH/BCL2* rearrangement (high-grade B-cell lymphoma, unclassifiable, with features intermediate between diffuse large B-cell lymphoma and Burkitt lymphoma, or "gray zone" lymphoma, or double-hit lymphoma).

Management Approach Intensive high-dose chemotherapy regimen designed for Burkitt lymphoma. Regimens including hyperfractionated cyclophosphamide, vincristine, doxorubicin and dexamethasone (hyper-CVAD) alternating with methotrexate and cytarabine (MTX/ AraC) or the Magrath protocol using cyclophosphamide, doxorubicin, vincristine and methotrexate (CODOX-M) alternating with ifosphamide, mesna, cytarabine and etoposide (IVAC). Prophylaxis against tumor lysis syndrome, using vigorous hydration and allopurinol should be used. If the patient has marrow involvement, intrathecal prophylaxis should be strongly considered as well. This patient received hyper-CVAD treatment and intrathecal methotrexate He achieved complete remission. For his iron deficiency, he was treated with ferrous sulfate 1 tablet 3 times a day, which normalized his MCV and his ferritin. However, his hemoglobin level increased only to 10.2 g/dL, most likely reflecting the chemotherapy effect.

General Discussion The so-called double-hit lymphomas are high-grade B-cell lymphoma that may arise either de novo or follow a prior history of low-grade follicular lymphoma. Usually middle age or older patients are affected. According to the current WHO classification scheme, these cases usually fall into the category of high-grade B-cell lymphoma, unclassifiable, with features intermediate between Burkitt lymphoma and diffuse large B-cell lymphoma. Strong BCL2 immunoreactivity and *IgH/BCL2* gene fusion are considered to be features not typical for classical or atypical Burkitt lymphoma. In many instances these lymphoma may be CD10+ or negative. The morphology of these cases sometimes is considered Burkitt like but shows more cell size variation and more large cells. Despite a germinal center immunophenotype in a subset of cases, double-hit lymphomas generally have a poor prognosis even with intensive high-dose chemotherapy regimen designed for Burkitt lymphoma. Novel therapies are needed.

T-Lymphoblastic Lymphoma

David S Bosler, Eric Hsi

Patient A 42-year-old male with a 1-month history of progressive dyspnea and chest discomfort.

Clinical History A CT scan of the chest and abdomen showed a large mediastinal mass, 15 cm in greatest dimension, as well as lymphadenopathy involving right perihilar, right paratracheal, and esophageal junction areas, with possible involvement of the liver and kidney.

Family History No known history of hematolymphoid neoplasm. Maternal history unknown, father died in an accident, 2 siblings alive and healthy.

Medications Metoprolol, hydrochlorthiazide, amlodipine.

Physical Examination Vital signs normal, healthy appearing male, essentially unremarkable physical exam. No palpable liver or spleen. No palpable lymph nodes.

Initial Work-Up

CBC		WBC Differential	%	# (×10³/μL)
WBC (×10³/μL)	6.2	Neutrophils	66	4.1
RBC (×10⁶/μL)	4.6	Bands	0	
HGB (g/dL)	14.0	Lymphocytes	25	1.6
HCT (%)	43.2	Monocytes	6	0.4
MCV (fL)	89	Eosinophils	3	0.2
MCH (pg)	30.4	Basophils	0	
MCHC (g/dL)	32.4			
PLT (×10³/μL)	248			
RDW-CV (%)	14.5			

Lymph node, prescalene, excisional biopsy: Sections showed effacement of lymph node architecture (**Figure 1**), which was replaced by a diffusely infiltrative population of intermediate-sized lymphocytes with a high nuclear to cytoplasmic ratio, round nuclei, an open, granular chromatin pattern, and indistinct nucleoli (**Figure 2**). Numerous mitotic figures were present.

Differential Diagnosis The differential diagnosis of this prescalene lymph node composed of diffusely infiltrating intermediate-sized lymphocytes and a high mitotic rate included Burkitt lymphoma, lymphoblastic lymphoma, and blastoid variant of mantle cell lymphoma. In a mediastinal biopsy, the differential will also include thymoma. Although the cells were smaller in this case than would be typical, the appearance might also raise the question of a small round blue cell tumor of nonlymphoid origin.

Additional Work-Up Immunohistochemistry: the neoplastic cells expressed CD45, and did not express cytokeratins, neuroendocrine markers, or neuron-specific enolase. Flow cytometry: the cells expressed CD2, CD4, CD5, CD7, cytoplasmic CD3, dim TdT, and CD1a, and were negative for surface CD3, CD34, CD19, and cytoplasmic myeloperoxidase.

Final Diagnosis T-lymphoblastic lymphoma.

Section E: Lymphomas and Their Mimics
T-Lymphoblastic Lymphoma

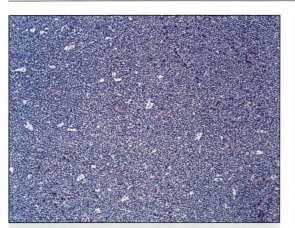

Figure 1 Prescalene lymph node biopsy (H&E, ×100) showing diffuse infiltrate of intermediate-sized lymphocytes.

Management Approach General therapeutic approaches have changed over time as standard induction regimens have proven suboptimal. Current approaches often involve intensive, multiagent induction therapy such as cyclophosphamide, vincristine, adriamycin, and dexamethasone (hyper-CVAD) alternating with high-dose methotrexate in combination with cytarabine (AraC/MTX). Induction therapy includes CNS prophylaxis and is followed by consolidation therapy with or without hematopoietic progenitor cell transplant. CNS prophylaxis is prevalent regardless of CNS involvement, since the CNS is a frequent site of relapse. This patient received 6 cycles of cyclophosphamide, doxorubicin, vincristine, and prednisone (CHOP) after diagnosis, and achieved complete remission. Five months after diagnosis however, he developed visual abnormalities including diplopia, progressing to include left facial droop, and CSF analysis ultimately confirmed that the CNS was involved by T-lymphoblastic lymphoma (T-LBL). He began receiving a regimen of intrathecal methotrexate alternating with systemic chemotherapy with methotrexate, vincristine, and procarbazine, but during this therapy developed recurrence in the left testis. After orchiectomy and completion of chemotherapy, the CNS was negative, then recurred. Upon transfer of his care, he received additional intensive systemic and CNS chemotherapy consisting of hyper-CVAD alternating with high-dose methotrexate and Ara-C, along with intrathecal methotrexate and Ara-C. He then underwent autologous stem cell transplant and, although he initially did well, ultimately his disease recurred in CNS and bone marrow and he was transferred to hospice care.

General Discussion The flow cytometric immunophenotyping analysis confirms the diagnosis in this case. The presence of cytoplasmic CD3 indicates T-cell lineage, and the coexpression of TdT and CD1a confirm the lymphoblastic nature of the T cells suspected based on their morphologic appearance. The other T-cell markers present

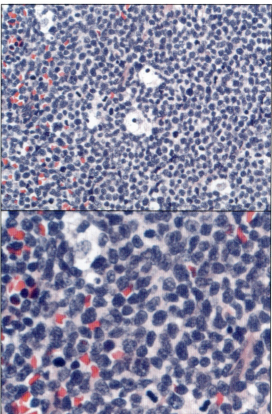

Figure 2 Prescalene lymph node biopsy (H&E, upper ×400; lower, ×1000) in which neoplastic cells have round nuclei, open chromatin, and indistinct nucleoli. Several mitoses are also present.

(CD2, CD4, CD5, CD7) are helpful, but not lineage defining. Although not present in this case, expression of myeloid markers such as CD13 or CD33 is common, and does not affect the diagnosis. Despite the lack of dual CD4 and CD8 staining in this case, the immunophenotype otherwise correlates most closely with the cortical T-cell stage of thymic differentiation (positive for cytoplasmic CD3, CD2, CD7, CD1a, and negative for surface CD3 and CD34). The lack of keratin staining and homogenous pattern of T-cell antigen expression in the lymphoblasts exclude the possibility of thymoma. In many ways this case is a prototypic presentation. Although T-LBL is less common overall than B-lymphoblastic leukemia/lymphoma, it is more common among cases that present as lymphoma. It is more common in males than females, and more common in adolescents and adults than younger children. T-LBL classically presents as a large mediastinal mass, and may also involve other sites including lymph nodes, liver, CNS and testis (as in this case) as well as skin, tonsil and spleen. This patient has several factors that appear to adversely influence response to therapy and prognosis, including age >40, bulky disease (>10 cm), and >2 extranodal sites of involvement.

Section E: Lymphomas and Their Mimics

Extranodal NK/T-Cell Lymphoma, Nasal Type

Jerald Z Gong, Alina Dulau Florea

Patient A 46-year-old Oriental man with 2 months of nasal stuffiness and intermittent epistaxis.

Clinical History The patient has a history of hypertension, hypercholesterolemia, and gastroesophageal reflux disease.

Family History No known family history of hematologic malignancies.

Medications Hydralazine, simvastatin, and esomeprazole.

Physical Examination The nasal mucosa was swollen and erythematous with extensive ulceration. No lymphadenopathy or hepatosplenomegaly were noted.

Initial Work-Up

CBC		WBC Differential	%	# (×10³/µL)
WBC (×10³/µL)	8.4	Neutrophils	62	5.2
RBC (×10⁶/µL)	3.46	Bands	6	0.5
HGB (g/dL)	10.2	Lymphocytes	20	1.7
HCT (%)	30.9	Monocytes	10	0.8
MCV (fL)	89.3	Eosinophils	1	0.1
MCH (pg)	29.5	Basophils	1	0.1
MCHC (g/dL)	33.0			
PLT (×10³/µL)	120			
RDW-CV (%)	13.8			

Peripheral blood smear revealed no abnormality.
Results of the basic metabolic panel including electrolytes, creatinine, BUN and glucose were normal, as were transaminases. Coagulation studies and urinalysis were also normal. Computed tomography of nasal sinus showed bilateral mucosal thickening and opacification of ethmoid and maxillary sinuses.
The nasal lesion was biopsied and the histologic examination showed diffuse infiltration of nasal mucosa with small lymphocytes (**Figure 1**). These lymphocytes had atypical nuclear morphology with cleaved and folded nuclei. There was a prominent angiocentric and angiodestructive growth pattern associated with frequent necrosis and ulceration (**Figure 2**).

Section E: Lymphomas and Their Mimics
Extranodal NK/T-Cell Lymphoma, Nasal Type

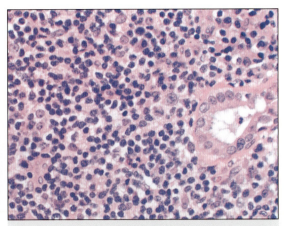

Figure 1 Nasal lesion biopsy (H&E, ×400) showing an infiltrate of small lymphocytes with irregular nuclear contour and scant cytoplasm in the nasopharyngeal mucosa.

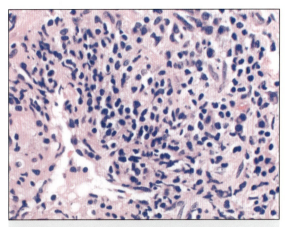

Figure 2 Nasal lesion biopsy (H&E, ×400) showing angiocentric and angiodestructive growth pattern of the neoplastic cells.

Differential Diagnosis Diagnostic considerations included reactive nasal congestion, nasopharyngeal carcinoma, T- and NK-cell lymphomas including lymphomatoid granulomatosis, blastic NK-cell leukemia/lymphoma, enteropathy-associated T-cell lymphoma, and subcutaneous panniculitic T-cell lymphoma.

Additional Work-Up Immunohistochemistry of the nasal lesion revealed an abnormal lymphoid population expressing CD2, CD3, CD7, CD56, TIA-1, and granzyme B. The tumor cells showed approximately 80% proliferation activity by Ki-67 stain. In situ hybridization of Epstein-Barr Early RNA (EBER) was positive for EBV infection in the tumor cells (**Figure 3**). Flow cytometry revealed a natural killer cell phenotype with expression of CD2, cytoplasmic CD3, CD7, CD56, and negative surface CD3, CD4, CD5, and CD8. T-cell receptor γ chain gene rearrangement by PCR was negative for T-cell clonal rearrangement. Staging procedures included computed tomography (CT) of head and neck, chest, and abdomen, whole body positive emission tomography (PET), and bone marrow biopsy and aspirate. CT and PET showed no additional lymphadenopathy. Examination of the bone marrow biopsy showed a normocellular marrow with mature trilineage hematopoiesis with no lymphoma involvement.

Final Diagnosis Extranodal NK/T-cell lymphoma, nasal type.

Management Approach For localized nasal disease, radiotherapy alone is used with good results. The best conventional treatment for more advanced disease combines radiotherapy with anthracycline-based chemotherapy. Hematopoietic progenitor cell transplantation (both autologous and allogeneic) may provide a survival benefit for patients with extranasal or advanced stages of nasal disease. With upfront radiotherapy and more intensive chemotherapy, the overall survival of extranodal NK/T-cell lymphoma has been improved in recent years. This patient was treated with radiation therapy of the nasal region only and

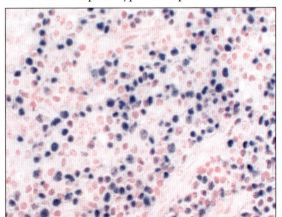

Figure 3 Nasal lesion biopsy (in situ hybridization for EBER, ×400) showing positive EBV staining in the lymphoma cells.

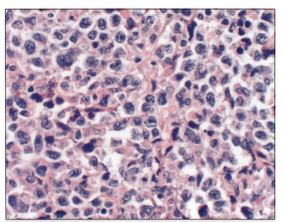

Figure 4 Biopsy of the recurrent nasal lesion (H&E, ×400) showing primarily large cell morphology. The lymphoma cells have highly irregular nuclear contour and variable pink cytoplasm.

achieved complete remission. The tumor recurred in the nasal cavity 4 years after the initial diagnosis. Biopsy of the tumor at the recurrence showed a predominance of large cells (**Figure 4**). Flow cytometry and immunohistochemistry confirmed recurrence of the NK/T-cell lymphoma.

General Discussion Extranodal NK/T-cell lymphoma is a rare type of non-Hodgkin lymphoma. Approximately 85% have been reported from Asian and Hispanic adults, while the remaining 15% have been seen in Western populations. The median age ranges from 44 years-52 years, with male to female ratio of approximately 2:1. Patients usually present with symptoms of nasal obstruction and epistaxis. More advanced cases present with expansion and distortion of nasal bridge due to destructive sinonasal or midline facial tumors. Sinonasal lesion is the primary presentation. Less frequently, the lymphoma may present outside the nasal cavity such as skin, GI tract, orbit, testis, brain, liver, spleen, and soft tissue. Bone marrow and lymph node involvement may occur but are uncommon at initial presentation. Cases with primary extra-nasal presentation are considered as the same disease as the primary nasal lesion, and the term "nasal type" includes lesions from both nasal and extra-nasal origins. Morphologically, tumor cells may vary from small cells to large cells. In South America and Asia, majority of the cases present with small cell morphology. In the United States, large cell morphology is more common. Angiocentric and angiodestructive growth pattern with invasion and destruction of blood vessels as well as mitosis, apoptosis, and necrosis are almost always present. Majority of the tumor cells show NK-cell phenotype with expression of CD2, cytoplasmic CD3 epsilon, and CD56. Other T/NK associated markers such as CD5, CD7, CD16, and CD57 are often negative. The tumor is usually double negative for CD4 and CD8, with a small percent expressing either CD4 or CD8. Cytotoxic markers TIA-1 and granzyme B are almost always positive. T-cell receptor genes are in germline configuration in NK cell type. A small number of the lesions show T-cell phenotype with surface CD3 and T-cell receptor α-β or γ-δ expression. In the T-cell type, clonal T-cell receptor rearrangement can be detected. EBV can be detected in up to 90% of the cases. However, the precise role of EBV in pathogenesis of this lesion is still not completely clear. EBV is present in clonal episomal form, indicating that EBV infection is an early event in tumor development. EBV is best detected by in situ hybridization of EBER (Epstein-Barr early RNA). Other genetic changes include deletion of 6q, isochromosome 6p, and methylation of p73 promotor. However, these changes were reported in sporadic cases and recurrent genetic abnormalities are yet to be discovered. The prognosis is generally poor with mean survival of 2 years-3 years. For the nasal cases, prognosis can be assessed using International Prognostic Index (IPI) and Korean Prognostic index (KPI). Bone marrow involvement is infrequent at diagnosis, but bone marrow involvement often is associated with very poor prognosis. Other adverse prognostic indicators include severe anemia, thrombocytopenia, elevated C-reactive protein, high level of circulating EBV DNA, high Ki67 proliferation rate in tumor cells, increased large tumor cells, and presence of EBV+ cells in bone marrow. The prognostic indicators of extranasal cases are less well defined. However, extranasal cases are generally associated with very poor prognosis.

Angioimmunoblastic T-Cell Lymphoma

Tahseen Al-Saleem, Essel Dulaimi-Al-Saleem, Michael M Millenson

Patient A 57-year-old Caucasian male with complaints of worsening fever and painful lymphadenopathy of 1-week duration.

Clinical History The patient also reported having drenching night sweats and some weight loss during the past year. He has a history of major depression, deep venous thrombosis, Guillain-Barré disease, hepatitis A and hepatitis B.

Family History There is no family history of cancer.

Medications Pantoprazole and enoxaparin.

Physical Examination Generalized lymphadenopathy, marked splenomegaly, mild hepatomegaly and generalized pruritic diffuse erythematous papular rash.

Initial Work-Up The CBC results were significant for normocytic normochromic anemia (HGB of 8.1 g/dL) and thrombocytopenia (PLT of $41 \times 10^3/\mu L$) with normal differential leukocyte counts Imaging studies were positive for generalized lymphadenopathy. Right groin lymph node excisional biopsy: there was complete effacement of the architecture with prominent arborization of small blood vessels. Also present were medium-large atypical cells with clear to pale cytoplasm and distinct cytoplasmic membranes (**Figure 1**).

Differential Diagnosis Differential diagnostic considerations included atypical hyperplasia, Hodgkin lymphoma, and non-Hodgkin lymphoma.

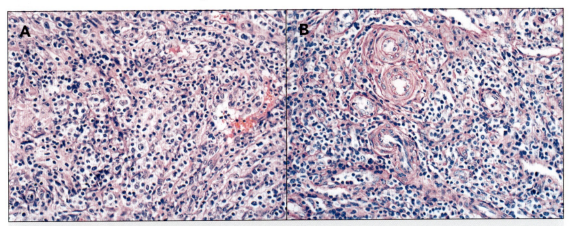

Figure 1 Lymph node **A** (PAS, ×200) and **B** (PAS, ×400) showing complete effacement of architecture, vascular arborization with prominent high endothelial venules, and medium to large atypical cells with pale cytoplasm.

Section E: Lymphomas and Their Mimics
Angioimmunoblastic T-Cell Lymphoma

Additional Work-Up By immunohistochemical staining of lymph node sections, most cells stained positive for CD3 (**Figure 2A**) and CD5. The medium-large atypical cells were CD4+. Many, including the large cells were CD10 (**Figure 2B**) and BCL6 positive. CD21 highlighted a network of dendritic follicular cells (FDCs) associated with the atypical T cells (**Figure 3**). The background B cells were positive with CD20 and latent membrane protein (LMP-1) for Epstein-Barr virus (**Figure 4**). PCR test detected a clonal T-cell population. Bone marrow biopsy was hypercellular with foci of fibrosis, granuloma-like formation and scattered atypical aberrant T cells. Flow cytometry of the marrow and peripheral blood showed rare T cells (4% of the lymphocytes) with an aberrant phenotype: CD2+, surface CD3−, CD4+, CD5+, CD7−, CD8− and CD10+. Atypical reactive processes may have CD3+ cells that might express CD10 but these are not aberrant phenotypically and are usually polyclonal. Angioimmunoblastic T-cell lymphoma (AITL) with EBV+ Reed-Sternberg-like B cells may simulate classic Hodgkin lymphoma but aberrant T cells and other features of AITL are usually diagnostic. Other peripheral T-cell lymphomas have a different morphology and the neoplastic T cells are CD10 and BCL6 negative.

Final Diagnosis Angioimmunoblastic T-cell lymphoma, stage IVB.

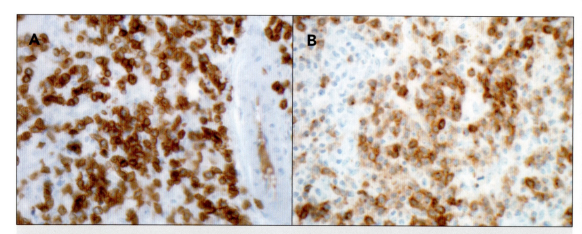

Figure 2 Lymph node **A** (cytoplasmic CD3, ×600) in which tumor cells are positive and **B** (CD10, ×600) in which tumor cells are positive.

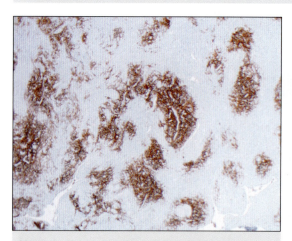

Figure 3 Lymph node (CD21, ×400) showing that follicular dendritic meshwork is highlighted.

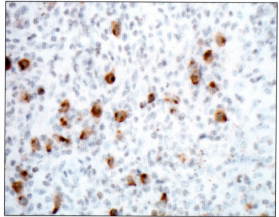

Figure 4 Lymph node (LMP-1 for EBV, ×600) showing B cells that are positive.

Management The disease has a rapid progression in most patients. Spontaneous remissions may occur, but the median survival is <3 years. It is usually treated with anthracycline containing regimens. Large B-cell lymphoma thought to be EBV driven can occur.

This patient received 4 cycles of chemotherapy with cyclophosphamide, doxorubicin, vincristine and prednisone (CHOP). Unfortunately, he relapsed quickly. Salvage therapy followed by hematopoietic progenitor cell transplantation was planned, but he expired with fulminant bacteremia.

General Discussion The cause of AITL is unknown. It most likely arises de novo as a peripheral T-cell lymphoma. AITL is rare (about 2% of all non-Hodgkin lymphomas). Lymph nodes are usually the primary site. Generalized lymphadenopathy is the most common presentation in addition to hepatosplenomegaly and anemia. Other clinical features are skin rash, pulmonary effusion, edema, ascites, polyarthritis and arthralgia. Anemia and polyclonal hyperγ-globulinemia are very common. Other laboratory findings might include circulating immune complexes, cold agglutinins, Coombs-positive hemolytic anemia, positive rheumatoid factor and antismooth muscle antibodies, lymphopenia, thrombocytopenia, hypereosinophilia, increased serum LDH and hypoalbuminemia.

The majority of AITL cases display a proliferaion of cells with the phenotypc of follicular dendritic cells (FDCs) localized outside the residual follicles (CXCL13+, PD1+, CD10+ CD4+ neoplastic T cells which typically line the high endothelial venules (HEVs). Occasionally only remnants of follicles remain with a "burned out" appearance. FDC proliferaton may be recognized only after immunohistochemical staining with CD21, CD23 or CD35. A key feature is the presence of numerous frequently arborizing postcapillary HEVs (**Figure 1**) The infiltrate may extend beyond the capsule but the cortical sinuses remain patent, which is an important diagnostic feature, The neoplastic lymphocytes are predominantly T cells (CD3+ and CD5+) (**Figure 2A**), usually with an admixture of CD4 and CD8, although CD4 predominates in most of the cases. CD21 highlights the disorganized and expanded meshwork of FDCs (**Figure 3**) which surrounds the HEVs. The neoplastic cells will also express CXCL13, CD10 and BCL6. EBV may be demonstrated in 50%-95% of cases by in situ hybridization. Bone marrow involvement is common, usually multifocal with a nodular pattern (78%). AITL in the BM may be difficult to assess due to the surrounding reactive microenvironment cells. PCR for T-cell receptor-γ chain rearrangement shows monoclonal pattern in 75%-90% of the cases. Immunoglobulin heavy chain gene rearrangement may be clonal even in the absence of a histological evidence of large B-cell lymphoma. The most frequent cytogenics abnormalities are trisomy 3, trisomy 5 and an additional X chromosome. Gains of chromosome 22q, 19 and 11q13 and losses of 13q were reported in a subset of patients.

Hepatosplenic T-Cell Lymphoma

David S Bosler, Eric D Hsi

Patient A 76-year-old male with a history of indolent systemic mastocytosis presented with cytopenias and severe acute illness following a cat scratch that resulted in a non-healing wound.

Clinical History His mastocytosis had primarily been managed by localized therapy for skin manifestations as needed. Clinically, he was thought to have disseminated intravascular coagulopathy.

Medications Lovastatin, aspirin.

Physical Examination Pale, acutely ill-appearing male. Significant findings included sinus tachycardia, hepatosplenomegaly, petechiae and delayed capillary refill.

Initial Work-Up

CBC		WBC Differential	%	# (×10³/μL)
WBC (×10³/μL)	10.0	Neutrophils	81	8.1
RBC (×10⁶/μL)	2.10	Bands	0	
HGB (g/dL)	6.0	Lymphocytes	8	0.8
HCT (%)	18.2	Monocytes	6	0.6
MCV (fL)	86.7	Eosinophils	0	
MCH (pg)	28.6	Basophils	0	
MCHC (g/dL)	33.0	Atypical cells	5	0.5
PLT (×10³/μL)	15			
RDW-CV (%)	13.9			

Peripheral blood smear revealed a few atypical cells with large irregular nuclei, smudged chromatin and occasional nucleoli. Bone marrow biopsy was slightly hypercellular with trilineage hematopoiesis. Clusters and sheets of large atypical cells representing approximately 30% of cellularity were noted (**Figure 1**). Small clusters of atypical mast cells were also present. Mild dyserythropoiesis was appreciated. Bone marrow aspirate smear also revealed an abnormal population of large cells characterized by a high nuclear to cytoplasmic ratio, irregular nuclear borders, vesicular chromatin, often multiple nucleoli, and basophilic cytoplasm with occasional cytoplasmic blebbing (**Figure 2**). The cells did not appear cohesive.

Differential Diagnosis The differential diagnosis for these morphologic findings includes large cell lymphoma (B-cell or less likely T-cell), anaplastic large cell lymphoma, a histiocytic or dendritic cell neoplasm, and metastatic malignancy including melanoma. Although cytoplasmic blebbing might also raise the possibility of acute myeloid leukemia of monoblastic, erythroblastic, or megakaryoblastic types, other cytologic features such as the nuclear irregularities and chromatin pattern, as well as the relatively normal background hematopoiesis and the clustered pattern of infiltration make these entities unlikely.

Section E: Lymphomas and Their Mimics
Hepatosplenic T-Cell Lymphoma

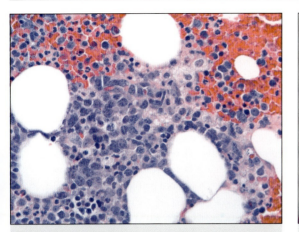

Figure 1 Bone marrow clot section (H&E, ×400) showing hypercellular marrow with a sheet of large atypical cells.

Figure 2 Bone marrow aspirate smear (Wright-Giemsa, ×1000) showing an abnormal population of large cells among normal hematopoietic cells.

Additional Work-Up Immunohistochemistry: the neoplastic cells expressed CD3 (**Figure 3**), CD7 and TIA-1 (**Figure 4**), but not CD2, CD5, CD4, CD8, TCR-BF1, granzyme B, CD20, PAX5, CD34, TdT, CD117, CD68, CD30, ALK-1, CD21, CD35, Clusterin, or any of the variety of hematopoietic markers or plasma cell markers tested. Molecular studies: T-cell receptor γ chain gene rearrangement studies by PCR detected a clonal rearrangement. The patient did very poorly, and died soon after presentation of complications from disseminated intravascular coagulopathy. An autopsy was performed, and showed involvement of the liver by the same process described in the bone marrow, with large lymphocytes expanding the hepatic sinusoids (**Figure 5**). Sections showed numerous mitotic and apoptotic figures. The spleen was enlarged, but too extensively autolyzed to evaluate for lymphoma.

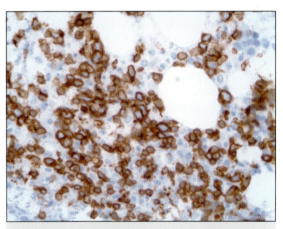

Figure 3 Bone marrow biopsy (CD3, ×400) in which neoplastic cells are positive, indicating T-cell lineage.

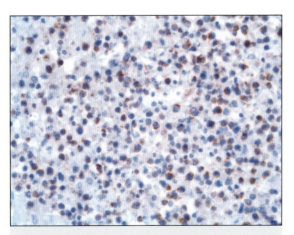

Figure 4 Bone marrow biopsy (TIA-1, ×400) in which neoplastic cells are positive for cytotoxic marker.

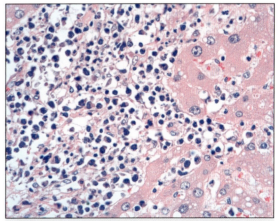

Figure 5 Liver tissue section (H&E, ×400) highlighting the intrasinusoidal pattern of infiltration.

Section E: Lymphomas and Their Mimics
Hepatosplenic T-Cell Lymphoma

Final Diagnosis Hepatosplenic T-cell lymphoma.

Management Approach The clinical course is aggressive. Although agents active in other non-Hodgkin lymphoma have activity against the disease and patients often respond initially, the prognosis is poor (median survival <2 years). Most patients are treated with combination therapies, but there is no specific standard for this disease. Enrollment on clinical trial should be pursued if that is an option.

General Discussion Hepatosplenic T-cell lymphoma (HSTCL) is a rare lymphoma of T cells usually with the γ-δ T-cell receptor type. The normal counterparts of these neoplastic cells are post-thymic, mature cytotoxic memory T cells of the innate immune system that express the γ-δ type of T-cell receptor. These cells normally account for only a small percentage of cells in the T-cell repertoire. As is seen in this case, the disease most often involves the liver, spleen and bone marrow without significant lymphadenopathy. Cytopenias, particularly thrombocytopenia, are frequently present at diagnosis. Circulating lymphoma cells are infrequent however, and are most often seen late in the disease course. A significant minority of HSTCL cases occur in the setting of immunosuppression, autoimmune disease or chronic antigen stimulation. Although not evaluated in this case, isochromosome 7q is present in a majority of HSTCL cases. Trisomy 8 is also frequent. The diagnosis often relies on the combined clinical, morphologic and immunophenotypic findings. The marked cytopenias and hepatosplenomegaly, while nonspecific, raise concern for a neoplastic process involving the spleen and/or bone marrow and are typical of HSTCL. Morphologically, the intrasinusoidal pattern of infiltration seen in the liver is also typical. Bone marrow involvement is nearly an invariant feature of HSTCL, but the infiltration is often subtle, sometimes requiring immunohistochemistry to aid in its recognition. Such recognition was not problematic in this case due to both the high number of tumor cells and the pronounced cytologic atypia. In fact, the neoplastic cells of HSTCL are most often monotonous and intermediate in size, with pronounced atypia and large cells such as seen in this case present in a minority of cases. Although the intrasinusoidal pattern often present in the bone marrow is not seen in this case, this pattern may be obscured by the relatively high burden of tumor cells in the bone marrow. The neoplastic cells of HSTCL, as in this case, express CD3, are double negative for CD4 and CD8, and can show loss of other T-cell associated antigens such as CD5. Characteristically, while they express the cytotoxic marker TIA-1, they lack granzyme B. Additionally, the lack of expression of TCR-BF1, an antigen associated with the chain of the T-cell receptor, further supports the γ-δ phenotype by inference. Several features in this case, including the severe cytopenias, circulating tumor cells, high bone marrow tumor burden, and pronounced cytologic atypia, suggest that the patient presented relatively late in the disease course, likely contributing to his precipitous clinical deterioration.

Primary Cutaneous T-Cell Lymphoma, γ-δ Type

Mingyi Chen, Maria Delioukina, Karen Chang

Patient A 25-year-old woman with a large lesion on the skin of her posterior calf.

Clinical History The skin lesion had been slowly increasing in size over the past 5 years. A biopsy was performed and showed panniculitis, with focal small vessel inflammation and necrosis. The patient received antibiotics and did not improve. Five months after the first biopsy, she had another biopsy, which showed T-cell lymphoma, and she underwent chemotherapy. After the chemotherapy, she was transferred to our hospital for consideration of hematopoietic progenitor cell transplantation (HPCT). Of note, approximately 7 years prior to the posterior calf lesion, she had been diagnosed with stage II melanoma of the right arm, with negative sentinel lymph nodes.

Family History The patient's father died from acute myeloid leukemia. Her maternal grandfather had glioblastoma multiforme and there was a history of "skin cancers."

Medications Antibiotics prescribed after the first biopsy were ineffective. Following the diagnosis of T-cell lymphoma, the patient completed 6 cycles of cyclophosphamide, doxorubicin, vincrisitne and prednisone (CHOP) chemotherapy.

Physical Examination The patient had a solitary, violaceous, plaque-like lesion in the left mid-posterior calf. The lesion measured 8 × 6 cm and was edematous, tender, and partially scaly. Within the same lesion, there was a darker pigmented portion that measured 2 × 2 cm. In addition, the patient had several small subcutaneous nodules in the right posterior calf. No palpable peripheral lymphadenopathy and organomegaly were detected. She had no constitutional symptoms.

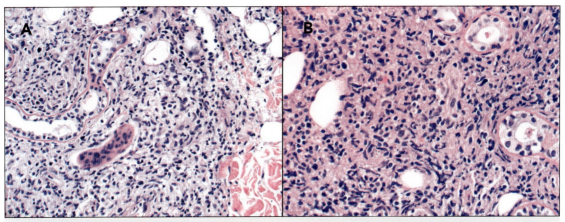

Figure 1 Skin **A** (H&E, ×20) showing a dense dermal lymphoid infiltrate that extends into the subcutaneous tissue. **B** (H&E, ×60) showing medium abnormal lymphocytes with dense clumped chromatin and irregular but not cerebriform nuclear contours.

Section E: Lymphomas and Their Mimics
Primary Cutaneous T-Cell Lymphoma, γ-δ Type

Initial Work-Up At the time of presentation, her WBC, hemoglobin, and platelet count were normal. Her WBC differential showed a mild left shift and no atypical lymphocytes. The skin biopsy showed an extensive nodular dermal lymphoid infiltrate that extended into the subcutaneous tissue, but spared the epidermis (**Figure 1A**). The infiltrate was composed of small to medium-sized atypical lymphocytes (**Figure 1B**). There was no rimming of fat spaces, karyorrhexis, or foamy histiocytes.

Differential Diagnosis Diagnostic considerations included cutaneous γ-δ T-cell lymphoma, subcutaneous panniculitis-like T-cell lymphoma, mycosis fungoides/Sézary syndrome, primary cutaneous CD30+ lymphoproliferative disorder, primary cutaneous peripheral T-cell lymphoma, unspecified, primary cutaneous CD4+ small- to medium-sized pleomorphic T-cell lymphoma, primary cutaneous aggressive epidermotropic CD8+ T-cell lymphoma, cutaneous NK-cell lymphoma, and lupus erythematosus profundus (lupus panniculitis). The key differentiating features of these conditions are outlined in **Table 1**.

Additional Work-Up By immunohistochemistry the tumor cells stained for CD3 (**Figure 2A**), CD43, CD45, and TIA-1, but not for CD4, CD8, βF1 (**Figure 2B**), or CD56. The tissue contained monoclonal TCR γ gene rearrangements and no TCR rearrangements.

A staging bone marrow biopsy showed a hypocellular marrow with trilineage hematopoiesis and no evidence of lymphoma involvement. CT scan showed mild pelvic, iliac, and inguinal lymphadenopathy.

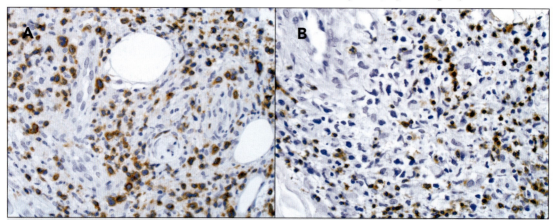

Figure 2 Skin **A** (CD3, ×60) showing cytoplasmic staining of the large atypical cells and **B** (βF1, ×60) showing only normal reactive T lymphocytes are positive and not the large atypical cells.

Final Diagnosis Cutaneous γ-δ T-cell lymphoma.

Management Approach There exists a large range of T-cell lymphoma subtypes, and thus treatments vary greatly. The treatment modalities include topical creams, systemic treatments such as corticosteroids, retinoids and methotrexate, systemic combinatorial chemotherapy regimens, light therapies, ultraviolet light, psoralen and ultraviolet A (PUVA) therapy, extracorporeal photopheresis (ECP), and radiation therapy. Some patients have an aggressive and stormy course and are resistant to multiagent chemotherapy and radiation.

This patient completed 6 cycles of CHOP chemotherapy. Because she subsequently developed systemic disease, she underwent fractionated total-body irradiation followed by matched-unrelated donor allogeneic HPCT.

The patient was in complete remission with complications of chronic graft-vs-host disease of the oropharynx 1 year after HPCT.

General Discussion The majority of skin lymphomas are derived from T cells (**Table 1**). Approximately 95% express the α-β TCR. The remainders express γ-δ TCR. Cutaneous γ-δ T-cell lymphoma (CGD-TCL) is a rare entity that has a unique immunophenotype and clinical course. The γ-δ T-cell lymphomas usually lack CD4 and CD8 surface markers; most of them express CD56 and TIA-1. Rare cases are CD8+. CGD-TCL may have a subcutaneous presentation, resembling the α/β variant of panniculitis-like T-cell lymphoma but with a more aggressive clinical course than its counterpart bearing the α-β receptor. CGD-TCL is derived from skin nonneoplastic γ-δ T cells with cytotoxic capabilities. Some patients have rapidly disseminated disease. Patients may develop the hemophagocytic syndrome.

Table 1. Diagnostic considerations with key differentiating features

Subcutaneous panniculitis-like T-cell lymphoma	• Generally confined to subcutaneous tissue with rare epidermal involvement • Frequent subcutaneous fat rimming, cytophagic histocytes, karyorrhexis, hyperchromatic lymphocytes • CD3+/CD8+, cytotoxic proteins+, (granzyme B, perforin and TIA1) /CD4−/CD30−/CD56− βF1+ • Indolent clinical course with 20% patients having underlying autoimmune disease, most commonly lupus erythematosus
Mycosis fungoides/Sézary syndrome	• Nodular ulcerative lesions with marked epidermotropism • Extensive involvement of the palms, soles, and oral mucosa • Derived from CD4+ T cells with loss of CD7 and low level of activation markers of CD25 and CD30
Hepatosplenic γ-δ T-cell lymphoma	• Marked hepatosplenomeglay and absence of lymphadenopathy. • Marked sinusoidal infiltrating pattern and sparing of portal triad and white pulp. • γ-δ T-cell origin with CD4 and CD8 double negative, negative for CD5, granzyme B and perforin, positive for CD56 and TIA1 • Recurrent chromosomal anomalies: i7q and trisomy 8
Primary cutaneous CD30+ lymphoproliferative disorders	• CD30+ cytotoxic markers • Often lack CD3
Primary cutaneous peripheral T-cell lymphoma, unspecified	• Localized but more frequently generalized plaques or nodules; may be associated with systemic lymphoma, especially on relapse • Diffuse, nodular, or bandlike pattern infiltrates occur in the dermis, in decreasing frequency; epidermotropism is generally mild or absent; medium to large pleomorphic or immunoblast-like >30% • CD4+/CD30−
Primary cutaneous CD4+ small- to medium-sized pleomorphic T-cell lymphoma	• Dense diffuse or nodular infiltrates within the dermis with a tendency to infiltrate the subcutaneous tissue with minimal or no epidermotropism. • Small to medium lymphocytes <30% large pleomorphic cells • CD3+/CD4+/CD8−/CD30− cytotoxic proteins (granzyme B, TIA)
Primary cutaneous aggressive epidermotropic CD8+ T-cell lymphoma	• Early lesions show intraepidermal pagetoid spread of atypical lymphocytes • Fully-developed lesions are characterized by a band-like, lichenoid, angiocentricity, pleomorphic blastic nuclei, small to large • βF1+/CD3+/CD8+/perforin+/ TIA−1+/CD45RA+/CD56−/CD45RO−/CD2−/CD4−/CD5−
Cutaneous NK cell lymphomas	• Chronic active EBV infection • CD56+ and CD4+
Lupus erythematosus profundus (lupus panniculitis)	• Benign lesion with typical serology finding and indolent clinical course • No T-cell receptor gene rearrangement

The biopsies show a striking diffuse and/or nodular infiltrate that usually spans the entire thickness of the dermis with frequent extension into fat and infrequent epidermotropism. Angiotropism and adnexotropism are frequently seen. The tumor cells are intermediate in size with significant nuclear irregularity. The degree of atypia exceeds that observed in mycosis fungoides. The cells usually manifest a double (CD4 and CD8) negative phenotype. There is variable deletion of pan-T-cell markers such as CD2, CD5, CD7 and CD62L. In addition, there is expression of the cytotoxic antigens including T cell intracellular antigen-1 (TIA-1), perforin and granzyme B.

Some cutaneous lymphomas, such as mycosis fungoides, hydroa vacciniforme-like lymphoma, primary cutaneous CD30+ lymphoproliferative disorders, subcutaneous panniculitis-like T-cell lymphoma and primary cutaneous CD4+ small or medium pleomorphic T-cell lymphoma, run an indolent course whereas others, such as Sézary syndrome, primary cutaneous peripheral T-cell lymphomas (subtypes include γ-δ, CD8+ aggressive epidermotropic cytotoxic, natural killer/T-cell (nasal-type), and unspecified), have an aggressive clinical behavior.

Nodal Marginal Zone Lymphoma

Tahseen Al-Saleem, Mitchell R Smith, Valentin Robu

Patient A 60-year-old white female of Ashkenazi Jewish descent visited her physician for a periodic check-up.

Clinical History The patient was recently found to carry the deleterious BRCA2 mutation, after a maternal first cousin was diagnosed with breast cancer and found to have the BRCA2 gene mutation. The patient receives appropriate screening by her primary care physician including mammography, colonoscopy and frequent physical examinations. She has also a history of asthma and hypertension.

Family History Mother with eye melanoma, father with pancreatic cancer, paternal aunt and maternal first cousin with breast cancer and malignant lymphoma in a maternal uncle.

Medications Diltiazem, enalapril, salmeterol, albuterol and ibuprofen.

Physical Examination Incidentally discovered 4-cm mobile mass in the abdominal wall of the left lower quadrant, otherwise no organomegaly, enlarged lymph nodes or other abnormal findings.

Initial Work-Up All laboratory investigations, including CBC and serum proteins were normal and CT scans otherwise were negative. The mass was clinically diagnosed as desmoid and excised, together with prophylactic bilateral tubo-oophorectomy and omentectomy.

The mass measured 4.5 × 3.5 × 2.7 cm and had a uniform, white/tan cut surface. Microscopically, the mass was a lymph node completely replaced by a monotonous proliferation of small lymphoid cells separated by thin fibrous septae producing a "macronodular" pattern (**Figures 1** and **2**). On higher power, most lymphocytes were small with scanty cytoplasm and nuclei containing fine chromatin with inconspicuous nucleoli (**Figure 3**). However, there were foci where the cells had more abundant cytoplasm

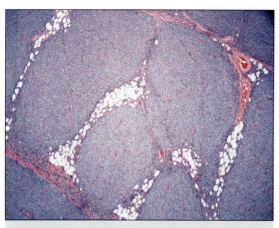

Figure 1 Abdominal mass/lymph node (H&E, ×400) showing macronodular pattern with thin fibrous septae.

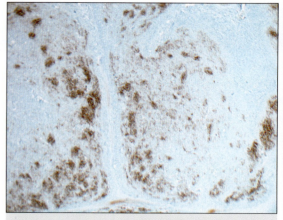

Figure 2 Abdominal mass/lymph node (CD23, ×400) showing fragmented expanded dendritic cell network.

producing a monocytoid appearance and other areas showing plasmacytic differentiation. Scattered throughout were large cells with prominent or multiple small nucleoli that represented about 5% of the cellular elements.

Differential Diagnosis Absence of hyalinized collagenous bands and sheets of neoplastic epithelial cells helped rule out the diagnoses of desmoid tumor and metastatic carcinoma, respectively. Other considerations included small lymphocytic lymphoma/chronic lymphocytic leukemia (SLL/CLL), mantle cell lymphoma, marginal zone lymphoma, lymphoplasmacytic lymphoma, follicular lymphoma and peripheral T-cell lymphoma.

Additional Work-Up By immunohistochemical stains the tumor cells were diffusely positive for CD20 and BCL2 and negative for CD3, CD5, CD10, cyclin D1 and CD23. CD5 and CD3-stained background T lymphocytes. CD23-stained follicular dendritic cells infiltrated by tumor cells. BCL6-stained scattered cells. Staging investigations, including peripheral blood and bone marrow flow cytometry were negative.

Final Diagnosis Nodal marginal zone lymphoma (NMZL), stage 1A (low-grade lymphoma).

Management Approach This tumor is generally indolent and 60%-80% of patients survive longer than 5 years. However, some cases may be aggressive being identified clinically by the international prognostic scoring index for non-Hodgkin lymphoma. Symptomatic patients are usually treated by radiotherapy (if early stage) or rituximab alone or with non-adriamycin containing regimens. Transformed cases are treated with R-CHOP. This patient was simply observed.

General Discussion NMZL is defined as "primary nodal B-cell neoplasm that morphologically resembles lymph nodes involved by marginal zone lymphoma of extranodal or splenic types, but without evidence of extranodal or splenic disease," NMZL is uncommon, comprising only 1.5%-1.8% of lymphoid neoplasms. It usually presents as an asymptomatic mass. It a disease of the elderly with a mean age of 60 years, though may occur in children. There is an equal sex incidence. Some reports, suggest a high association with hepatitis C (20%-24%). The overall pattern of NMZL lymph node involvement is generally described as diffuse in 75% of cases, nodular/ follicular in 10%, interfollicular in 14%

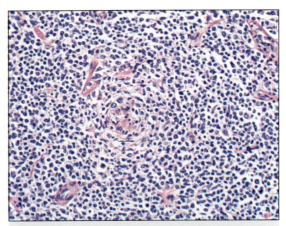

Figure 3 Abdominal mass/lymph node (H&E, ×400) showing sheets of small lymphocytes with occasional large forms, with invasion of and colonization of a germinal center producing a focal "interfollicular pattern."

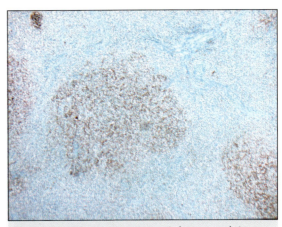

Figure 4 Abdominal mass/lymph node (CD21, ×200) showing a residual follicular dendritic cell network.

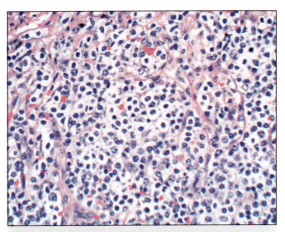

Figure 5 Axillary lymph node from another case of NMZL with monocytoid cells (H&E, ×600) showing abundant clear cytoplasm and folded nuclei, monocytoid appearance. Foci of similar morphology were seen in our case.

and perifollicular in 2% of cases. This case describes another pattern characterized as macronodular due to the enlargement of the germinal centers colonized by the proliferating neoplastic margin zone cells with the expansion of the residual follicular dendritic reticulum cell network (**Figures 1**, **2** and **4**). A mixed pattern is common. The tumor cells can be small or medium size lymphoid (**Figure 3**), monocytoid (**Figure 5**), or plasmacytoid with scattered blast cells, but not in sheets (**Figure 6**). Some consider the presence of >20% large cells as evidence of transformation to large B-cell lymphoma whereas others require 50% large cells, and/or sheets of large cells. Immunoglobulin heavy chains are clonally arranged with the predominance of mutated VH3 and VH4 families. Trisomy 3, 18, and 7 have been observed and trisomy 12 is described in about 20% of cases. Small lymphocytic lymphoma may mimic NMZL, but is CD5 and CD23+ with dim CD20. Mantle cell lymphoma is also CD5+ but is cyclin D1+. Follicular lymphoma with marked marginal cell proliferation, usually have some CD10+ BCL6+ residual neoplastic follicles. However, in some extreme cases FISH or molecular analysis for t(14;18) can be helpful. Cases of NMZL with marked plasma cell proliferation may be very difficult to differentiate from lymphoplasmacytic lymphoma. The latter can be ruled out by serum protein studies, and bone marrow examination which is usually diffusely involved by lymphoplasmacytic lymphoma and mostly nodular in NMZL. Bone marrow is positive in about 50% of NMZL cases. The presence of extranodal MZL has to be also carefully ruled out.

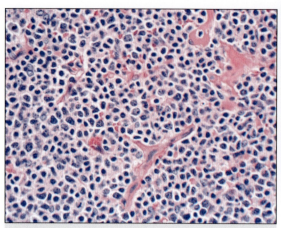

Figure 6 Axillary lymph node from another case of NMZL with plasmacytic cells in a patient with hepatitis C (H&E, ×600) showing diffuse pattern, centroblast-like cells 30%-40%, but not in sheets, plasmacytoid features present. Foci of similar morphology were seen in our case.

Peripheralization of Follicular Lymphoma

Javed Gill

Patient A 54-year-old male with generalized lymphadenopathy (mediastinal, paratracheal and retroperitoneal) noted on CT scans performed after a motor vehicle accident.

Clinical history Follicular lymphoma (FL), diagnosed 3 years earlier; received no therapy.

Family History Noncontributory.

Medications None.

Physical examination Notable for bilateral cervical lymphadenopathy, spleen palpable 2 cm below subcostal margin and accident-related injuries involving the arms, legs and chest.

Initial Work-Up

CBC

WBC (×10³/μL)	10.3
RBC (×10⁶/μL)	4.48
HGB (g/dL)	11.7
HCT (%)	37.9
MCV (fL)	84.6
MCH (pg)	26.1
MCHC (g/dL)	30.9
PLT (×10³/μL)	154
RDW-CV (%)	15.0
MPV (fL)	9.6

WBC Differential

	%	# (×10³/μL)
Neutrophils	27	2.8
Bands	2	0.2
Lymphocytes	63	6.5
Monocytes	5	0.5
Eosinophils	2	0.2
Basophils	0	
Metamyelocyte	1	0.1

Serum chemistries including LDH were normal.
Peripheral blood smear revealed many lymphocytes, some with irregular and/or cleaved nuclei (**Figure 1**).

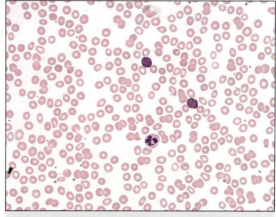

Figure 1 Blood smear (Wright stain, ×500) showing 1 lymphoma cell with nuclear cleft.

Differential Diagnosis Diagnostic considerations included chronic lymphocytic leukemia, peripheralized lymphoma, and reactive conditions (such as infectious mononucleosis).

Additional Work-Up An excised left cervical lymph node (LN) touch preparation revealed many small lymphocytes with nuclear cleaves and a few large immature cells (**Figure 2**). The biopsy sections showed many follicles (**Figure 3**) comprised mostly of centrocytes (small cells) and rare (about 3/hpf) centroblasts (large transformed cells). The

Section E: Lymphomas and Their Mimics
Peripheralization of Follicular Lymphoma

immunohistochemical stains displayed CD20 and BCL2+ cells predominating within the follicles (**Figures 4** and **5**). No tingible body macrophages and only rare mitoses were noted. Flow cytometric analysis on LN demonstrated mostly κ restricted small sized CD20 and CD10+ cells; a phenotype consistent with B-cell lymphoma of follicle center cell origin. Bone marrow (BM) examination revealed 50% cellularity, trilineage hematopoiesis and multiple (4) para trabecular lymphoid aggregates, occupying about 20% of marrow (**Figure 6**).

Final Diagnosis (a) Peripheralization of follicular lymphoma (FL). (b) Left cervical LN excisional biopsy: follicular lymphoma, grade 1-2/3.

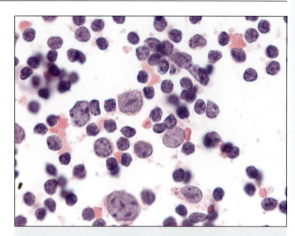

Figure 2 Lymph node, touch preparation (Wright, ×1000), showing many small lymphoid cells with nuclear irregularities/cleaves and few large immature cells.

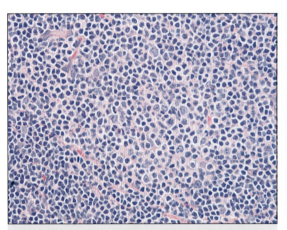

Figure 3 Lymph node (H&E, ×400) showing a neoplastic follicle mostly comprised of small lymphoid cells with irregular nuclear outlines.

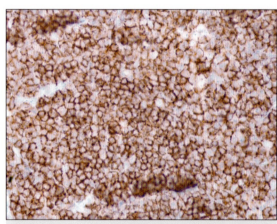

Figure 4 Lymph node (CD20, × 400) showing most cells within follicle are CD20+ B cells.

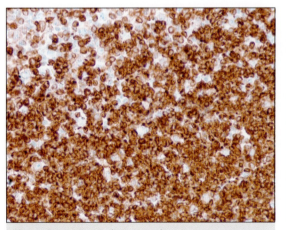

Figure 5 Lymph node (BCL2, ×400) in which most cells within follicular structure express BCL2.

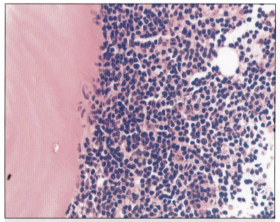

Figure 6 Bone marrow biopsy (H&E, ×400) showing paratrabecular lymphoid aggregate.

Management Approach Generally, a palliative approach has been adopted, cycling through "watchful waiting," radiotherapy (for localized disease), immunotherapy (such as rituximab), oral alkylating agents and combination chemotherapy (for symptomatic advanced disease). Allogeneic stem cell transplantation may be considered for younger patients. This patient received rituximab plus chemotherapy (cyclophosphamide, vincristine and prednisone) and achieved a complete remission.

General Discussion Most patients present with widespread disease including generalized lymphadenopathy and splenomegaly. The bone marrow (BM) is involved in 40%-70% of cases. FL is a neoplasm of germinal center B cells, displays follicular pattern, back to back follicles effacing the LN architecture. Neoplastic follicles are often poorly defined and unlike polarized centroblasts in reactive follicles, show randomly distributed centroblasts. Similarly, tingible body macrophages and mitoses present in reactive or normal follicles are usually absent. FL is graded by counting or estimating the absolute number of centroblast (large or small) in 10 representative follicles expressed per 40× high-power field (hpf). Grade 1 and 2 are comprised mostly of centrocytes (grade 1 = 0 to 5 centroblasts, grade 2 = 6 to 15/hpf). Since grade 1 and 2 are both clinically indolent, distinction between them is not encouraged, and a grade 1-2 of 3 can be reported. Grade 3 cases have >15 centroblasts/hpf, and is subdivided into grade 3A where centrocytes are present, while 3B follicles are composed entirely of centroblasts. If distinct areas of grade 3 are present in an otherwise grade 1-2, a separate diagnosis of Grade 3 should also be made, and the approximate amount of each grade reported. Diffuse areas, completely lacking follicles may be present, and if comprised predominantly of centroblasts is equivalent to diffuse large B-cell lymphoma (DLBCL), and a separate DLBCL diagnosis should be made. However, significance of diffuse areas predominantly comprised of small cells is not clear. Nevertheless, it is recommended that the relative proportions (%) of follicular and diffuse areas be noted in the pathology report. The tumor cells usually express clonal surface immunoglobulin, B cell markers (CD19, CD20, CD22), BCL2, BCL6, CD10, and are negative for CD5 and CD43. Some cases especially Grade 3B may lack CD10 but retain BCL6 expression. BCL2 protein can be useful in distinguishing neoplastic from reactive follicles, although absence of BCL2 does not exclude the diagnosis. However, "in situ" FL is essentially identified by overexpression of BCL2 on CD10 and BCL6 expressing cells in some of the follicles (partial nodal involvement). Immunoglobulin heavy and light chain genes are clonally rearranged in the neoplastic cells, detectable by PCR in about 80% of cases. Cytogenetically a t(14;18)(q32;q21) is detected in up to 90% of the cases, by FISH (fluorescent in situ hybridization); the most sensitive and specific method. This translocation results in rearrangement of the BCL2 proto-oncogene (at 18q21) to Ig heavy chain gene (at 14q32), with gains/amplifications of BCL2 locus; normally switched off in follicle center cells. This causes constitutional expression of "anti-apoptosis" BCL2 protein. A comparison of gene expression profiles show a germinal center B-cell-associated signatures in t(14;18)+ FL, but activated B-cell-associated signatures in t(14;18)– FL. However, overall survival does not appear to differ between FL with and without t(14;18).

Mycosis Fungoides/Sézary Syndrome

Tsieh Sun

Patient A 75-year-old man with a 2-week history of a whole-body pruritic, scaling erythematous rash.

Clinical History The patient had no history of psoriasis or other dermatologic problems.

Family History Noncontributory.

Medication None.

Physical Examination Generalized exfoliative erythroderma involved the whole body. Lymphadenopathy involving the posterior auricular, axillary and inguinal regions was noted. Hepatosplenomegaly was not present.

Initial Work-Up

CBC		WBC	%	# ($\times 10^3$/μL)
WBC ($\times 10^3$/μL)	10.0	Neutrophils	26	2.6
RBC ($\times 10^6$/μL)	3.50	Bands	5	0.5
HGB (g/dL)	11.3	Lymphocytes	45	4.5
HCT (%)	34.0	Monocytes	1	0.1
MCV (fL)	97.2	Eosinophils	8	0.8
MCH (pg)	32.3	Basophils	0	
MCHC (g/dL)	33.2	Atypical lymphs	15	1.5
PLT ($\times 10^3$/μL)	79			
RDW-CV (%)	14.1			

Peripheral blood smear revealed atypical lymphocytes with cerebriform nuclei (**Figure 1**).
Skin biopsy showed a band-like lymphocytic infiltrate occupying the dermis and extending into the overlying epidermis (**Figure 2**). The infiltrate was composed of irregular-shaped medium-sized lymphoid cells. Multiple intraepidermal lymphoid aggregates, consistent with Pautrier microabscesses, were present (**Figure 3**). Immunohistochemical stains revealed that the malignant cells were immunoreactive to CD3, CD4 and CD45RO, but were negative for CD8 and CD20.

Differential Diagnosis It included exfoliative psoriasis and cutaneous T-cell lymphoma

Additional Work-Up A right axillary lymph node biopsy revealed total replacement of the normal architecture by extensive tumor cell infiltration. Flow cytometric analysis of the peripheral blood and lymph node revealed high percentages of CD3, CD4, CD5, but low percentages of CD7, CD8 and B-cell antigens (CD19, CD20, κ and λ). T-cell-receptor gene rearrangement analysis of the blood specimen demonstrated a clonal T-cell population.

Final Diagnosis Sézary syndrome (SS).

Management Approach The clinical course of mycosis fungoides (MF) is usually indolent and is frequently preceded by a premalignant phase for several years. SS, on the other hand, is an aggressive disease from the onset with an overall survival rate at 5 years of 10%-20%. General approaches to systemic treatment include phototherapy with ultraviolet radiation (UVA or UVB), chemotherapy (doxorubicin, methotrexate, pentostatin, fludarabine, etc), and immunotherapy (eg, alemtuzumab), either singly or in combination.

Section E: Lymphomas and Their Mimics
Mycosis Fungoides/Sézary Syndrome

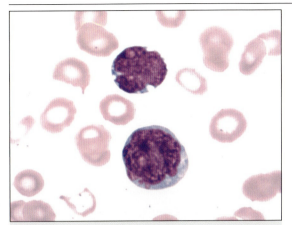

Figure 1 Blood smear (Wright-Giemsa, ×1000) showing 2 cerebriform Sézary cells.

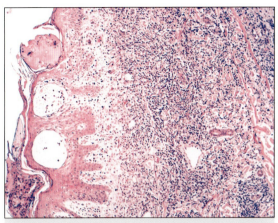

Figure 2 Skin biopsy (H&E, ×100) showing a bandlike lymphoid infiltration in the upper dermis. Lymphoid infiltration is also seen in the epidermis.

Skin-directed therapeutic agents include glucocorticoids, retinoids, and tacrolimus. This patient was treated with psoralen plus ultraviolet A (PUVA) and interferon α, which he tolerated poorly. The treatment was switched to local application of low-dose topical steroids. The patient died 3 months after the diagnosis due to congestive heart failure and renal insufficiency.

General Discussion Mycosis fungoides (MF) accounts for 50%-65% of primary cutaneous lymphoma. Clinically, patients usually present with the patch, plaque and tumor stages. Previously, the erythroderma stage was also included as the terminal stage of MF, but it is now considered to be the clinical presentation of a distinct entity, Sézary syndrome (SS). MF and SS were considered 2 phases of a same disease before, but the International Society for Cutaneous Lymphoma (ISCL) and the cutaneous lymphoma task force of the European Organization for Research and Treatment of Cancer (EORTC) classify them as 2 separate diseases, partly because their prognoses are markedly different. The histologic features vary in different clinical stages of MF. In the patch stage, there is only patchy lymphocytic infiltration in the upper dermis. It is usually perivascular. Intraepidermal lymphoid infiltration (Pautrier microabscesses) is rare or absent. Cytologic atypia is minimal. In the plaque stage, a dense, bandlike infiltrate of atypical lymphoid cells is present in the upper dermis. Pautrier microabscesses are often seen. The atypical lymphoid cells show hyperchromatic and convoluted nuclei and scant cytoplasm. The deep dermis and subcutis are seldom involved. In the tumor stage, the atypical lymphoid infiltrate may extend into the lower dermis and subcutis. At the same time, the tumor cells increase in number and in size, so that many large cerebriform cells and blasts are coexistent with small and medium tumor cells. Pautrier microabscesses, on the other hand, gradually disappear. In the ISCL classification, SS is defined by the following criteria: (a) an absolute Sézary cell count of >1,000/μL; (b) demonstration of im-

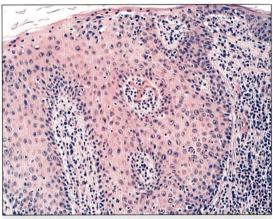

Figure 3 Skin biopsy (H&E, ×200) showing several Pautrier microabscesses in the epidermis.

munophenotypic abnormalities: CD4/CD8 ratio of >10 or aberrant loss of pan-T-cell markers by flow cytometry; and (c) demonstration of a T-cell clone in the peripheral blood by molecular or cytogenetic techniques. The 2008 WHO classification further requires the presence of the neoplastic T cells not only in the peripheral blood, but also in the skin and the lymph node. The current case shows the tumor cells in all 3 sites and they express the typical immunophenotype and genotype, so that it is a typical case of SS. SS accounts for only about 5% of all cutaneous T-cell lymphomas Most patients are adults, elderly, and male. Patients with SS generally present with erythroderma, pruritus, alopecia, ectropion, hyperkeratoses, onychodystrophy and generalized lymphadenopathy. The histologic features in the lymph node of MF/SS are those of dermatopathic lymphadenopathy. It is characterized by the presence of sinus histiocytosis, an abundance of pigment-laden macrophages, and various numbers of atypical lymphocytes, depending on the stage of the disease.

Follicular Hyperplasia

Stefania Pittaluga, Joo Y Song

Patient A 39-year-old woman, who presented with an enlarged submandibular mass.

Clinical History The patient has a history of salivary gland pleomorphic adenoma. She has not felt ill recently. She has had no constitutional symptoms. She has not noted any other enlarged lymph nodes.

Family History Noncontributory.

Medications None.

Physical Examination Left submandibular triangle lymphadenopathy measuring 1.5 cm in largest dimension.

Initial Work-Up		
CBC		
WBC ($\times 10^3/\mu L$)	5.9	
RBC ($\times 10^6/\mu L$)	4.74	
HGB (g/dL)	8.7	
HCT (%)	30.7	
MCV (fL)	64.7	
MCH (pg)	18.4	
MCHC (g/dL)	28.4	
PLT ($\times 10^3/\mu L$)	421	
RDW-CV (%)	17.1	
MPV (fL)	7.2	
WBC Differential	**%**	**# ($\times 10^3/\mu L$)**
Neutrophils	65	3.9
Bands	0	
Lymphocytes	33	2.0
Monocytes	2	0.1

Sections from the submandibular lymph node excisional biopsy showed an enlarged lymph node with an intact non-thickened capsule. The nodal architecture was intact with enlarged follicles varying in size and shape and patent sinuses (**Figure 1**). The enlarged secondary follicles showed a distinct mantle cuff with polarization of the germinal centers and scattered tingible-body macrophages giving a "starry-sky" appearance (**Figure 2**). The paracortical areas of the lymph node showed mostly small mature lymphocytes with scattered immunoblasts.

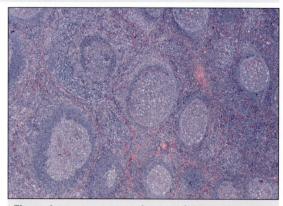

Figure 1 Lymph node biopsy (H&E, ×40) showing expanded follicles that vary in size and shape.

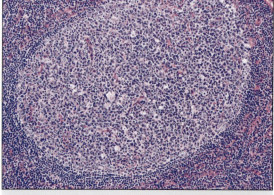

Figure 2 Lymph node biopsy (H&E, ×100) showing a germinal center with sharply defined mantle and heterogeneous populations of cells.

Differential Diagnosis Based on the location and the patient's prior history of a pleomorphic adenoma, the possibility of a metastasis was entertained clinically. However, the histological sections confirmed that the lesion was an enlarged lymph node. The differential diagnostic considerations for lesions involving the lymph node included reactive conditions such as follicular hyperplasia or infectious lymphadenitis as well as neoplastic conditions such as follicular lymphoma, or marginal zone lymphoma.

Additional Work-Up Immunohistochemical stains performed on the lymph node showed that the CD20+ B cells were restricted to the follicles and CD3 highlighted the paracortical T cells. IgD highlighted the sharply defined mantle cuffs around the germinal centers (**Figure 3**). Ki-67 (MIB-1) showed a brisk proliferation index within the germinal centers which were well polarized (**Figure 4**). BCL2 was negative within the germinal centers. Flow cytometric analysis showed 70% of the events were small to medium-sized B cells that expressed CD20, CD23, and FMC-7. No light chain restriction was noted with κ and λ. T lymphocytes showed no aberrant phenotype and a normal CD4 to CD8 ratio.

Final Diagnosis Reactive follicular hyperplasia.

Management Approach These benign lesions are usually self-limited but may result from an autoimmune disease or infection. Therefore, therapy focused on the underlying condition is preferred.

General Discussion Reactive follicular hyperplasia (FH) is commonly seen in children and adolescents, and its cause is mostly unknown. Lymph nodes constantly respond to stimuli. During T-cell-dependent responses, B cells upon antigen interaction differentiate into germinal center B cells and in about 2 weeks give rise to secondary B follicles. The low-power architecture can be very helpful in the diagnosis of FH. There is usually preservation of the architecture and the sinuses are patent. The secondary B follicles are usually enlarged, varying in size and shape and are unevenly distributed. The hyperplasia may be florid, particularly in the younger age groups, with follicles occupying both cortex and paracortex, and even medullary areas. Similar features can also be observed in HIV-related lymphadenopathy. The germinal centers are usually sharply demarcated from the mantles. Both components, mantles and germinal centers, are polarized. The germinal center is often composed of a heterogeneous

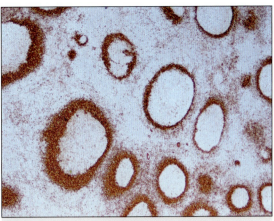

Figure 3 Lymph node biopsy (IgD, ×40) showing distinct mantle cuffs surrounding the expanded germinal centers.

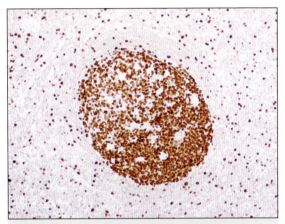

Figure 4 Lymph node biopsy (MIB-1, ×100) showing polarization of the germinal centers with proliferating cells accumulating in the dark zone

population of cells; large centroblasts, small cleaved centrocytes, tingible-body macrophages with associated apoptotic bodies, and inconspicuous follicular dendritic cells.

In the germinal centers, the area corresponding to the clonal expansion of activated B cells is known as the dark zone and it is composed predominantly of centroblasts, which are actively proliferating. Centrocytes with low to no affinity undergo apoptosis, and cellular debris are phagocytosed by macrophages, giving rise to the so-called starry-sky pattern. Occasionally monocytoid B-cell hyperplasia can be associated with the FH (especially with toxoplasmosis and HIV infection) and monocytoid B cells accumulate in the perisinusoidal space. Aggregates of monocytoid B cells are easily appreciated at low power due to their pale cytoplasm and also their association with

Section E: Lymphomas and Their Mimics
Follicular Hyperplasia

neutrophils. The main differential diagnosis of follicular hyperplasia is from follicular lymphoma (FL) and other low-grade B-cell lymphomas with a follicular/nodular growth pattern. It is important to rely on multiple criteria such as the distribution of the follicles, their density, variation in size and shape and their cellular composition. The follicles in FL are usually back-to-back and are more uniformly shaped and evenly distributed. The interfollicular areas are usually compressed or nonexistent (back-to-back). Excisional biopsy or non-invasive procedures such as a fine-needle aspiration with flow cytometric analysis is helpful in ruling out a neoplastic process. The immunohistochemical pattern for FH is also helpful in differentiating from a neoplastic process. Pan B-cell markers highlight the follicles (centrocytes, centroblasts, and mantle cells) with only scattered positive cells in the interfollicular areas. BCL2 is negative in the germinal centers (as opposed to follicular lymphoma), while CD10 and BCL6 are expressed in the reactive germinal centers as well as in the majority of follicular lymphomas. IgD stains the sharply demarcated mantle cuffs around the germinal centers. Ki-67 (MIB-1) shows often a high proliferation rate in the germinal centers and highlights the prominent polarization. CD21 and CD23 stain the follicular dendritic cell meshwork.

Rosai-Dorfman Disease

Kathryn Foucar, Douglas W Kingma

Patient A 59-year-old female, in otherwise good health, developed isolated painless cervical adenopathy.

Clinical History Noncontributory.

Family History Unremarkable.

Medications None.

Physical Examination Significant for submandibular adenopathy.

Initial Work-Up The biopsy sections of a lymph node revealed capsular fibrosis and reactive follicular hyperplasia with expanded paracortical spaces containing proliferations of large histiocytes with enlarged nuclei, vesicular chromatin, and abundant pink-staining granular cytoplasm (**Figure 1**). The histiocytes demonstrated prominent emperipolesis of lymphocytes, neutrophils and plasma cells (**Figure 2**). A background of cytologically unremarkable lymphocytes and plasma cells was noted.

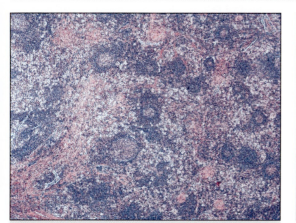

Figure 1 Lymph node biopsy (H&E, ×100) showing reactive appearance, intact architecture, and an expanded interfollicular zone populated primarily by abundant pale-staining histiocytes.

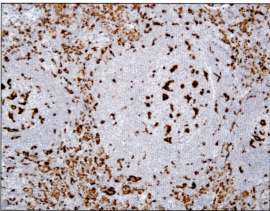

Figure 2 Lymph node biopsy (H&E, ×400) in which lymphocytes are seen within the cytoplasm of many histiocytes (emperipolesis).

Differential Diagnosis Lymphoma (non-Hodgkin lymphoma and Hodgkin lymphoma), metastatic malignancy, and reactive lymphadenopathy. The age of the patient and painless adenopathy favor a neoplastic process.

Additional Work-Up By immunohistochemical stains the histiocytes stained positive for CD68 (**Figure 3**) and S100 (**Figure 4**). Immunophenotyping by flow cytometry revealed no evidence of a monoclonal B-cell population or an aberrant T-cell population. There were 35% polytypic B cells with 57% T cells (CD4:CD8 ratio of 5.7:1). Plasma cells were polytypic for cytoplasmic light chain by in situ hybridization.

Section E: Lymphomas and Their Mimics
Rosai-Dorfman Disease

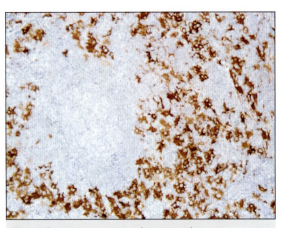

Figure 3 Lymph node biopsy (CD68, ×200) showing histiocytes are positive.

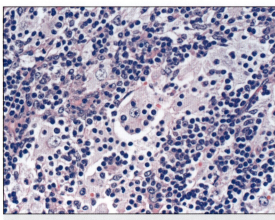

Figure 4 Lymph node biopsy (S100, ×200) showing histiocytes that are positive.

Final Diagnosis Sinus histiocytosis with massive lymphadenopathy (Rosai-Dorfman Disease).

Management The disease typically has a prolonged course, and many cases showing eventual spontaneous resolution. Some patients develop progressive disease which can be manifested by the development of systemic adenopathy, involvement of extranodal sites, and CNS disease. Such cases have been managed by chemotherapy, radiation therapy, steroid therapy, and/or rituximab. Overall, responses in these cases have generally been inferior to those expected with malignant hematopoietic neoplasms. Follow-up records for this patient showed no additional therapeutic intervention, including additional excision biopsies or therapy.

General Discussion Sinus histiocytosis with massive lymphadenopathy (SHML), or Rosai-Dorfman disease, was first described by Rosai and Dorfman in 1969. This rare disorder is a benign condition that primarily affects cervical lymph nodes, but can involve extranodal sites (up to 25% of cases) including skin, upper respiratory tract, eyelid and orbit, salivary gland and bone. Lymph nodes in other areas may be enlarged, but often to a lesser degree. Most patients are in good health at presentation, with the majority having a polyclonal elevation of IgG (though there are documented cases of monoclonal gammopathy). The erythrocyte sedimentation rate is elevated in almost 90% of cases. A low-grade fever at presentation is not unusual. The distinctive histologic features include capsular/pericapsular fibrosis and conspicuous dilatation of lymph node sinuses filled with S100+ histiocytes exhibiting emperipolesis. Although these histiocytes most commonly engulf lymphocytes within their cytoplasm, plasma cells and erythrocytes (hemophagocytosis) can also be seen. The remaining lymph node usually demonstrates a background follicular hyperplasia with variably sized reactive appearing follicles. Interfollicular plasma cells are polytypic and can show intracytoplasmic inclusions (Russell bodies). The differential diagnosis includes sinus histiocytosis, Langerhans cell histiocytosis (LCH), metastatic carcinomas and melanomas. Carcinomas and melanomas can be identified by appropriate immunohistochemical stains. Sinus histiocytosis can be distinguished from SHML by the absence of emperipolesis and immunohistochemical staining for S100 by histiocytes. Langerhans cell histiocytosis, in contrast to SHML, is typically associated with a prominent eosinophilia. The histiocytes of LCH also show characteristic nuclear features (smaller nuclei, nuclear groves, and indistinct nucleoli) and uniquely stain for CD1a, which is negative in SHML.

Kikuchi-Fujimoto Disease (Histiocytic Necrotizing Lymphadenitis)

Stefania Pittaluga, Qingyan Liu

Patient A 32-year-old female, who presented to the emergency room with enlarged right neck "lumps."

Clinical History The patient had noted gradually enlarging lymph nodes on the right side of her neck over the prior several weeks. She recalled no trauma or recent infections. She has had no constitutional symptoms.

Family History Noncontributory.

Medications Cephalexin monohydrate.

Physical Examination She was afebrile with a normal blood pressure and pulse. She had a few enlarged lymph nodes (2 cm-3 cm each) in the right anterior cervical region, tender to palpation. There was no evidence of airway compromise or infection in the oropharynx. She had no other palpable lymph nodes and no hepatosplenomegaly.

Initial Work-Up

CBC		WBC Differential	%	# (×10³/μL)
WBC (×10³/μL)	4.6	Neutrophils	50.5	2.30
RBC (×10⁶/μL)	4.69	Bands	0	
HGB (g/dL)	13.8	Lymphocytes	39.8	1.81
HCT (%)	42.1	Monocytes	8.8	0.40
MCV (fL)	89.8	Eosinophils	0.7	0.03
MCH (pg)	29.4	Basophils	0.2	0.01
MCHC (g/dL)	32.8			
PLT (×10³/μL)	264			
RDW-CV (%)	12.6			

Other laboratory tests including renal and liver functions were essentially normal. The right cervical lymph node was biopsied. Histologically, the biopsy showed largely preserved nodal architecture with patchy, irregular shaped areas of necrosis distributed in the interfollicular areas. The necrosis mainly consisted of a histiocytic proliferation, numerous karyorrhectic debris, and eosinophilic fibrinoid deposits (**Figure 1**). Some histiocytes actively phagocytosed the cellular debris, forming compressed, crescentic nuclei, resembling signet ring cells. Small lymphocytes, immunoblasts, and scattered plasma cells were also present in the necrotic areas; however, neutrophils and eosinophils were absent. In areas, clusters of plasmacytoid dendritic cells were noted (**Figure 2**).

Differential Diagnosis Systemic lupus erythematosus (SLE) associated lymphadenopathy, herpes simplex virus (HSV)-associated lymphadenopathy, and lymphoma.

Additional Work-Up By immunohistochemical stains the histiocytes were positive for CD68 and MPO (**Figure 3**); the lymphocytes were mainly CD3/CD8+ T cells and CD20+ B cells were scarce (**Figure 4**); CD30 highlighted the immunoblasts. The plasma cells were polyclonal as demonstrated by κ and λ light chain stains. Epstein-Barr virus (EBV) was negative by in situ hybridization using EBER probe. Flow cytometry analysis showed no evidence of non-Hodgkin lymphoma.

Section E: Lymphomas and Their Mimics
Kikuchi-Fujimoto Disease (Histiocytic Necrotizing Lymphadenitis)

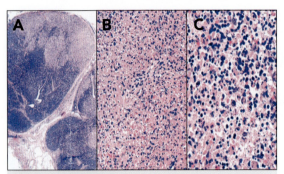

Figure 1 Lymph node biopsy showing **A** (H&E, ×20) areas of patchy necrosis made-up of histiocytes, karyorrhexis, and eosinophilc fibrinoid deposits, **B** (H&E, ×100) histiocytes with phagocytosis of cellular debris and eccentric nuclei, resembling signet ring cells, and **C** (H&E, ×400) absence of neutrophils.

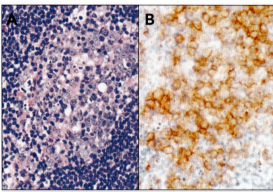

Figure 2 Lymph node biopsy **A** (H&E, ×400) showing plasmacytoid dendritic cells seen among histiocytes. **B** (CD123, ×400) plasmacytoid dendritic cells are positive.

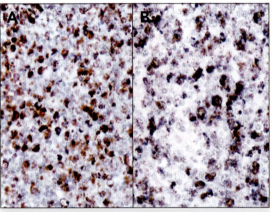

Figure 3 Lymph node biopsy **A** (CD68, ×400) and **B** (MPO, ×400) in which histiocytes are positive.

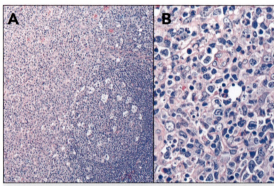

Figure 4 Lymph node biopsy from a different case of Kikuchi-Fujimoto disease **A** (H&E, ×100) and **B** (H&E, ×400) showing cytologic atypia among the immunoblasts mimicking lymphoma.

Final Diagnosis Histiocytic necrotizing lymphadenitis (Kikuchi-Fujimoto disease).

Management Approach Histiocytic necrotizing lymphadenitis is a self-limited disease with low recurrence rate (3%-4%). Care of these patients is generally supportive and includes the use of nonsteroidal anti-inflammatory agents. In more severe cases, including those lasting >2 weeks, those with neurologic or liver involvement, or those with a severe lupus-like syndrome, steroids may be used. Steroids are also used in the rare patients with recurrent disease. Other immune suppressants may be used in rare life-threatening disease. This patient was asked to take ibuprofen as needed for symptomatic relief. Her lymph nodes gradually returned to normal after several weeks.

General Discussion Histiocytic necrotizing lymphadenitis, so-called Kikuchi-Fujimoto disease, is a benign and self-limited disease, which was first described by Kikuchi and by Fujimoto almost simultaneously in 1972. The disease has a worldwide distribution with a high prevalence in Asia. It commonly affects young females, presenting with unilateral swollen cervical lymph nodes without constitutional symptoms. Generalized lymphadenopathy is rare. Etiology of this disease is unclear. The hallmark histologic features are patchy necrosis with histiocytic proliferation, karyorrhexis or pyknotic cells, fibrinoid deposits, and the absence of neutrophils. The nodal architecture is usually preserved. Recent studies have shown that the histiocytes coexpress CD68 and MPO, suggesting that the peripheral blood MPO+/CD68+ monocytes might be attracted into tissue because of the lack or paucity of granulocytes. Clusters of plasmacytoid dendritic cells positive for CD68 and CD123, and negative for MPO, can also be observed. Important differential diagnosis includes lupus lymphadenopathy, viral lymphadenopathy (HSV, EBV), and non-Hodgkin lymphomas. The histologic features of lupus lymphadenopathy are overlapping with histiocytic necrotizing lymphadenitis, careful clinical history and laboratory tests to rule out systemic lupus erythematosus are necessary. HSV-associated lymphadenopathy usually has mucosal or skin lesions near the sites of lymphadenopathy, and the lymph node biopsy usually shows necrosis with neutrophils and virally induced cytopathic effect can be seen often at the edge of the necrosis. EBV-associated lymphadenopathy (infectious mononucleosis) shows follicular and paracortical hyperplasia with numerous immunoblasts often resembling Reed-Sternberg cells, areas of necrosis and numerous EBV+ cells by in situ hybridization. In Kikuchi lymphadenitis when numerous immunoblasts, occasionally forming sheets, are present associated with the necrosis, it can be confused with non-Hodgkin lymphoma (**Figure 4**). It is essential to rule out the latter diagnosis, since the therapeutic implications are quite different. The correct diagnosis is achieved usually by combining careful histologic examination with immunophenotyping and molecular studies for T-cell receptor gene rearrangement.

Progressive Transformation of Germinal Centers

Mehmet I Goral

Patient A 44-year-old male with a painless enlargement in the neck.

Clinical History The patient was otherwise healthy. He had noticed the swelling in the neck several weeks earlier. It had grown slowly to its current size. It was not sore. He didn't recall any recent illness. He had not had any fevers, chills, sweats or weight loss.

Family History Noncontributory.

Medications None.

Physical Examination An enlarged lymph node was noted in the right neck, which was mobile and nontender. No additional lymphadenopathy was detected. Liver and spleen were nonpalpable.

Initial Work-Up Results of CBC, differential leukocyte count, and routine serum chemistries were within normal limits. The patient was taken to the operating room and the enlarged lymph node was excised. The lymph node measured 4.5 cm in maximal dimension, and the cut surface was uniformly tan-white in color, without any gross evidence of hemorrhage, necrosis or nodularity. On microscopic examination the lymph node revealed open sinuses with reactive follicular hyperplasia. A few follicles were significantly enlarged, about 3 to 4 times the size of the reactive follicles, and showed infiltration of small round lymphocytes (**Figures 1** and **2**). Rare immunoblasts and histiocytes were also present. No Reed-Sternberg cells or its variants were identified. A portion of the lymph node was submitted for flow cytometry studies.

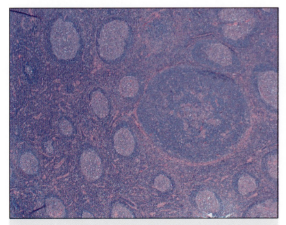

Figure 1 Lymph node (H&E, ×40) showing an enlarged nodule representing progressive transformation of germinal center in the background follicular hyperplasia.

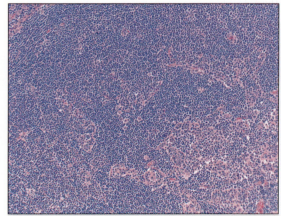

Figure 2 Lymph node (H&E, ×400) showing numerous small lymphocytes infiltrating progressively transformed germinal center, note lack of tangible body macrophages, small cleaved cells, large transformed cells, Reed-Sternberg cells and its variants.

Differential Diagnosis The diagnostic considerations included progressive transformation of germinal centers (PTGC), nodular lymphocyte-predominant Hodgkin lymphoma (NLPHL), classical Hodgkin lymphoma (lymphocyte rich) and follicular lymphoma.

Additional Work-Up Flow cytometry studies showed that B cells were polyclonal and T cells did not show any abnormal phenotype.

Final Diagnosis Reactive hyperplasia with progressive transformation of germinal centers.

Management Approach Surgical excision of involved lymph nodes is sufficient for treatment of PTGC. Long-term close follow-up with excision of persistent or recurrent lymphadenopathy is generally recommended based on possible association with NLPHL. Also, pathologists should be aware of this association and not mistake PTGC as recurrent disease in patients with history of NLPHL. In this patient also, no additional treatment was deemed necessary. The association of PTGC with NLPHL was stated, and sampling of any recurrent and/or persistent lymphadenopathy was recommended.

General Discussion PTGC was originally described in reactive lymph nodes with follicular hyperplasia and appears to represent a morphological step in progression of follicular hyperplasia. Reported incidence ranges between 3.5% and 12% in reactive lymph nodes, although the higher percentages may be related to sampling bias of consultative material. The etiology of PTGC is unknown. PTGC occurs in all age groups, more commonly in adults, with male predominance; recurrent disease is more common in children. Usually a single group of lymph nodes are involved, generalized disease is rare. Cervical lymph nodes are the most commonly involved site, followed by axillary and inguinal lymph nodes. Lymph nodes involved by PTGC show reactive follicular hyperplasia with 1 or a few enlarged germinal centers that show infiltration of small lymphocytes. These follicles show loss of polarization as well as lack of distinct mantle zones. Tingible body macrophages are usually absent, a few scattered histiocytes and/or immunoblasts may be present. A florid form of PTGC with numerous progressively transformed germinal centers has also been described. Progressively transformed germinal centers comprise of a mixture of B and T cells. While the lymphocytes in reactive germinal centers are mostly B cells with germinal center phenotype (pan-B cell markers-positive, express CD10, BCL6, and BCL2 negative); in PTGC the infiltrating lymphocytes are predominantly mantle zone B cells (pan-B cell-positive, express IgD, BCL2, and are negative for CD10 and BCL6) and few scattered T cells (**Figure 3**). Unlike NLPHL, rosette formation with CD57+ T cells is only rarely seen. Immunohistochemical staining with antibodies to follicular dendritic cells show enlarged and disturbed follicular dendritic network (**Figure 4**). The neoplastic nodules in NLPHL and lymphocyte rich classic Hodgkin lymphoma morphologically may resemble the nodules in PTGC. These neoplastic conditions usually involve the entire lymph node with effaced architecture and do not show background follicular hyperplasia. Presence of Reed-Sternberg cells or L&H (popcorn) cells is key to diagnosis of Hodgkin

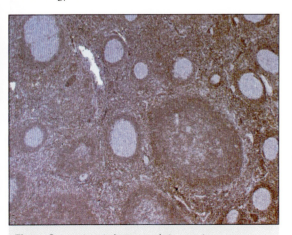

Figure 3 Lymph node (BCL2, ×40) showing that reactive germinal centers in the background are negative but infiltrating lymphocyte in progressively transformed germinal center are positive.

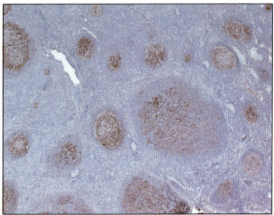

Figure 4 Lymph node (CD21, ×40) highlighting expanded follicular dendritic meshwork.

lymphoma, and a panel of immunohistochemistry studies may help confirm presence of neoplastic cells. The clinical association of PTGC with NLPHL is intriguing, but not clear cut; while most cases of PTGC have no clinical consequences, PTGC has been shown to precede, coexist and follow NLPHL. The elapsed time between diagnosis of PTGC and NLPHL may be as long as 13 years; thus long-term follow-up in these patients is recommended. In an early paper, based on morphologic similarities and coexistence of 2 conditions in same patients, Poppema et al suggested that PTGC represents a precursor lesion for NLPHL. Later studies have failed to show a prospective association of NLPHL with PTGC and it is now accepted that PTGC is not a preneoplastic condition. Lymph nodes involved by follicular lymphoma usually show complete effacement of normal architecture with back-to-back follicles; these follicles may spread to surrounding adipose tissue. Neoplastic follicles in follicular lymphoma consist of mixture of small-cleaved cells and/or large transformed cells instead of small lymphocytes seen in PTGC. Presence of polarization, tingible body macrophages and lack of BCL2 expression indicate reactive germinal centers. These features may not be discernible in cases of florid PTGC, where the differential diagnosis becomes more difficult morphologically. PTGC show a heterogeneous infiltrate of lymphocytes into the expanded germinal centers without small cleaved cells or large transformed cells; while BCL2 immunohistochemistry is not helpful, flow cytometry or gene rearrangement studies fail to show a clonal population.

Castleman Disease

Stefania Pittaluga, Ryan M Gill

Patient A 52-year-old woman was found to have enlarged inguinal lymph nodes during a routine annual physical.

Clinical History The patient was asymptomatic and had no known infectious disease history. She has had no fever, chills or weight loss.

Family History Noncontributory.

Medications None.

Physical Examination Localized left inguinal lymphadenopathy. There was no other palpable adenopathy, splenomegaly or hepatomegaly.

Initial Work-Up Sections of the left groin lymph node excisional biopsy showed an enlarged lymph node with an intact thin capsule and relatively preserved architecture, though lymph node sinuses were lacking within the lesion. Follicles were abnormal with small and sclerotic germinal centers (**Figure 1**); some were penetrated by hyalinized vessels and had prominent mantle cell expansion with an "onion-skin" appearance (**Figure 1**). Several examples of 2 sclerotic germinal centers in close proximity, surrounded by a single mantle zone (ie, "twinning"), were noted (**Figure 2**). There was expansion of the interfollicular compartment with vascular proliferation (**Figure 3**) and clusters of plasmacytoid dendritic cells were noted (**Figure 4**). Occasional interfollicular plasma cells were also evident, but they were not a predominant finding. Concurrent flow cytometric analysis was negative for monoclonal B-cell or aberrant T-cell populations.

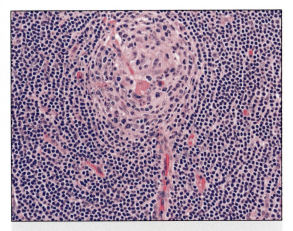

Figure 1 Lymph node (H&E, ×200) showing a representative regressively transformed germinal center with a characteristic expanded mantle zone and penetrating hyalinized vessel.

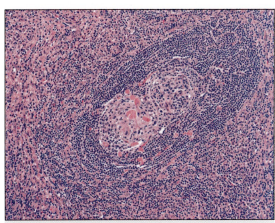

Figure 2 Lymph node (H&E, ×100) showing characteristic follicle within follicle "twinning."

Section E: Lymphomas and Their Mimics
Castleman Disease

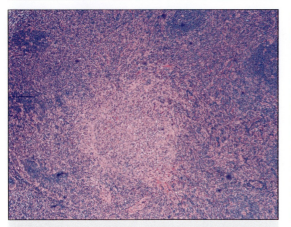

Figure 3 Lymph node (H&E, ×100) showing focal vascular proliferation.

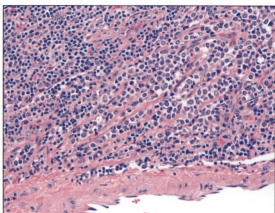

Figure 4 Lymph node (H&E, ×200) showing clusters of interfollicular plasmacytoid dendritic cells.

Differential Diagnosis Nonspecific follicular hyperplasia, progressive transformation of germinal centers, HIV lymphadenitis, and Castleman lymphadenopathy, hyaline vascular variant (CD-HV) could be considered in the differential diagnosis, based on the above initial findings.

Additional Work-Up Immunohistochemical stains performed on the lymph node sections demonstrated CD20+ cells largely restricted to widely spaced follicles with only rare larger cells also staining in the interfollicular regions (consistent with immunoblasts). CD3 was negative in larger cells and highlighted a normal T-cell component. CD138, κ and λ highlighted the slight interfollicular plasmacytosis noted above, but no light chain restriction was appreciated and plasma cells did not form sheets. CD21 highlighted a network of follicular dendritic cells, with overall intense staining of germinal centers and mantle zones (**Figure 5**). CD34 and CD31 highlighted a focal vascular proliferation as well as slightly increased interfollicular capillary density, but were negative in larger cells. CD123 was positive in numerous cells, often forming clusters, consistent with plasmacytoid dendritic cells (**Figure 6**). HHV8 was negative.

Final Diagnosis Castleman lymphadenopathy, hyaline vascular variant.

Management Approach Unicentric Castleman disease is most typically associated with the hyaline vascular variant (80%-90% of all unicentric cases), as in this case. Most unicentric patients are asymptomatic and surgical excision is curative, as it was for this patient.

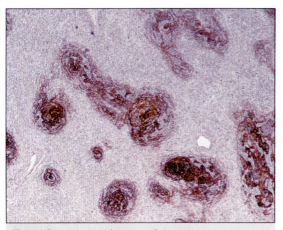

Figure 5 Lymph node (CD21, ×40) showing positive follicular dendritic cell meshwork.

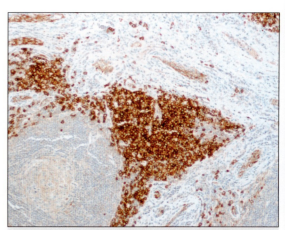

Figure 6 Lymph node (CD123, ×100) highlighting CD123+ interfollicular plasmacytoid dendritic cells.

General Discussion The morphologic findings seen in Castleman disease are not entirely specific and can be seen in reactive lymph nodes. Therefore, correct diagnosis relies on observation of multiple characteristic features and correlation with clinical findings. Castleman disease may present in a unicentric or multicentric fashion. The former may demonstrate either hyaline vascular or, less commonly, plasma cell variant histology. The hyaline vascular variant is not restricted by gender, age, or lymph node location and typically presents as a large mass (the mediastinum is a particularly common site). The plasma cell variant accounts for <20% of unicentric Castleman disease and, like the hyaline vascular variant, it is not restricted by gender, age or location, though the mediastinum is less commonly involved. The distinction between unicentric plasma cell variant Castleman disease and multicentric Castleman disease is problematic given that some patients with unicentric disease are symptomatic and reportedly progress to a multicentric form (typically in patients with HIV infection). In any event, symptomatic patients most often have the plasma cell variant of Castleman disease and there is evidence to suggest a role for IL-6 (so-called IL-6 syndrome) in this etiology. The hyaline vascular variant characteristically demonstrates an enlarged lymph node distorted by abnormal follicles (small sclerotic lymphocyte-depleted germinal centers with hyaline deposits and broad mantle zones), some with penetration by hyalinized vessels ("lollipop lesion"). The follicular component can be predominant in some cases and follicle within follicle architecture (ie, 2 follicles surrounded by a mantle zone, also known as "twinning") is a particularly characteristic finding. Follicular dendritic cells can be large and may appear dysplastic in some cases. The interfollicular regions typically demonstrate some degree of vascular hyperplasia and vessels may be sclerotic; this hyperplasia is particularly prominent in the stroma rich variant, which is defined as Castleman lymphadenopathy with >50% interfollicular tissue. Plasmacytoid dendritic cell clusters are frequently encountered in the interfollicular compartment, as is a mixed population of plasma cells, immunoblasts, small lymphocytes, and eosinophils. Given that the morphologic findings of hyaline vascular Castleman disease are not entirely specific, the differential diagnosis can be problematic. In considering causes of isolated lymphadenopathy, nonspecific follicular hyperplasia should be considered; however, in this entity the lymph node will not demonstrate the above described characteristic abnormal follicles throughout the lymph node, as seen in our case. HIV related follicular hyperplasia is another consideration, but again the follicles are not typically characterized by small and sclerotic germinal centers with broad mantle zones, as in CD-HV and instead more often demonstrate hyperplastic germinal centers with mantle zone attenuation, and evidence of follicular lysis. Progressive transformation of germinal centers, with its influx of mantle cells into a germinal center, is not typically mistaken for Castleman disease. A variety of interfollicular stromal proliferations have been described in Castleman disease and this finding can raise concern for a vascular neoplasm such as Kaposi sarcoma or angiosarcoma, but the interfollicular endothelial cells in Castleman disease are not markedly atypical and lack expression of HHV-8 (unlike the cells of Kaposi sarcoma).

Section F: Plasma Cell Disorders

Monoclonal Gammopathy of Undetermined Significance

Joanne Filicko-O'Hara, Ryan Gentzler, Gene Gulati

Patient A 68-year-old male was noted to be more confused in the past several days by his family.

Clinical History The patient has a history of hypertension, end-stage liver disease secondary to non-alcoholic steatohepatitis (NASH), chronic renal insufficiency, diabetes mellitus, and hypothyroidism.

Family History Significant for a father with coronary artery disease; no history of liver disease; no history of malignancy.

Medications Metoprolol XL, paricalcito, levothyroxine, spironolactone, and tamulosin.

Physical Examination Notable only for hypertension (BP 164/69 mm/Hg), mild tachycardia (HR 108 bpm) and temperature 95.9° F, and 1+ pitting edema in bilateral lower extremities.

Initial Work-Up

CBC			Chemistry Panel	
WBC ($\times 10^3/\mu L$)	3.3		Na$^+$ (mmol/L)	140
RBC ($\times 10^6/L$)	4.67		K$^+$ (mmol/L)	5.5
HGB (g/dL)	13.1		Cl$^-$ (mmol/L)	111
HCT (%)	41.0		CO_2 (mmol/L)	23
MCV (fL)	88		BUN (mg/dL)	74
MCH (pg)	28.1		Cr (mg/dL)	3.4
MCHC (g/dL)	32.0		Ca^{2+} (mg/dL)	8.7
PLT ($\times 10^3/\mu L$)	32		Protein (g/dL)	7.8
RDW-CV (%)	18.7		Albumin (g/dL)	3.5
WBC			Bilirubin, total (mg/dL)	1.5
Differential	%	# ($\times 10^3/\mu L$)		
Neutrophils	84.4	2.8	Bilirubin, direct (mg/dL)	0.5
Lymphocytes	8.7	0.3	Alk phos (IU/L)	90
Monocytes	5.7	0.2	AST (IU/L)	23
Eosinophils	0.9	0.0	ALT (IU/L)	19
Basophils	0.3	0.0	B_2-microglobulin (ml/L) (normal 1.42-3.41)	17.15

Section F: Plasma Cell Disorders
Monoclonal Gammopathy of Undetermined Significance

Serum Protein Electrophoresis (SPEP) with Immunofixation		
		Normal
Total protein	7.8 g/dL	(6.0-8.5)
Albumin	3.5 g/dL	(3.3-5.2)
α-1 globulin	0.2 g/dL	(0.1-0.3)
α-1 globulin	0.4 g/dL	(0.5-0.9)
β-globulin	0.5 g/dL	(0.5-1.2)
γ-globulin	1.6 g/dL	(0.6-1.6)
IgG	3,270 mg/dL	(723-1,685)
IgA	95 mg/dL	(69-382)
IgM	82 mg/dL	(63-277)

Serum Free Light Chain Analysis		
Free κ	23.60 mg/dL	(normal 0.33-1.94)
Free λ	24.60 mg/dL	(normal 0.57-2.63)
κ:λ	0.96	(normal 0.26-1.65)

Coagulation Studies	
PT (sec)	18.9 (normal 12-15)
INR	1.55 (normal 0.8-1.2)
PTT (sec)	41 (normal 20-35)

Urinalysis	
Specific gravity	1.012
pH	6.0
Protein	2+
Blood	2+
Hyaline casts	3

Urine Protein Electrophoresis (UPEP)	
Urine albumin	81%
Prot:Cr	6.8
Cr	172 mg/dL
Protein	724 mg/dL
Total 24-hr protein	4,851 mg/TV

As part of the work-up for his acute and chronic renal failure, urinalysis was performed and it revealed moderate proteinuria. A monoclonal band was detected in the γ region. Immunofixation identified this band as IgG κ. 24-hr protein measurement identified severe proteinuria (>3.5g/day).

Differential Diagnosis Monoclonal gammopathy of undetermined significance (MGUS), smoldering myeloma, multiple myeloma, lymphoproliferative disease, non-Hodgkin lymphoma, primary amyloidosis, plasmacytoma.

Additional Work-Up
- Bone marrow biopsy: normocellular marrow containing all normal hematopoietic elements. No evidence of malignancy
- Flow cytometry performed on bone marrow aspirate revealed no evidence of lymphoid monoclonality. CD45–/CD38+ plasma cells accounted for <1% of all analyzed cells
- Skeletal survey: negative for lytic lesions or fractures

Final Diagnosis Monoclonal gammopathy of undetermined significance (MGUS).

Management Approach The diagnosis of MGUS requires no specific treatment, but knowing that MGUS has the tendency to progress to multiple myeloma or other malignant plasma cell disorders at a rate of 1% per year, careful monitoring of these patients is recommended. Annual laboratory work for patients with MGUS should include serum protein electrophersis with immunofixation (SPEP/IEP), urine protein electorphoesis (UPEP), complete blood count, and basic metabolic panel to monitor for increasing serum protein levels, renal failure, anemia, or hypercalcemia. Should the serum monoclonal protein increase over 3 g/dL, a repeat marrow aspiration and biopsy should be considered to evaluate the patient for progression to smoldering myeloma, which would require more frequent monitoring, or to overt multiple myeloma. This patient was followed with laboratory evaluation (SPEP/IEP and quantitative immunoglobulins) every 3 months and subsequently on a yearly basis. His paraprotein has been stable and his IgA and IgM have remained in the normal range. He continues to be followed closely by nephrology for chronic renal insufficiency.

General Discussion It is important to distinguish MGUS from smoldering myeloma and multiple myeloma. The diagnostic criteria for MGUS includes:
- bone marrow biopsy demonstrates <10% plasma cells
- serum monoclonal protein <3 g/dL
- absent clinical manifestations of multiple myeloma

Smoldering myeloma has either >10% plasma cells in the marrow *or* serum monoclonal protein >3 g/L. Multiple myeloma has the same laboratory criteria as smoldering myeloma in addition to clinical manifestations of multiple myeloma. Patients with multiple myeloma and MGUS often have translocations at chromosome 14q32, which is the immunoglobulin heavy chain locus, and 1 of several other loci including 11q13 (CCND1), 4p16.3 (FGFR-3 and MMSET), 6p21 (CCND3), 16q23 (c-maf), and 20q11 (mafB).

Plasmacytoma

Robert A Kyle, Curtis A Hanson

Patient A 32-year-old white male with a swelling in his left neck.

Clinical History The patient also complained of discomfort in the right upper chest.

Family History Noncontributory.

Medications None.

Physical Examination Small 1-cm painless node in left cervical area. No other abnormalities were found.

Initial Work-Up

CBC	
WBC (×10³/μL)	3.4
RBC (×10⁶/μL)	4.67
HGB (g/dL)	14.5
HCT (%)	41.0
MCV (fL)	87.9
MCH (pg)	31.1
MCHC (g/dL)	35.4
PLT (×10³/μL)	197

WBC Differential	%	# (×10³/μL)
Neutrophils	52	1.8
Lymphocytes	33	1.1
Monocytes	7	0.2
Eosinophils	7	0.2
Basophils	1	0.0
Calcium (mg/dL)	9.4	(normal 8.5-10.5)
Creatinine (mg/dL)	1.2	(normal 0.6-1.2)

Biopsy of the cervical node and rib lesion both showed a plasmacytoma, images of this case were not available but representative images from another case are shown in **Figures 1** and **2**.

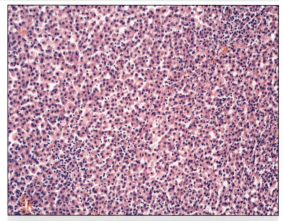

Figure 1 A representative bone biopsy (H&E, ×100) showing bone marrow replacement by a monomorphous population of atypical plasma cells. A few scattered small lymphocytes are also present.

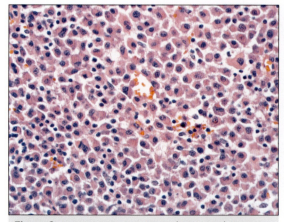

Figure 2 A representative bone biopsy (H&E, ×600) showing bone marrow replacement by a monomorphous population of atypical plasma cells.

Differential Diagnosis Diagnostic considerations included multiple myeloma, POEMS syndrome, and metastatic carcinoma.

Additional Work-Up
- Serum protein electrophoresis: normal
- Immunofixation of serum: negative
- IgG: 1,240 mg/dL; IgA 183 mg/dL; IgM 186 mg/dL
- Immunofixation of urine: negative
- Metastatic bone survey: destructive lesion in the anterior right third rib
- Bone marrow aspirate and biopsy: no increase in plasma cells

Final Diagnosis Solitary plasmacytoma of bone and solitary extramedullary plasmacytoma.

Management Approach The patient was given radiation therapy (50 Gy) for the nodal lesion and then received 40 Gy over 4 weeks for the rib lesion. Eleven years later, he developed midback pain, difficulty in walking and numbness of his anterior thighs. He also had urinary incontinence. An MRI revealed severe cord compression at T9. There was replacement of the entire body, pedicles, and posterior neural arch and transverse process of T9. No evidence of multiple myeloma was found. He was treated with 3,000 cGy in 14 fractions. He has had no recurrence of plasmacytoma or development of multiple myeloma during 10 additional years of follow-up.

General Discussion
Solitary plasmacytoma of bone: Most patients present with bone pain or a fracture of the affected bone. In some instances, the plasmacytoma can extend into the surrounding soft tissue, which may appear as a palpable mass. The axial skeleton is more commonly involved than is the appendicular skeleton. Multiple myeloma must be excluded in the differential diagnosis. POEMS syndrome and metastatic carcinoma are also included in the differential diagnosis. Treatment consists of tumorcidal radiation to the plasmacytoma. There is no proof that adjuvant or prophylactic chemotherapy is of benefit. Overt multiple myeloma develops in about half of patients with solitary plasmacytoma of bone. The majority of patients who progress do so within 5 years. The median overall survival of patients with solitary plasmacytoma of bone is approximately 10 years. Progression is more likely in older patients and in those with axial skeletal lesions. Patients with an abnormal free light chain assay, larger solitary lesion (>5 cm), reduction of uninvolved immunoglobulins and the presence of high-grade angiogenesis in the tumor have increased risk of progression.

Extramedullary plasmacytoma: Approximately 80% of extramedullary plasmacytomas involve the upper respiratory tract (oronasopharynx and paranasal sinuses). This may produce epistaxis, nasal obstruction or airway compromise. Occasionally, the lymph nodes, gastrointestinal tract, liver, skin, lung or testes may be the site of initial involvement. Multiple myeloma must be excluded. Treatment consists of radiation therapy in a dose of 40 Gy-50 Gy over a 4-week period. Occasionally, complete surgical resection may be possible and in that setting, radiation therapy may not be needed. There is no compelling evidence that chemotherapy in addition to radiation is of value. Approximately 5%-10% of patients will develop local or regional recurrence. This is more likely if the plasmacytoma is ≥ 5 cm in maximum diameter. Only 10%-15% of patients will develop symptomatic multiple myeloma. The median survival of patients with extramedullary plasmacytoma is 10 years-12 years. A comprehensive work-up of such patients should include a thorough history and physical examination. A complete blood count, calcium, creatinine, electrophoresis and immunofixation of serum and urine, free light chain assay, skeletal roentgenograms, and bone marrow aspiration and biopsy should be performed. In addition, an MRI of the spine and pelvis is recommended for a patient with a solitary plasmacytoma of bone.

Section F: Plasma Cell Disorders

Multiple Myeloma

Joanne Filicko-O'Hara, Ryan Gentzler, Gene Gulati

Patient A 74-year-old male with the complaints of bilateral lower extremity weakness, low back pain, and shoulder pain that was getting progressively worse for the past 2 months-3 months.

Clinical History The patient had a history of type 2 diabetes mellitus and hypertension. He also reported that he had been having more difficulty with maintaining his activities of daily living due to generalized fatigue, lethargy and some associated shortness of breath. He experienced some numbness and tingling in his toes on and off for several years and denied bowel or bladder incontinence.

Family History The patient's brother and sister had lung cancer. He also had 2 brothers with stomach cancer.

Medications Amlodipine, aspirin, ferrous sulfate, furosemide, glyburide, insulin 70/30, metformin, metoprolol.

Physical Examination He appeared tired but in no distress. The lung exam was significant for coarse breath sounds bilaterally, but no rhonchi or wheezes were appreciated. The area over his lower thoracic spine was tender on touch. The neurologic exam was significant for 4/5 strength in bilateral upper extremities and 3/5 strength in bilateral lower extremeties. Reflexes were symmetric throughout. Cranial nerves II through XII and position sense and sensation to both light touch and pinprick were intact.

Initial Work-Up

CBC		Serum Protein Electrophoresis with Immunofixation		
WBC (×10³/μL)	9.9			Normal
RBC (×10⁶/μL)	4.02	Total protein	7.5 g/dL	(6.0-8.5)
HGB (g/dL)	11.7	α-1 Globulin	0.3 g/dL	(0.1-0.3)
HCT (%)	35.0	α-1 Globulin	0.9 g/dL	(0.5-0.9)
MCV (fL)	87	β-Globulin	2.5 g/dL	(0.5-1.2)
MCH (pg)	33.4	γ-Globulin	0.4 g/dL	(0.6-1.6)
PLT (×10³/μL)	406	IgG	437 g/dL	(723-1,685)
RDW-CV (%)	12.8	IgA	2,360 g/dL	(69-382)
MPV (fL)	9.9	IgM	17 g/dL	(63-277)
WBC Differential	%	# (×10³/μL)	**Basic metabolic panel (BMP)**	
Neutrophils	76.9	7.60	Na⁺ (mmol/L)	136
Bands	0	0	K⁺ (mmol/L)	4.2
Lymphocytes	15.4	1.52	Cl⁻ (mmol/L)	95
Monocytes	6.1	0.60	CO₂ (mmol/L)	28
Eosinophils	1.4	0.14	BUN (mg/dL)	16
			Cr (mg/dL)	1.2
			Ca⁺⁺ (mg/dL)	11.7

Immunofixation identified a monoclonal IgA band
Urine protein electrophoresis: moderate proteinuria, IgA κ band. Bone marrow was hypercellular with 25% plasma cells, some of which were mature and some immature (**Figure 1**). By immunostaining, all plasma cells were κ-restricted.

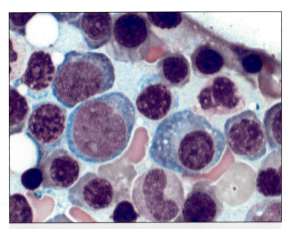

Figure 1 Bone marrow aspirate smear (Wright-Giemsa, ×1000) showing a mature plasma cell and an immature plasma cell.

Differential Diagnosis Diagnostic considerations included osteoarthritis/degenerative disc disease, vertebral disc herniation, spinal cord compression, primary or metastatic cancer involving the spine or thoracic cavity, and multiple myeloma.

Additional Work-Up
- X-rays: multilevel degenerative disc disease of the lumbar spine. Lytic lesions in the right glenoid and right humeral head
- CT chest/abdomen/pelvis: multiple lytic bone lesions. Specifically, the T12 lesion destroys the posterior elements and encroaches on the spinal cord
- MRI lumbar spine: large enhancing expansile lesion within the spinous process, posterior elements and posterior soft tissues of T12 causing near complete obliteration of the central canal

Final Diagnosis Multiple myeloma with impending spinal cord compression.

Management Approach Patients with symptomatic multiple myeloma should be started on therapy soon after diagnosis. Significant findings that are indications for treatment include end organ damage, such as renal insufficiency and anemia, hypercalcemia, lytic bone lesions, and/or evidence of extramedullary plasmacytoma. The absence of these findings in the setting of >10% plasma cells in the bone marrow is considered smoldering multiple myeloma, and treatment with chemotherapy should be delayed until symptoms develop. The choice of therapeutic agent depends upon whether the patient will eventually be a candidate for hematopoietic progenitor cell transplant. Recent advances in myeloma therapy have led to multiple options for front line therapy including steroids in combination with lenalidomide, thalidomide, or bortezomib. These agents have also been given in combination with improved response rates in some studies (eg, thalidomide + bortezomib). Those patients who are transplant candidates may receive induction therapy for 3 months-4 months, or until "best response" followed by high-dose melphalan and stem cell rescue. Alkylating agents should be avoided as they may have damaging effects on stem cells. For patients who are not candidates for stem cell transplantation, the standard therapy includes either the new agents noted above or a combination of one of these agents with melphalan and prednisone. Standard low-dose melphalan and prednisone given over a 7-day period and repeated every 6 weeks until there is stable disease is still a reasonable option. This patient received high-dose dexamethasone and radiation to the involved area with improvement in pain and some improvement in weakness. He went on to receive 4 months of induction therapy with bortezomib and dexamethasone with excellent response. He received mobilization chemotherapy with cyclophosphamide, had autologous stem cells collected and proceeded to high-dose therapy with melphalan followed by autologous stem cell rescue. He was in a very good partial remission at the time he received cyclophosphamide, and in complete remission prior to stem cell transplant and until 3 years following transplant.

General Discussion It is important to distinguish multiple myeloma from monoclonal gammopathy of undetermined significance (MGUS) and smoldering myeloma, both of which lack bone lesions and end organ damage.

The diagnostic criteria of multiple myeloma include:
- monoclonal protein in serum
- bone marrow biopsy demonstrates >10% plasma cells which are monoclonal (typically CD138+)
- lytic bone lesions and/or clinical manifestations of multiple myeloma including anemia, hypercalcemia, renal failure, extramedullary plasmacytomas

Diagnosis of MGUS requires <10% plasma cells in the bone marrow, serum M protein <3g/dL, and lack of end organ damage. Smoldering myeloma may have either >10% plasma marrow cells or M protein >3g/dL, but also lacks end organ damage as is seen in MGUS. Patients with multiple myeloma and MGUS often have translocations at chromosome 14q32, which is the immunoglobulin heavy chain locus, and 1 of several other loci including 11q13 (CCND1), 4p16.3 (FGFR-3 and MMSET), 6p21 (CCND3), 16q23 (c-maf), and 20q11 (mafB).

Section F: Plasma Cell Disorders

IgM-Secreting Myeloma

Pei Lin

Patient A 58-year-old woman with pain in the back of the head, lower lumbar area, and the rib cage.

Clinical History The patient reported having the lower back pain for 2 years. Because of worsening pain, she spent the past 3 months in bed and was unable to stand for >20 minutes at a time. She also felt new onset rib pain that radiated to her back.

Family History Noncontributory.

Medications Aspirin, lorazepam, and famotidine.

Physical Examination She was unable to lie down on the examination table due to severe back pain. She was tender over her thoracic and lumbar spine and over lower ribs bilaterally. She had no neurological deficits. Otherwise, the examination was unremarkable.

Initial Work-Up		
CBC		
WBC (×10³/μL)	4.9	
RBC (×10⁶/μL)	2.20	
HGB (g/dL)	6.3	
HCT (%)	18.3	
MCV (fL)	83	
MCH (pg)	28.6	
MCHC (g/dL)	34.4	
PLT (×10³/μL)	141	
RDW-CV (%)	14.1	
WBC Differential	**%**	**# (×10³/μL)**
Neutrophils	67	3.3
Lymphocytes	27	1.3
Monocytes	4	0.2
Eosinophils	2	0.1

Further work-up at the hospital revealed renal failure with creatinine of 3.4 mg/dL (normal range: 0.7-1.3 and BUN 29 mg/dL (normal range: 8-20), she was also found to have hypercalcemia with a serum calcium level: 10.3 mg/dL (normal range: 8.4-10.2).

Differential Diagnosis Plasma cell myeloma vs other causes of acute renal failure such as systemic lupus erythematosus.

Additional Work-Up
Serum protein electrophoresis:
- Total protein 12.4 g/dL (normal 6-8.5)
- Albumin 2.6 g/dL (normal 3.2-4.9)
- M protein 9.8 g/dL

Immunoglobulin quantitation:
- IgG 168 g/dL (normal: 700-1,600)
- IgM 8,050 g/dL (normal: 40-230)
- IgA 38 g/dL (normal 70-400)

- Urine immunofixation studies detected λ Bence-Jones proteinuria
- Radiographic imaging: bone survey revealed diffuse demineralization, mild to moderate compression fractures in the lumbar spine, T6, T11 and T12
- MRI of the thoracic spine showed a loss of height of T6, T8-12. T10 showed biconcave compression fractures, and T11-12 showed mild height reduction
- Bone marrow aspirate and biopsy: approximately 90% cellularity with > 90% of plasma cells with a small cell morphology resembling plasmacytoid lymphocytes (**Figures 1** and **2**). By immunohistochemical staining these cells were positive for cyclin D1 (**Figure 3**)
- Flow cytometry immunophenotyping: the plasma cells were positive for CD38 bright, CD138, and immunoglobulin λ light chain and negative for CD19, CD20, CD33, CD56 and CD52

Section F: Plasma Cell Disorders
IgM-Secreting Myeloma

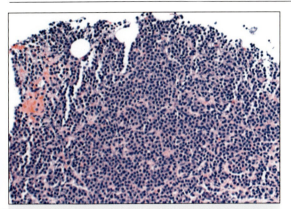

Figure 1 Bone marrow biopsy (H&E, ×200) showing sheets of plasma cells.

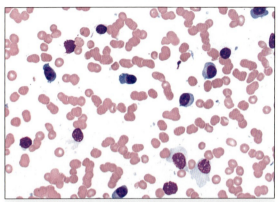

Figure 2 Bone marrow aspirate smear (Wright-Giemsa, ×500) showing numerous plasma cells, many of which resembled plasmacytoid lymphocytes.

Cytogenetics:
- 45, X, –X, t(11;14)(q13;q32), del(12)(p11.2p13)[2]
- 45, X, –X, del(6)(q15q25), t(11;14)(q13;q32), del(12)(p11.2p13), –16, +mar[1]
- 46, XX[17]
- Fluorescence in situ hybridization detected IGH/CCND1 gene fusion

Final Diagnosis IgM-secreting myeloma with t(11;14) translocation.

Management Approach In 2010, multiple options for therapy are available for patients with multiple myeloma. In the past, patients had been treated with chemotherapy melphalan and prednisone (MP), or vincristine and doxorubicin plus intermittent high-dose dexamethasone (VAD). More recently newer agents including immunomodulating agents (thalidomide and lenalidomide) and the proteosome inhibitor bortezomib are being increasingly used, particularly in combination therapy. Myeloablative chemotherapy with high-dose melphalan is usually followed by autologous hematopoietic progenitor cell transplantation (HPCT). The patient was initially treated with intravenous dexamethasone which controlled the hypercalcemia and renal failure. She was subsequently treated with lenalidomide and dexamethasone for 2 cycles and achieved partial remission. She then underwent high-dose therapy on a clinical trial, using bortezomib with arsenic trioxide, ascorbic acid and high-dose melphalan followed by autologous HPCT. She subsequently died of progressive disease.

General Discussion Although other causes of renal failure should be considered, the general symptoms (bone pain) along with serum M protein and lytic bone lesions point to myeloma. IgM myeloma comprises <1% of myeloma cases. Despite a small cell morphology, these cases have

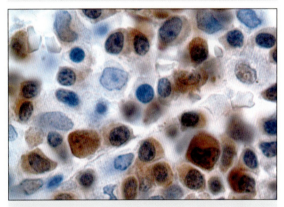

Figure 3 Bone marrow biopsy (cyclin D1, × 500) showing the neoplastic cells are positive for cyclin D1 in a nuclear and cytoplasmic pattern.

clinical features of myeloma instead of lymphoplasmacytic lymphoma/Waldenström macroglobulinemia (LPL/WM). Lytic bone lesions, renal failure, anemia, hypercalcemia may be present, as seen in this case. The t(11;14) positive myeloma is often associated with a small cell morphology. The tumor cell may express CD20. Cyclin D1 is consistently expressed and tends to be stronger than myeloma cases that express cyclin D1 without the translocation. The pattern of both nuclear and cytoplasmic staining distinguishes myeloma from mantle cell lymphoma. Identification of t(11;14) essentially confirms the diagnosis of myeloma and rule out LPL/WM. The International Staging System uses serum β2 microglobulin (B2M) and albumin levels to stratify patients into 3 stages. High B2M and lower albumin levels indicate a high stage of disease and shorter survival. In addition, an abnormal karyotype by conventional cytogenetic analysis also predicts a poorer prognosis. Myeloma used to be considered an incurable disease. With the newer agents and more targeted therapy, long-term survival of myeloma patient appears to be achievable.

POEMS Syndrome (Polyneuropathy, Organomegaly, Endocrinopathy, Monoclonal Protein and Skin Changes)

Robert A Kyle, Curtis A Hanson

Patient A 50-year-old white female with complaints of numbness in the feet and calves bilaterally.

Clinical History The patient noted tingling of her toes 1 year before admission. The paresthesias increased and she was started on prednisone without benefit. She was found to have an IgG λ monoclonal protein of 1.26 g/dL in her serum and a CSF protein level of 104 mg/dL. Further studies revealed thrombocytosis and mixed lytic and sclerotic lesions in the left pelvis. She also developed weakness of her feet. There was no involvement of her hands.

Family History Noncontributory.

Medications Lisinopril, estrogen patch, and ranitidine.

Physical Examination The liver was palpable 2 cm below the costal margin (span 11 cm) and the spleen tip was palpable on deep inspiration. Cherry angiomas were present on her chest and upper back. There was no lymphadenopathy, hyperpigmentation, or hypertrichosis. Neurologic examination revealed sensorimotor peripheral neuropathy involving her feet and lower legs.

Initial Work-Up

CBC		WBC Differential	%	# ($\times 10^3/\mu L$)
WBC ($\times 10^3/\mu L$)	8.8	Neutrophils	61	5.4
RBC ($\times 10^6/\mu L$)	5.11	Bands	6	0.5
HGB (g/dL)	13.9	Lymphocytes	24	2.1
HCT (%)	40.8	Monocytes	4	0.4
MCV (fL)	79.9	Eosinophils	3	0.3
MCH (pg)	27.2	Basophils	2	0.2
MCHC (g/dL)	34.1			
PLT ($\times 10^3/\mu L$)	651	Calcium (mg/mL)	9.5	(normal 8.5-10.5)
		Creatinine (mg/dL)	0.9	(normal 0.6-1.2)
		Serum Protein Elecrophoresis and Immunofixation		
		IgG λ (mg/dL)	1,350	(normal 0.57-2.63)
		IgG (mg/dL)	1,150	(normal 723-1,685)
		IgA (mg/dL)	139	(normal 69-382)
		IgM (mg/dL)	132	(normal 63-277)
		Vitamin B_{12} (pg/mL)	321	(normal 180-900)
		Folate (ng/mL)	8.7	(normal 3-18)

X-ray findings: a bone survey showed a mixed sclerotic and lytic lesion near the left acetabulum

Section F: Plasma Cell Disorders
POEMS Syndrome (Polyneuropathy, Organomegaly, Endocrinopathy, Monoclonal Protein and Skin Changes)

Differential Diagnosis
- Monoclonal gammopathy of undetermined significance (MGUS): sensorimotor peripheral neuropathy may be seen in patients with MGUS, but osteosclerotic lesions, endocrinopathy, organomegaly and skin changes are not found
- Multiple myeloma: sensorimotor peripheral neuropathy is rare in multiple myeloma unless the patient has AL amyloidosis. The presence of anemia, renal failure, hypercalcemia, pathologic fractures and a high percentage of plasma cells in the bone marrow which are characteristic of multiple myeloma help to differentiate myeloma from POEMS syndrome
- Solitary plasmacytoma of bone: this is characterized by a single osteolytic bone lesion (plasmacytoma) without evidence of neuropathy, anemia, renal insufficiency or hypercalcemia. No osteoblastic changes are seen
- Primary AL amyloidosis: the diagnosis is made by demonstration of amyloid in the fat aspirate, bone marrow biopsy or biopsy of other tissue which shows positive staining with Congo red and the presence of amyloid fibrils on electron microscopy. No osteosclerotic lesions, skin changes or papilledema are seen

Additional Work-Up Biopsy of the left acetabular lesion revealed plasma cell myeloma (**Figures 1** and **2**).

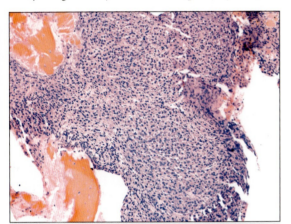

Figure 1 Left hip biopsy (H&E, ×100) showing bone marrow replacement by a monomorphous population of atypical plasma cells.

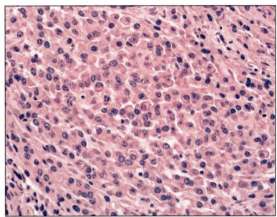

Figure 2 Left hip biopsy (H&E, ×600) showing bone marrow replacement by a monomorphous population of atypical plasma cells; occasional plasma cells with nucleoli are present.

Final Diagnosis POEMS syndrome (osteosclerotic myeloma).

Management Approach Single or multiple osteosclerotic lesions in a limited area should be treated with radiation in a dose of 40 Gy-50 Gy. More than half of patients show substantial improvement of the neuropathy. The improvement may be very slow and if there is no evidence of progression of neuropathy, the individual should be followed patiently. If the patient has widespread osteosclerotic lesions, systemic therapy is necessary. Melphalan and prednisone as well as various combinations of alkylating agents have produced some benefit. Autologous hematopoietic progenitor cell transplantation is another consideration for patients who are eligible for this procedure. Stem cells must be collected before the patient is exposed to alkylating agents. In our experience, all patients have had some neurologic improvement or stabilization of their neuropathy. The procedure is associated with significant morbidity. This patient received radiation therapy and responded but slowly. 6 years later, she had absent ankle jerk reflexes and was unable to walk on her heels. She had a mild bilateral footdrop. Sensory examination revealed mild bilateral decreased sensation for touch and temperature of the lower extremities. She had no other symptoms.

General Discussion POEMS syndrome (<u>p</u>olyneuropathy, <u>o</u>rganomegaly, <u>e</u>ndocrinopathy, <u>m</u>onoclonal protein and <u>s</u>kin changes) is characterized by osteosclerotic myeloma, Castleman disease, organomegaly, endocrinopathy, edema, skin changes or papilledema. Almost all patients have an osteosclerotic lesion. The cause of POEMS syndrome is unknown. Interleukin-6, interleukin-1β and tumor necrosis

Section F: Plasma Cell Disorders
POEMS Syndrome (Polyneuropathy, Organomegaly, Endocrinopathy, Monoclonal Protein and Skin Changes)

factor α are frequently elevated. Thrombocytosis is not uncommon and a mistaken diagnosis of a myeloproliferative disorder may be made. All patients have peripheral neuropathy and a monoclonal plasma cell disorder. Symptoms of peripheral neuropathy usually begin in the feet and are symmetric and progressive. Severe weakness is often a prominent feature and the patient may be confined to a wheelchair. Cranial nerves are not affected and autonomic symptoms are not seen. Papilledema is present in ⅓ of patients. The cerebrospinal fluid protein level is increased in almost all persons. Electromyographic studies show slowing of nerve conduction. The sural nerve demonstrates both axonal degeneration and demyelination. Approximately ½ of patients have hepatomegaly, splenomegaly or lymphadenopathy. Biopsy of enlarged lymph nodes often reveals Castleman disease. Hypogonadism, hypothyroidism and pituitary insufficiency may be seen. All patients have a monoclonal plasma cell disorder. Nearly 90% have a monoclonal protein in the serum and/or urine. The type of light chain is almost always λ. The plasma cell infiltration of the bone marrow is modest with >80% of patients having fewer than 10% plasma cells. Hyperpigmentation and/or hypertrichosis occurs in >½ of patients. Osteosclerotic lesions appeared in 97% of our patients. Bone lesions are solitary in almost ½ of patients. Castleman disease is frequently associated. Renal insufficiency is uncommon. Thrombotic events are not uncommon. Pulmonary hypertension may be seen. Anemia is an infrequent finding while erythrocytosis is present in about a sixth of patients. Thrombocytosis occurs in approximately half. Diagnosis of POEMS syndrome requires the presence of polyneuropathy and a monoclonal plasma cell disorder along with osteosclerotic lesions, Castleman disease, organomegaly, endocrinopathy, edema, skin changes or papilledema.

Primary Amyloidosis

Pei Lin

Patient A 51-year-old woman, who presented with lower extremity edema.

Clinical History The patient reported progressively worsening edema of the lower extremity over the past 1 year-2 years. She was being followed by her primary care physician who subsequently referred her to a nephrologist for evaluation. On evaluation, the patient was found to have proteinuria and subsequently a kidney biopsy was performed.

Family History Noncontributory.

Medications None.

Physical Examination She appeared tired. Lung exam showed a few rales at both bases. Cardiac exam included an S3. She had 2+ bilateral peripheral edema. The rest of her exam was unremarkable.

Initial Work-Up

CBC		WBC Differential	%	# (×10³/µL)
WBC (×10³/µL)	5.2	Neutrophils	73	3.8
RBC (×10⁶/µL)	4.86	Lymphocytes	25	1.3
HGB (g/dL)	14.4	Monocytes	2	0.1
HCT (%)	42.9			
MCV (fL)	88	Urine protein (mg/dL)		56 (normal 1-14)
MCH (pg)	29.6	Urine protein in total volume (mg)		2,436 (normal 50-100)
MCHC (g/dL)	33.6	Urine albumin (%)		79.2 (normal 33-50)
PLT (×10³/µL)	155	Urine globulin (%)		20.8 (normal 50-66)
RDW-CV (%)	13.2	Urine IFE: free κ light chain Bence-Jones protein		

Serum Chemistry		Urine protein electrophoresis: nonspecific proteinuria without monoclonal peak	
Phosphorus (mg/dL)	4.6	(normal 2.5-4.5)	
BUN (mg/dL)	36	(normal 8-20)	Serum protein electrophoresis and immunofixation electrophoresis no M-protein
Creatinine (mg/dL)	2.4	(normal 0.8-1.5)	
Uric acid (mg/dL)	8.1	(normal 2.6-7.1)	Serum free κ light chain (mg/L)	474 (normal 3.30-19.40)
B2M (mg/L)	6.4	(normal 0.7-1.8)	Serum free λ light chain (mg/L)	29.30 (normal 5.71-26.30)
ALK (IU/L)	161	(normal 38-126)	Serum free κ/λ ratio	16.18 (normal 0.26-1.65)
ASP (IU/L)	57	(normal 15-46)	PT (sec)	16.1 (normal 10.6-13.3)
CKMB (ng/mL)	10.1	(normal 0.6-6.3)	PTT (sec)	36.6 (normal: 24.7-35.9)
Troponin-I/CTNI (ng/mL)	0.05	(normal 0.00-0.03)		
B-type natriuretic peptide (pg/mL)	500	(normal 0-100)		

Section F: Plasma Cell Disorders
Primary Amyloidosis

Differential Diagnosis Renal insufficiency due to primary amyloidosis vs other causes of amyloidosis vs immunoglobulin light or heavy chain deposition disease.

Additional Work-Up A renal biopsy showed amyloidosis (**Figures 1** and **2**) with κ light chain restriction. Bone marrow biopsy showed amyloidosis (**Figure 3**) and approximately 5% of plasma cells positive for CD138 (**Figure 4**) and κ light chain predominance. Flow cytometry immunophenotyping identified 3% of monoclonal κ immunoglobulin light chain-restricted plasma cells positive for CD138, CD38, CD56 and κ light chain and negative for CD19, CD20 and CD33. Bone survey showed no focal lytic lesions.

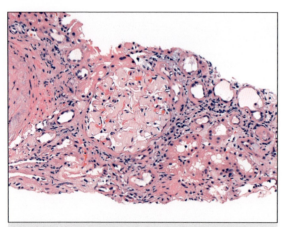

Figure 1 Kidney biopsy (H&E, ×200) showing glomerulosclerosis with amorphous eosinophilic material deposited in the glomerulous and the vessels.

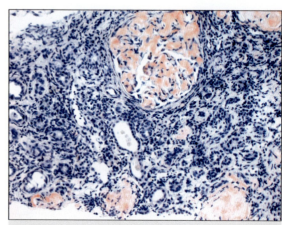

Figure 2 Kidney biopsy (Congo red, ×200) showing the amorphous eosinophilic materials seen on H&E section is positive staining.

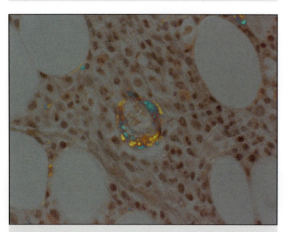

Figure 3 Bone marrow biopsy (Congo red, polarized ×200) showing amyloid deposition in a vessel that appears to be apple-green birefringent.

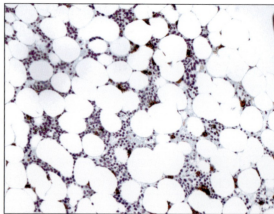

Figure 4 Bone marrow biopsy (CD138, ×200) highlighting the scattered plasma cells in the interstitium.

Final Diagnosis Primary amyloidosis associated with κ light chain restriction.

Management Approach Treatment of primary amyloidosis usually aims at eliminating monoclonal plasma cells. Chemotherapy (melphalan and prednisone) or immunomodulating agents (thalidomide and lenalidomide) with or without steroids have been used. Bortezomib, a proteosome inhibitor has shown promising results in recent trials. Autologous hematopoietic progenitor cell transplantation (HPCT) using high-dose melphalan can be used in selected patients, but is associated with higher mortality in this patient population compared to other patients with plasma cell dyscrasias, due to compromised organ functions. This patient was treated with melphalan and bortezomib and responded well. Due to cardiac involvement, the patient was considered ineligible for autologous HPCT.

General Discussion Primary amyloidosis is caused by deposition of amyloid fibers consisting of monoclonal immunoglobulin light chain secreted by neoplastic plasma cells. The amyloid fibers are composed of abnormal λ light chain in ¾ of cases and κ light chain in ¼ of cases. In contrast, light or heavy chain deposition diseases are usually composed of κ light chain. Monoclonal plasma cells in the bone marrow are usually <10%. It is essential to confirm that the amyloid fibers are composed of the same light chain type as those produced by the monoclonal plasma cells in the bone marrow since conditions such as monoclonal gammopathy of unknown significance coexisting with secondary amyloidosis may give similar clinical presentations. Amyloid fibers appear apple green birefringent on Congo red staining when viewed under polarized light. Congo red reactivity distinguishes primary amyloidosis from immunoglobulin deposition diseases. Immunostains can be used to confirm presence of amyloid P component and immunoglobulin light chain. Proteinomics (mass spectrometry) can be used to further type amyloid fibers. Clinical presentations of amyloidosis are usually nonspecific and high index of suspicion is needed for the diagnosis. Symptoms largely depend on organs involved. Usually heart, kidney, nerve system and gastrointestinal tract are involved causing organ dysfunction or failure. Coagulopathy with factor X deficiency can also occur. Although no coagulopathy work-up was done, mild prolongation of both PT and PTT in this case could be potentially attributed to acquired factor X deficiency secondary to binding of the factor to amyloid protein. Cardiac damage can be assessed by CKMB, troponin-I and B-type natriuretic peptide. Patients with kidney involvement usually present with proteinuria in the range of nephrotic syndrome.

Light Chain Deposition Disease

Joanne Filicko-O'Hara, Ryan Gentzler, John Krause

Patient A 53-year-old female with mild swelling of her both ankles.

Clinical History The patient has a history of hypothyroidism and hypertension. She has had hypertension for approximately 5 years, which has been well-controlled with medications. She denied any recent changes to medications. There were no complaints concerning urinary frequency, dysuria, or changes in the color of her urine. She did report that the swelling in her ankles at times got worse in the evening and occasionally she felt transient light-headedness when standing from a recumbent position. The laboratory studies revealed renal insufficiency, which was new since her last visit 6 months prior.

Family History Her mother died from lung cancer. Her father had diabetes and heart failure.

Medications Levothyroxine, amlodipine, hydrochlorothiazide.

Physical Examination Her vital signs are normal with a blood pressure of 110/65 and a heart rate of 90. Her exam is only remarkable for 1+ bilateral lower extremity edema.

Initial Work-Up

CBC			Chemistry	
WBC ($\times 10^3$/L)	5.4		Na+ (mmol/L)	143
RBC ($\times 10^6$/µL)	4.52		K+ (mmol/L)	4.6
HGB (g/dL)	13.6		Cl- (mmol/L)	109
HCT (%)	38.5		CO_2 (mmol/L)	27
MCV (fL)	86		BUN (mg/dL)	34
MCH (pg)	30.0		Cr (mg/dL)	1.7
MCHC (g/dL)	35.3		Ca^{++} (mg/dL)	9.8
PLT ($\times 10^3$/µL)	192			
RDW-CV (%)	11.6			

WBC Differential	%	# ($\times 10^3$/µL)	Urinalysis	
Neutrophils	63.2	3.4	Specific gravity	1.015
Lymphocytes	26.6	1.4	pH	5.0
Monocytes	7.7	0.4	Blood	1+
Eosinophils	2.1	0.1	Protein	Negative
Basophils	0.4	0.0	Hyaline casts	2+

Section F: Plasma Cell Disorders
Light Chain Deposition Disease

		Normal
β2-Microglobulin (mg/L)	6.4	(1.42-3.41)
ANA	negative	
P-ANCA	negative	
C-ANCA	negative	
Hepatitis B surface antigen	negative	
Hepatitis C antibody	negative	

Quantitative Immunoglobulins:

		Normal
IgA (mg/dL)	40	(69-382)
IgG (mg/dL)	455	(723-1,685)
IgM (mg/dL)	97	(63-277)

Serum Protein Electrophoresis with Immunofixation

		Normal
Total protein (g/dL)	5.7	(6.0-8.5)
Albumin (g/dL)	4.0	(3.3-5.2)
α-1 globulin (g/dL)	0.2	(0.1-0.3)
α-2 globulin (g/dL)	0.6	(0.5-0.9)
β-globulin (g/dL)	0.6	(0.5-1.2)
γ-globulin (g/dL)	0.5	(0.6-1.6)

A faint band was seen in the γ region. This band was identified as IgG κ by immunofixation. Immunoglobulin quantitation by nephelometry showed IgG concentration of 398 mg/dL.

Urine Protein Electrophoresis

Urine albumin (%)	87
Prot:Cr ratio	0.7
Cr (mg/dL)	64
Protein (mg/dL)	42
Total 24-hr protein (mg/TV)	546

Moderate proteinuria in this 24-hr specimen. Albumin is the predominant urinary protein. No monoclonal paraproteins were identified.

Urine free κ light chains (mg/dL)	10.20 (0.33 – 1.94)
Urine free λ light chains (mg/dL)	1.12 (0.57-2.63)
κ:λ ratio	9.11 (0.26-1.65)

Differential Diagnosis The patient has a monoclonal protein in the serum which could be related to a monoclonal gammopathy of undetermined significance (MGUS), multiple myeloma, primary light chain amyloidosis, light chain deposition disease or a lymphoproliferative disease. The associated renal failure, although mild, makes a plasma cell dyscrasia more likely, although she could simply have mild renal insufficiency due to hypertensive disease. The decreased immunglobulins, associated with the IgG κ paraprotein is also more consistent with a plasma cell dyscrasia. Further evaluation is warranted with tissue biopsy. It would be reasonable to start with either marrow aspiration and biopsy or kidney biopsy. This patient had a kidney biopsy first.

Additional Work-Up Kidney biopsy: the non-sclerotic glomeruli had a lobular appearance with diffuse mesangial cell proliferation and thickened basement membranes (**Figure 1**). An increase in PAS-positive mesangial matrix-like material was noted. There was patchy tubular atrophy with interstitial fibrosis (visualized with trichrome stain) and chronic inflammation. In these areas the atrophic tubules had prominently thickened basement membranes (visualized with PAS stain). The media of the intralobular arteries was thickened by an accumulation of amorphous PAS+ deposits that replaced the normal smooth muscle cells. Congo red stain was negative. Electron microscopy showed punctate, granular electron-dense deposits on the interstitial side of the tubular basement membranes, in the subendothelial side of the glomerular baement membranes, in the mesangium, and in Bowman's capsule. In addition, there were amorphous, electron-dense deposits in the sub-endothelial space of the glomeruli, and in the media of blood vessels. Bone marrow: normocellular with 10% atypical plasma cells (**Figure 2**). Skeletal survey: negative for fractures or lytic lesions

Section F: Plasma Cell Disorders
Light Chain Deposition Disease

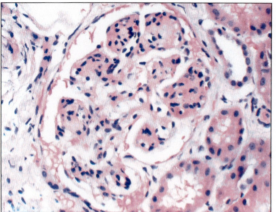

Figure 1 Kidney biopsy (H&E, ×200) showing lobular appearance of glomeruli, with diffuse mesangial cell proliferation and thickened basement membranes.

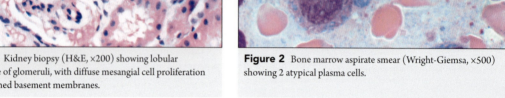

Figure 2 Bone marrow aspirate smear (Wright-Giemsa, ×500) showing 2 atypical plasma cells.

Final Diagnosis Light chain deposition disease.

Management Approach Light chain deposition disease (LCDD) is 1 of several plasma cell dyscrasias that can involve the kidney. It is often associated with multiple myeloma, but may also present without diagnostic criteria of myeloma. Like primary amyloidosis, it can lead to renal failure, but the light chain deposits in the kidney are not amyloid. Survival from time of diagnosis can range from a few months to >10 years. Patients are usually treated in a similar fashion as those with multiple myeloma. In the current era, this would include agents such as lenalidomide or thalidomide, or bortezomib as first line agents. High-dose therapy with melphalan followed by autologous hematopoietic progenitor cell transplantation (HPCT) has prolonged survival and reversed kidney failure in some patients. This patient was started on thalidomide. She had slight improvement in her blood and urine studies and a decrease in the clonal plasma cell burden to <5% after several months of therapy. Thalidomide was discontinued after 1 year. During the next 2 years her disease progressed, with increasing light chains in her urine, increased creatinine, and increased clonal plasma cells (20%) in her marrow. Following cyclophosphamide mobilization and stem cell collection, she received high-dose melphalan and autologous hematopoietic progenitor cell transplantation (HPCT). Her renal failure improved and the clonal protein in blood and urine disappeared. She remains in complete remission 18 months following transplant.

General Discussion Light chain deposition disease (LCDD) is 1 of the less common plasma cell dyscrasias. A variable degree of plasmacytosis in the bone marrow is present in 50%-60% of cases. It manifests as light chain deposition in the glomeruli, as opposed to classic "myeloma kidney" with light chain deposition in the renal tubules. Patients with true multiple myeloma may present with renal insufficiency due to light chain deposition in the glomeruli (light chain deposition disease), light chain deposition in the renal tubules (myeloma kidney), amyloid deposition or rarely plasma cell infiltration of the kidneys. The diagnosis of LCCD is usually made by examination of kidney biopsy using anti-light chain antibodies and by electron microscopy. The characteristic findings are smooth, ribbon-like linear peritubular deposits of monotypic immunoglobulin (primarily κ) by immunoflourescence and as dense punctuate, nonfibrillary deposits by electron microscopy. Therapy for patients with multiple myeloma is improving with newer agents, and thus it is hoped that therapy for related diseases will improve as well. Often in light chain deposition disease, as with other nonmyeloma plasma cell dyscrasias, there may be only a small percentage of clonal plasma cells. Thus it is hoped that intensive anti-myeloma therapy including autologous HPCT may eradicate these smaller clones, providing long-term remissions.

Multiple Myeloma and Acquired von Willebrand Disease

Joanne Filicko-O'Hara, Ryan Gentzler, John R Krause

Patient A 57-year-old female with pain in her right arm and elbow that began shortly after walking her dog 3 days prior.

Clinical History The patient reported that her dog pulled at his leash and pulled her arm forward, but she did not fall or sustain direct trauma to the arm. The pain had gotten progressively worse over the last 3 days, and was accompanied by swelling of the arm. She had multiple episodes of gastrointestinal bleeding over the past year and also reported an increase in the frequency and size of bruises she gets after bumping into something around the house over the past 2 months-3 months. She denied any past history of nosebleeds or other problems with bleeding. She has 2 healthy children who were delivered at full term by cesarean section without complications or excessive bleeding 7 and 10 years earlier.

Family History She denied any family history of bleeding disorders.

Medications Sertraline and buprorion.

Physical Examination Her vital signs were unremarkable except for mild hypertension (BP 174/89). Her HEENT exam showed no evidence of mucosal bleeding. Her right upper extremity showed marked edema, tender to palpation over the medial aspect of the biceps femoris and severely limited range of motion due to pain. Her neurologic exam was normal except in the right upper extremity where her strength was 0/5 for hand grasp and biceps testing. She had multiple eccyhymoses on her lower extremities at various stages of healing.

Initial Work-Up CBC was normal except for mild anemia with hemoglobin 11.1 g/dL, hematocrit 33.5%, and MCV 97 fL. Serum chemistry panel was also normal. The liver and renal function test results were within normal limits.

X-ray of Humerus Mild degenerative acromioclavicular joint osteoarthritis. No fracture. No lytic lesions.

CT of Right Upper Extremity Right mid and proximal biceps intramuscular hematoma with element of active intramuscular hemorrhage.

Coagulation Studies

PT (sec)	15.9 (normal 12-15)
INR	1.21 (0.8-1.2)
APTT(sec)	59 (normal 20-35)

Differential Diagnosis Acquired von Willebrand disease, acquired factor VIII inhibitor, other acquired disorders of hemostasis, malignancy, or autoimmune disease as underlying cause of acquired bleeding disorder.

Urine Protein Electrophoresis (UPEP) 24-hour urine specimen showed 1,723 mg protein that was predominantly albumin, but with a monoclonal band detected in the γ region. Immunofixation identified this band as IgA λ.

Bone Marrow Hypercellular marrow diffusely infiltrated by a population plasma cells (**Figure 1**).

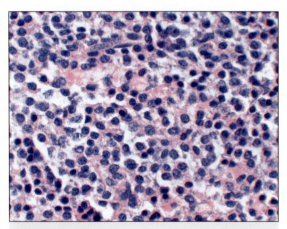

Figure 1 Bone marrow biopsy (H&E, ×400) showing diffuse infiltration by plasma cells.

Final Diagnosis Multiple myeloma with acquired von Willebrand disease (AvWD).

Management Approach For patients with active bleeding secondary to acquired von Willebrand disease (AvWD), treatment options are similar to that for inherited von Willebrand disease (vWD), including desmopressin (DDAVP) and infusions of von Willebrand factor (vWF). Depending on the possible mechanism causing the AvWD, there may also be a role for intravenous immunoglobulins, since the half-life of transfused vWF may be reduced by an inhibitor. Ultimately, the first goal of treatment should be to treat the associated disease to prevent recurrent bleeding in the long term. In general, DDAVP is the drug of choice for first line treatment of active bleeding in AvWD. If this fails to work, the next line of therapy depends on the associated disease causing AvWD. If the suspected mechanism is high levels of antibodies, such as in SLE or other autoimmune disease, IgG monoclonal gammopathies, or lymphoproliferative diseases, IV Ig should be the second line therapy of choice, followed by vWF concentrate infusions as a third-line therapy. Conversely, if the associated disease

Additional Work-Up

		Normal
vWF activity	<0.20	(0.44-1.52)
von Willebrand Ag	<0.10	(0.51-1.63)
Factor VIII level	0.08	(0.47-1.26)

Serum Protein Electrophoresis (SPEP) with Immunofixation

		Normal
Total protein	7.5 g/dL	(6.0-8.5)
Albumin	3.9 g/dL	(3.3-5.2)
α-1 globulin	0.2 g/dL	(0.1-0.3)
α-1 globulin	0.4 g/dL	(0.5-0.9)
β-globulin	0.5 g/dL	(0.5-1.2)
γ-globulin	2.6 g/dL	(0.6-1.6)

A monoclonal band was identified in the γ region. Immunofixation demonstrated a monoclonal IgA λ band.

		Normal
IgG	342 mg/dL	(723-1,685)
IgA	4,790 mg/dL	(69-382)
IgM	14 mg/dL	(63-277)

Serum Free Light Chain Analysis

		Normal
Free κ	0.40 mg/dL	(0.33-1.94)
Free λ	597 mg/dL	(0.57-2.63)
κ:λ	0.00	(0.26–1.65)

is a monoclonal IgM gammopathy, IV Ig has been shown to be less effective and transfusion of vWF concentrate should be used as the second-line therapy. This patient was treated with DDAVP and then IV Ig which led to stabilization and her bleeding stopped. She then had several months of recovery for the neurologic dysfunction resulting from the intramuscular bleed and compartment syndrome. She did not respond to therapy with bortazomib or combination chemotherapy with vincristine and liposomal doxorubicin, but subsequently did respond to therapy with lenalidomide with normalization of her coagulation studies, von Willebrand antigen, factor VIII and ristocetin cofactor activities. She subsequently underwent therapy with high-dose melphalan followed by autologous stem cell rescue. Her AvWD went into remission concurrently with her myeloma.

General Discussion Diagnosis of acquired von Willebrand syndrome is difficult to make on laboratory testing alone. It is often based on clinical suspicion in the setting of an associated disorder, as well as on a history that fits with an acquired bleeding disorder as opposed to an inherited one. Moreover, there is no family history of vWD in patients with AvWD. Associated diseases include lymphoproliferative, myeloproliferative, neoplastic, immune-related, and congenital cardiovascular diseases. Several possible mechanisms include specific antibodies to vWF, nonspecific antibodies that form circulating complexes with vWF, absorption of vWF into malignant cells, or loss of vWF due to high shear stress. Work-Up for AvWD should include prothombin time, activated partial thromboplastin time, vWF antigen, ristocetin cofactor activity or vWF collagen binding assay, and factor VIII activity. The most sensitive laboratory tests for AvWD are the functional assays for vWF, including ristocetin cofactor activity or collagen binding activity. These assays typically show decreased activity in similar range to those seen in patients with inherited vWD. In patients with abnormal vWF functional assays, analysis of vWF multimers may be beneficial to help confirm the diagnosis. Therapy must be directed at the underlying malignancy or autoimmune disease. In some cases, long-term remissions are obtained with aggressive treatment, but often these are cases that are refractory to standard therapies.

Immune Thrombocytopenic Purpura (ITP)

Michael J Berger, Robert W McKenna

Patient A 39-year-old female with heavy vaginal bleeding.

Clinical History The patient had noted an increase in her menstrual bleeding with passage of clots over the past few months. She denied nosebleeds and gum bleeding.

Family History No history of hematologic or autoimmune disorders.

Medications Fluoxetine, fexofenadine, omeprazole, aminocaproic acid and lorazepam.

Physical Examination She appeared pale and pertinent findings included some lesions in her left upper oropharynx which appeared to be blood blisters, small scattered petechiae on her abdomen, and some bruising in her antecubital areas bilaterally.

Initial Work-Up

CBC

WBC ($\times 10^3/\mu L$)	8.4
RBC ($\times 10^6/\mu L$)	3.34
HGB (g/dL)	9.5
HCT (%)	27.9
MCV (fL)	83
MCH (pg)	28.5
MCHC (g/dL)	34.2
PLT ($\times 10^3/\mu L$)	11
RDW-CV (%)	13.2

WBC Differential

	%	# ($\times 10^3/\mu L$)
Neutrophils	61	5.1
Bands	1	0.1
Lymphocytes	32	2.7
Monocytes	3	0.3
Eosinophils	2	0.2
Basophils	1	0.1

Peripheral blood smear was unremarkable except for decreased number of platelets and occasional giant forms (**Figure 1**).

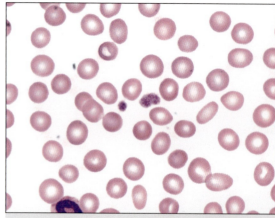

Figure 1 Blood smear (Wright, ×1000) demonstrating thrombocytopenia with rare large, but well-granulated platelets.

Differential Diagnosis Clinically the patient was suspected to have immune thrombocytopenic purpura (ITP) and the laboratory finding of isolated thrombocytopenia supported it.

Additional Work-Up A bone marrow biopsy was performed 3 weeks after presentation to confirm the diagnosis of ITP in light of the lack of response to multiple therapies and to assess the degree of megakaryopoiesis before instituting rituximab therapy. Marrow cellularity was 70%-90% with trilineage hematopoietic maturation and increased megakaryocytes (**Figures 2**-**4**).

Final Diagnosis Immune thrombocytopenic purpura (ITP), treatment refractory.

Management Approach

Adults: Patients generally respond to glucocorticoids. Nonresponders may be treated with intravenous immunoglobulin (IV Ig), splenectomy, Rho(D) Immune globulin, antineoplastic drugs such as rituximab and vincristine and alternative immune modulators (azathioprine).

Children: Children may be treated with glucocorticoids depending on symptoms. The course in this age group rarely becomes chronic and spontaneous remissions are the rule. This patient initially received 2 doses of intravenous immunoglobulin (IV Ig, 2 g/kg total dose) and prednisone (1 mg/kg/day). A lack of response prompted the addition of Rho(D) immune globulin 40 mcg/kg (reduced dose due to low hemoglobin). Steroids, in the form of pulse dexamethasone, were continued upon discharge with a rapid taper planned. The patient's platelet count remained below $10 \times 10^3/\mu L$ despite the steroids, IV Ig and Rho(D) immune globulin. The clinical team planned the use of weekly rituximab until response was achieved.

General Discussion Immune (autoimmune, idiopathic) thrombocytopenic purpura generally results in a severe acquired thrombocytopenia caused by antiplatelet antibodies that lead to increased platelet destruction. Classification can be based on the presence or absence of underlying associated disease (primary or secondary), rapidity of onset (acute or chronic) and age (childhood or adult ITP). In adults, ITP is usually insidious in onset, chronic in duration, more commonly seen in women, and rarely resolves without treatment. In contrast, young boys and girls are affected equally, the onset is usually acute often following a viral illness, and remits within weeks to months. Incidence of ITP ranges from 3.2-5.5/100,000/year depending on the platelet cutoff. Incidence increases with age. Antibodies directed against the GpIIB-IIIa complex (80% of cases) are recognized by splenic (primarily) and liver macrophages and result in platelet clearing in these organs. Antibodies directed against the GpIb-IX, GpIV and GpIa-IIa surface molecules characterize the bulk of the remaining cases. A variable

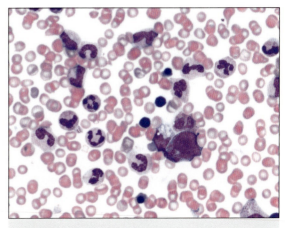

Figure 2 Bone marrow aspirate smear (Wright, × 500) showing normal trilineage hematopoiesis.

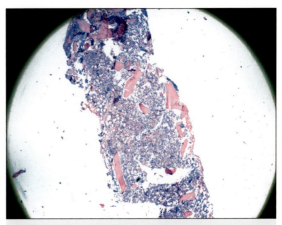

Figure 3 Bone marrow biopsy (H&E, ×100) showing 70%-90% cellularity.

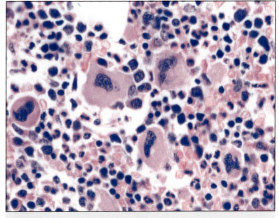

Figure 4 Bone marrow biopsy section (H&E, ×500) highlighting increased megakaryopoiesis.

Section G: Platelet Disorders
Immune Thrombocytopenic Purpura (ITP)

degree of bleeding in the form of purpura (eccymoses and petechiae), epistaxis, gingival bleeding and/or menorrhagia typifies the clinical manifestation of ITP, specially in those with platelet count below $30 \times 10^3/\mu L$. Constitutional symptoms are rarely seen and reflect underlying/concurrent conditions. Peripheral blood smear usually demonstrates isolated thrombocytopenia. There is increased platelet anisocytosis. Occasional large platelets can be seen, but if the population is uniformly large or giant a search for inherited disorders should be entertained. Bone marrow examination, though neither routinely performed nor considered necessary for diagnosis, usually reveals a normocellular marrow with trilineage hematopoiesis, including increased megakaryopoiesis; morphologic dysplasia is not a feature of this disease. Accurate history, complete blood count, and peripheral blood film usually provide the information necessary for diagnosis. Additional diagnostic work-up may include antiplatelet antibody testing, search for a lupus anticoagulant, direct antiglobulin test and mean platelet volume.

Glanzmann Thrombasthenia

A Koneti Rao

Patient A 23-year-old woman of Asian Indian origin with a lifelong history of easy bruising, excessive bleeding following injury and cuts, epistaxis and menorrhagia.

Clinical History The patient has a history of longstanding microcytic hypochromic anemia for which she has been on oral iron therapy.

Family History Noncontributory.

Medications Iron supplementation.

Physical Examination Bruises (1 inch-2 inches) on extremities. Rest of the examination was unremarkable.

Initial Work-Up	
Hemoglobin	7.4 g/dL
MCV	57 fL
MCH	16.7 pg
PT	11 sec
PTT	27 sec
Platelet count	340 × 10³/µL
Bleeding time	>15 min

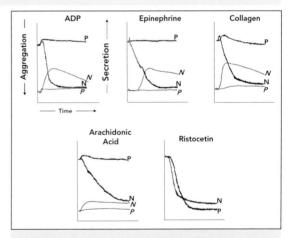

Differential Diagnosis The history of longstanding mucocutaneous bleeding symptoms in the setting of normal PT, PTT and platelet count and prolonged bleeding time suggests a disorder of platelet function, including von Willebrand disease.

Additional Work-Up
- Factor VIII coagulant activity 110% (normal 50-150)
- von Willebrand factor antigen 120% (normal 50-150)
- Ristocetin cofactor 98% (normal 50-150)

Platelet aggregation and secretion studies (**Figure 1**) Platelet aggregation in response to ADP, epinephrine,

Figure 1 Platelet aggregation and ATP secretion tracings of studies performed using a lumi-aggregometer on platelet-rich plasma (PRP) in the patient (P) and a healthy normal subject (N). Shown are responses to ADP (7.5 µM), epinephrine (7.5 µM), collagen (1 µg/mL), ristocetin (1.5 µg/mL) and arachidonic acid (1 µM). Aggregation (P patient; N normal control); secretion (patient P; normal control N). With all of the agonists except ristocetin neither the primary wave nor the secondary wave of aggregation are noted.

collagen, and arachidonic acid was absent; neither a primary nor a secondary wave present. Aggregation in response to ristocetin 1.2 mg/mL was normal. Secretion of dense granule ATP (measured using a

Section G: Platelet Disorders
Glanzmann Thrombasthenia

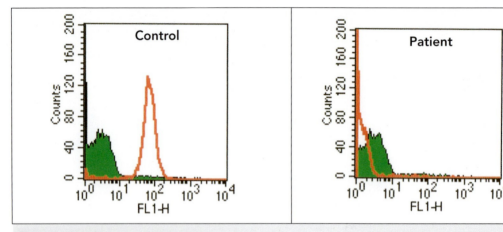

Figure 2 Flow cytometric evaluation of platelet membrane glycoproteins on platelet surface. Platelets from the patient and a control subject were incubated with an antibody against GPIIb. The patient's platelets show a virtual absence of the GPIIb-IIIa complexes.

lumiaggregometer) was markedly decreased with ADP, epinephrine, collagen, and arachidonic acid.

Additional Studies The diagnosis of Glanzmann thrombasthenia (GT) was established in this patient using flow-cytometry. These studies showed a virtual absence of binding of an anti-GPIIb antibody (**Figure 2**) consistent with the absence GPIIb-IIIa complexes on her platelets.

Final Diagnosis Glanzmann thrombasthenia.

Management Approach Transfusion of platelets remains the major therapy for serious bleeding in thrombasthenia and as prophylaxis prior to surgery or other major hemostatic challenges. These patients may develop antibodies against the GPIIb or IIIa that compromise the efficacy of subsequent transfusions. Recombinant factor VIIa is a non-blood product alternative that has been shown to control bleeding episodes in GT, especially in patients with antibodies. Antifibrinolytic agents epsilon aminocaproic acid or tranexamic acid are useful in patients with mucosal bleeding.

General Discussion Glanzmann thrombasthenia is severe, rare, autosomal recessive disorder characterized by a severe reduction in, or absence of, platelet aggregation in response to multiple physiologic agonists due to qualitative or quantitative abnormalities of platelet GPIIb and/or GPIIIa. GPIIb and GPIIIa are distinct gene products. The platelet GPIIB-IIIa receptor is required for platelet aggregation induced by all physiologic agonists; therefore, abnormalities in the receptor result in a failure of hemostatic plug formation and excessive bleeding. This receptor is also responsible for clot retraction and it is abnormal in these patients. Heterozygotes have normal platelet aggregation responses and do not have bleeding disorder. Patients with congenital afibrinogenemia also have absent aggregation in platelet studies with tracings essentially identical to those in thrombasthenia; however, in contrast to patients with GT, PT and APTT are prolonged.

Gray Platelet Syndrome

Craig M Kessler

Patient An 18-year-old female with worsening menorrhagia.

Clinical History The patient presented to a hematologist for further evaluation of menorrhagia prior to pelvic laparoscopy for endometriosis. In addition, she reported easy bruising and recurrent epistaxis. The patient had a history of mild thrombocytopenia (ranging from $95 \times 10^3/\mu L$-$115 \times 10^3/\mu L$). She had experienced excessively prolonged bleeding with loss of her deciduous teeth but she had never undergone any previous major surgery.

Family History Her father and her paternal uncle both have mild thrombocytopenia (ranging from $90 \times 10^3/\mu L$ to $100 \times 10^3/\mu L$), lifelong easy bruising, and abnormal surgical bleeding, her father after a tonsillectomy and her paternal uncle after a colon resection for a localized adenocarcinoma. Both were successfully treated with platelet transfusions empirically because of their mild thrombocytopenia.

Medications None.

Physical Examination Unremarkable except for scattered small ecchymoses over all extensor surfaces. No splenomegaly, petechiae, lymphadenopathy, or anatomical deformities, eg, absent radius, were detected.

Initial Work-Up The CBC was remarkable only for a reduced platelet count to $95 \times 10^3/\mu L$ and an increased mean platelet volume to 15.2 fL. Assessment of the peripheral blood smear revealed quantitatively reduced but large platelets with agranular, pale cytoplasm (**Figure 1**). No platelet aggregates or Döhle bodies were noted. Screening coagulation laboratory studies, including the PT, APTT, thrombin time, and fibrinogen, were completely normal.

Differential Diagnosis Diagnostic considerations included pseudothrombocytopenia, Glanzmann thrombasthenia, von Willebrand disease variant 2B, autoimmune thrombocytopenic purpura, hereditary thrombotic thrombocytopenic purpura, Bernard-Soulier syndrome, gray platelet syndrome, May-Hegglin anomaly, Fechtner syndrome, Epstein syndrome, and Sebastian syndrome.

Additional Work-Up FVIII:C activity = 120% with von Willebrand factor activities (vWF:RCof and vWF:Ag) and VWF multimeric analysis all normal. Platelet aggregation was normal with ristocetin but suboptimal second phase aggregation responses were noted with adenosine diphosphate and epinephrine. The bleeding time was prolonged (>15 minutes before being terminated). The bone marrow aspirate and biopsy revealed morphologically normal trilinear precursors and quantitively normal megakaryocytes.

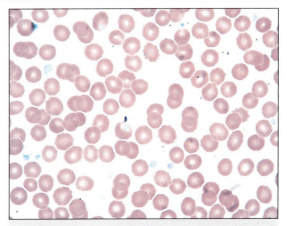

Figure 1 Blood smear (Wright-Giemsa, ×1000) showing large pale (gray) platelets.

There was +3 increased fibrosis on the biopsy. Because of the pale or gray appearance of the platelets on peripheral smear, the patient's bone marrow aspirate and peripheral blood in EDTA were subjected to electron microscopy (EM) at a nearby university pathology laboratory. EMs demonstrated quantitatively normal mitochondria, dense bodies, peroxisomes and lysosomes in platelets and megakaryocytes but few or no *a*-granules. The laboratory analysis for the presence of the platelet surface membrane glycoproteins Ib/IX and IIb/IIIa was normal.

Final Diagnosis Gray platelet syndrome (GPS).

Management Approach The treatment of gray platelet syndrome (GPS) is primarily aimed toward normalization of platelet function. Most individuals with GPS are minimally symptomatic except during surgical or traumatic challenges. In these situations, prevention and reversal of bleeding complications are best achieved by platelet transfusions. Alternatively, intravenous or intranasal administration of DDAVP (1-deamino-8-arginine vasopressin) prior to minor surgeries (tooth extractions, etc.) can be considered as a way to minimize host exposure to transfused blood components. DDAVP stimulation testing should be performed on GPS patients in advance of urgent clinical situations in order to test its potential utility. Corticosteroid administration has anecodotally raised platelet counts temporarily, but has limited clinical usefulness and would not be expected to reverse platelet dysfunction to a significant degree. For mucocutaneous bleeding the adjunctive use of antifibrinolytic agents, eg, ε-aminocaproic acid or tranexamic acid, may help to stabilize clot formation. Finally, if all standard treatment methods fail to reverse active bleeding, one may consider the administration of recombinant factor VIIa concentrate, which has demonstrated effectiveness in qualitative and quantitative platelet disorders. The patient's hematologist and gynecologist were concerned about taking the patient to surgery in view of the laboratory abnormalities and her personal history of excessive bleeding after trauma and surgical challenges. The preoperative IV DDAVP challenge did not normalize the platelet aggregation or bleeding time. Ultimately, she was transfused with single donor platelets immediately prior to surgery, which was completed without excessive bleeding. On postoperative follow-up, the consequences of her myelofibrosis was discussed; however, in the absence of splenomegaly and cytopenias, a longitudinal surveillance posture was assumed. The patient was advised to avoid aspirin and other nonsteroidal anti-inflammatory agents. An estrogen-containing oral contraceptive was prescribed to reduce menorrhagia and the symptoms of endometriosis found on laparoscopy.

General Discussion GPS is an uncommon autosomal-dominant inherited macrothrombocytopenia with associated platelet dysfunction. Some cases with autosomal recessive inheritance pattern been reported. Mutations in the *NBEAL2* (Neurobeachin-like 2) gene on chromosome 3 (3p21) have recently been reported as the cause of GPS (*Nature Genetics*, published online 17 July 2011; doi:10.1038/ng. 883-885). The definitive diagnosis of this specific α-storage pool disorder depends on the presence of a uniform population of large platelets (increased MPV), which are pale (gray) in appearance on the peripheral blood smear. Electron microscopy reveals markedly reduced numbers of intact cytoplasmic α granules in platelets and megakaryocytes. The functional expression of the qualitative defect is demonstrated by the abnormal platelet aggregation studies and prolonged bleeding time, consistent with the fact that the α granules contain many hemostatically important proteins. Individuals with GPS are clinically heterogeneous and laboratory assessments of their platelet function may be variable. Their clinical and laboratory phenotypes may correlate with the degree of thrombocytopenia and the amount of hemostatic proteins contained in the α granules of their platelets. The pathophysiologic basis of GPS is predicated on quantitatively and qualitatively defective α granules, which cannot "store" constituent proteins. Thus, the myelofibrosis, which is observed in many GPS patients may be due to the persistent "leak" of platelet derived growth factor and PF4 (a collagenase inhibitor) from megakaryocytes into the bone marrow milieu with subsequent fibroblast activation and reticulin collagen accumulation. The myelofibrosis is not progressive and treatment for this appears unnecessary. The thrombocytopenia is probably caused by splenic sequestration of the abnormally enlarged platelets. Splenectomy may be followed by a modest increase in platelet count from baseline but the hemostatic defect does not improve. Comprehensive laboratory assessment is critical to documenting GPS as the specific megathrombocytopenic state responsible for the patient's signs and symptoms. Global hemostatic testing is neither specific nor sensitive (prothrombin time, activated partial thromboplastin test, fibrinogen, thrombin time, bleeding time, etc.) and a more focused approach to platelet function is required. Use of the PFA-100 apparatus will not be discriminatory due to the normal levels of VWF protein in the plasma. Lumiaggregometry rules out the dense body variant of GPS if ATP release is normal. Bernard-Soulier syndrome can be eliminated if platelet aggregation responses to ristocetin (1.2 mg/mL) are normal and platelet surface glycoprotein Ib/IX analysis by flow cytometry is normal. von Willebrand disease variant 2B can be ruled out by demonstrating abnormal VWF multimeric composition with loss of the highest molecular weight multimers and also by observing platelet aggregation hyperresponsiveness to low-dose ristocetin (0.6 mg/mL). Glanzmann thrombasthenia is not associated with thrombocytopenia and the first wave platelet aggregation responses to ADP and epinephrine are blunted or absent. Hereditary thrombotic thrombocytopenic purpura can be diagnosed by the presence of ultra high molecular weight multimers of VWF on SDS-gel chromatography and by decreased plasma VWF protease activity. These individuals frequently present with hypercoagulable events rather than bleeding and have schistocytosis on their peripheral blood smears. The other differential diagnoses above can be ferreted out by close examination of the peripheral smear, eg, inclusion Döhle bodies in the neutrophils in May-Hegglin anomaly.

Wiskott-Aldrich Syndrome

Lakshmanan Krishnamurti, Nidhi Aggarwal, Raymond E Felgar

Patient A 3-year-old male with eczema and petechiae scattered throughout the body.

Clinical History The infant was born at term with low platelet count and has been thrombocytopenic since then. He has a history of recurrent skin and ear infections and history of blood in the stools.

Family History The child has a 6-year-old sister who is healthy; a 4-year-old brother, who has asthma, infections, thrombocytopenia and eczema; and a 19-month-old half brother with the same mother who also has thrombocytopenia, eczema and ear infections. There is no history of consanguineous marriage.

Medications None at presentation. He had been treated in the past with steroids and intravenous immune globulin (IV Ig).

Physical Examination Alert and active young child. Weight 14.2 kg, height 91.5 cm. Left tympanic membrane was inflamed. Lungs had bilateral scattered rhonchi. There was a palpable lymph node in the left axilla. Examination of the skin revealed multiple scattered petechiae and dry eczematous rash.

Initial Work-Up

CBC	Value	Normal
WBC (×10³/μL)	7.4	5.0-17.0
RBC (×10⁶/μL)	4.36	3.90-5.30
HGB (g/dL)	12.1	11.5-13.5
HCT (%)	34.4	34.0-40.0
MCV (fL)	78.8	75.0-87.0
MPV (fL)	5.8	6.8-10.4
PLT (×10³/μL)	18	156-369
Neutrophils (×10³/μL)	3.68	1.50-8.50

Peripheral blood smear confirmed thrombocytopenia. The platelets were small. The red blood cells were normocytic normochromic. White blood cells were normal in number and morphology (**Figure 1**).

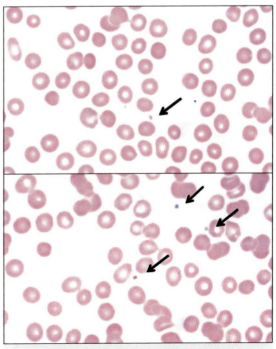

Figure 1 Blood smear (Wright-Giemsa, ×1000) showing thrombocytopenia with small platelets.

Differential Diagnosis The differential diagnoses for thrombocytopenia, infections and eczema include X-linked hyper IgM syndrome, X-linked thrombocytopenia and human immunodeficiency virus infections.

Additional Work-Up
- HIV and HTLV antibody screens were negative
- IgA 245 mg/dL (normal 15-241), IgE total 168 IU/mL
- IgG 645 Mg/dL (normal 559-1,116), IgM<25 mg/dL (normal 23-99)
- A point mutation was identified in the WAS gene (Xp11.23-p11.22), exon 1a, c.116T>C that causes a single amino acid substitution at codon 39 (p.Leu39Pro)

Final Diagnosis Wiskott-Aldrich syndrome.

Management Approach Treatment options depend on an individual's predicted disease burden and consist of topical steroids for eczema; antibiotics for infected eczema; judicious use of immunosuppressants for autoimmune disease; granulocyte colony stimulating factor (G-CSF) and appropriate antibiotics for neutropenia antibiotic prophylaxis, intravenous immunoglobulin (IV Ig) replacement therapy every 3 to 4 weeks by age 6 months and judicious use of platelet transfusions. Allogeneic hematopoietic progenitor cell transplantation (HPCT) is the only known curative treatment. This patient required repeated treatment for thrombocytopenia with steroids and IV Ig. He was treated for asthma exacerbations. Eczema was treated with topical steroids. He received pneumocystis carinii prophylaxis with trimethoprim/sulfamethoxazole. He underwent HPCT from an HLA-identical sibling and has made a complete hematologic recovery.

General Discussion The WAS-related disorders are X-linked disorders and include Wiskott-Aldrich syndrome (WAS), X-linked thrombocytopenia (XLT), and X-linked *congenital* neutropenia (XLN). These are a spectrum of disorders of hematopoietic cells, with predominant defects of platelets and lymphocytes caused by *mutations* in the WAS *gene*. WAS usually presents in infancy with thrombocytopenia, intermittent mucosal bleeding, bloody diarrhea, intermittent or chronic petechiae and purpura, eczema, and recurrent bacterial and viral infections, particularly recurrent ear infections. Patients may develop autoimmune manifestations such as hemolytic anemia, immune thrombocytopenic purpura (ITP), immune-mediated neutropenia, arthritis, vasculitis of small and large vessels, and immune-mediated damage to the kidneys and liver. Patients have an increased risk of developing lymphomas, which often occur in unusual, extranodal locations such as the brain, lung, or gastrointestinal tract. Patients with XLT have thrombocytopenia with small platelets, but eczema and immune dysfunction, are mild or absent. The diagnosis is confirmed in the presence of mutations in WAS gene by sequence analysis.

δ-Storage Pool Deficiency (Hermansky-Pudlak Syndrome)

A Koneti Rao, Gauthami Jalagadugula

Patient A 43-year-old Hispanic man from Puerto Rico, who presented with a lifelong history of easy bruising, excessive bleeding following injury and cuts, and epistaxis.

Clinical History The patient had a history of albinism and nystagmus since childhood and a 20-year history of colitis. There was no history of hemarthrosis.

Family History No other family members have a bleeding diathesis or history of albinism.

Medications None at the time of presentation.

Physical Examination He was noted to have albinism involving his hair and eyes, and nystagmus. A few bruises (1 inch-2 inches) were noted on his extremities.

Initial Work-Up	
Hemoglobin	12.4 g/dL
PT	10.1 sec (normal 9.8-14.0)
PTT	25.3 sec (normal 25-36)
Platelet count	376 × 10³/μL
Bleeding time	>15 min

Differential Diagnosis The history of longstanding mucocutaneous bleeding symptoms in the setting of normal PT, PTT and platelet count and prolonged bleeding time suggests a disorder of platelet function, including von Willebrand disease.

Additional Work-Up
- Factor VIII coagulant activity >200% (normal 50-150)
- von Willebrand factor antigen 112% (normal 50-150)
- Ristocetin cofactor 143% (normal 50-150)
- Platelet aggregation and secretion studies (**Figure 1**)

Platelet aggregation in response to ADP and epinephrine were abnormal with presence of the primary wave, but not the secondary wave of

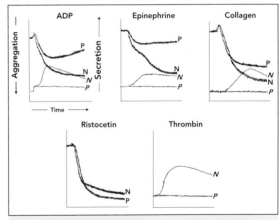

Figure 1 Aggregation and ATP secretion tracings of studies performed using a lumi-aggregometer on platelet-rich plasma (PRP) in the patient (P) and a healthy normal subject (N). Shown are responses to ADP (7.5 μM), epinephrine (7.5 μM), collagen (1 μg/mL), ristocetin (1.5 mg/mL) and thrombin (2 μg/mL). With thrombin only secretion is shown because addition of thrombin induces clotting of PRP and does not permit recording of aggregation. Aggregation (P patient; N normal control); secretion (P patient; N normal control).

aggregation. In response to collagen, the aggregation response was decreased. Aggregation in response to ristocetin 1.2 mg/mL was normal. Secretion of dense granule contents was absent with ADP, epinephrine

Section G: Platelet Disorders
δ-Storage Pool Deficiency (Hermansky-Pudlak Syndrome)

and collagen. In response to thrombin no secretion was noted.

Additional Studies Measurement of ATP and ADP content of platelets revealed decreased levels. The ATP:ADP ratio was increased, consistent with a diagnosis of dense granule storage pool deficiency (SPD). The diagnosis of SPD can also be made using electron microscopy to show decreased number of dense granules.

Final Diagnosis Storage pool deficiency, associated with the Hermansky-Pudlak syndrome. The combination of oculocutaneous albinism, nystagmus and platelet dysfunction with δ-storage pool deficiency suggests the diagnosis of the Hermansky-Pudlak syndrome (HPS).

Management Approach Transfusion of platelets remains the major therapy for serious bleeding in SPD and as prophylaxis prior to surgery or other major hemostatic challenges. In some studies, some SPD patients have responded to intravenous administration of desmopressin (DDAVP) with a shortening of the bleeding time.

General Discussion Storage pool deficiency is a heterogeneous group of disorders involving deficiency of platelet granules or their contents. These patients may have defects affecting dense granules (δ-storage pool deficiency), α-granules (α-storage pool deficiency, or the Gray platelet syndrome), or both dense bodies and α granules (αδ-storage pool deficiency). δ-SPD is a heterogeneous disorder characterized by a bleeding tendency, abnormalities in the second wave of platelet aggregation, and variable deficiencies of the contents of platelet dense granules. δ-storage pool deficiency can be a primary, inherited platelet disorder or a component of a multisystem (syndromic) disorder, such as the Hermansky-Pudlak syndrome (HPS) (variable oculocutaneous albinism, excessive accumulation of ceroid-like material in lysosomes in monocyte-macrophage cells in bone marrow and other tissues, variable pulmonary fibrosis and inflammatory bowel disease, and a hemorrhagic diathesis), the Chédiak-Higashi syndrome (partial oculocutaneous albinism, giant lysosomal granules, and frequent pyogenic infections), and the Wiskott-Aldrich syndrome. Patients with the δ-SPD have decreased dense granules on electron microscopy and are characterized by an impaired platelet secretion of dense granule contents on activation. Dense granules contain ATP, ADP, calcium and serotonin, and all of these are reduced in δ-SPD. The etiology of primary human δ-SPD is unclear, but studies in patients with the syndromic variants indicate that defects in biogenesis of lysosome-related organelles (which includes melanosomes and dense granules) form the basis of the disorders. Hermansky-Pudlak syndrome, an autosomal recessive disorder, is unusually common in patients from northwest Puerto Rico, and linkage analysis of patients from this area led to the identification of the gene abnormal in these patients (HPS1). δ-SPD can be established by direct measurement of platelet ATP and ADP showing decreased content or by electronic microscopy.

Inherited Platelet Secretion Defect/Signal Transduction Defect

A Koneti Rao

Patient A 43-year-old Caucasian woman, who was referred to our institution for evaluation of longstanding easy bruising.

Clinical History The patient presented with a lifelong history of easy bruising, excessive bleeding from gums when brushing her teeth and menorrhagia. She appeared otherwise healthy.

Family History Her brother, paternal aunt and grandmother had history of excessive bleeding following surgical procedures. The paternal aunt had been diagnosed as having a platelet function abnormality.

Medications None.

Physical Examination Notable only for few small bruises on extremities.

Initial Work-Up		
Hemoglobin	12.4 g/dL	
PT	11 sec	(normal 10-14)
PTT	27 sec	(normal 25-36)
Platelet count	250 ×10³/μL	
Bleeding time	10 min	(normal 2-7)

Differential Diagnosis The history of mucocutaneous bleeding symptoms and the laboratory findings (normal PT, PTT and platelet count and prolonged bleeding time) indicate an inherited disorder of platelet function.

Additional Work-Up
- Factor VIII coagulant activity 74% (normal 50-150)
- von Willebrand factor antigen 82% (normal 50-150)
- Ristocetin cofactor activity 104% (normal 50-150)

Platelet aggregation in response to ADP, epinephrine, collagen, and thromboxane A$_2$ analog (U46619) was decreased in the patient and her son (**Figure 1**). Primary wave of aggregation was present but the secondary wave was decreased or absent with ADP and epinephrine. Aggregation in response to collagen and U44619 was decreased. Secretion of 14C-serotonin from dense granules was markedly decreased with

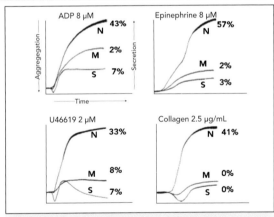

Figure 1 Aggregation tracings and secretion studies (monitored with 14C-serotonin) performed using platelet-rich plasma (PRP) in the propositus (M), her son (S) and a healthy control (N). Shown are responses to ADP (8 μM), epinephrine (8 μM), collagen, and a thromboxane A$_2$ analog (U46619 [8 μM]). The numerals next to the tracings are the percent 14C-serotonin secreted. Both aggregation and secretion in response to the above agonists are impaired in mother and son. The response to ristocetin (1.5 mg/mL) was normal in the patient and her son (not shown).

these agonists. Aggregation was normal with ristocetin (1.2 mg/mL) (not shown). Platelet ADP and ATP content of platelets was measured and found to be normal in both the mother and the son, thereby excluding dense granule deficiency. The presence of the primary wave of aggregation excludes thrombasthenia and the normal response to ristocetin excludes the Bernard-Soulier Syndrome. The findings on aggregation studies noted in this patient are not uncommon among patients with a bleeding disorder and a platelet defect. The impaired dense granule secretion is an important feature of the platelet abnormality. The normal ADP and ATP content of platelets in this patient excludes δ-storage pool disease. Patients with such findings may have abnormalities in events that occur following platelet activation leading to aggregation and secretion. They have been lumped for convenience under the rubric of platelets secretion defects, platelet activation defects or signal transduction defects. Patients with these findings constitute a large proportion of patients commonly encountered with inherited platelet defects. In the vast majority, the underlying abnormalities remain unknown.

Final Diagnosis Inherited platelet function defect; platelet secretion activation defect.

Management Approach Transfusion of platelets remains the major therapy for serious bleeding and as prophylaxis prior to surgery or other major hemostatic challenges. Other options in selected patients include administration of DDAVP (Desmopressin) and recombinant factor VIIa, both non-blood products. Neither is FDA approved for this indication.

General Discussion Disorders of platelet secretion and signal transduction: patients lumped in this remarkably heterogeneous group generally manifest impaired secretion of dense granule contents and absence of the second wave of aggregation upon stimulation of platelet-rich plasma with ADP or epinephrine along with impaired responses to other agonists. Conceptually, platelet function is abnormal in these patients either when the granule contents are diminished (storage pool deficiency, SPD) or when there is an aberration in the mechanisms governing aggregation and secretion. Signal transduction mechanisms encompass processes initiated by the interaction of an agonist with specific platelet receptors and include responses such as G-protein activation and activation of phospholipase C and phospholipase A_2. If the key components in signal transduction are the surface receptors, the G-proteins, and the effector enzymes, evidence now exists for specific human platelet abnormalities at these levels. Patients with receptor defects have impaired responses because of an abnormality in the platelet surface receptor for a specific agonist. Such defects have been documented for ADP, thromboxane A_2, collagen, and epinephrine. G-proteins link surface receptors and intracellular effector enzymes. Patients with defects in G-protein activation due to deficiencies in Gαq, Gαi1 and Gαs have been described. Patients have been reported with impaired signal transduction and defects in phospholipase C activation, calcium mobilization and pleckstrin phosphorylation. Some have had specific deficiencies of phospholipase C-β2 and protein kinase C-ε enzymes. Lastly, a major platelet response to activation is liberation of arachidonic acid from phospholipids and its subsequent oxygenation to thromboxane A_2. Patients with impaired thromboxane synthesis due to congenital deficiencies of cyclooxygenase and thromboxane synthase and phospholipase A_2 have been documented. Many of the commonly encountered patients with impaired aggregation and secretion are likely to have similar defects in the above-mentioned processes rather than membrane glycoprotein deficiencies or storage pool deficiency. Detailed studies in the patient described above showed a deficiency in the enzyme phospholipase C-β2, which plays a major role in platelet activation.

Acquired Platelet Function Defect-Induced by Selective Serotonin-Reuptake Inhibitor

David Essex, A Koneti Rao

Patient A 74-year-old female, who was referred for preoperative evaluation.

Clinical History The patient had fallen at home and fractured the left femur in multiple sites a year prior to this presentation. Massive bleeding was encountered at surgery for fixation of the fracture sites with the hemoglobin falling to 6 g/dL. A year later, she was being scheduled for a hip replacement with comminuted left femur fracture. The orthopedic surgeon felt strongly that the bleeding following the initial surgery was unusually excessive and was reluctant to reoperate. The patient reported easy bruisability on the arms for 2 years but otherwise had no prior history of abnormal bleeding. The patient was not on aspirin at the time of the initial surgery. She had been on a selective serotonin reuptake inhibitor (SSRI) for several years for depression.

Family History There is no family history of bleeding diathesis.

Medications Escitalopram; esomeprazole; simvastatin; vitamin D.

Physical Examination Ecchymoses were noted on her arms and legs.

Initial Work-Up

PT	11.4 sec	(normal 11–13)
INR	1.0	(normal 0.9–1.1)
PTT	32 sec	(normal 27–32)
Platelet count	326 ×10³/µL	

Differential Diagnosis The patient was investigated for a bleeding disorder. A drug-induced acquired disorder of platelet function was considered.

Additional Work-Up A von Willebrand disease work-up was normal: Factor VIII antigen >200% (high); vWF:ristocetin cofactor activity >200% (high); vWF antigen >200% (high).

Platelet aggregation and secretion studies were performed while the patient was on the selective serotonin reuptake inhibitor (SSRI), escitalopram (**Figure 1**). The results showed decreased aggregation with ADP (5.0 µM) and decreased secretion with all doses of ADP tested. There was decreased aggregation

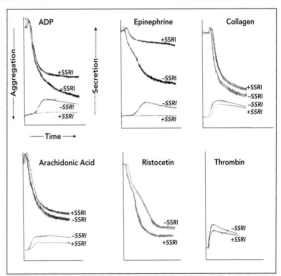

Figure 1 Aggregation and ATP secretion tracings of studies performed using platelet-rich plasma (PRP) when the patient was on the SSRI (+SSRI) and after the SSRI was discontinued (−SSRI). Shown are responses to ADP (5 µM), epinephrine (7.5 µM), collagen (5µg/mL), arachidonic acid (5.0 mM), ristocetin (1.5 mg/mL) and thrombin (1 µg/mL). With thrombin only secretion is shown because addition of thrombin induces clotting of PRP and does not permit recording of aggregation. Secretion studies are labeled in italics (*SSRI*).

and no secretion with all doses of epinephrine. There was decreased secretion with collagen and arachidonic acid relative to the normal control. Aggregation to ristocetin was normal. Secretion induced by thrombin (1 U/mL) was normal. The results of the aggregation and secretion studies performed while the patient was on the SSRI (+SSRI) and 2 weeks after the SSRI was discontinued (–SSRI) are shown in the figure. The responses to ADP and epinephrine as well as the abnormal secretion responses to collagen and arachidonic acid completely normalized when she was off the medication.

Final Diagnosis SSRI-induced platelet function defect. This likely contributed to the excess bleeding with orthopedic surgery for the comminuted fracture of the left femur.

Management Approach The SSRI was discontinued for 2 weeks at which time repeat platelet aggregation studies were found to be normal. The patient underwent left hip replacement without the enormous amount of bleeding found following the first surgery. She had a subsequent orthopedic procedure, again without excess bleeding.

General Discussion A large number of disease states are associated with acquired defects in platelet function including renal failure, myeloproliferative diseases, and a host of medications. Acquired defects in platelet function are induced by selective serotonin release inhibitors (SSRIs) which are widely used antidepressant medications worldwide with a greatly reduced side effect profile compared to the older antidepressant medications. These include (with common trade names): fluoxetine (Prozac), setraline (Zoloft), paroxetine (Paxil), fluvoxamine (Luvox), citalopram (Celexa) and the drug our patient was on, escitalopram (Lexapro). SSRIs inhibit the reuptake serotonin pump of the presynaptic neuron, increasing the amount of serotonin (also known as 5-hydroxytryptamine) in the synapse and increasing postsynaptic receptor occupancy. Serotonin in plasma is taken up into platelets where it is stored in the dense granules accounting for the vast majority of whole blood serotonin being found in the platelets. Serotonin released by platelets at sites of vascular injury amplifies the platelet aggregation response and thrombus formation. SSRIs inhibit the uptake of serotonin by platelets and have been shown to decrease cellular serotonin by 80%. The decrease in platelet serotonin results in the inhibition of platelet function and is associated with an increased bleeding risk. Epidemiological studies found an increased risk of gastrointestinal bleeding in patients on SSRIs. This risk is substantially potentiated in patients by concomitant nonsteroidal anti-inflammatory drugs (NSAID) therapy. Bleeding episodes requiring hospital admission are also increased by the use of SSRIs. Additionally, blood loss with orthopedic procedures is double in patients on an SSRI (500 mL excess blood loss) compared to those not on a non-SSRI antidepressant. This results in a 4-fold increase in requirement for blood transfusions. Postoperative drainage is also slightly but significantly increased in patients on SSRIs. In our patient we found evidence of platelet dysfunction and this was associated with life threatening surgical bleeding while the patient was on a SSRI. With removal of the SSRI the in vitro platelet dysfunction resolved and the bleeding with repeat orthopedic surgeries was not excessive. A study comparing the use of platelet aggregation and secretion studies with the platelet function analyzer-100 (PFA-100) method to detect the effect of SSRIs on platelet function found that platelet aggregation/secretion studies were the better method for detecting platelet function abnormalities caused by SSRIs. Levels in the therapeutic range of the specific SSRI our patient was on, escitalopram, have been shown to inhibit platelet aggregation (secretion was not studied).

Babesiosis

Brian R Smith, Alexa J Siddon, Christopher A Tormey

Patient A 76-year-old man, who presented to the emergency department with fever (100°F-101°F) and dyspnea on exertion.

Clinical History The patient reported that he had been feeling weak over the past few weeks and that the weakness had progressed considerably during the past few days to the point where he fell at home. His past medical history is significant for hypertension, chronic obstructive pulmonary disease and a splenectomy following a motor vehicle accident at the age of 22. The patient lives in rural Connecticut. He is a hunter who last went hunting about 6 weeks prior to presentation. He has a 20 pack/year smoking history, although he quit smoking 10 years prior to presentation.

Family History Noncontributory.

Medications Verapamil, tiotropium bromide (inhaler), and budesonide-formoterol (inhaler).

Physical Examination Notable for lethargic appearance and slightly diminished breath sounds. No organomegaly and no rashes. Temperature 99.9°F, blood pressure 112/78, pulse 103, respiration 29 (93% SaO_2 on room air).

Initial Work-Up

CBC		WBC Differential	%	# (×10³/µL)
WBC (×10³/µL)	4.9	Neutrophils	51	2.5
RBC (×10⁶/µL)	3.26	Bands	17	0.8
HGB (g/dL)	11.1	Lymphocytes	11	0.5
HCT (%)	31.0	Monocytes	15	0.7
MCV (fL)	95	Eosinophils	5	0.2
MCH (pg)	34.0	Basophils	1	0.1
MCHC (g/dL)	35.8	**Serum Chemistry**		
PLT (×10³/µL)	102	AST (U/L)	250	(normal 5-40)
RDW-CV (%)	13.4	ALT (U/L)	159	(normal 5-40)
		Alkaline phosphatase (U/L)	17	(normal 30-130)
		Total bilirubin (mg/dL)	3.41	(normal 0.2-1.2)
		Direct bilirubin	2.21	(normal <0.2 mg/dL)
		Creatinine (mg/dL)	1.5	(normal 0.5-1.2)
		Blood urea nitrogen (mg/dL)	31	(normal 8-18)

Peripheral blood smear revealed extracellular and intraerythrocytic organisms (7%), Howell-Jolly bodies, and occasional nucleated red cells (**Figure 1**).

Section H: Hematologic Infectious Diseases
Babesiosis

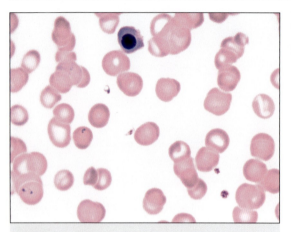

Figure 1 Blood smear (Wright-Giemsa, ×1000) showing multiple red blood cells harboring parasites and occasional extracellular ring forms. A nucleated red blood cell is also pictured.

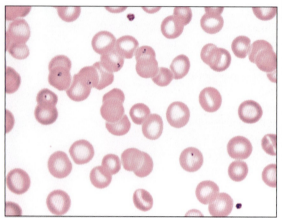

Figure 2 Blood smear (Wright-Giemsa, ×1000) showing multiple red blood cells harboring parasites, suggestive of a high parasite burden.

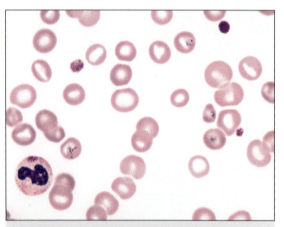

Figure 3 Blood smear (Wright-Giemsa, ×1000) showing a red blood cell at the lower left that harbors 4-5 small ring forms and nearly forms a "Maltese cross."

Differential Diagnosis Diagnostic considerations included tick-borne illness (babesiosis vs anaplasmosis) and an occult malignancy. Malaria was considered unlikely based on clinical presentation and no history of travel to endemic areas.

Additional Work-Up
– Lyme antibody titers: negative
– Routine blood culture: negative after 5 days incubation
– Chest/abdominal CT scan: negative for malignancy; confirmation of asplenia
– *Babesia microti* DNA PCR: positive

Final Diagnosis Babesiosis (*Babesia microti*).

Management Approach Treatment generally consists of a 2-drug therapy—atovaquone and azithromycin for mild cases, or clindamycin plus quinine for more severe cases. For patients that are asplenic, those that demonstrate evidence of end-organ damage, or those with a parasite load >10%, erythrocytapheresis (red blood cell exchange) is an important therapeutic option. In this procedure, the red blood cell parasite burden can be rapidly reduced with the simultaneous replenishment of fresh red blood cells; all of this can be accomplished without the risk of volume overloaded associated with simple red cell transfusion. Despite these therapeutic options, many healthy patients with functioning spleens may not even be aware of a *Babesia* infection and typically do not require treatment. However, there is some evidence to suggest that such patients may continue to harbor very small numbers of parasites for long periods of time. As such, should these individuals become immunocompromised or lose splenic function, it is possible for the disease to reemerge, often with very high parasite counts. Clindamycin plus quinine was the initial antibiotic regimen chosen for this patient. Red blood cell transfusions were also provided to overcome the hemolytic anemia. After the patient continued to demonstrate hemolysis and general refractoriness to antibiotics over a period of 2 days, erythrocytapheresis (red blood cell exchange transfusion) was performed to reduce the circulating parasite load and to replenish red blood cells. Following red blood cell exchange the patient showed marked improvement with a reduction in parasitemia to <1% of total red blood cells. He was maintained on antibiotic therapy for several more days with resolution of hemolysis and no detectable increase in circulating parasite burden.

General Discussion *Babesia microti* is a tick-borne illness common in the coastal New England region of the United States. In Europe, the most common babesia species is *Babesia divergens*, which has a similar clinical presentation to its American counterpart. *Babesia microti* is transmitted via the *Ixodes scapularis* tick, the same tick vector as *Borrelia burgdorferi* (the spirochete agent of Lyme disease) and *Anaplasma phagocytophilum* (the parasitic agent of human granulocytic anaplasmosis). For this reason, it is not uncommon for a patient to be co-infected with these diseases. While ticks are the most common source of transmission, blood transfusion is also a risk factor for an infection with *Babesia* species. While many cases of babesiosis are mild and can go unnoticed in healthy hosts, *Babesia microti* can also cause more severe disease, particularly in patients with asplenia or those with immunodeficiency/immunosuppression. Common symptoms associated with babesiosis are fevers, shaking chills, fatigue, and hemolytic anemia. Laboratory testing will confirm the hemolytic anemia, typically with rises in parameters such as lactate dehydrogenase (LDH) and total bilirubin. Patients may even demonstrate increases in creatinine due to the hemolysis. Of note, patients do not demonstrate positive Coombs tests because the hemolysis in these cases is due to mechanical clearance and/or disruption of the red cell membrane by the parasitic organism and not an auto- or alloantibody. The diagnosis of babesiosis is typically made by examination of a peripheral blood smear, which demonstrates parasitic forms within the red blood cells. The classic image is the "Maltese cross" of a parasitic tetrad made of 4 merozoites. This finding and the identification of extracellular parasites may help a pathologist distinguish between babesiosis and malarial infection; in malaria, ring forms are uniformly intracellular and typically manifest as only 1 form-2 forms/cell. For a more definitive diagnosis of babesia infection, PCR-based tests can be utilized to identify *Babesia*-specific nucleic acids. Serologic tests to identify anti-*Babesia* antibodies may also be of use in difficult cases.

Section H: Hematologic Infectious Diseases

Anaplasmosis

Brian R Smith, Alexander Finkelstein, Christopher A Tormey

Patient A 55-year-old woman with fever, myalgias, headache, and malaise of 4 days duration.

Clinical History The patient has a history of hypertension and coronary artery disease. She did not recall a particular provoking or exacerbating factor. She denied any runny nose, throat pain, wheezing, cough, shortness of breath, orthopnea, syncope, chest pain, joint pain, diarrhea, or dysuria. The patient also denied any sick contacts. Although she spends much time outdoors, she had not hiked in the last few months and could not recall having been bit by a tick. She had not sought medical attention until the current presentation.

Family History Noncontributory.

Social history The patient is lives in rural Connecticut with her husband and 1 child; she has many outdoor hobbies including gardening and hiking.

Medications Enalapril, metoprolol, aspirin, and multivitamin.

Physical Examination The patient appeared mildly lethargic, but otherwise was unremarkable. Temperature 102.2°F, blood pressure 106/66, pulse 110, respiration 22 (97% SaO_2 on room air).

Initial Work-Up

CBC		WBC Differential	%	# (×10³/μL)
WBC (×10³/μL)	4.5	Neutrophils	54	2.4
RBC (×10⁶/μL)	3.8	Bands	30	1.4
HGB (g/dL)	11	Lymphocytes	8	0.4
HCT (%)	33	Monocytes	7	0.3
MCV (fL)	82	Eosinophils	1	0.1
PLT (×10³/μL)	87	Basophils	0	
RDW-CV (%)	12.8			

Cardiac enzymes (troponin I, CK-MB): within normal limits. AST (U/L) 204 (normal 5-40), ALT (U/L) 360 (normal 5-40). Bilirubin (mg/dL): total 1.46 (normal 0.2-1.2); Direct 0.26 (normal <0.2 mg/dL). Routine blood culture: no growth after 5 days incubation. EKG: nonspecific ST changes. Chest X-ray: mild elevation of left hemidiaphtragm, no other acute cardiopulmonary abnormality. Cardiomediastinal silhouette was normal.

Differential Diagnosis Diagnostic considerations included viral syndrome (influenza/parainfluenza viruses, reovirus, adenovirus, hepatitis group, etc), malaria, babesiosis, human anaplasmosis (human granulocytic ehrlichiosis), human monocytic ehrlichiosis, and Rocky Mountain spotted fever.

Additional Work-Up
- Peripheral blood smear revealed granulocytes with small purple inclusions in the cytoplasm (**Figure 1**). There were no inclusions noted in monocytes or red blood cells
- Viral cultures: negative
- *Anaplasma phagocytophilum* DNA PCR: positive

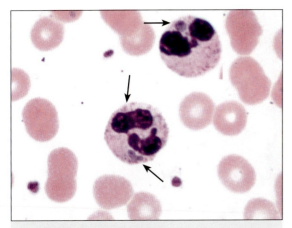

Figure 1 Blood smear (Wright-Giemsa, ×1000) composite of 2 different areas: *Anaplasma phagocytophilum* morulae (arrows) located in the peripheral cytoplasm of granulocytes.

Final Diagnosis Anaplasmosis or human granulocytic anaplasmosis (formerly known as human granulocytic ehrlichiosis).

Management Approach Treatment typically consists of antibiotic therapy with either doxycycline or rifampin. Doxycycline is generally considered a first-line therapy while rifampin is an acceptable alternative for pregnant women or children younger than 8 years of age. This patient was treated with oral doxycycline and intravenoue hydration with significant improvement in symptoms and laboratory parameters. She became afebrile on day 2 of antibiotic therapy. Repeat blood smears performed on days 4 and 5 of antibiotic therapy were negative for intracellular organisms.

General Discussion Human granulocytic anaplasmosis (HGA) is a tick-borne rickettsial infection of neutrophils caused by *Anaplasma phagocytophilum*. The human disease was first identified in 1990, although the pathogen was defined as a veterinary agent in 1932. HGA was first identified in 1990 in a Wisconsin patient who died with a severe febrile illness 2 weeks after a tick bite. During the terminal phases of the infection, clusters of small bacteria, assumed to be phagocytosed gram-positive cocci, were noted within neutrophils in the peripheral blood. A careful review of the blood smear suggested the possibility of human ehrlichiosis. All blood cultures were unrevealing, and specific serologic and immunohistochemical tests for *Ehrlichia chaffeensis*, the causative agent of human monocytic ehrlichiosis (HME) were negative. Within the next 2 years, 13 cases with similar intraneutrophilic inclusions were identified in the same region of northwestern Wisconsin and eastern Minnesota. Common features among these patients included fever, headache, myalgias, malaise, absence of skin rash, leukopenia, thrombocytopenia, and mild transaminitis. In 1994, through application of broad range molecular amplification and DNA sequencing, the causative agent was recognized as distinct from *E chaffeensis*. HGA is increasingly recognized as an important and frequent cause of fever after tick bite in the upper Midwest, New England, parts of the mid-Atlantic states, northern California, and many parts of Europe. The bacterium is maintained in a transmission cycle with *Ixodes* complex ticks, including *I scapularis* in the eastern United States and *I pacificus* in the western United States. Infection is established after a tick blood meal involving a human host. The major mammalian reservoir for *A phagocytophilum* in the eastern United States is the white-footed mouse, although other small mammals and white-tailed deer (*Odocoileus virginianus*) can also be infected. White-footed mice have transient (1-4 weeks) bacteremia; deer are persistently and subclinically infected. HGA is clinically variable, but most patients have a moderate-to-severe febrile illness associated with headache, myalgias, and malaise. Frequent laboratory abnormalities identified include thrombocytopenia (~71% of infected patients), leukopenia (~49% of infected patients), anemia (~37% of infected patients), and elevated transaminases (~71% of infected patients). Approximately 5%-7% of patients require intensive care, and at least 7 deaths have been identified; in those cases with the worst outcome delayed diagnosis and treatment were the most important risk factors. Severe complications include a septic or toxic shock–like syndrome, coagulopathy, atypical pneumonitis/acute respiratory distress syndrome (ARDS), acute abdominal syndrome, rhabdomyolysis, myocarditis, acute renal failure, hemorrhage, demyelinating polyneuropathy, and opportunistic infections. At least 3 of the deaths resulted from opportunistic fungal or viral infections or hemorrhage that occurred immediately after HGA. Unlike results of animal observations, no evidence has shown *A phagocytophilum* persistence in humans.

A diagnosis of HGA can be made based on the following tests/modalities: (1) examination of a peripheral blood smear or of a buffy coat preparation to maximize granulocyte content; purple inclusions (morulae) should be found within neutrophils, (2) serologic examination for anti-anaplasma antibodies, and (3) PCR amplification of the 16S rRNA gene or amplification of the major surface protein gene *msp2*.

Malaria (*Plasmodium vivax*)

Joan E Etzell, Christian P Nixon

Patient A 64-year-old man, who presented with fever (103°F) and shaking chills of 1-week duration.

Clinical History The patient had returned from a trip to Belize 2 weeks prior where he had traveled both overland and along the coast. During the trip he was asymptomatic. Upon returning he complained of general malaise. One week prior to presentation he began to experience shaking chills each night. These awakened him from sleep around midnight and were partially responsive to acetaminophen. He described his appetite as poor and stated that food had tasted bland for the last 10 days. The patient denied nausea, vomiting, dyspnea, cough, chest pain, sore throat, ear/sinus pain, abdominal or genitourinary pain. He had previously been vaccinated for hepatitis A, hepatitis B and yellow fever, but did not take antimalarial medication during his trip. He is a Vietnam veteran who currently works as a dentist and travels extensively on scuba diving trips.

Family History Noncontributory.

Medications Efudix 5% cream, sildenafil citrate, sertraline, omeprazole.

Physical Examination He was in no acute distress, currently afebrile. He had a postural blood pressure drop with syncope and associated decline in systolic blood pressure to the high 70s. He had no jaundice, and no splenomegaly. The remainder of the examination was normal. Pulse 63/minute, respirations 20/minute, temperature 97.3°F, blood pressure 84/53 lying down, 72/50 standing, pulse oximetry on room air 98%, and BMI 26.6.

Initial Work-Up

CBC		WBC Differential	%	# (×10^3/μL)
WBC (×10^3/μL)	3.8	Neutrophils	60	2.3
RBC (×10^6/μL)	4.37	Bands	0	
HGB (g/dL)	13.9	Lymphocytes	28	1.1
HCT (%)	41.1	Monocytes	8	0.3
MCV (fL)	94.0	Eosinophils	3	0.1
MCH (pg)	31.8	Basophils	1	0.0
MCHC (g/dL)	33.8	**Serum Chemistry**		
PLT (×10^3/μL)	230	Bilirubin, total (mg/dL)	1.5	
RDW-CV (%)	16.9	Bilirubin, direct (mg/dL)	0.3	
		Urea nitrogen (mg/dL)	25	
		Creatinine (mg/dL)	1.5	
		Alkaline phosphatase (U/L)	227	
		AST (U/L)	81	
		ALT (U/L)	111	

Section H: Hematologic Infectious Diseases
Malaria (Plasmodium vivax)

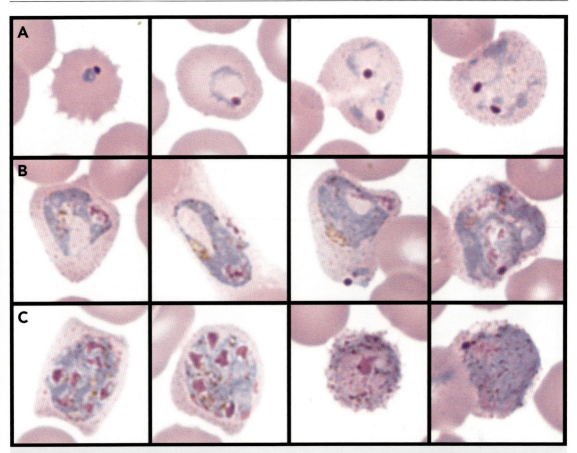

Figure 1 Blood smear (Wright-Giemsa, ×1000) with a composite of various parasitic forms: **A** ring forms (trophozoites) with a subset showing a large ameboid appearance (upper and center rows), **B** schizonts containing several merozoites (lower left and lower left center), and **C** gametocytes filling the red cell cytoplasm (lower right center and lower right).

Differential Diagnosis A prodromal flu-like illness followed 7 days-14 days later by cyclical fevers interspersed with shaking chills/defervescence after travel of a malaria-naïve individual to an endemic country, is highly suggestive of blood stage infection with a *Plasmodium* species (*P falciparum, P vivax, P ovale, P malariae*, and more recently *P knowlesi*). Acute febrile illness associated with Dengue fever should be considered after an individual has traveled to the tropics; however the absence of the characteristic bright red petechial rash makes this diagnosis less likely. Infectious mononucleosis caused by Epstein-Barr virus or cytomegalovirus, and enteric fever associated with typhoid and paratyphoid fever are also considerations in the traveler with systemic fever. Other infectious organisms that could be responsible for high relapsing fever include common *Rickettsia, Anaplasma, Coxiella* and *Borrelia burgdorferi*. However, the diseases caused by these organisms are typically associated with tick bites, pathognomic skin lesions or exposure to animals such as cattle or sheep (*Coxiella*) and are typically acquired in the United States.

Additional Work-Up The Wright-Giemsa-stained blood smear demonstrated malarial parasitic organisms infecting mostly enlarged red blood cells (**Figure 1**). Parasitic forms included (a) ring forms (trophozoites) with a subset showing a large ameboid appearance, (b) schizonts containing several merozoites, and (c) gametocytes filling the red cell cytoplasm.

Diagnosis *Plasmodium vivax*. Infectivity rate was approximately 1.0% (infected red blood cells/100 RBC count).

Section H: Hematologic Infectious Diseases
Malaria (Plasmodium vivax)

Management Approach Chloroquine has historically been the drug of choice to treat infection with *P vivax*; however, chloroquine resistance has become an increasingly prevalent problem in many endemic countries, such as the Papua province of Indonesia. *P vivax* isolates that remain chloroquine-sensitive can be initially treated with chloroquine 10 mg base/kg (maximum 600 mg base) orally, followed by 5 mg base/kg (maximum 300 mg base) 6, 24, and 48 hours later, with cure rates exceeding 95%. Chloroquine-resistant *P vivax* isolates have been successfully treated with mefloquine, quinine sulfate plus doxycycline, or atovaquone-proguanil. Dormant *P vivax* liver hypnozoites should also be empirically treated to prevent relapse. Primaquine phosphate, one of the few currently licensed drugs capable of eradicating liver hypnozoites, is administered at a dose of 30 mg/day for 14 days immediately after the completion of a course of chloroquine. Prior to initiating treatment with primaquine, patients should always be screened for glucose-6-phosphate dehydrogenase deficiency (G6PD) to prevent severe oxidant hemolysis. Mild G6PD deficiency can be compensated for by reducing the dose of primaquine to 0.8 mg base/kg/week for 8 weeks. This patient was treated with choroquine and primaquine phosphate, which completely resolved his *P vivax* infection.

General Discussion Malaria is the most important parasitic infection of humans, resulting in over 1 million deaths worldwide each year. It is most often transmitted by the bite of a female *Anopheles* sp mosquito. *P falciparum* and *P vivax* are the most common causes of malaria. *P falciparum* predominates in Africa, New Guinea, Haiti, and the Dominican Republic. *P falciparum* is often associated with life-threatening infection. In addition, chloroquine-resistant *P falciparum* is common in some regions of the world; thus, rapid identification may be important for therapeutic decisions. *P vivax* is endemic in Africa, Asia, Central and South America, and the south Pacific, and may be chloroquine sensitive or resistant. *P vivax* presents as a febrile illness; other signs and symptoms can include chills, fatigue, malaise, headache, tachypnea, tachycardia, abdominal pain, anorexia, nausea/vomiting, diarrhea, cough, arthralgias, and myalgias. Physical examination may reveal jaundice, hepatomegaly and/or splenomegaly. In a subset of patients, *P vivax* infection can be associated with severe pulmonary disease (eg, acute lung injury, acute respiratory distress syndrome), splenic rupture, severe anemia, disseminated intravascular coagulation, renal failure, and/or cerebral malaria. Detection of parasites on Giemsa-stained thin and thick blood smears remains the gold standard for diagnosis. The sensitivity of microscopy is quite good, with experts able to detect as few as 5-10 parasites/µL. Microscopy also allows semi-quantitation of parasite load and speciation. Additionally, other organisms, such as filariasis, trypanosomiasis, babesiosis, and borreliosis can be detected by this method. Microscopy should be performed whenever possible even if rapid diagnostic tests are also used.

In the rapid assays, antibodies are used to detect a variety of proteins, including proteins seen across all human malarial parasites (eg, aldolase), as well as those specific to *P falciparum* (eg, histidine-rich protein-2; HRP2). The sensitivity of these rapid assays depends on the patient population they are used in as semi-immune individuals may not become symptomatic until the parasite load is high, thus increasing the sensitivity of the assay in this patient population. One rapid detection kit has a reported sensitivity of 95% for *P falciparum* and 69% for *P vivax* with specificity of 94% for *P falciparum* and 100% for *P vivax*. Generally, negative results must be confirmed by microscopy of blood smears. (We wish to thank Paul Viduya, CLS, MBA of Department of Microbiology at Veterans' Affairs Medical Center in San Francisco, California, for providing us with the blood smear of the case.)

Relapsing Fever Secondary to *Borrelia hermsii*

Cordelia Sever

Patient A 14-year-old Native American male living on the Indian Reservation in a Western State came to the clinic because of a waxing and waning fever.

Clinical History The patient also reported having abdominal pain for the past 3 weeks.

Family History Noncontributory.

Medications None.

Physical Examination Notable for a temperature of 102.2°F and tachycardia.

Initial Work-Up

CBC	
WBC (×10³/μL)	13.2
RBC (×10⁶/μL)	3.77
HGB (g/dL)	11.8
HCT (%)	34.7
MCV (fL)	92.1
MCH (pg)	31.3
MCHC (g/dL)	34.0
PLT (×10³/μL)	206
RDW-CV (%)	12.8
MPV (fL)	9.7

WBC Differential	%	# (×10³/μL)
Neutrophils	73	9.6
Bands	5	0.7
Lymphocytes	16	2.1
Monocytes	4	0.5
Eosinophils	1	0.1
Basophils	0	0.0

Peripheral blood smear revealed spirochetes (**Figure 1**).

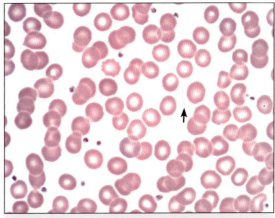

Figure 1 Blood smear (Wright-Giemsa, ×1000) showing a spirochete (arrow).

Differential Diagnosis Once the spirochetal organisms are recognized, the specific subtype needs to be identified. In most spirochetal diseases seen in the US, such as Lyme disease or syphilis, the organisms are either extremely scant or not found in the peripheral blood. Since spirochetes were quite easy to find in this patient's peripheral blood, averaging 1 organism/10 hpf, the tick-borne (*Borrelia hermsii, B parkeri*) and louse-borne (*B recurrentis*) recurrent fevers were highest on the list.

Additional Work-Up Serologic testing was positive for high titers of IgM (≥1:256) and IgG (>1:256) antibody to *Borrelia hermsii*, indicative of an acute infection. No antibodies to *Borrelia burgdorferi* (Lyme disease) and *Treponema pallidum* were detected.

Final Diagnosis Relapsing fever secondary to *Borrelia hermsii*.

Management Approach Tick-borne relapsing fevers are usually treated with doxycycline in adults. Children and pregnant women who should not receive tetracyclines are generally treated with erythromycin. There is in vitro sensitivity to azithromycin which may be better tolerated than erythromycin, but clinical data are lacking. *Borrelia* meningitis, which is uncommon, can be treated with ceftriaxone for a prolonged course of 14 days. Louse-borne fever can usually be treated with a single dose of either doxycycline or erythromycin. A major concern with therapy is the Jarisch-Herxheimer reaction, believed to be caused by antigen release after the first dose or therapy, which occurs in up to 50% of cases and may cause fatal shock. For this reason patients should be observed for 2 hours after initiation of therapy. This patient was treated with doxycycline as outlined for the tick-borne relapsing fevers.

General Discussion Peripheral blood findings are very nonspecific and are characterized by moderate degrees of neutrophilic leukocytosis which may be associated with left shift especially in febrile episodes. Relapsing fever secondary to *B hermsii* in the United States is mainly seen in endemic areas in mountainous regions of the Western United States. It is transmitted by a tick whose natural reservoir is small rodents. Exposure is characteristically traceable to overnight stays in rodent-infested log cabins. Since it is uncommon, the greatest difficulty in clinical diagnosis is usually thinking of the possibility. In this case, an astute medical technologist found the organisms, eliciting appropriate serologic testing and clinical examination. The other arthropod-transmitted organism, *B recurrentis*, is exclusively transmitted by the human body louse and is largely seen in Africa and travelers from Africa. The diagnostic distinction is important since untreated louse-borne relapsing fever carries a mortality rate of 30%-70%, in part because it usually affects malnourished patients. With treatment the mortality rate is <1%.

Disseminated *Histoplasma capsulatum*

Powers Peterson, Scott Weisenberg

Patient A 48-year-old African-American male with dyspnea.

Clinical History The patient reported having fever for the prior 10 days. He was seen at a local urgent care clinic twice, and was noted to have increased liver function test results. A test for influenza was negative. He was treated with a course of azithromycin. His past history was significant for diabetes mellitus, hypertension, atherosclerotic cardiovascular disease (ASCVD), and a renal transplant 7 years prior to current presentation. He recently traveled to Trinidad and Cancun, Mexico. His HIV status has been repeatedly negative.

Family History Noncontributory.

Medications Prednisone, mycophenolate mofetil, tacrolimus, metoprolol XL, nifedipine XL, pioglitazone, and baby aspirin.

Physical Examination Temperature 100.6°F; BP 120/80 mmHg; heart rate 130/min, respiratory rate 30/min; oxygen saturation 95% on 2 liters oxygen. His sclerae were icteric. His chest was clear to auscultation and percussion. His abdomen was soft and slightly distended with normal bowel sounds present.

Initial Work-Up

CBC

WBC ($\times 10^3/\mu L$)	1.8
RBC ($\times 10^6/\mu L$)	4.52
HGB (g/dL)	13.5
HCT (%)	40.0
MCV (fL)	88.4
MCH (pg)	32.1
MCHC (g/dL)	33.8
PLT ($\times 10^3/\mu L$)	44
RDW-CV (%)	15.0
MPV (fL)	10.6

WBC Differential	%	# ($\times 10^3/\mu L$)
Neutrophils	82	1.5
Immature granulocytes	8	0.1
Lymphocytes	7	0.1
Monocytes	3	0.1

Peripheral blood smear revealed intracytoplasmic organisms within monocytes and neutrophils (**Figure 1**). Chest X-ray: interstitial prominence without focal infiltrates.

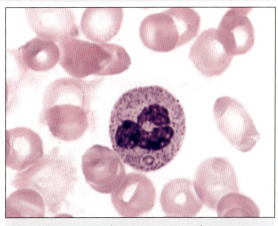

Figure 1 Blood smear (Wright-Giemsa, ×1000) showing an *Histoplasma* organism within a neutrophil.

Differential Diagnosis Diagnostic considerations included *Candida* species, *Histoplasma capsulatum*, *Toxoplasma gondii*, and *Leishmania donovani*.

Section H: Hematologic Infectious Diseases
Disseminated Histoplasma capsulatum

Additional Work-Up

Alkaline phosphatase (U/L)	444 (normal 29-92)
Total bilirubin (mg/dL)	6.5 (normal 0.2-1.2)
Direct bilirubin (mg/dL)	4.5 (normal 0-0.4)
AST (U/L)	143 (normal 7-42)
ALT (U/L)	48 (normal 1-45)

Bone marrow aspirate and biopsy: Intracellular organisms measuring 2 μm-4 μm within macrophages in both the aspirate and biopsy (**Figures 2** and **3**). The organisms in the biopsy stained positively with Gomori methanamine silver (GMS) stain (**Figure 4**). Urine *Histoplasma* antigen: positive blood culture: *Histoplasma capsulatum* (results not immediately available).

Final Diagnosis Disseminated *Histoplasma capsulatum*.

Management Approach The first line treatment for disseminated histoplasmosis is the lipid form of amphotericin-B at 3-5 mg/kg/day for 1 week-2 weeks. This is followed by itraconazole (200 mg orally TID for 3 days, then BID) to complete at least 12 weeks of therapy. Duration of therapy is longer in immunosuppressed patients, who should continue itraconazole as long as they remain immunosuppressed. For this patient, liposomal amphotericin, 5 mg/kg/day, was initiated immediately. Initially, he experienced hypotension, tachycardia, and fever but improved considerably and recovered fully. Therapy was changed to itraconazole after 2 weeks, and he remains on itraconazole at 200 mg PO BID.

General Discussion Histoplasmosis is caused by the pathogenic fungus *Histoplasma capsulatum*. The initial infection is pulmonic with hilar lymph node involvement; disseminated disease, as in this case, involves other lymph nodes, spleen, liver and marrow. *H capsulatum* is acquired by inhalation of mold microconidia found in soil contaminated by bird or bat droppings. Interestingly, the infection is not transmitted from person to person. After the initial pulmonary infection the organism converts to the yeast form, attaches to CD18 integrin receptors, and is ingested by polymorphonuclear leukocytes and tissue macrophages. The organisms can be seen within macrophages at very high magnifications on H&E stains and are usually easily identified with appropriate fungal stains, specifically methenamine silver. The yeast forms measure 2.5 μm-5 μm, such that the differential based on size includes *Candida* species, toxoplasmosis and

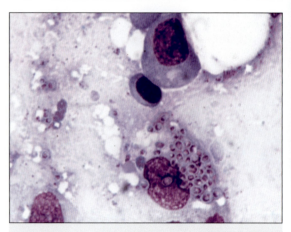

Figure 2 Bone marrow aspirate smear (Wright-Giemsa, ×1000) showing intracellular and free *Histoplasma* organisms.

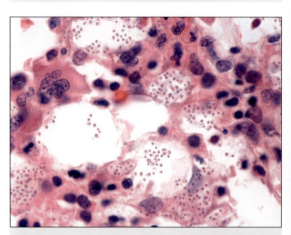

Figure 3 Bone marrow biopsy (H&E, ×1000) showing *Histoplasma* organisms.

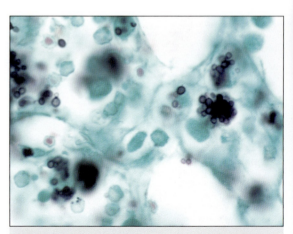

Figure 4 Bone marrow biopsy (GMS stain, ×1000) showing *Histoplasma* yeast forms.

L donovani. This patient's presentation with prolonged fever, increasing dyspnea and altered LFT's indicated disseminated disease. The diagnosis in such cases is made by demonstration of the organisms, usually in marrow. Special stains are required for diagnosis. Since a positive silver stain may not differentiate *Histoplasma* from *Candida* in tissue sections, a recommended test for disseminated disease is the EIA urine *Histoplasma* antigen. In this case, examination of the peripheral blood smear revealed the diagnosis. The cytology of the *H capsulatum* organisms identified within both neutrophils and monocytes, specifically the "halo," largely eliminates *Candida* from the differential. In Romanowsky stains the yeast forms are 2 μm-5 μm in diameter, have a round body with a basophilic center, and are surrounded by a clear halo. The halo is caused by shrinking of the capsule. A cardinal feature of *Candida* that distinguishes it from *Histoplasma* is that *Candida* exhibits dimorphism, with both yeast forms and hyphae and pseudohyphae. Neither *Toxoplasma gondii* nor *Leishmania* stain with silver stains, and *Leishmania* is also excluded clinically by the lack of travel to endemic areas.

Persistent Polyclonal B-Lymphocytosis

Lydia Contis

Patient A 44-year-old female with an absolute lymphocytosis noted on routine blood work performed as part of an annual physical.

Clinical History Significant only for a 20-year history of smoking, otherwise asymptomatic.

Family History Noncontributory.

Medications None.

Physical Examination Notable for splenomegaly only. She had no palpable lymphadenopathy.

Initial Work-Up		
CBC		
WBC (×10³/μL)	22.0	
RBC (×10⁶/μL)	5.16	
HGB (g/dL)	14.2	
HCT (%)	40.9	
MCV (fL)	79.2	
MCH (pg)	27.5	
MCHC (g/dL)	34.7	
PLT (×10³/μL)	225	
RDW-CV (%)	14.6	
WBC Differential	**%**	**# (×10³/μL)**
Neutrophils	30	6.6
Bands	1	0.2
Lymphocytes	61	13.4
Monocytes	8	1.8
Eosinophils	0	
Basophils	0	

Blood smear revealed numerous atypical lymphocytes that were medium to large with moderate amounts of basophilic cytoplasm, condensed nuclear chromatin and binucleation (**Figure 1**). Internuclear bridging was seen in the majority of these cells. Nucleoli were variably prominent. Monocytes were also increased but did not demonstrate nuclear atypia or immaturity.

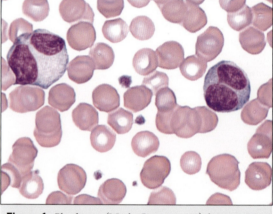

Figure 1 Blood smear (Wright-Giemsa, ×1000) showing atypical lymphoid cells with bilobed nuclei.

Differential Diagnosis Benign lymphocytosis vs malignant lymphocytosis.

Additional Work-Up Bone marrow biopsy revealed normocellular marrow (50%-60% cellular) with trilineage hematopoiesis. There were few scattered variably sized nonparatrabecular lymphoid aggregates (**Figure 2**). These were composed of small lymphoid cells with mostly rounded nuclear contours (**Figure 3**). Bone marrow aspirate: the myeloid to erythroid ratio was 2.3:1 with a normal differential count, including 17% lymphocytes which were mostly small with rounded nuclear contours and with very

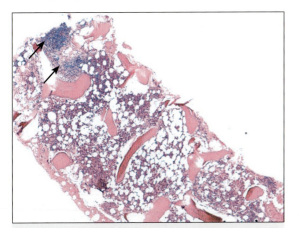

Figure 2 Bone marrow biopsy (H&E, ×40) showing normocellular marrow with lymphoid aggregates (arrows).

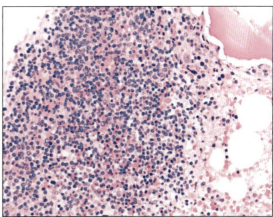

Figure 3 Bone marrow biopsy (H&E, ×400) showing lymphoid aggregate composed of small lymphoid cells.

rare binucleated forms, similar to those seen in the peripheral blood (**Figure 4**). Immunohistochemistry performed on bone marrow biopsy demonstrated few scattered polytypic κ+ and λ+ plasma cells. Most lymphoid aggregates were absent on immunostained sections and demonstrated the following: CD20: scattered positive lymphoid cells, some in an apparent intrasinusoidal pattern (**Figure 5**); CD3: moderate number of scattered positive lymphoid cells and within few small aggregates (**Figure 6**); CD5: B cells appeared negative; cyclin D1: negative; EBV-ISH (EBER): negative; CD10: some nonspecific staining, lymphoid cells appeared negative; TdT: negative. Flow cytometry studies performed on the bone marrow demonstrated approximately 31% B cells with a κ:λ ratio of 1.3:1 and the following phenotype: κ+, λ+, CD5–, CD10–, CD20+, CD22+, CD23+, FMC7+; 14% T cells

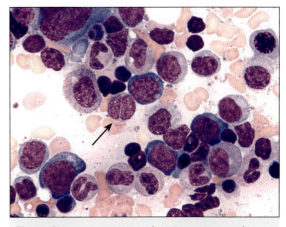

Figure 4 Bone marrow aspirate (Wright-Giemsa, ×1000) showing normal myelopoiesis and erythropoiesis with a rare bilobed lymphoid cell (arrow).

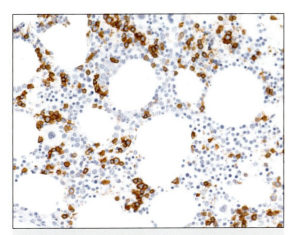

Figure 5 Bone marrow biopsy (CD20, ×400) demonstrates scattered positive cells, some in an intrasinusoidal pattern.

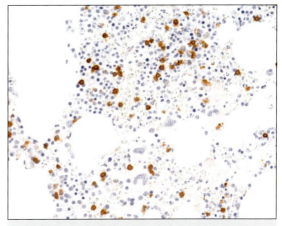

Figure 6 Bone marrow biopsy (CD3, ×400) demonstrates scattered positive cells.

without phenotypic aberrancy and a CD4:CD8 ratio of 2.1, granulocytes, and 1% CD34+ myeloblasts.

Cytogenetics 46, XX [20].

Molecular Analysis of Bone Marrow
Immunoglobulin heavy chain gene rearrangement was not detected by PCR and Southern blot. BCL2 gene rearrangement (Mbr region)(t14;18) was not detected by PCR.

Final Diagnosis Persistent polyclonal B-lymphocytosis.

Management Approach Close clinical observation without therapy. This patient remained asymptomatic and continued to demonstrate an absolute lymphocytosis. A repeat bone marrow examination performed 4 years after diagnosis demonstrated largely similar findings without morphologic, immunophenotypic or genotypic evidence of malignant lymphoma.

General Discussion First described in 1982, persistent polyclonal B-lymphocytosis (PPBL) is a rare lymphoid disorder characterized by a persistent lymphocytosis with binucleated or bilobated lymphoid cells. There is an associated polyclonal increase in serum IgM immunoglobulin, as well as reduced IgA and IgG levels. This disorder occurs mostly in young to middle-aged females with a median age of 40 years. The majority of patients have a history of heavy smoking and are asymptomatic. Physical examination is usually unremarkable, although mild to moderate splenomegaly can be present. The lymphoid cells in the peripheral blood are small to large in size with abundant basophilic cytoplasm. The nuclei may be rounded with a slight indentation or bilobed with an internuclear bridge. Nuclear chromatin is dense and nucleoli can be visible. The proportion of binucleated lymphoid cells in the blood can range from 1%-25%. Bone marrow examination can indicate variable cellularity and can demonstrate an interstitial lymphoid infiltrate, small lymphoid aggregates or an intravascular pattern of infiltration. Immunohistochemical staining of the lymphoid infiltrates typically indicate few T cells and many B cells. Few binucleated or bilobed cells are present in the marrow. Flow cytometry studies demonstrate polytypic B cells with expression of CD19, CD20, CD22, CD79, FMC7, rarely CD5 and CD23, and lack expression of CD10, CD43, CD11c or myeloid antigens. PPBL is often associated with chromosomal abnormalities which include +i(3q), trisomy 3 and chromosomal instability. Normal karyotypes have also been reported. Genotypic studies have demonstrated multiple BCL2/IgH gene rearrangements by polymerase chain reaction, while the t(14;18) translocation has been reported in a number of PPBL patients. A genetic predisposition has been suggested by the association of this entity with HLA-DR7, its presence in monozygotic twins and multiple BCL2/IgH gene rearrangements among first-degree relatives. The majority of patients remain stable with an indolent clinical course. The lymphocytosis has been reported to decrease in association with smoking cessation. There are few reports of patients who develop non-Hodgkin lymphoma, such as diffuse large B-cell lymphoma or marginal zone lymphoma, or non-hematopoietic tumors. Whether this entity represents a benign or a premalignant condition with a long latency period remains uncertain. Recognition of this entity is important in order that aggressive therapy for a lymphoid neoplasm is not instituted.

Infectious Mononucleosis

Linda Sandhaus

Patient A 22-year-old college student with fatigue.

Clinical History The patient reported having sore throat and mild fever for the week prior.

Family History Noncontributory.

Medications None.

Physical Examination 2 small lymph nodes were palpated in the cervical area bilaterally.

Initial Work-Up

CBC		WBC Differential	%	# (×10³/µL)
WBC (×10³/µL)	11.3	Neutrophils	31	3.5
RBC (×10⁶/µL)	4.99	Bands		
HGB (g/dL)	14.4	Lymphocytes	25	2.8
HCT (%)	42.4	Atypical lymphocytes	35	4.0
MCV (fL)	85	Monocytes	9	1.0
MCHC (g/dL)	34	Eosinophils		
PLT (×10³/µL)	235	Basophils		
RDW-CV (%)	12.4			

Peripheral blood smear revealed lymphocytosis with many atypical (reactive) lymphocytes (**Figures 1-4**).

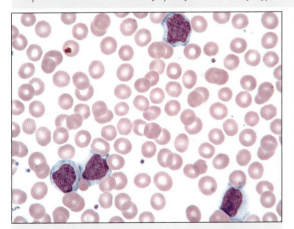

Figure 1 Blood smear (Wright-Giemsa, ×1000) showing 4 atypical lymphocytes.

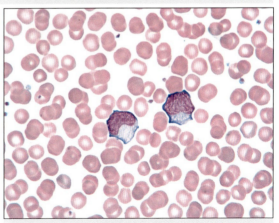

Figure 2 Blood smear (Wright-Giemsa, ×1000) showing 2 atypical lymphocytes.

Section I: Miscellaneous Hematologic Conditions
Infectious Mononucleosis

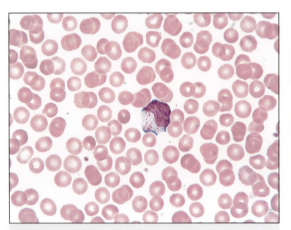

Figure 3 Blood smear (Wright-Giemsa, ×1000) showing an atypical lymphocyte with prominent azure granules.

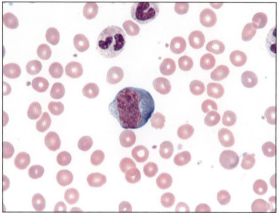

Figure 4 Blood smear (Wright-Giemsa, ×1000) showing an immunoblast.

Differential Diagnosis There is a mild lymphocytosis with many atypical lymphocytes. The atypical morphology favors a reactive lymphocytosis and is suggestive of an acute viral infection. Other causes of reactive lymphocytosis include autoimmune and connective tissue disorders, postvaccination, toxoplasmosis, acute stress reaction, and some drug reactions, such as dilantin. A chronic lymphoproliferative disorder, such as chronic lymphocytic leukemia or a marginal zone lymphoma would be extremely unlikely in this age group. Some of the lymphoid cells are large and have a prominent nucleolus, features that might suggest a malignancy, such as acute leukemia or a large cell lymphoma.

Additional Work-Up Heterophile antibody test was positive.

Final Diagnosis Acute infectious mononucleosis due to acute Epstein-Barr virus (EBV) infection.

Management Approach No specific medical therapy is indicated. Patients are asked to rest and "take it easy" during the acute illness. Symptomatic relief with antipyretics and antiemetics is helpful in some patients.

General Discussion The clinical history, lymphocyte morphology, and positive heterophil antibody test are sufficient to confirm a diagnosis of acute infectious mononucleosis (IM) due to EBV infection. Recognition of the spectrum of reactive lymphocytes in the blood smear is important to the prompt diagnosis of infectious mononucleosis. Reactive lymphocytes are generally larger than normal lymphocytes, with nuclei that are round, ovoid, or irregularly indented. The chromatin is generally dense and homogeneous but may be finely granular and open as in a blast cell or in between the dense and finely granular. Cytoplasm is variably abundant, usually pale blue and often has a peripheral zone that stains deeply basophilic. Azurophilic granules may be prominent in some of the reactive lymphocytes (**Figure 3**). A frequent feature is the "amoeboid" cytoplasm that appears to partially wrap around adjacent erythrocytes. The presence of a nucleolus and deeply basophilic cytoplasm are features of reactive immunoblasts (**Figure 4**). Circulating large lymphoma cells may be indistinguishable from immunoblasts; however, the presence of a heterogenous lymphocyte population and the clinical history are usually sufficient to make this distinction. In general, the marked heterogeneity of the reactive lymphocyte proliferation contrasts with the more monotonous, homogeneous appearance of lymphocytes in the chronic lymphoproliferative disorders, such as chronic lymphocytic leukemia and marginal zone lymphoma/leukemias. The magnitude of the lymphocytosis is also helpful in the differential diagnosis of reactive and neoplastic lymphocytoses. Reactive lymphocytoses rarely exceed $30 \times 10^3/\mu L$, whereas malignant lymphoproliferative disorders are frequently higher at presentation. Large granular lymphocytic leukemias, which are clonal proliferations of cytotoxic/suppressor cells or NK cells, may share some morphologic resemblance to reactive lymphocytes. However, these disorders also display a striking homogeneity of the lymphocyte morphology and are typically associated with neutropenia or other cytopenia(s).

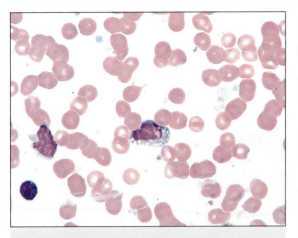

Figure 5 Blood smear (Wright-Giemsa, ×1000) showing an apoptotic lymphocyte.

Another clue to the diagnosis of IM is the presence of apoptotic/pyknotic lymphocytes (**Figure 5**). The majority of reactive lymphocytes are CD8+ cytotoxic/suppressor T cells. Natural killer (NK) cells are also increased. The deeply basophilic immunoblasts may correspond to EBV-infected B cells. Flow cytometric immunophenotyping is rarely indicated in the evaluation of a reactive lymphocytosis, but can be useful in selected cases to exclude a lymphoproliferative disorder. The findings of a reversed CD4/CD8 ratio with expression of lymphocyte activation antigens and presence of polyclonal B cells are consistent with a reactive lymphocytosis. T-cell lymphoproliferative disorders usually have abnormal expression or loss of one or more pan-T-cell markers. T-cell clonality can be established by T-cell receptor Vβ analysis. IM affects patients of all ages, but is most common in adolescents and young adults. Patients typically have fatigue, fever, sore throat, and lymphadenopathy. The lymphadenopathy is usually symmetrical and posterior-cervical. Splenomegaly, usually mild, is present in >50% of patients, while hepatomegaly is much less common (about 20%). There is usually an absolute lymphocytosis that rarely exceeds $20 \times 10^3/\mu L$. Mild thrombocytopenia is not uncommon, while severe thrombocytopenia is rare and appears to be autoimmune.

Although most cases of IM are self-limited and require no treatment, serious complications can occur. In 1%-3% of cases, hemolytic anemia due to anti-i antibodies may occur. Splenic rupture is another rare, but serious complication. In patients with marked lymphadenopathy, clinical concern for lymphoma may lead to a lymph node biopsy. It is important for pathologists to be familiar with the extreme reactive changes that may be occur in IM and which can mimic Hodgkin lymphoma or non-Hodgkin lymphoma.

The diagnosis of IM is confirmed by the detection of heterophil antibodies, usually by a rapid agglutination test. In older children and young adults, positive heterophil antibody titers are detected in the vast majority of those with EBV-induced IM. In infants and the elderly, the incidence of heterophil positivity is much lower. When the rapid slide test is negative and the blood smear suggests IM, the diagnosis should be pursued with additional serologic studies. Repeating the heterophil antibody test may yield a positive test in 1 week-2 weeks. EBV-specific serologic tests that are based on the detection of antibodies produced against specific viral antigens may also be diagnostic. Antibodies against different viral components have characteristic patterns that rise and fall with the course of the infection and provide evidence for acute or past infection. Anti-viral capsid antigen (anti-VCA) of both IgG and IgM type appears early in the course of IM. Elevated IgM anti-VCA is useful in diagnosis of acute IM, since its titers diminish rapidly during convalescence and it is usually undetectable at 12 weeks. Persistence of IgG anti-VCA is indicative of past infection. Anti-early antigen (anti-EA) is another marker of acute, as well as chronic or reactivated, infection. Anti-Epstein-Barr nuclear antigen (EBNA) does not appear until after resolution of symptoms, and then persists for life. In infants, VCA-IgM and EA responses may not be detected during acute EBV infection.

Alloimmune Neonatal Neutropenia

Suba Krishnan

Patient A 2-day-old male infant with severe neutropenia.

Clinical History The baby was born at 34 weeks gestational age by normal delivery, with a birth weight of 2.4 kg, with APGAR scores of 8 and 10 at 1 and 5 minutes respectively. His initial CBC showed a low WBC count of $3 \times 10^3/\mu L$, with severe neutropenia (absolute neutrophil count [ANC] was 150/µL) on the first day of life (DOL). There was no anemia, neonatal jaundice or thrombocytopenia. He was placed on prophylactic broad spectrum antibiotic coverage with ampicillin and gentamicin and transferred to a tertiary care pediatric center for work-up of neonatal neutropenia and appropriate management. Within 24 hours of admission, he became hypothermic (temperature dropped to 96.8°F-97.7°F) with the only pertinent finding on clinical examination being mild erythema around the umbilical cord site. As a result antibiotic coverage was expanded to add oxacillin for possible oomphalitis. Hematology was consulted for the work-up of neonatal neutropenia (detailed below). He received 1 dose of filgrastim (G-CSF) on DOL-4 to which he had a robust response within 24 hours. He remained clinically stable without any documented infection (blood and urine cultures were negative) and continued to thrive with satisfactory weight gain. He was discharged after a week upon completion of his diagnostic work-up.

Maternal History Significant for gestational diabetes. There was no history of pregnancy-induced hypertension.

Family History Family is of south Asian Indian origin. Both parents are healthy. There is no history of anemia, bleeding disorders, or autoimmune disorders in first- or second-degree relatives. Child has a 5-year-old brother who is healthy with normal WBC and no history of neonatal neutropenia. Mother has 2 sisters; neither of them has had any children so far. There is no history of congenital bone marrow failure syndromes.

Medications Antibiotics, as noted above.

Physical Examination Unremarkable, except for mild erythema around the umbilical cord site.

Differential Diagnosis Neonatal neutropenia due to deceased neutrophil production is very commonly associated with sepsis, and less commonly associated with drug-induced or immune-mediated mechanisms. Conditions that result from decreased neutrophil production include the commonly seen neutropenia related to maternal hypertension, the somewhat less common though not rare situations such as drug-induced or Rh hemolytic disease-related neutropenias, and the rarer conditions such as Kostmann severe congenital neutropenia, cyclic neutropenia, Schwachman-Diamond syndrome, reticular dysgenesis, Chédiak-Higashi syndrome, severe congenital immunodeficiency among others. The 2 main forms of hereditary or nonsyndromic variants of congenital

Section I: Miscellaneous Hematologic Conditions
Alloimmune Neonatal Neutropenia

Initial Work-Up and Pertinent Serial Labs

Date	DOL2 5/27/09	5/28/09	5/30/09	6/3/09	4 weeks 6/24/09	7/21/09	7/28/09	9 weeks 8/1/09	8/2/09	8/9/09	23 weeks 11/10/09
WBC (x10^3/μL)	3.7	4.7	5.4	16.7	13.4	10.8	8.9	8	10.4	15.6	9.3
ANC (x10^3/μL)	0	25	54	3,340	3,216	1,296	534	322	4,222	2,652	3,232
Neutrophils (/μL)	0				3,216						3,200
Bands (/μL)	0				5						0
Lymphocytes (/μL)	3,400				9,619						5,600
Monocytes (/μL)	250				450						360
Eosinophils (/μL)	50				110						140
HGB (g/dL)	15.4	13.8	12.2	11.7	9.7	9.0	9.8	10.0	8.9	11.0	9.8
MCV (fL)	100	98.0	98.0	98.8	93.0	84.0	81.9	80.0	79.1	78.0	80.0
PLT (x10^3/μL)	208	235	222	316		359	442	472	397	542	320
Reticulocytes (%)	5.5	3.0	1.1	1.2	3.0	3.4	1.8	1.8		1.4	1.1
Blood group Coombs	O+ Neg										
Blood culture	No growth x5 days										
Urine culture	No growth x5 days										
G-CSF (μg/Kg)				5				5			

neutropenia are cyclic neutropenia and severe congenital neutropenia, which are most commonly associated with specific mutations in *ELA2*, and *HAX1* genes (additional gene mutation studies if these are negative are usually dictated by the clinical picture). A detailed clinical examination for dysmorphic features can also help to identify syndromes in which neutropenia occurs as a component, eg, abnormal thumbs associated with Fanconi anemia, or oculocutaneous albinism seen in Chédiak-Higashi syndrome. In this patient, maternal history was negative for pregnancy-induced hypertension. There was no history of maternal autoimmune disease or maternal neutropenia or other cytopenia. The baby's clinical examination was completely unremarkable. Hence an expanded work-up was carried out.

Additional Work-Up

Tests in Baby: Bone marrow examination (aspirate and biopsy) revealed normocellular marrow with trilineage hematopoiesis and relative myeloid hyperplasia. There was no maturation arrest suggestive of severe congenital neutropenia/Kostmann Syndrome. Importantly, there were no dysplastic changes or evidence of acute leukemia. Chromosomal analysis revealed normal karyotype (46XY). Mutations more commonly associated with severe congenital neutropenia (ELA-2 and HAX-1) were negative. No antineutrophil antibody was detected by flow cytometry in baby's serum, suggesting the absence of an unlikely autoimmune neutropenic process in the baby. Quantitative immunoglobulin panel was normal for age.

Tests in Mother: Neutrophil antibody screen on mother's serum was positive for neutrophil specific antibodies to HNA-1a (NA1). Maternal HLA antibody screen was also positive. Neutrophil crossmatching between maternal serum and paternal neutrophils resulted in aggregation; however no aggregation occurred between maternal serum and maternal neutrophils. This implied that maternal serum contained antibodies that were directed against specific antigens on father's neutrophils but not against her own (self) neutrophils. This was very supportive of a diagnosis of alloimmunization in the mother resulting from fetal neutrophil antigens (inherited from father) that are absent in mother. This situation is analogous to Rh hemolytic disease but involves neutrophils rather than red cells. Because HLA antibody screen was positive, monoclonal antibody immobilization of neutrophil antigens (MAINA) was carried out to differentiate between HLA antibodies and neutrophil antigen-specific antibodies. Extended antibody testing in the MAINA assay detected reactivity to the CD16 molecule (FcγRIII). Specificity for HNA-1a (NA1) was identified (differentiating presence of neutrophil-specific antibodies from HLA antibodies). Additionally, maternal granulocyte antibody direct assay was negative (ie, maternal autocontrol was negative) providing indirect evidence of absence of HNA-1a on maternal neutrophils. Taken together, these results suggested alloimmunization against paternal neutrophil antigens that were absent in mother and presented to her by fetal neutrophils, with subsequent passive transplacental transfer of IgG antibodies from the mother to the fetus.

Diagnosis Findings are suggestive of alloimmune neonatal neutropenia with specificity for HNA-1a epitope, well known to be associated with neutrophil isoimmunization.

Management Approach Although the majority of infants with alloimmune neonatal neutropenia may have minor or no symptoms, significant infection-related morbidity and mortality have been known to occur in these patients. The issue of the choice and efficacy of specific therapy to increase the blood neutrophil count in the management of alloimmune neonatal neutropenia is not fully defined. Most neonates and infants are treated empirically with prophylactic antibiotic therapy. Clinical literature documents the use of both intravenous immunoglobulin and recombinant human granulocyte colony-stimulating factor (r-G-CSF). Additionally, parents should be counseled regarding subsequent pregnancies that may be affected. Early serological detection in those cases will therefore allow for surveillance and management of affected offspring of future pregnancies. This patient received G-CSF on 2 occasions: (1) at the age of 4 days, he was given 1 dose of G-CSF for suspected oomphalitis, along with empiric antibiotic coverage and (2) at 9 weeks of age he once again received 1 dose of G-CSF with empiric antibiotic coverage for fever (104.4°F) with neutropenia (absolute neutrophil count of 322/µL). On both occasions robust increments in WBC and ANC counts were achieved. He has been followed in the outpatient clinic up to the age of 23 weeks. His ANC has remained in the normal range without G-CSF support for several weeks and he has not experienced any serious infections.

General Discussion Alloimmune neonatal neutropenia is caused by maternal sensitization to paternally inherited neutrophil antigens on fetal neutrophils that are missing on her own neutrophils. The passive transfer of these neutrophil-specific maternal IgG antibodies across the placenta occurs during pregnancy. These antibodies then bind to fetal neutrophils and may result in severe neutropenia. Immediately after birth some affected neonates have very low absolute neutrophil counts and may become symptomatic as a result with cutaneous infections, oomphalitis, otitis, fever, and respiratory or urinary tract infections. Often the bacterial infections are mild; however, serious infections do occur with a mortality rate of approximately 5%. In this case, no documented bacterial infection occurred, and the child was managed with empiric antibiotic coverage and administration of G-CSF. Alloimmune neonatal neutropenia as a cause for neonatal neutropenia occurs rarely; the reported incidence is less than or equal to 0.1%, but it is involved in 1.5% of all admissions to a neonatal special care unit. However, it is likely to be underdiagnosed and advances in techniques for antineutrophil antibody screening could lead to increased diagnosis of the condition. Hence confirmatory serological testing is advisable especially in unexplained neonatal neutropenia as in this case. In confirmed cases of alloimmune neonatal neutropenia, the following neutrophil-specific antibodies, HNA-1a, HNA-1b and HNA-2a, have been implicated in over 50% of these cases. Other neutrophil-specific antibodies such as HNA-1c, HNA-3a and HNA-4a can also lead to alloimmune neonatal neutropenia. Serological work-up and confirmation of this diagnosis is usually done in conjunction with a specialized laboratory (usually associated with specialized blood banks or the Red Cross). Confirmation of the diagnosis usually involves step-wise testing in the order outlined below:

- Neutrophil antibody screen—no single technique can detect all clinically relevant neutrophil antibodies; thus, a combination of granulocyte agglutination (GA) and granulocyte immunofluorescence (GIF) assays are used
- HLA antibody screen

Leukemoid Reaction Associated with Growth Factor Therapy

Linda Sandhaus

Patient A 62-year-old male with diarrhea.

Clinical History The patient had recently completed a second course of induction chemotherapy for B-precursor acute lymphoblastic leukemia. He was readmitted to the hospital.

Family History Noncontributory.

Medications Pegfilgrastim.

Physical Examination The patient appeared acutely ill, febrile and dehydrated.

Initial Work-Up

CBC		WBC Differential	%	# (×10³/µL)
WBC (×10³/µL)	33.7	Neutrophils	43	14.9
RBC (×10⁶/µL)	2.39	Bands	22	7.4
HGB (g/dL)	7.1	Lymphocytes	8	2.7
HCT (%)	21.3	Monocytes	4	1.4
MCV (fL)	89	Eosinophils	0	0
MCHC (g/dL)	33.3	Basophils	0	0
PLT (×10³/µL)	89	Metamyelocytes	9	3.0
RDW-CV (%)	16.8	Myelocytes	3	1.0
Promyelocyes	7 2.4	Blasts	4	1.4

Peripheral blood smear revealed immature granulocytes at various stages of maturation and prominent toxic granulation and Döhle bodies in neutrophils and bands (**Figures 1-4**).

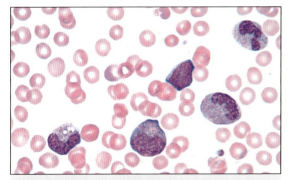

Figure 1 Blood smear (Wright-Giemsa, ×1000) showing a blast, a cell in transition from promyelocyte to myelocyte, 2 bands and a neutrophil.

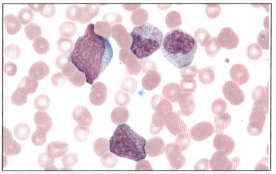

Figure 2 Blood smear (Wright-Giemsa, ×1000) showing 2 promyelocytes and 2 myelocytes.

Section I: Miscellaneous Hematologic Conditions
Leukemoid Reaction Associated with Growth Factor Therapy

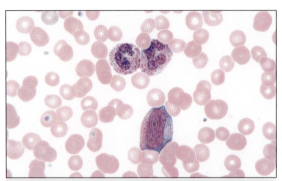

Figure 3 Blood smear (Wright-Giemsa, ×1000) showing 1 promyelocyte and toxic granulation in neutrophils/bands.

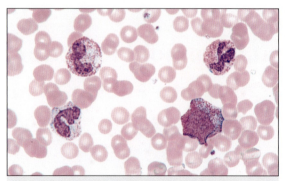

Figure 4 Blood smear (Wright-Giemsa, ×1000) showing 1 promyelocyte and toxic granulation and Döhle bodies in neutrophils/bands.

Differential Diagnosis The patient was recovering from recent chemotherapy for acute leukemia and presented with an acute febrile illness. The CBC was remarkable for normocytic anemia, thrombocytopenia, and a neutrophilia with marked left shift. The clinical history and neutrophila with left shift suggested an infectious etiology for the leukocytosis. However, given the history of acute leukemia, the presence of circulating blasts raises the question of recurrent acute leukemia. The patient was receiving Neulasta, a long-acting granulocytic growth factor, which could also explain the neutrophilic shift and circulating blasts.

Additional Work-Up Flow cytometry was performed on the peripheral blood. Approximately 3% of the leukocytes were CD13+, CD34+, CD117+ consistent with normal myeloblasts.

Final Diagnosis Leukemoid reaction secondary to growth factor effect.

Management Approach The patient underwent gastrointestinal evaluation and cultures were taken to search for a source of infection, which was never identified. He received antibiotics and antifungal agents and was discharged after resolution of the acute illness.

General Discussion Granulocyte colony stimulating factor (G-CSF) and granulocyte-macrophage colony stimulating factor (GM-CSF) are commonly used to shorten the period of neutropenia in patients who have received myelotoxic chemotherapy for cancer and following bone marrow transplantation. These agents are often used in other diseases associated with severe neutropenia, such as aplastic anemia and congenital neutropenias. Growth factors are also used to increase the number of circulating stem cells for stem cell collections. The use of these growth factors is associated with predictable changes in the peripheral blood and bone marrow granulocyte composition. Typically, there is a marked granulocytic hyperplasia in the marrow and a marked left shift in the peripheral blood. In the blood, the granulocytes display prominent "toxic" changes with prominent azurophilic granules and Döhle bodies. The left shift may include a relatively high percentage of early precursors, even when the WBC count is extremely low. It can be difficult to distinguish promyelocytes from myelocytes due to nuclear/cytoplasmic asynchrony and the prominence of the primary granules. GM-CSF also causes an eosinophilia and monocytosis. Patients who receive these agents to mobilize peripheral blood stem cells for autologous bone marrow transplantation may achieve very high WBC counts after a few days of treatment. Hypersegmented and hyposegmented neutrophils and occasional neutrophils with ring nuclei may be seen. These morphologic variants may reflect decreased marrow maturation time. Other morphologic findings that have been described with growth factor therapy include immature monocytes with prominent vacuolization and leukoerythroblastic reaction as the WBC count increases. Myeloblasts usually account for <2% of the WBC; however, rarely patients may exhibit significantly higher blast counts, which can be problematic, especially in patients whose underlying disease is acute leukemia or myelodysplastic syndrome. In patients with ALL, flow cytometry can readily distinguish between leukemic lymphoblasts and growth factor-induced myeloblasts by their distinctly different immunophenotypes. For patients with AML, flow cytometry is also useful, particularly when the immunophenotype of the patient's known leukemic blast population is known. Leukemic blasts usually have some aberrant phenotypic expression that allows distinction from normal myeloblasts. Not uncommonly, pathologists review peripheral blood and bone marrow samples from patients who are receiving growth factors, but this history is not provided. The presence of a marked toxic left shift in a known oncology patient, particularly in the presence of neutropenia, should alert the pathologist to the likelihood of growth factor therapy. Another scenario that is becoming increasingly frequent is the patient with undiagnosed neutropenia who has already received growth factor therapy prior to the performance of a diagnostic bone marrow. A high index of suspicion for growth factor therapy and a phone call to confirm it may be necessary for correct interpretation of the morphologic findings.

Chronic Benign Neutropenia

Suba Krishnan

Patient A 17-month-old female child with a low absolute neutrophil count (ANC).

Clinical History This toddler was born full-term by normal delivery. There were no perinatal complications (no neutropenia, no jaundice, no anemia). At 8 months of age, she was seen in the emergency room with fever and treated for otitis media. At 12 months of age, she was noted to be neutropenic on a routine blood count. Before she could be evaluated further by hematology, she was admitted with fever and neutropenia and treated with prophylactic antibiotics and subsequently discharged when blood culture and urine culture remained negative, with satisfactory increase in ANC. She has not suffered from skin infections such as cellulitis or recurrent abscesses. She had diaper rash once, which resolved with local application of diaper ointment. She has never developed oral ulcers or mucositis. There is no history of documented pneumonia, bacteremia or sepsis.

Family History Both parents are in good health. This is their first child. Both parents are of Hispanic ethnicity (from Puerto Rico).

Medications None.

Physical Examination Unremarkable. Height is 50th percentile for age; weight is 75th percentile for age. No organomegaly noted.

Initial Work-Up and Pertinent Serial Laboratory Results

Date	10/22/09	10/14/09	10/13/09	10/12/09	7/23/09	6/17/09	5/26/09	3/26/09
WBC ($\times 10^3/\mu L$)	4.7	5.3	3.9	2.9	4.6	4.7	5.9	6.3
ANC ($\times 10^3/\mu L$)	235	689	78	116	138	752	767	378
APC (ANC + absolute monocyte count)	752	1,219	546	667	506	1,316	885	819
HGB (g/dL)	12.7	12.5	11.7	11.8	12.9	12.1	11.7	12.3
MCV (fL)	74.9	76.3	77	75.6	76	75	75	76
PLT ($\times 10^3/\mu L$)	273	240	182	220	314	303	305	306
Reticulocytes (%)	0.8		0.4	0.5				
Blood culture			Neg ×5 days					

Section I: Miscellaneous Hematologic Conditions
Chronic Benign Neutropenia

Differential Diagnosis Conditions associated with chronic absolute neutropenia include hypersplenism, viral suppression, primary autoimmune neutropenia, secondary neutropenia (including HIV, Evan syndrome), primary immunodeficiency disorder with cytopenias, drug-induced neutropenia, and severe congenital neutropenia including Kostmann syndrome and cyclic neutropenia. Bone marrow failure syndromes, particularly Schwachman-Diamond syndrome, could also present with isolated neutropenia as a hematologic abnormality in the setting of a constellation of other clinical features including growth failure.

Additional Work-Up

Coombs	Negative
ANA panel	Negative
Parvo B19 IgG/IgM	Negative
EBV panel	Negative for recent or past infection
CMV IgG/IgM	Negative
Immunoglobulin panel	Normal for age
HIV	Negative
Antineutrophil antibody by flow cytometry. (Granulocyte immunofluorescence and granulocyte agglutination)	Positive for neutrophil-specific antibodies to HNA-1b
Monoclonal antibody immobilization of neutrophil antigens (MAINA)	Extended antibody testing in the MAINA assay detected reactivity to the CD16 molecule (FcγRIIIb)
Granulocyte antibodies (cANCA, pANCA)	Negative
Bone marrow aspiration and biopsy	Trilineage maturation; mature neutrophils noted but decreased in number, with compensatory increase in immature forms (promyelocytes, metamyelocytes and bands) No dysplastic neutrophil precursors noted No blasts No immunophenotypically abnormal cells seen Normal karyotype: 46XX

This toddler has had neutropenia for over 6 months since it was first noted. During this period, her ANC has ranged between 100-800/μL and her APC (absolute phagocyte count = absolute neutrophil count + absolute monocyte count) has ranged between 500 and 1,300/μL. She has not had any significant infection despite these low absolute neutrophil counts and after a documented episode of fever, her ANC and APC both increased within 24 hours of onset of fever, suggesting that she does have some bone marrow reserve capacity that is able to support her through infectious episodes. Additionally, her platelet count also appears to have decreased during her recent febrile illness and sometimes that can be an indication of the presence of antiplatelet antibodies as well. Absence of splenomegaly ruled out hypersplenism as a cause of neutropenia. The viral serologies were all negative and the chronic nature of her neutropenia ruled out viral suppression. She is growing well and does not have GI symptoms suggestive of Schwachman-Diamond syndrome. Her HIV status was negative. Her ANA screen was negative, ruling out secondary autoimmune neutropenia; additionally Coombs test was negative, ruling out the possibility of an Evan syndrome. Her immunoglobulin levels were normal, ruling out underlying immunodeficiency disorder, and she is not on any medication to suggest a drug-induced process. She was advised to have serial weekly CBCs measured for 6 weeks to assess for possible cyclic neutropenia, but her mother has not been compliant so far in following through with this. However, she has not had any documented serious infection in the 7 months since neutropenia was noted.

Final Diagnosis The clinical picture (age of onset: 11 months-12 months of age and benign clinical course so far) and work-up are consistent with a diagnosis of chronic benign neutropenia or primary autoimmune neutropenia of childhood.

Management Approach Most children do not have significant or serious infections. All parents are advised to seek immediate medical attention should the child develop fever (>101.5°F) or any features of a severe infection. Treatment of presenting infection with appropriate antibiotics is sufficient in most instances. Filgrastim (G-CSF), corticosteroids, and intravenous immunoglobulin have all been demonstrated to raise the neutrophil count. G-CSF is used even when there is a temporary need to raise the neutrophil count, for example in severe infection or before surgery. This child has not been treated with G-CSF so far. She has only received antibiotics for an episode of fever with neutropenia.

General Discussion Chronic benign neutropenia of infancy and childhood, also known as primary autoimmune neutropenia, is caused by neutrophil specific antibodies. It is 10-fold more common than severe congenital neutropenia (associated with much more serious infections) with an incidence of 1:100,000. It is a condition that occurs predominantly in infancy (median age of diagnosis is 8 months; majority are diagnosed by 15 months of age). Most children present with febrile episodes associated with minor infections of the skin, respiratory and urinary tracts, or otitis media. Despite severe neutropenia (ANC <500 is commonly seen), serious or life threatening infections occur very rarely, with the vast majority of cases suffering only minor infections that do not require long-term treatment. Additionally, most children undergo spontaneous remission 6 months-2 years after diagnosis. Once a positive antineutrophil antibody has been demonstrated, in the absence of other clinical features, the diagnosis of primary autoimmune neutropenia can be made without the need for bone marrow examination. However, repeated testing is often required before positive antineutrophil antibodies can be demonstrated in the patient. If bone marrow examination is performed, the marrow is usually normocellular or hypocellular with a reduction in segmented neutrophils. However, trilineage maturation is noted without any dysplastic cells or blasts.

Acute Graft-vs-Host Disease

Neal Flomenberg, Dolores Grosso, George Murphy

Patient A 62-year-old Caucasian female presents with rash, nausea, vomiting and diarrhea 6 months after hematopoietic progenitor cell transplant (HPCT).

Clinical History She had originally presented with asymptomatic lymphocytosis during routine yearly history and physical exam, and was diagnosed with chronic lymphocytic leukemia (CLL). Fluorescent in situ hybridization of her CLL cells demonstrated deletion of 17p. Her absolute lymphocyte count was about 40,000/μL at presentation and rose to 150,000/μL over the next 8 months. She did not have appreciable adenopathy. A spleen tip was palpable at the costal margin. Because of her high-risk status (including deletion 17p) and family history as noted below, the decision was made to proceed to HPCT, after initial control of her disease with alemtuzumab. Because of her strong family history of CLL, an unrelated donor was deemed to be her preferred donor option rather than a transplant from a first-degree relative. Following 4 months of alemtuzumab therapy, she was transplanted using a regimen consisting of fludarabine, cytosine arabinoside, cyclophosphamide, and alemtuzumab, and received prophylaxis against graft-vs-host disease with mycophenolate mofetil and tacrolimus. Her counts recovered promptly without CD5+ B lymphocytes in the peripheral blood. Marrow and blood chimerism revealed that about 50% of the cells were of donor origin and 50% were of host origin. Her mycophenolate mofetil was stopped 28 days post-transplant, and her tacrolimus was tapered off by about 4 months after transplant, following institutional guidelines. About a month later (5 months after HPCT), her chimerism showed a shift to 92% donor-derived cells. 3 weeks later, at a routine follow-up appointment, she noted onset of several new symptoms over the last few days prior to the visit. These included rash, 1-2 loose stools per day, nausea and 1 episode of vomiting, and dark urine. As a consequence, the decision was made to admit her to the hospital.

Family History There was a family history of CLL in several relatives, which in several of these cases was associated with a short duration of survival, including her father, paternal grandmother, and a paternal uncle.

Medications Valacyclovir.

Physical Examination It was remarkable for obvious scleral icterus. Skin exam revealed jaundice and an erythematous maculopapular rash over 75% of her body with some vesicles and bullae (**Figure 1**). There were some lacey, whitish, lichenoid changes over the buccal mucosa. There was no adenopathy or hepatosplenomegaly. The rest of the exam was unremarkable.

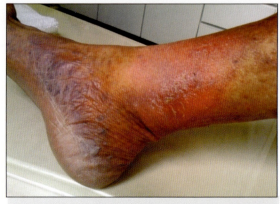

Figure 1 Acute GVHD clinical appearance (clinical photo courtesy of Arturo Saavedra).

Section I: Miscellaneous Hematologic Conditions
Acute Graft-vs-Host Disease

Initial Work-Up				
CBC		WBC Differential	%	# (×10³/µL)
WBC (×10³/µL)	2.3	Neutrophils	51	1.2
RBC (×10⁶/µL)	3.09	Bands	1	0.0
HGB (g/dL)	9.9	Eosinophils	7	0.2
HCT (%)	30.5	Basophils	1	0.0
MCV (fl)	99	Lymphocytes	32	0.7
MCH (pg)	32	Monocytes	8	0.2
MCHC (%)	33.4			
PLT (×10³/µL)	106			
	Day of admission	10 days prior to admission		
Total bilirubin (mg/dL)	11.7	0.7		
Direct bilirubin (mg/dL)	7.0	0.2		
Alkaline phosphatase (mg/dL)	468	84		
AST (SGOT) (mg/dL)	441	35		
ALT (SGPT) (mg/dL)	538	26		

Differential Diagnosis The triad of skin rash, loose or diarrheal stools, and jaundice is consistent with acute graft-vs-host disease (GVHD). GVHD of the upper gastrointestinal tract can also cause anorexia, nausea, and emesis. The major items to rule out include drug eruptions (unlikely on valacyclovir alone), a variety of viral diseases, including cytomegalovirus, viral hepatitis, adenovirus, and others, and enteric infection with *Clostridium difficile*. These agents may represent alternative or contemporaneous diagnoses. Biliary tract stone disease was less likely given her prior cholecystectomy. Autoimmune hemolysis secondary to her CLL was also deemed unlikely as her CLL was in complete remission. Microangiopathic hemolysis due to calcineurin inhibitors was thought unlikely to have begun after the tacrolimus had already been tapered off.

Additional Work-Up Stool cultures were negative for *Clostridium difficile* and other enteric pathogens. Viral loads and serologies for relevant pathogens were negative. Ultrasound of the biliary tree was unremarkable. Biopsies of skin, liver, upper gut, and colon were obtained and were consistent with acute GVHD (**Figures 2**, **3**, and **4**). Coombs test was negative. There were no schistocytes or spherocytes on peripheral blood smear.

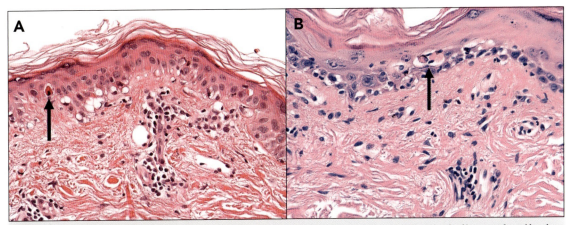

Figure 2 Skin biopsy **A** (H&E, ×200) showing early acute GVHD in skin, showing sparse superficial lymphoid infiltrate, epidermal basal cell layer vacuolization, and scattered apoptotic keratinocytes (arrow). **B** (H&E, ×400) An area of more advanced cutaneous acute GVHD, showing increased number of apoptotic cells associated with lymphocytes in apposition (satellitosis; arrow). Note the sparse lymphoid infiltrate, yet the substantial epidermal injury, a characteristic feature of this condition.

Section I: Miscellaneous Hematologic Conditions
Acute Graft-vs-Host Disease

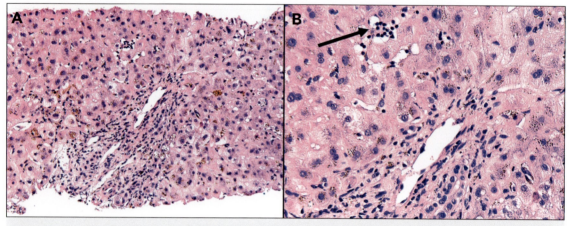

Figure 3 Liver biopsy **A** (H&E, ×200) and **B** (H&E, ×400) with acute GVHD; there is a prominent periportal lymphoid infiltration with distortion and destruction of the bile duct epithelium, evidence of cholestasis, and scattered necrotic hepatocytes associated with lymphocyte apposition (arrow).

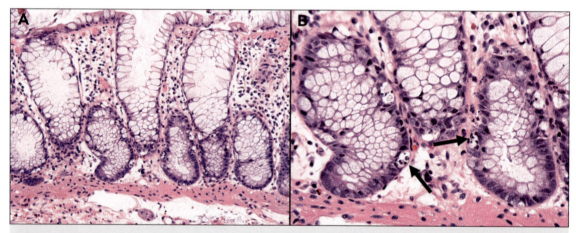

Figure 4 Colon biopsy **A** (H&E, ×200) and **B** (H&E, ×400) showing colorectal mucosa in acute GVHD; there is a sparse lymphoid infiltrate involving the crypts, with scattered apoptotic cells flanking the lateral borders of the lowermost portions of the crypts (arrows).

Final Diagnosis Acute GVHD of skin, GI tract, and liver.

Management Approach The patient was started on methylprednisolone 1mg/kg intravenously every 12 hours. Skin and gastrointestinal manifestations resolved. However, liver function tests continued to worsen. Tacrolimus and mycophenolate mofetil were added, but liver function tests continued to worsen, ultimately peaking at a bilirubin of 40.9, alkaline phosphatase 597 mg/dL, AST 616 mg/dL, ALT 1,021 mg/dL. Lympholytic therapy with muromonab-CD3 was administered for 14 days, and liver function studies slowly improved. Corticosteroids were slowly tapered off. Tacrolimus was slowly tapered off, and mycophenolate mofetil was discontinued. Most recent liver chemistries were total bilirubin 0.8, alkaline phosphatase 205 mg/dL, AST 57 mg/dL, ALT 47 mg/dL.

General Discussion GVHD is a major cause of morbidity and mortality after allogeneic HPCT. The process is initiated by allogeneic lymphocytes capable of recognizing minor or major histocompatibility antigens present in the recipient but lacking in the donor. Depletion of T cells from the graft inoculum can dramatically reduce the incidence and severity of graft-vs-host disease, but at the price of increased rates of graft rejection, immunoincompetence, opportunistic infections, and relapse. Acute GVHD typically involves skin, gut, and liver in varying combinations. Other organs may be involved less frequently. Lymphocyte-mediated inflammation and apoptosis of skin or gut epithelium and the small bile ducts of the liver characterize the process. The percentage of the body involved with skin rash, the volume of diarrhea, and the degree of bilirubin elevation are used to assess the overall grade of acute GVHD. The incidence of severe acute GVHD is influenced by age, graft source (marrow vs peripheral blood vs umbilical cord blood), donor type (matched sibling, unrelated donor, mismatched donor), sex matching and donor parity, and other factors. In HLA-identical sibling transplantation, the incidence of severe GVHD is around 10%. Higher incidences are seen in unrelated donor transplantation. In the past acute and chronic GVHD were separated based on the time of onset. As the number of different sources of stem cells has increased, time of onset has proved to be a poor distinguishing characteristic and these 2 entities are now separated based on clinical and pathologic characteristics. In cases of severe GVHD, it is not uncommon for skin manifestations to resolve while visceral manifestations persist or worsen. Rarely, liver failure or intestinal perforation will directly contribute to the death of a patient from acute GVHD. More often, it is the severe immunoincompetence caused by the condition itself and its treatment that leads to the patient's demise.

Chronic Graft-vs-Host Disease

Neal Flomenberg, Dolores Grosso, George Murphy

Patient A 42-year-old Caucasian female, who had previously undergone allogeneic hematopoietic progenitor cell transplantation (HPCT), presented with stiff fingers and hands.

Clinical History The patient had undergone allogeneic HPCT for mantle cell lymphoma in second remission. Her original diagnosis had been made 3 years earlier when she was treated with rituximab, cyclophosphamide, doxorubicin and prednisone (R-CHOP) and involved field radiation. She relapsed 3 years later, achieved a second remission with R-CHOP and underwent a nonmyeloablative HPCT from her HLA-identical sister. Chimerism assays performed 28 days after transplant by analyzing short tandem repeat polymorphisms in genomic DNA demonstrated 96% of cells in blood and marrow were of donor origin, increasing to over 99% by the end of the second month after transplant. Her immune suppression was tapered off by 4 months after transplant. Marrow and CT studies 3 and 6 months after transplant showed continued complete remission. At her 9-month visit, she reported stiffness in her fingers and hands. She indicated that she had seen her primary care physician and had been advised to take nonsteroidal anti-inflammatory drugs for arthritis. She reported difficulty turning door knobs because of her inability to extend her wrists. On further questioning, she reported that her eyes were dry and she also noted vaginal dryness. Within the prior few weeks, she had developed ulcerations over her shins at the sites of minor trauma.

Family History Noncontributory.

Medications Valacyclovir, ibuprofen, sumatriptan.

Physical Examination The exam was remarkable for stiffness and thickening of her fingers. Her skin was taut with reduction in the fine skin creases and markings. She could no longer fully extend her digits or wrists fully. Ulcerations were noted over both shins (**Figure 1**). Her conjunctivae were injected. Her mouth was dry but was without other changes in the gums or buccal mucosa. There was no adenopathy or organomegaly. The rest of her exam was unremarkable.

Initial Work-Up

CBC		WBC Differential	%	# ($\times 10^3/\mu L$)
WBC ($\times 10^3/\mu L$)	7.3	Neutrophils	49	3.6
RBC ($\times 10^6/\mu L$)	4.13	Eosinophils	33	2.4
HGB (g/dL)	13.2	Lymphocytes	7	0.5
HCT (%)	39.1	Monocytes	11	0.8
MCV (fl)	94.8			
MCH (pg)	31.9			
MCHC (%)	33.7			
PLT ($\times 10^3/\mu L$)	295			

Liver enzymes were normal.

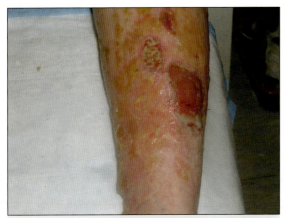

Figure 1 Clinical appearance, chronic (sclerodermoid) GVHD thickened, indurated skin with ulceration is noted (clinical photo courtesy of Arturo Saavedra).

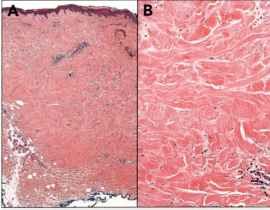

Figure 2 Skin biopsy **A** (H&E, ×40) showing diffuse replacement of reticular dermis by thickened collagen bundles, producing a characteristically 'squared-off' biopsy contour; **B** (H&E, ×400) showing thickened, pale collagen bundles with attenuation of intervening spaces. These changes are indistinguishable from morphea.

Differential Diagnosis The skin findings, conjuctival inflammation, mucosal dryness, and eosinophilia are consistent with sclerodermatous chronic graft-vs-host disease (GVHD).

Additional Work-Up Rodnan skin score (assessing the extent of sclerodermatous skin change) was 22. Schirmer test demonstrated a moderate decrease in tear production. Skin biopsy was consistent with chronic GVHD (**Figure 2**).

Final Diagnosis Chronic GVHD of skin and eyes.

Management Approach The patient was started on methylprednisolone and cyclosporine. Physical therapy was consulted and prepared splints for her wrists and hands to maintain them in a more functional position. Range-of-motion exercises were also initiated. Ophthalmology provided preservative-free eye moistening drops, placed plugs in her tear ducts, and initiated a brief trial of cyclosporine ophthalmic emulsion eye drops. Over the next 6 months, the skin in the hands and wrists softened, resulting in a gradual return to normal range of motion and functional utility. Immune suppression was tapered off over the next 6 months without reappearance of the skin manifestations. Her eyes remain a bit dry so she continues to use tear duct plugs and eye drops. She returned to work and has remained without recurrence for 7 years after transplant.

General Discussion GVHD is a major cause of morbidity and mortality after allogeneic bone marrow or peripheral blood stem cell transplantation. The process is initiated by allogeneic lymphocytes capable of recognizing minor or major histocompatibility antigens present in the recipient but lacking in the donor. Chronic GVHD, as described here, may evolve from acute GVHD or may develop de novo. Chronic GHVD has a wide range of manifestations. Skin manifestations may resemble lichen planus or scleroderma. Sun exposure may trigger exacerbations. Liver abnormalities typically manifest in a cholestatic pattern. Though abnormalities may persist for years, portal hypertension and cirrhosis are rare. Ocular sicca syndrome and oral dryness are common. Patients may experience oral pain or discomfort related to spicy or acidic foods. Lichenoid changes in the oral mucosa may be confused with candidiasis. Obstructive lung disease, dysphagia, and weight loss can also be manifestations. Patients are commonly immunodeficient and hypogammaglobulinemic. Antibiotic prophylaxis for encapsulated organisms and *Pneumocystis carinii* pneumonia and replacement intravenous immune globulin (IV Ig) are often important adjuncts to the primary GVHD therapy. Chronic GVHD has been associated with a graft vs tumor effect, most noticeable in patients transplanted with relapsed disease. However chronic GVHD contributes to transplant related mortality and to a diminished quality of life. In that regard, the patient presented here did well.

Donor Lymphocyte Infusion Therapy

Neal Flomenberg, Dolores Grosso, Alina Dulau Florea

Patient A 42-year-old Caucasian female with fatigue 1 year after allogeneic hematopoietic progenitor cell transplantation (HPCT).

Clinical History The patient has a history of Philadelphia chromosome-positive (Ph+) chronic myelogenous leukemia (CML) in accelerated phase and had undergone HPCT after demonstrating intolerance of tyrosine kinase inhibitor therapy. Her HLA-identical brother was her donor. Following transplant, blood counts recovered promptly and bone marrow morphology appeared normal on an aspirate and biopsy 30 days post-transplant. Cytogenetic studies revealed that 20 of 20 cells showed a normal male (XY) karyotype without the Philadelphia chromosome. BCR/ABL transcripts were not detected by PCR analysis. She had no clinically evident graft-vs-host disease (GVHD) throughout her post-transplant course. At the time of her 1-year anniversary visit, she reported that she had felt a bit more tired over the past 3 months. No other new symptoms were elicited on a thorough review of systems.

Family and Social History Noncontributory.

Medications Valayclovir.

Physical Examination It was remarkable only for a palpable spleen. The spleen had not been palpable during the prior 6 months. There was no clinical evidence of GVHD and no evidence of a localized or systemic infection.

Initial Work-Up

CBC		WBC Differential	%	# (×10³/µL)
WBC (×10³/µL)	45.3	Neutrophils	65	29.4
RBC (×10⁶/µL)	3.44	Bands	9	3.6
HGB (g/dL)	10.3	Metamyelocytes	5	2.3
HCT (%)	31.5	Myelocytes	3	1.4
MCV (fl)	82	Promyelocytes	2	0.9
MCH (pg)	29.9	Blasts	1	0.5
MCHC (%)	33.3	Eosinophils	3	1.4
PLT (×10³/µL)	550	Basophils	2	0.9
		Lymphocytes	2	0.9
		Monocytes	8	3.6

Differential Diagnosis Based on peripheral blood findings the diagnostic considerations included recurrent/relapsed CML or leukemoid reaction. It would be unlikely that she would have developed a different myeloproliferative disorder in the post-transplant setting.

Additional Work-Up There were no infectious symptoms or signs to suggest that this was a leukemoid reaction. Bone marrow was hypercellular and showed trilineage hematopoiesis with full maturation and small megakaryocytes (**Figure 1**). The M:E ratio was

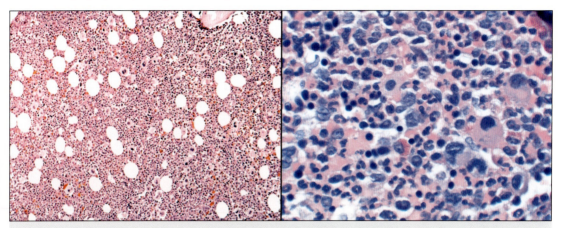

Figure 1 Bone marrow biopsy at presentation **A** (H&E, ×100) and **B** (H&E, ×400) showing hypercellular marrow with granulocytic hyperplasia and small megakaryocytes, consistent with chronic myelogenous leukemia in chronic phase.

significantly increased due to granulocytic hyperplasia. These findings were consistent with CML.

Cytogenetics and Molecular Studies 20/20 cells demonstrated a female (XX) karyotype with the Philadelphia chromosome. By fluorescent in situ hybridization (FISH), 190 of 200 cells were XX, 7 XY and 3 XO. (Note that normal male cells may occasionally lose the Y chromosome producing an XO karyotype.) Approximately 95% of the cells revealed fusion signal for BCR-ABL.

Final Diagnosis Relapsed chronic myelogenous leukemia.

Management Approach Her counts were controlled with 500 mg hydroxyurea twice a day. The patient received 3 donor lymphocyte infusions (DLI) from her HPCT donor to deliver a dose of T cells of 1×10^8/kg. Little happened over the next 2 months until the patient abruptly became neutropenic and thrombocytopenic 9 weeks-10 weeks after the donor lymphocyte infusions. A repeat bone marrow specimen was now completely aplastic (**Figure 2**). Within a few weeks, the patient slowly recovered normal counts. A follow-up marrow obtained shortly after recovery of normal blood counts was normocellular with trilineage normal hematopiesis (**Figure 3**). Cytogenetic studies revealed that 20 of 20 cells demonstrated a normal male karyotype (XY, Ph–). FISH revealed 92% XY cells, 5% XO cells and 3% XX cells. FISH analyses for BCR-ABL fusion were negative, but PCR analysis revealed that BCR-ABL transcripts could be amplified from the patient's marrow. A routine marrow study was performed 3 months later (approximately 6 months-7 months after donor lymphocyte therapy). 20 of 20 cells demonstrated a normal male karyotype (XY, Ph–). FISH studies revealed 95% XY cells and 5% XO cells without BCR-ABL fusion signal. PCR studies could no longer detect BCR-ABL transcripts. The patient developed mild GVHD responsive to a short course of corticosteroids. She remains in molecular remission, 7 years after her donor lymphocyte therapy. Her performance status is 100%.

General Discussion Allogeneic hematopoietic progenitor cell transplantation can eradicate hematologic malignancies through 2 mechanisms. Myeloablative transplants utilize dose intensive treatment in an effort to ablate the malignancy. The transplant of hematopoietic progenitor cells serves as rescue of the patient from the aplastic state that would result from simultaneous ablation of the normal

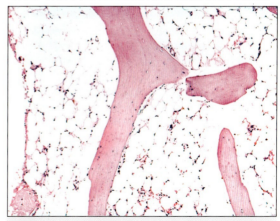

Figure 2 Bone marrow biopsy obtained 10 weeks after donor lymphocyte infusion (H&E, ×100) showing aplastic marrow with few hematopoietic precursors evident.

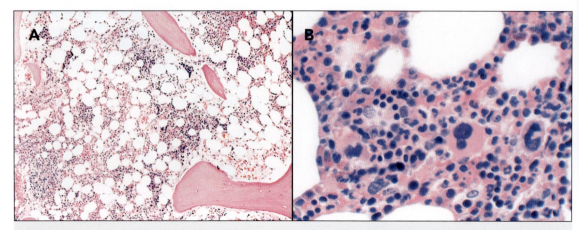

Figure 3 Bone marrow biopsy **A** (H&E, ×100) and **B** (H&E, ×400) normocellular marrow with trilineage hematopoiesis and normal cellular maturation, consistent with hematologic remission and complete recovery. Note: **Figures 1A** and **2** were originally published in *Blood* 82:2,310-2,318, 1993. They are reproduced with the permission of William Drobyski and the American Society of Hematology.

marrow elements. Allogeneic transplants also eradicate malignancy through graft-vs-tumor effects. One of the best examples of clinically relevant graft-vs-tumor effects is the demonstration that, in a number of hematologic malignancies, relapse rates are higher in recipients of transplants from identical twin donors than in recipients of similar transplants from HLA-identical siblings. The relative contributions of dose intensity and graft-vs-tumor effects varies amongst different hematologic malignancies. In CML, the donor immune system is important for the long-term control of the disease. If one T cell depletes transplants for CML in an effort to control GVHD, relapse rates increase appreciably. Conversely, most patients who relapse after transplant respond to donor lymphocyte therapy if their disease is still in a chronic phase. Response rates are lower in patients with accelerated or blast phase disease. As in this case, when the patient has reverted to almost all host-type hematopoiesis, a period of aplasia may ensue after donor lymphocyte therapy. The frequency and severity of this may be less if patients still have a significant component of donor derived hematopoiesis at the time of lymphocyte infusion. Fewer transplants are now performed in CML because of the availability of tyrosine kinase inhibitor therapy. Most transplants for CML now occur in patients who are intolerant of the tyrosine kinase inhibitors or who acquire resistance to these drugs, usually through mutations in the BCR-ABL gene. Indolent lymphoproliferative disorders are also exquisitely sensitive to graft-vs-tumor effects. Many centers will approach indolent lymphoproliferative disorders with reduced intensity approaches relying on the donor immune system, rather than ablative radiochemotherapy, to cure the patient. The degree of eradication of the underlying malignancy may be quite profound after DLI therapy such that no evidence of residual malignancy can be detected even using the most sensitive techniques available. Many CML patients who have relapsed after transplant have had longstanding remissions (and presumed cure) after DLI. Although donor T cells may persist in these patients at the time of relapse after transplant, these cells appear to have become tolerant of the CML, while the newly infused donor lymphocytes instead mount an effective immune response capable of controlling the disease.

Transient Abnormal Myelopoiesis

John Kim Choi

Patient A 6-week-old boy with Down syndrome (DS).

Clinical History Normal vaginal delivery at 38-week gestation. A CBC performed at day 3 of life revealed a WBC of $15 \times 10^3/\mu L$ with 12% blasts.

Family History Noncontributory.

Medications None.

Physical Examination He has facial features consistent with Down syndrome, and hepatosplenomegaly on abdominal examination.

Initial Work-Up

CBC		Normal
WBC (×10³/µL)	153.4	(5.0-19.5)
RBC (×10⁶/µL)	1.64	(3.0-5.4)
HGB (g/dL)	6.4	(10.0-18.0)
HCT (%)	16.6	(31.0-55.0)
MCV (fL)	101.8	(85.0-123.0)
MCH (pg)	38.9	(28.0-40.0)
MCHC (g/dL)	38.2	(29.0-37.0)
PLT (×10³/µL)	134	(150-400)
RDW-CV (%)	20.4	(11.5-14.5)
MPV (fL)	7.6	(7.4-10.4)
WBC Differential	**%**	**# (×10³/µL)**
Neutrophils	14	21.5
Bands	0	
Lymphocytes	8	12.3
Monocytes	1	1.5
Eosinophils	0	
Basophils	0	
Blasts	77	118.1

Peripheral blood smear revealed many blasts (**Figure 1**).

Differential Diagnosis Transient abnormal myelopoiesis (TAM), DS-associated acute myeloid leukemia (DS-AML), non-DS-associated AML or acute lymphoid leukemia (ALL).

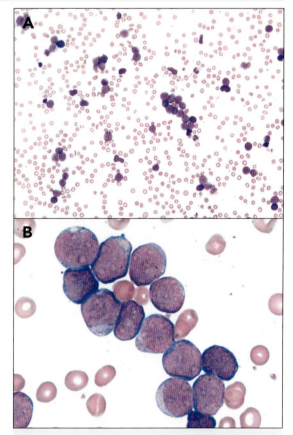

Figure 1 Blood smear **A** (Wright-Giemsa, ×400) **B** (Wright-Giemsa, ×1000) showing many blasts.

Additional Work-Up By flow cytometry the blasts were positive for CD45 (dim), CD34, CD33 and CD61 and negative for B cell (CD19, cytoplasmic CD79a), T cell (CD3, CD5), granulocytic (cytoplasmic MPO), monocytic (CD4, CD14) and erythroid (Glycophorin A) antigens. Cytogenetic karyotyping demonstrated constitutional trisomy 21 and additional chromosome 19 and 21: 49XY,+19,+21,+21c[19].

Final Diagnosis Transient abnormal myelopoiesis.

Management Approach Typically, TAM spontaneously resolves within 2 days-194 days with a mean of 58 days. However, 11%-52% of TAM cases are associated with neonatal death secondary to liver failure, heart failure, sepsis, hemorrhage, hyperviscosity, and disseminated intravascular coagulation. Some patients with leukocytosis, ascites, preterm delivery, or bleeding respond favorably to low dose cytosine arabinoside therapy. This patient was managed conservatively with hydration, red cell transfusions, and observation. WBC and blast percentage decreased such that by 4 months of age, the WBC was $8.0 \times 10^3/\mu L$ with 0% blasts. The patient was surveyed closely for occurence of AML and ALL that have increased incidence in DS children.

General Discussion Transient abnormal myelopoiesis (TAM) has been also designated transient myeloproliferative disorder (TMD) and transient leukemia (TL). TAM is defined as the morphologic detection of blasts in a DS patient <3 months of age. This disease is unique to DS patients and usually detected in the 1st week of life and spontaneously resolves by 3 months of age. Occasional cases are detected in the fetus. The incidence of TAM is 3%-6% of all DS patients. The blasts in TAM are of megakaryocytic origin in the vast majority of cases and can be equal to or >20% of the white blood cells in the peripheral blood. The morphology and immunophenotype of the blasts are virtually identical to both DS and non-DS-associated acute megakaryoblastic leukemia (DS-AMKL and non-DS-AMKL) and their distinction requires clinical and cytogenetic information (**Table 1**).

Table 1 Distinguishing characteristics among TAM, DS-AMKL, and non-DS-AMKL

	TAM	DS-AMKL	Non-DS-AMKL
DS/trisomy 21	+	+	–
GATA1 mutation	+	+	–
t(1;22)	–	–	±
Age	<3 months	>6 months	Any

At <3 months of age, the diagnosis in a patient with DS is almost always TAM. However, the possibility that blasts are unrelated to DS cannot be completely excluded and other diagnoses such as congenital acute leukemia (myeloid or lymphoid) need to be excluded. TAM should be considered even in a patient without apparent DS because the infant could be mosaic for trisomy 21 and may not display the characteristic physical features. The bone marrow findings in TAM ranges from increased blasts with a percentage similar or less than that seen in the peripheral blood. Occasional cases show few to no blasts despite the presence of numerous blasts in the peripheral blood. Other bone marrow findings include megakaryocytic hyperplasia, dyspoietic megakaryocytes and dyspoietic erythroid precursors. Blast infiltration has been also reported in skin and liver with the latter showing increased extramedullary hematopoiesis, dysplastic megkaryocytes, and megakaryoblasts, associated with diffuse lobular fibrosis. The blasts in TAM can have typical megakaryoblastic morphology (occasional binucleation, slightly round condensation of the chromatin, scant basophilic cytoplasm, occasional fine azurophilic granules consistent with platelet granules, and cytoplasmic blebbing). In some TAMs, the blasts resemble lymphoblasts, erythroblasts, myeloblasts, and even monoblasts. Hence, the blasts in TAM are often difficult to distinguish from blasts in AML and even some ALL cases. By cytochemistry, the TAM blasts are negative for Sudan black B, negative for myeloperoxidase, negative for chloroacetate esterase, occasionally granular to block positive for periodic acid-Schiff (PAS), and strongly positive for acid phosphatase. The nonspecific esterase staining, depending on substrate used and reaction conditions, varies from negative to multi-punctate pattern that is partially resistant to fluoride inhibition but not a diffuse cytoplasmic pattern that is typical of monocytic differentiation. By ultrastructural cytochemistry, the peroxidase activity is limited to the nuclear envelope and the endoplasmic reticulum, a pattern is typically referred as platelet peroxidase (PPO). Immunophenotyping by flow cytometry demonstrates that the TAM blasts are megakaryoblasts and express CD45, CD34, CD33, CD38, CD36, CD56, HLA-DR, CD7, and at least 1 of the megakaryocytic markers CD41, CD42a, or CD61. Less frequently, the TAM blasts express CD13, CD11b, CD265 (glycophorin A), CD4, or CD15. In general, flow cytometry detection of CD41, CD42b, or CD61 reactivity on blasts indicates megakaryocytic lineage. However, this reactivity can be seen on non-megakaryoblasts with platelet satellitosis that can be excluded by examining the Wright-stained cytospin of the flow cytometry specimen or immunohistochemstry for CD61 on cytospin preparations. All TAM blasts contain extra copies of chromosome 21. In some patients, the TAM blasts have additional karyotypic abnormalities consisting of complex karyotypes or non-recurrent aberrations. All TAM blasts have various somatic mutations in the X-linked gene GATA1 that encodes a transcription factor that is critical for normal erythroid and megakaryocytic development. Trisomy 21 and GATA1 mutations are also present in TAMs that present in neonates who are mosaic for trisomy 21 and lack the clinical feature of DS. A subset of TAM also has mutations in the tyrosine kinase JAK3. Following resolution of TAM, 13%-29% of the DS children develop acute megakaryocytic leukemia (AMKL) after 6 months of age. TAMs presenting with other cytogenetic abnormalites in addition to trisomy 21, pleural effusion, and thrombocytopenia ($<100 \times 10^3/\mu L$) have an increased risk of developing AMKL; in contrast, CBC indices other than platelet count, percentage of blasts, AST, ALT, age, and sex have no prognosis in predicting the occurrence of DS-AMKL.

Pelger-Huët Anomaly

Sandra Hollensead, Nancy Kubiak

Patient A 46-year-old Caucasian female, who was brought to the emergency room after police found her sitting on the side of the road, unable to speak.

Clinical History The patient was alert, but initially verbally unresponsive to questions. When able to give a history, she related decreased appetite and oral intake for several days, but denied hallucinations, delusions, suicidal or homicidal ideation. She has a history of paranoid schizophrenia.

Family History Patient stated she was adopted as a newborn and raised by the "wrong family."

Medications None.

Physical Examination Temperature 97.8°F, respirations 18/minute, blood pressure 108/71, and pulse 91/minute. The patient appeared disheveled; examination was otherwise unremarkable.

Initial Work-Up		
CBC		
WBC (×10³/µL)	10.2	
RBC (×10⁶/µL)	4.86	
HGB (g/dL)	10.2	
HCT (%)	35.4	
MCV (fL)	72.8	
MCH (pg)	21.0	
MCHC (g/dL)	28.8	
PLT (×10³/µL)	329	
RDW-CV (%)	19.2	
MPV (fL)	9.8	
WBC Differential	**%**	**# (×10³/µL)**
Neutrophils	16	1.6
Bands	50	5.1
Lymphocytes	20	2.0
Monocytes	8	0.8
Eosinophils	1	0.1
Metamyelocytes	5	0.5

Basic metabolic panel: all results within normal limits. Peripheral blood smear review revealed >50% of neutrophils having bilobed nuclei that were counted as band forms. Although the nuclear shape of the granulocytes suggested immaturity, nuclear chromatin was dense and mature appearing (**Figure 1**).

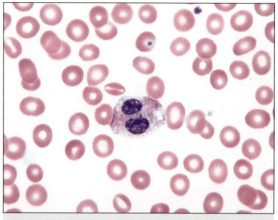

Figure 1 Blood smear (Wright-Giemsa, ×1000) showing a neutrophil with symmetrical bilobed nucleus and dense nuclear chromatin.

Differential Diagnosis The patient presented with an acute psychotic episode manifested by bizarre behavior, which could have been precipitated by medication noncompliance, toxic ingestion or illicit drug use, or infection, particularly herpes encephalitis, or HIV/AIDS. Her normal vital signs, chemistries, and prior history of schizophrenia with medication noncompliance suggested that this episode was an exacerbation of her underlying psychiatric disease. From the peripheral blood findings, additional diagnostic possibilities included leukemoid reaction, Pelger-Huët anomaly, myeloproliferative disorder, and myelodysplastic syndrome.

Additional Work-Up The peripheral smear was reviewed by the pathologist, and the differential was repeated with bilobed neutrophils counted as mature neutrophils rather than bands. Optimally, family members (parents and siblings) should have blood smears reviewed to confirm the hereditary nature of the disorder. The patient refused diagnostic work-up for her anemia.

Final Diagnosis Pelger-Huët anomaly (PHA), and microcytic hypochromic anemia.

Management PHA is a benign condition not requiring treatment. Recognition of this abnormality is paramount to avoid unnecessary clinical work-up that might delay more urgent care, and to differentiate from pseudo-Pelger-Huët anomaly (pseudo-PHA), which may be a manifestation of an underlying hematologic malignancy.

General Discussion In the heterozygous state, PHA is benign with only the altered white blood cell nuclear morphology. In the homozygous state clinical presentation is variable, with psychomotor retardation, disproportionate body stature, macrocephalus with prominent forehead, ventricular septal defect, polydactyly and short metacarpals being described. A mutant defect in the lamin B receptor (LBR) gene has been recognized as the etiology of PHA. The LBR is an integral membrane protein of the nuclear envelope that controls the shape of the nuclear membrane by regulating the trafficking of heterochromatin and nuclear lamins. The PHA cells are characterized by low nuclear:cytoplasmic ratio, and nuclear chromatin that is densely clumped, coarse, and dark. In the heterozygous phenotypes, 55%-93% of the neutrophils show a bilobed nucleus, described as "dumbbell" or "pince-nez" in appearance. Lobes are connected by a thin chromatin filament. A small population of neutrophils has a nonlobulated or peanut-shaped nucleus, known as

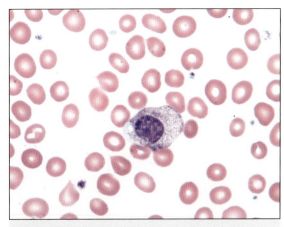

Figure 2 Blood smear (Wright-Giemsa, ×1000) showing a unilobed neutrophil.

Stodtmeister cells. The cell size, cytoplasm, and granular pattern are comparable to normal neutrophils. In homozygous PHA, the nucleus is often single, round, or slightly indented, eccentrically placed in the granulocyte with little or no nuclear segmentation (**Figure 2**). Distinction from myelocytes or metamyelocytes is made by observing the small size of the nucleus and the markedly dense chromatin pattern. Cells with this morphology make up 94%-96% of the total neutrophils in homozygous PHA, and 0%-4% in heterozygous PHA. The nuclei of all leukocytes (neutrophils, lymphocytes, monocytes, eosinophils and basophils are affected in PHA. Bilobed and unilobed neutrophils are also seen in acquired conditions and are known as pseudo-PHA cells. These acquired conditions include leukemoid reactions during severe bacterial infections, HIV, tuberculosis and *Mycoplasma pneumoniae* infections, some medications, myelodysplastic syndromes, myeloproliferative neoplasms, and acute myeloid leukemia. Thus the distinction of PHA from pseudo-PHA is clinically important. Knowledge of morphology can allow this distinction in most cases. Döhle bodies, vacuolations, and toxic granulations, common to granulocytes in leukemoid reactions, are not present in PHA. Pseudo-PHA cell nuclei in the myeloproliferative/myelodysplastic syndromes have marked heterogeneity in nuclear lobations; those that are bilobed often lack the nuclear symmetry seen in PHA (**Figure 3**). Other findings of dysplasia are also present in the granulocytes, including hypogranulation, and increased nuclear:cytoplasmic ratio. The pseudo-PHA cells are in the minority, and hypersegmented neutrophils may be seen. The nuclear chromatin is not as dark and condensed as in PHA. In the myelodysplastic syndromes, anemia and cytopenias are often present, with circulating blasts and nucleated red blood cells at times seen on peripheral blood smear. In the patient described above, the peripheral smear white blood cell morphology could be a red herring if interpreted as a left-shifted granulocyte count. The distinction can be troublesome at times, leading to erroneous differential counts containing high numbers of bands and metamyelocytes that can lead to unnecessary clinical work-ups or treatment for infection. For preservation of optimal white blood cell morphology, a carefully prepared peripheral blood smear should be examined within 3 hours of collection, as older specimens (>12 hours from collection) can show changes of neutrophils related to apoptosis, further confounding the recognition of PHA.

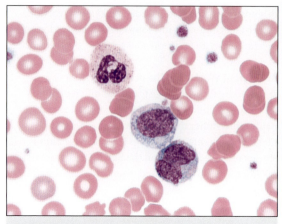

Figure 3 Blood smear from another case of chronic monomyelocytic leukemia (Wright-Giemsa, ×1000) showing a pseudo-Pelger-Huët neutrophil with asymmetrical bilobed nucleus and sparse granules, accompanied by a dysplastic myelocyte and a monocyte.

May-Hegglin Anomaly

Matthew T Hurford

Patient A 25-year-old Hispanic male with multiple fractures and compartment syndrome of the left foot secondary to trauma from a falling garage door.

Clinical History Noncontributory.

Family History Hypercholesterolemia (maternal).

Medications None.

Physical Examination Notable for marked swelling, ecchymosis and discoloration of the mid foot.

Initial Work-Up

CBC		WBC Differential	%	# (×10³/µL)
WBC (×10³/µL)	5.0	Neutrophils	74	3.7
RBC (×10⁶/µL)	4.73	Bands	0	
HGB (g/dL)	12.5	Lymphocytes	17	0.9
HCT (%)	38.5	Monocytes	6	0.3
MCV (fL)	81	Eosinophils	2	0.1
MCH (pg)	26.4	Basophils	1	0.1
MCHC (g/dL)	32.4			
PLT (×10³/µL)	91*	PT (sec)	11.5	(normal 11-15)
RDW-CV (%)	15.5	PTT (sec)	28.0	(normal 20-35)

Flagged for: large/giant platelets.

Differential Diagnosis The differential diagnosis of macrothrombocytopenia includes chronic autoimmune thrombocytopenia (chronic ITP), Bernard-Soulier syndrome (BSS), Paris-Trousseau syndrome/Jackson syndrome, X-linked macrothrombocytopenia, gray platelet syndrome (GPS), Mediterranean macrothrombocytopenia, macrothrombocytopenia associated with velocardiofacial syndrome, and MYH9-related disorders (May-Hegglin anomaly, Epstein syndrome, Fechtner syndrome and Sebastian platelet syndrome). In ITP, usually <10% of platelets are "giant" platelets. If another family member demonstrates thrombocytopenia, the diagnosis of ITP is unlikely. Bernard-Soulier syndrome (BSS) is characterized by giant platelets caused by reduced or absent expression of the glycoproteins Ib-IX-V receptor complex. Platelet aggregation studies demonstrate absent aggregation with ristocetin in BSS. The diagnosis is confirmed with quantitative analysis of GP Ib-IX-V complex expression on platelets or by genetic studies. The Paris-Trousseau syndrome/Jackson syndrome demonstrates large platelets with giant α granules. The disorder is differentiated from the MYH9 disorders by mental retardation and facial-cardiac abnormalities. The disorder is caused by a heterozygous deletion of part of chromosome 11q23. X-linked Macrothrombocytopenia is characterized by anemia with reticulocytosis, splenomegaly and thrombocytopenia with platelet function defects including decreased aggregation with ristocetin and weak aggregation with collagen. It is caused by a mutation in the GATA-1 gene Xp11-12, a transcription factor involved with erythropoiesis and megakaryopoiesis. GPS is characterized by moderate thrombocytopenia with giant platelets containing empty α granules. It is an hereditary bleeding disorder with an unknown defect.

Additional Work-Up Peripheral blood smear revealed thrombocytopenia with a few giant platelets and large Döhle body-like inclusions in neutrophils and eosinophils (**Figure 1**) narrowing the diagnostic list to primarily MYH9-related disorders. No additional studies (on proband or family members) were performed to confirm the diagnosis at the request of the family.

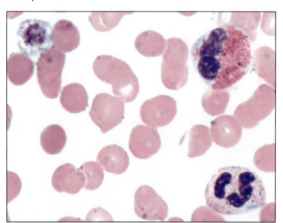

Figure 1 Blood smear (Wright, ×1000) showing a giant platelet (left) and a spindled Döhle-like inclusion in both a neutrophil and an eosinophil.

Final Diagnosis May-Hegglin anomaly, a MYH9-related platelet disorder.

Management Approach Patients with May-Hegglin anomaly may be asymptomatic or may have various bleeding abnormalities (easy bruising, epistaxis, gingival bleeding, menorrhagia, and excessive bleeding with surgical procedures). No treatment is usually required in asymptomatic patients. In cases with significant bleeding manifestations or at risk of excessive bleeding, transfusions of platelets may be necessary. The use of intravenous administration of desmopressin acetate (DDAVP) preoperatively has also been reported. This patient received 1 unit of pooled platelets prior to surgery and 2 units of pooled platelets postoperatively.

General Discussion May-Hegglin anomaly is characterized by the triad of thrombocytopenia, giant/large platelets, and leukocyte inclusion bodies that resemble Döhle bodies. The Döhle body-like inclusions are large, prominent and spindle-shaped, and appear blue in Wright-Giemsa-stained blood smears. The inclusions are generally found in granulocytes (neutrophils, eosinophils and basophils) but may also be found in lymphocytes and monocytes. There may be 1-4 inclusions per cell. The syndrome was first described by Richard May in 1909 and Robert Hegglin in 1945. The May-Hegglin anomaly is caused by a mutation in the MYH9 gene encoding a cytoskeletal contractile protein, the nonmuscle myosin heavy chain IIA (NMMHC-IIA). The NMMHC-IIA proteins play a functional role in cell motility, cytokinesis, phagocytosis and maintanence of cell shape. The bleeding is caused by reduced clot stability due to impaired clot retraction by abnormal platelet cytoskeleton. The bleeding manifests as bruising and hematomas and menorrhagia in women. Petechiae are rare. Major bleeding episodes and fatal spontaneous intracranial bleeding are rare. On blood smears, the giant platelets are usually the size of a red blood cell. The giant platelets change the shape of the platelet histogram to a broad shape and may also be counted as leukocytes. Platelet aggregometry and platelet function studies using the PFA-100 (Siemens Healthcare Diagnostics, Marburg, Germany) do not show major defects. The shape change in the aggregation curve is typically absent in platelet aggregometry tests; however, an absent shape change may also be found in other platelet disorders. The bone marrow shows normal or moderately elevated megakaryocytes with normal morphology. This finding may lead to misdiagnosis of autoimmune thrombocytopenia. The disorder rarely requires platelet transfusions. May-Hegglin is a member of the MYH9-related platelet disorders. The 4 autosomal dominant disorders with macrothrombocytopenia include the May-Hegglin syndrome, Fechtner syndrome, Epstein Syndrome, and Sebastian syndrome. The Fechtner syndrome is characterized by Döhle body-like inclusions, an Alport-like syndrome of hearing loss, nephritis and presenile cataracts. The Epstein syndrome is characterized by deafness and nephritis and absence of Döhle body-like inclusions and cataracts. The Sebastian syndrome is characterized by small leukocyte inclusions.

HIV/Therapy-Related Myelodysplasia

Powers Peterson, Scott Weisenberg

Patient A 45-year-old premenopausal African-American female, who presented for routine HIV follow-up.

Clinical History The patient had been previously diagnosed with and treated for HIV and *Mycobacterium avium* complex. The chief complaint at this time was fatigue.

Family History Noncontributory.

Medications Ritonavir, emticitabine/tenofovir disoproxil fumarate, and atazanavir sulfate (highly active antiretroviral therapy [HAART]).

Physical Examination Temperature 98°F, BP 120/80 mmHg, respiratory rate 14/min. His chest was clear to auscultation and percussion. His neurologic examination showed 4+/5 right upper extremity strength.

Initial Work-Up		
CBC		
WBC (×10³/μL)	3.4	
RBC (×10⁶/μL)	2.37	
HGB (g/dL)	8.1	
HCT (%)	25.1	
MCV (fL)	105.7	
MCH (pg)	34.2	
MCHC (g/dL)	32.2	
PLT (×10³/μL)	111	
RDW-CV (%)	16.8	
WBC Differential	**%**	**# (×10³/μL)**
Neutrophils	74	2.6
Lymphocytes	12.1	0.4
Monocytes	13.4	0.5
Eosinophils	0.7	0
Basophils	0.2	0

Peripheral blood smear revealed dysplastic nucleated red cells, hypogranular neutrophils, hypersegmented neutrophils, and abnormally granulated platelets (**Figures 1** and **2**).

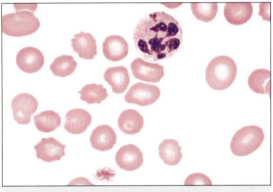

Figure 1 Blood smear (Wright, ×1000) showing a hypersegmented neutrophil, macro-ovalocytes, and a large platelet with abnormal granulation.

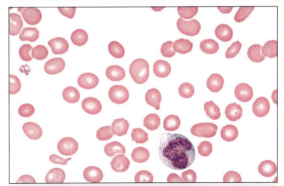

Figure 2 Blood smear (Wright, ×1000) showing a hypogranular metamyelocyte, an abnormally granulated large platelet, and dysmorphic, anisotic red cells.

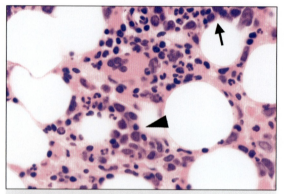

Figure 3 Bone marrow biopsy (H&E, ×400) showing dysplastic erythro- and granulopoiesis. The arrow points to a cluster of megaloblastic erythroid precursors. The arrowhead points to a cluster of primitive myeloid elements in the central marrow spaces (ALIP).

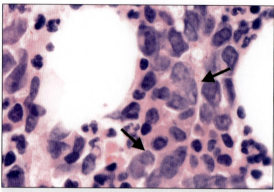

Figure 4 Bone marrow biopsy (H&E, ×1000) in which arrows point to foci of ALIP. The location of these early myeloid precursors would normally be paratrabecular.

Differential Diagnosis The list of conditions associated with pancytopenia is quite large, but the clinical history and peripheral blood findings led us to consider myelodysplasia secondary to HIV and/or HIV therapy, myelodysplastic syndrome, and megaloblastic anemia associated with folate and/or vitamin B_{12} deficiency as the most likely possibilities.

Additional Work-Up
- Serum B_{12} 317 pg/mL (normal 210-600)
- Serum folate 7.4 ng/mL (normal 2.8-16.4)
- CD4+ T cells 210/mL
- HIV viral load <48 copies/mL

Bone Marrow Aspirate and Biopsy Hypercellular marrow with dysplastic erythroid hyperplasia (**Figure 3**); increased iron stores; and atypical localization of immature myeloid precursors or ALIP (**Figures 3** and **4**) but no increase in percentage of blasts. Immunophenotypic analysis (flow cytometry) on peripheral blood: No suspicious lymphoid or blast population identified. Immunophenotypic analysis (flow cytometry) on marrow: inverted CD4/CD8 ratio of 0.5-1:1.

Final Diagnosis Anemia secondary to HIV infection. Myelodysplasia secondary to HIV infection and/or HAART.

Management Approach Antiretroviral therapy may improve HIV-associated anemia by 1- 2 g/dL over 6 months. The cornerstone of HAART is using multiple drugs that differently target viral replication in order to prevent the development of resistance. Atazanavir is a protease inhibitor that inhibits the viral processing of viral Gag and Gag-Pol proteins in HIV-1 infected cells. Ritonavir is another protease inhibitor typically added in low dose to other "primary" protease inhibitors in order to decrease metabolism of the "primary" protease inhibitor. Tenofovir is a nucleotide analogue of deoxyadenosine 5'-monophosphate. Dose reduction is indicated for patients with renal insufficiency. Emtricitabine is a well tolerated nucleoside reverse transcriptase inhibitor. Toxicity is a concern with all HIV medications. HIV-associated fat redistribution, lactic acidosis, and dyslipidemia have been associated with almost all of the HIV medications. Drug interactions must be sought, particularly for the protease inhibitors. Finally, in the months after starting HAART, immune reconstitution inflammatory syndromes may occur, as the result of renewed immune activity against latent or clinically silent infections. This patient responded well to HAART. The most recent HGB level was 11.8 g/dL. The CD4 cell count increased to 357/mL, and viral load remains undetectable.

General Discussion The etiology of cytopenias in HIV+ patients is multifactorial, and in patients on HAART the issue is complicated. Anemia was well documented in the pre-HAART period, as was HIV-related myelodysplasia. Direct infection of megakaryocytes may be responsible for thrombocytopenia. Although HAART improves many cytopenias, many of the drugs are also toxic to the marrow. The cytopenias are often accompanied by dysplasia. The dysplastic features in the peripheral blood of this patient included aniso- and poikilocytosis (enlarged and irregularly shaped red cells, elliptocytes, rare nucleated red cells, target cells, and fragmented red cells). The granulocytes displayed hypogranularity with abnormal granulations, nuclear hypersegmentation, occasional ring nuclei, and apoptotic-appearing nuclei. Platelet abnormalities included giant forms and abnormally granulated platelets. The marrow aspirate and biopsy both showed erythroid hyperplasia with megaloblastic features including nuclear-cytoplasmic asynchrony and atypical mitoses. Iron stores were increased.

Hemophagocytic Lymphohistiocytosis

Kathryn Foucar, Christine N Sillings

Patient A 14-month-old Hispanic male with an 8-day history of fever, nausea, and vomiting.

Clinical History The patient had no significant past medical history. He had received his 1-year immunizations, including MMR and *Varicella* vaccines, 1 week prior.

Family History No history of genetic or hematologic disorders.

Medications Amoxicillin/clavulanic acid, acetaminophen as needed.

Physical Examination The patient was febrile (102.7°F). Mild cervical and groin lymphadenopathy was present. The remainder of the exam was unremarkable.

Initial Work-Up

CBC		WBC Differential	%	# (×10³/µL)
WBC (×10³/µL)	3.8	Neutrophils	56	2.4
RBC (×10⁶/µL)	3.39	Bands	7	0.2
HGB (g/dL)	9.0	Lymphocytes	24	0.9
HCT (%)	24	Monocytes	8	0.3
MCV (fL)	72	Eosinophils	1	0.0
MCHC (g/dL)	34.7	Basophils	0	
PLT (×10³/µL)	149	Metamyelocyte	1	0.0
RDW-CV (%)	15.7			

Differential Diagnosis The clinical differential diagnosis included sepsis, a systemic viral infection, and neoplastic conditions, such as acute leukemia.

Additional Work-Up An extensive infectious disease work-up, including EBV and CMV serologies, turned up negative. Other pertinent laboratory values included elevated ferritin (8,100 ng/mL), elevated triglycerides (290 mg/dL), and a markedly elevated soluble IL-2 receptor α level (CD25) (19,795 pg/mL). Fibrinogen was not elevated. An NK function assay was within normal limits, and a perforin and granzyme B assay showed decreased perforin expression in NK cells. Perforin (PRFI) and Munc13-4 (UNC13D) mutational gene analyses were negative. A bone marrow biopsy revealed a mildly hypocellular marrow with left-shifted myelopoiesis, megakaryocytic hyperplasia, and hemophagocytosis (**Figures 1** and **2**). A CT scan of the abdomen/pelvis revealed hepatosplenomegaly. An MRI of the brain was negative.

Section I: Miscellaneous Hematologic Conditions
Hemophagocytic Lymphohistiocytosis

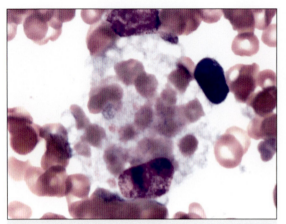

Figure 1 Bone marrow aspirate smear (Wright-Giemsa, ×1000) showing a histiocyte that has phagocytosed mature red blood cells and platelets.

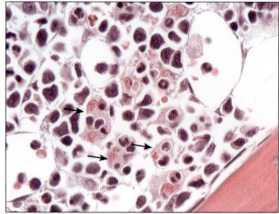

Figure 2 Bone marrow biopsy (H&E, ×100) in which several histiocytes are identified (arrows) with hemophagocytosis of hematopoietic bone marrow elements. Findings may be subtle.

Final Diagnosis Hemophagocytic lymphohistiocytosis (HLH).

Management Approach The patient was started on an 8-week treatment regimen of etoposide, dexamethasone, and cyclosporine A, in accordance with hemophagocytic lymphohistiocytosis (HLH)-2004 treatment guidelines. Per this protocol, for primary HLH or severe, persistent, or relapsed secondary HLH, continuation therapy with the above regimen is recommended until the patient is stable enough to undergo hematopoietic progenitor cell transplantation (HPCT). If patients with secondary HLH achieve clinical remission after 8 weeks, treatment may be discontinued. Intrathecal therapy with methotrexate with or without corticosteroids may be given in patients with persistent active or relapsed CNS disease. The patient did achieve clinical remission after 8 weeks, and therapy was discontinued.

General Discussion HLH represents a heterogenous group of disorders characterized by a spectrum of clinical and laboratory findings that result from a systemic hyperinflammatory response to an underlying stimulus. This sepsis-like picture is the result of dysfunctional NK and/or cytotoxic T cells, which lead to an inability of the immune response to be downregulated, causing unregulated stimulation of macrophages and lymphocytes and consequent high levels of circulating cytokines. Activated lymphohistiocytic cells infiltrate many organs including bone marrow, spleen, liver, lymph nodes, and CNS. Upregulation of major histocompatibility complex (MHC) and adhesion molecules on macrophages promotes hemophagocytosis. HLH is subdivided into primary and secondary HLH. Primary HLH includes familial histiocytic lymphohistiocytosis (FLH) and HLH associated with specific immunodeficiencies, such as Chédiak-Higashi syndrome, Griselli syndrome type 2, Hermansky-Pudlak syndrome type II, and X-linked lymphoproliferative syndrome. Patients with FLH usually present in infancy, although a wide range of ages has been reported. Genetic mutations in perforin 1 (PRF1), Munc13-4 (UNC13D), and syntaxin 11 (STX11) have been identified in some cases of FLH. Secondary causes of HLH include infection and malignancies. Patients are typically older at presentation than those with primary HLH. EBV and CMV are the most common viral etiologies, although many other inciting viral and bacterial agents have been reported. Neoplasms associated with secondary HLH include lymphoproliferative disorders, especially T- and NK-cell neoplasms. Other HLH associations include metabolic syndromes and autoimmune diseases, most notably systemic juvenile rheumatoid arthritis and adult-onset Still disease. Common presentations include prolonged fever (>7 days), cytopenias, and hepatosplenomegaly. Additional signs and symptoms may include lymphadenopathy, skin rash, neurological symptoms, jaundice, and edema. Characteristic laboratory values are seen, which are reflected in the diagnostic criteria (**Table 1**). Histologic exam of bone marrow and other involved organs shows an infiltrate of benign-appearing histiocytes, many of which display hemophagocytosis of hematopoietic cells. The histiocytes generally lack atypia; significant atypia suggests an alternative neoplastic process. Associated hypoplasia of granulocytic and erythroid lineages and occasionally megakaryocytic hyperplasia can be seen. Accompanying inciting neoplastic cells may be identified. Importantly, the absence of hemophagocytosis by morphology does not preclude the diagnosis if sufficient other diagnostic criteria are met. Untreated, HLH leads to multiorgan failure and can be rapidly fatal. Prior to the institution of chemotherapy and immunosuppressive therapy, the prognosis was dismal, with only a reported 5% overall survival at 1 year in patients with FLH. With current therapies, many patients can be brought into remission, although relapses in patients with primary HLH inevitably occur. Currently, the only potential for cure for FLH is HPCT. The prognosis for patients after HPCT has significantly improved over the years, with the reported overall survival ranging from 53%-75% depending on the series.

Table 1. Diagnostic criteria for HLH (HLH-2004 guidelines)

1. A molecular diagnosis consistent with HLH
2. Presence of 5 of 8 of criteria listed below:
Fever
Splenomegaly
Cytopenias affecting at least 2 of 3 lineages in the peripheral blood
Hemoglobin <9 g/dL (<10 g/dL in infants <4 weeks of age)
Platelets <100 × $10^3/\mu L$
Neutrophils <1.0 × $10^3/\mu L$
Hypertriglyceridemia and/or hypofibrinogenemia
Fasting triglycerides ≥3.0 mmol/L (≥265 mg/dL)
Fibrinogen ≤150 mg/dL
Hemophagocytosis in bone marrow, spleen, or lymph nodes
Low or absent NK-cell activity (according to local laboratory reference)
Ferritin ≥500 ng/mL
Soluble CD25 (ie, soluble IL-2 receptor) ≥2,400 U/mL

A spectrum of characteristic laboratory findings with or without genetic evidence of HLH are required to make an accurate diagnosis of HLH. HLH: hemophagocytic lymphohistiocytosis; NK: natural killer

# Alveolar Rhabdomyosarcoma of the Bone Marrow

Matthew T Hurford

Patient A 19-year-old African-American female with a right gluteal/perineum mass.

Clinical History She had noted the "lump" a few weeks earlier. When it did not resolve on its own, she presented to her primary care doctor for evaluation. She had not noted any other "lumps." She felt bloated but had not noted any change in her bowel or bladder habits. She had no other medical history.

Family History Noncontributory.

Medications None.

Physical Examination Significant abdominal distention and a 3 cm soft tissue mass of the right gluteal/perineum.

Initial Work-Up

CBC		
WBC (×10³/µL)	9.6	
RBC (×10⁶/µL)	4.71	
HGB (g/dL)	13.3	
HCT (%)	40.1	
MCV (fL)	85	
MCH (pg)	28.2	
MCHC (g/dL)	33.1	
PLT (×10³/µL)	363	
RDW-CV (%)	13.9	
MPV (fL)	7.6	

WBC Differential	%	# (×10³/µL)
Neutrophils	68.1	6.5
Lymphocytes	23.5	2.3
Monocytes	6.8	0.7
Eosinophils	1.5	0.1
Basophils	0.1	0.0

A CT scan demonstrated a 6.6cm heterogeneous mass. There was no evidence of an abscess or cyst. An excisional biopsy of the soft tissue mass demonstrated sheets of small round blue cells with eosinophilic to clear cytoplasm (**Figure 1**). No cross striations or strap cells were identified.

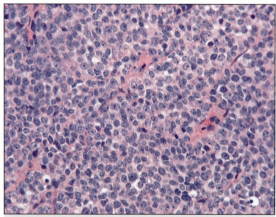

Figure 1 Gluteal/perineum soft tissue mass biopsy (H&E, ×400) showing sheets of small to medium cells with round nuclei, immature chromatin, small nucleoli and moderate eosinophilic cytoplasm.

Differential Diagnosis Diagnostic considerations included small round blue cell tumors (lymphoblastic leukemia/ lymphoma, neuroblastoma, Ewing sarcoma/primitive neuroectodermal tumor [PNET], lymphoma, desmoplastic small round cell tumor, Wilms tumor, and osteosarcoma) and acute myeloid leukemia.

Additional Work-Up Immunohistochemical studies performed on the soft tissue mass were positive for vimentin, desmin (focal) and MyoD1. There was no significant expression for cytokeratins (CAM5.2, AE1/AE3, CK7, CK20, & KER 903) and hematopoietic markers (CD45, CD20, CD22, PAX-5, CD2, CD3,

CD4, CD5, CD10, CD30, CD43, CD45RO, CD34, CD38, CD56, CD117, BCL2, BCL6, ALK-1, TdT, CD31, CD99, SMA, MSA, synaptophysin, NF, NSE, S-100, HMB-45, EMA, PLAP and WT1). Electron microscopy studies demonstrated a poorly differentiated small round cell tumor without sarcomeres. Molecular studies on the frozen soft tissue mass were positive for PAX3-FKHR and PAX7- FKHR rearrangements. The bone marrow biopsy performed for staging demonstrated a diffuse proliferation of small round blue cells. There were sheets of small to medium cells with round to ovoid nuclei, small eosinophilic nucleoli and moderate eosinophilic cytoplasm (**Figures 2** and **3**). By immunohistochemical staining, the marrow was positive for MyoD1 (**Figure 4**).

Final Diagnosis Alveolar rhabdomyosarcoma.

Management Approach Patients with good risk disease that is discovered while still operable, have surgical resection of the tumor. Most patients receive chemotherapy as well, either in the adjuvant setting or, as in this case, for metastatic disease. The estimated 3-year overall survival with metastatic disease is 30%. This patient received systemic chemotherapy with irinotecan and vincristine.

General Discussion Rhabdomyosarcoma is the most common soft tissue sarcoma of childhood/adolescence. It accounts for 50% of pediatric soft tissue sarcomas. The most common presentations include paratesticular, trunk and abdominal neoplasms in adolescence. Approximately 15% of children present with metastatic disease, frequently involving the lung and bone marrow. Massive bone marrow involvement is uncommon. The 2 major subtypes of rhabdomyosarcoma are alveolar (80%) and embryonal (20%). Alveolar rhabdomyosarcoma is most common in early to mid teens and affects deep muscles of the extremities, axial muscles or perineum. They are rapidly growing neoplasms with often high stage of presentation. Rhabdomyosarcoma with marrow involvement may present with fever, weakness, weight loss, anemia, bleeding manifestations, lymphadenopathy or hepatosplenomegaly and DIC. It may be confused with acute leukemia, especially acute lymphoblastic leukemia. Many cases are misdiagnosed as undifferentiated leukemia since cytochemical and immunophenotypic studies are not helpful. Immunohistochemical studies with desmin, muscle-specific actin and myoglobin are the most reliable markers. Myogenin and MyoD1 are also helpful. In

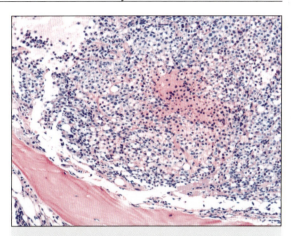

Figure 2 Bone marrow biopsy (H&E, ×100) showing sheets of medium cells with clear cytoplasm.

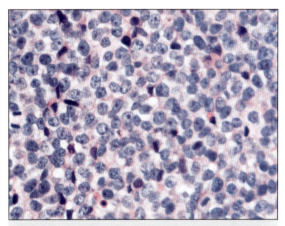

Figure 3 Bone marrow biopsy (H&E, ×400) showing sheets of small to medium cells with round nuclei, immature chromatin and moderate clear cytoplasm.

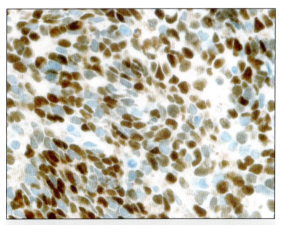

Figure 4 Bone marrow biopsy (Myo D1, ×400) showing strong nuclear staining confirming the muscle differentiation of rhabdomyosarcoma.

cases with bone marrow involvement, the aspirate smears usually demonstrate intermediate to large cells with round nuclei, fine chromatin, single or multiple small to prominent nucleoli and basophilic cytoplasm with vacuoles. There are no cytoplasmic granules or Auer rods. The bone marrow biopsy often demonstrates sheets or clusters of small to medium cells with round nuclei, immature chromatin and eosinophilic cytoplasm. The tumor cells are negative for periodic acid-Schiff (PAS) with and without diastase. The tumor cells are diffusely positive for vimentin and usually positive for markers of early muscle differentiation, myogenin and MyoD1, and focally positive for markers of late muscle differentiation, muscle specific actin and desmin. They are usually negative for CD45, CD99, NB84, S-100, chromogranin, α-fetoprotein, low molecular weight cytokeratin, human chorionic gonadotrophin and placental alkaline phosphatase. Ultrastructural studies with electron microscopy may reveal bundles of thick and thin filaments with well formed Z-bands characteristic of skeletal muscle differentiation. Cytogenetic studies by GTG banding, fluorescence in situ hybridization (FISH) or RT-PCR demonstrate a t(2:13)(q35;q14) translocation involving PAX3 and FKHR and less frequently t(1:13) translocation involving PAX7 and FKHR.

Lobular Carcinoma of the Breast, Metastatic to the Bone Marrow

John Anastasi

Patient A 50-year-old female with slowly progressive fatigue over the prior 2 months-3 months.

Clinical History She had been treated with lumpectomy and radiation for breast cancer of the lobular type, followed by adjuvant chemotherapy with doxorubicin and cyclophosphamide, followed by paclitaxel and traztuzumab. She had completed therapy 2 years earlier and had no evidence of disease on the most recent imaging studies 6 months prior.

Family History No known family history of breast cancer.

Medications None.

Physical Examination Noncontributory.

Initial Work-Up

CBC	
WBC (×10³/µL)	0.6
RBC (×10⁶/µL)	3.66
HGB (g/dL)	11.0
HCT (%)	33.1
MCV (fL)	90.4
MCH (pg)	30.1
MCHC (g/dL)	33.2
PLT (×10³/µL)	238
RDW-CV (%)	14.5

WBC Differential	%	# (×10³/µL)
Neutrophils	61	0.4
Bands	1	0.0
Lymphocytes	26	0.2
Monocytes	8	0.0
Eosinophils	4	0.0
Basophils	0	

Differential Diagnosis Diagnostic considerations included metastatic disease, myelodysplastic syndrome and acute leukemia related to prior therapy.

Additional Work-Up Bone marrow examination at low power appeared normocellular with trilineage hematopiesis (**Figure 1**). At high power; however, scattered metastatic tumor cells intermixed with normal marrow elements were appreciated (**Figures 2** and **3**). These tumor cells stained positive with keratin AE1/AE3 (**Figure 4**).

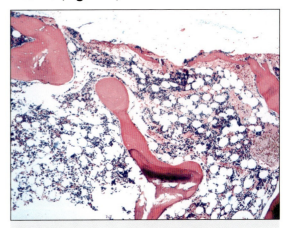

Figure 1 Bone marrow biopsy (H&E, ×100) showing normocellular marrow with intact architecture.

Section I: Miscellaneous Hematologic Conditions
Lobular Carcinoma of the Breast, Metastatic to the Bone Marrow

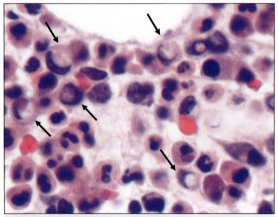

Figure 2 Bone marrow biopsy (H&E, ×400) showing scattered metastatic tumor cells (arrows) intermixed with normal marrow elements. Note the absence of cohesion of the cells and the lack of any desmoplastic reaction to them.

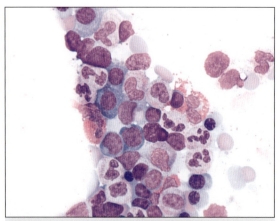

Figure 3 Bone marrow aspirate smear (Wright stain, ×1000) showing rare tumor cell (center) with a cytoplasmic globule, intermixed with normal bone marrow elements.

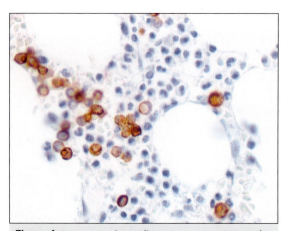

Figure 4 Bone marrow biopsy (keratin stain, AE1/AE3, ×400) showing scattered metastatic tumor cells made obvious by their positive staining.

Final Diagnosis Lobular carcinoma of the breast metastatic to the bone marrow.

Management Approach It is notable that while bone marrow or hematopoietic progenitor cell transplantation were once used for the treatment of metastatic breast cancer, they are no longer recommended outside the clinical trial setting since they did not fare better than standard treatments. Patients with solid tumors that are metastatic to bone marrow should be treated for the underlying malignancy. With the advent of newer therapies, it is possible that patients will be able to achieve long-term remissions in some cases. This patient was diagnosed with metastatic breast cancer in her marrow. Further staging did not show evidence of disease elsewhere. She received further chemotherapy with capecitabone and lapatinib, with improvement in her lab parameters but also with several admissions for complications from therapy. 18 months later, she developed progression of her disease and opted for hospice care at home.

General Discussion When metastatic lobular carcinoma of the breast involves the bone marrow it does so with little to no desmoplastic reaction. Typically, other types of metastatic disease, like prostate cancer or ductal adenocarcinoma of the breast, cause marrow fibrosis, effacement of the architecture and frequently bony changes such as osteosclerosis or lytic lesions. In lobular carcinoma of the breast, the tumor cells infiltrate the bone marrow cavity without effacing the marrow and without the accompanying fibrosis, vascular proliferation and desmoplasia. The tumor cells might be in small clusters or groups, or can even be present singly, but in either case they infiltrate among normal hematopoietic cells with little to no stromal reaction and without interrupting the marrow architecture. By examining the marrow at low power, one may be completely unaware of tumor infiltration. If not for the typical cytoplasmic inclusions in this case, which are not always present, the tumor cells might go completely unrecognized. They would simply appear as if they were immature marrow elements such as pronormoblasts or myelocytes on the biopsy section. Only with keratin staining do the inconspicuous cells become quite obvious. Renal cell carcinoma with minimal involvement might also give this inconspicuous result as the metastatic cells can have the appearance of foamy histiocytes on the biopsy specimen, especially when present singly. Metastatic neuroblastoma in tiny clusters can also be easily overlooked without immunostaining. The superiority of the biopsy over the aspirate in detecting metastatic tumor is related to the desmoplastic reaction, as the associated fibrosis prevents aspiration of tumor cells from the metastatic foci. Due to the lack of desmoplasia in lobular carcinoma of the breast, tumor cells may indeed be seen on the aspirate. However, again, they can be insidious and difficult to recognize among the immature hematopoietic elements. Thus, the best approach to evaluate involvement of the marrow for metastatic disease is obtaining bone core biopsy specimens of sufficient length and performing immunohistochemical stains. These are critical if the bone marrow appears negative histologically on the H&E sections.

Paroxysmal Nocturnal Hemoglobinuria

Emmanuel Besa, Ajay Kandra

Patient A 70-year-old female with abdominal pain, nausea, vomiting, and diarrhea.

Clinical History The patient has a history of fibromyalgia.

Family History Her father died from complications of cerebrovascular accident. Her brother has cardiac problems.

Medications Docusate.

Physical Examination Conjunctivae and skin were icteric. Severe right upper quadrant tenderness was noted on palpation. There was no splenomegaly or lymphadenopathy.

Initial Work-Up

CBC		WBC Differential	%	# ($10^3/\mu L$)
WBC ($\times 10^3/\mu L$)	12.1	Neutrophils	70.4	8.5
RBC ($\times 10^6/\mu L$)	3.85	Bands	0	
HGB (g/dL)	11.0	Lymphocytes	15.4	1.9
HCT (%)	33.6	Monocytes	13.6	1.6
MCV (fL)	87.0	Eosinophils	0.4	0.1
MCH (pg)	28.6	Basophils	0.2	0.0
MCHC (g/dL)	32.7			
PLT ($\times 10^3/\mu L$)	89			
MPV (fL)	12.3			

Peripheral smear revealed thrombocytopenia, normocytic, normochromic red cells and mild polychromasia.
Ultrasound of the abdomen revealed thrombosis in the portal vein suggestive of Budd-Chiari syndrome. MRI of abdomen showed main portal vein thrombosis with minimal filling of the main right and main left portal veins, non-occlusive splenic vein thrombus, spontaneous left splenorenal shunt and hepatomegaly.

Differential Diagnosis Conditions associated with hepatic vein thrombosis include primary myeloproliferative disorders (eg, polycythemia vera and essential thrombocythemia), paroxysmal nocturnal hemoglobinuria (PNH), thrombophilias (eg, factor V Leiden mutation, antiphospholipid antibody syndrome, protein C deficiency, protein S deficiency and antithrombin deficiency), anatomical lesions (membranous webs), and extrinsic compression (eg, tumor).

Additional Work-Up

Reticulocyte count 4% (absolute $131 \times 10^3/\mu L$)

Chemistries
- Total bilirubin (mg/dL)   2.8
- Direct bilirubin (mg/dL)   0.9
- AST (IU/L)   2,004
- ALT (IU/L)   1,368

- Alk phos (IU/L)   114
- Albumin (g/dL)   3.0
- LDH (U/L)   269
- PT (seconds)   24   (normal 11.5-15.5)
- INR   2.09
- PTT (seconds)   28   (normal 19-39)

Ferritin (ng/mL)   1,257

The patient's abnormal liver enzymes and prothrombin time were presumably related to portal vein thrombosis.

Urine hemoglobin: positive.

Hypercoaguability Work-Up Evaluation for factor V Leiden mutation, antiphospholipid antibody syndrome, protein C deficiency, protein S deficiency and antithrombin deficiency were negative. Flow cytometry evaluation of peripheral blood granulocytes and monocytes for expression of CD55 and CD59 was performed. The expression of CD55 and CD59 was reduced in both cell types (**Figure 1**). CD55 and CD59 were expressed in 45% of granulocytes. CD55 was expressed in 50% of monocytes and CD59 expression was seen in 56% of monocytes. Bone marrow was hypercellular with erythroid hyperplasia. There was no evidence of myeloproliferative process, aplastic anemia, or myelodysplastic syndrome.

Final Diagnosis Paroxysmal nocturnal hemoglobinuria (PNH).

Management Approach The primary therapy for patients with PNH who present with thrombosis is anticoagulation. Folate supplementation and replenishment of iron stores may be required. Eculizumab is now being used to treat hemolysis as well as provide symptomatic improvement in PNH. This patient was started on anticoagulation with heparin. Her liver enzyme results and platelet count gradually improved. After 5 days of heparin, anticoagulation was switched to warfarin. She was started on folate supplements. Once the liver enzyme results became normal, she was started on eculizumab. She received pneumococcal and meningococcal vaccines prior to initiation of eculizumab. Her haptoglobin prior to the initiation of treatment was <6. It improved to 36 within a week of initiating treatment. It has continued to stay in the 30s and 40s during the treatments. Her symptoms of fatigue, abdominal pain and headache improved.

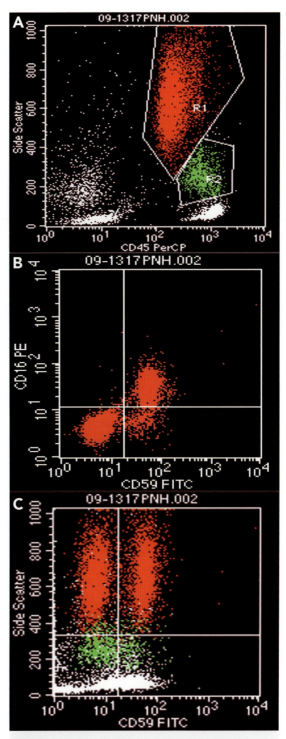

Figure 1 Peripheral blood flow cytograms. **A** CD45 vs side scatter: elucidating granulocyte (R1-red) and monocyte (R2-green) populations. **B** CD59 vs CD16 showing dual negative (CD59−/CD16−), single negative (CD59−) and dual positive granulocytes (CD59+/CD16+). **C** CD59 vs side scatter showing 2 distinct populations of granulocytes (red) and monocytes (green), each showing a CD59-deficient population.

Section I: Miscellaneous Hematologic Conditions
Paroxysmal Nocturnal Hemoglobinuria

General Discussion Paroxysmal nocturnal hemoglobinuria (PNH) is an acquired clonal hematopoietic stem cell disorder caused by a somatic mutation of the phosphatidylinositol glycan-complementation class A (PIG-A) gene, an X-linked gene. The PIG-A gene product is required for the synthesis of glycophosphatidylinositol anchored proteins (GPI-AP's), which serve as anchors for many cell surface proteins. 2 of these GPI-anchored complement regulatory proteins—CD55 (decay accelerating factor, DAF) and CD59 (membrane inhibitor of reactive lysis, MIRL)—normally inhibit the activation and destructive functions of alternative pathway of complement (APC). CD55 inhibits C3 convertases, and CD59 blocks formation of the membrane attack complex (MAC). PNH occurs in 1 to 10 individuals per million. Deficiency of CD55 and CD59 on RBCs in PNH makes these cells susceptible to both intravascular and extravascular hemolysis. Patients have a mixture of normal and PIG-A deficient cells in peripheral blood. Depending on the expansion of the PIG-A mutant clone, there is variability in the proportion of GPI-AP–deficient cells. The main clinical manifestations of PNH are hemolysis, anemia, thrombophilia, and bone-marrow failure. Poor quality of life due to symptoms of fatigue, lethargy, asthenia, dysphagia, odynaphagia, abdominal pain, and male erectile dysfunction are also common. Nocturnal hemoglobinuria is a presenting symptom in only about a quarter of patients. The median survival in PNH is 10 years-15 years, but with a wide variation. Thromboembolism is the leading cause of morbidity and mortality in PNH. There is overpresentation of venous thrombosis at unusual locations including hepatic (Budd-Chiari syndrome), mesenteric, dermal, or cerebral veins. PNH carries a high risk of thrombosis among pregnant females, requiring prophylactic anticoagulation. Others causes of mortality include complications of bone marrow failure, myelodysplastic syndrome (MDS) and leukemia. Traditional testing methods to detect PNH, which included the Ham acidified hemolysis test, the sucrose hemolysis test, and the complement lysis assay, have now been replaced by flow cytometric detection of CD55– and CD59– cells. Quantification of CD55– and CD59– white cells provides a more reliable clone size than that of red cells, since the red cell clone size decreases after each paroxysm of hemolysis resulting in underestimation. Typical laboratory findings include elevated serum lactate dehydrogenase (LDH) and reticulocytosis. Leukopenia and thrombocytopenia may also be seen. PNH presents in 2 forms: (1) the classical PNH, which is predominantly hemolytic without overt marrow failure and (2) the aplastic anemia PNH syndrome (AA-PNH), which presents with marrow failure. An association between PNH and acquired immune-mediated bone marrow failure syndromes (eg, aplastic anemia) is well known. Recent studies have reported that roughly a quarter to over a third of patients with PNH have an antecedent diagnosis of aplastic anemia. PNH has been found in association with low-risk myelodysplastic syndrome (MDS), more specifically with the refractory anemia (RA) subtype. Features of MDS found to have an association with PNH include a hypocellular marrow, HLA-DR15 positivity, normal cytogenetics, 5q– syndrome, and a potential response to immunosuppressive therapy. Eculizumab was approved for treatment of the hemolysis in PNH by the FDA in 2007. It is a humanized monoclonal antibody that blocks the activation of terminal complement at C5 and prevents the formation of C5a and the terminal complement complex, C5b-9 (MAC). It inhibits complement-mediated intravascular hemolysis, reduces or eliminates transfusion requirements, improves quality of life and may also reduce the risk of thromboembolism. Patients presenting with thrombosis need to be on lifelong anticoagulation. Prophylactic anticoagulation for other patients is controversial. In patients with AA/PNH, treatment should be focused on the underlying bone marrow failure. Hematopoietic progenitor cell transplantation is the only curative therapy for PNH.

Chédiak-Higashi Syndrome

John Kim Choi

Patient A 10-year-old female of Norwegian descent with a fever.

Clinical History The patient had been previously diagnosed with Chédiak-Higashi syndrome (CHS). She had had an episode of pneumonia at age 3.

Family History Father is healthy but has large granules in his platelets on EM studies.

Medications Prophylatic antibiotics (trimethoprim/sulfamethoxazole) for neutropenia associated with CHS.

Physical Examination She has fair skin and hair. Her physical exam is completely normal except for hepatosplenomegaly on abdominal examination.

Initial Work-Up

CBC		Normal	WBC Differential	%	# (×10³/µL)
WBC (×10³/µL)	1.3	(4.5-13.5)	Neutrophils	24	0.3
RBC (×10⁶/µL)	4.19	(4.0-5.2)	Bands	0	
HGB (g/dL)	12.7	(11.5-15.5)	Lymphocytes	74	1.0
HCT (%)	36.7	(35.0-45.0)	Monocytes	2	0.0
MCV (fL)	87.6	(77.0-95.0)	Eosinophils	0	
MCH (pg)	30.2	(25.0-33.0)	Basophils	0	
MCHC (g/dL)	34.5	(31.0-37.0)			
PLT (×10³/µL)	55.0	(150-400)			
RDW-CV (%)	17.9	(11.5-14.5)			
MPV (fL)	9.6	(7.4-10.4)			

Peripheral blood smear revealed neutropenia with large cytoplasmic inclusions in the neutrophils (**Figure 1**).

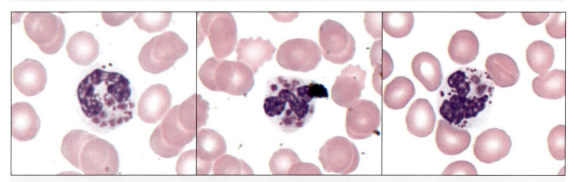

Figure 1 Blood smear (Wright-Giemsa, ×1000) showing neutrophils with giant granules.

Differential Diagnosis Chédiak-Higashi syndrome (CHS) with histiocytic lymphohistiocytosis (HLH) or infection-associated hemophagocytic syndrome (IAHS). Even without the clinical history of CHS, the presence of large cytoplasmic neutrophil inclusions should raise CHS high in the differential. However, CHS in this patient is not sufficient to explain the new onset of fevers, neutropenia, and thrombocytopenia. These findings suggested the occurrence of CHS-associated HLH that might require treatment by allogeneic bone marrow transplantation. Although less likely, these findings could also represent IAHS since patients with CHS have propensity for infections. The IAHS usually resolves with the treatment of the underlying infection.

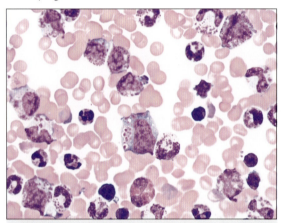

Figure 2 Bone marrow aspirate smear (Wright-Giemsa, ×500) showing many cells with giant granules (image generously provided by Marybeth Helfrich).

Additional Work-Up Fibrinogen 155 mg/dL (normal 172-471), triglyceride 439 mg/dL (normal 28-129), ferritin 2,216 ng/mL (normal 7-142). Bone marrow aspirate smear also showed cytoplasmic inclusions similar to those seen in the granulocytes of the peripheral blood (**Figure 2**). In addition, occasional macrophages with hemophagocytosis were present.

Final Diagnosis Chédiak-Higashi syndrome, childhood form, and associated histiocytic lymphohistiocytosis (accelerated phase of CHS).

Management Approach As in this case, the management of childhood form of CHL is with prophylactic antibiotics and aggressive management of opportunistic infections (most frequently cutaneous and pulmonary). Approximately 85%-90% of childhood forms of CHL develop HLH, also referred to as accelerated phase of CHL. HLH is characterized by uncontrolled activation of macrophages and T cells secondary to defective activity of NK/cytotoxic T cells, with the severe cases requiring allogeneic transplantation. The prognosis in accelerated phase of CHL is poor with mean survival of 3.1 years without allogeneic bone marrow transplantation. With allogeneic transplantation, overall survival is increased to 62%. This patient was treated with high-dose steroids and etoposide to control the HLH. Once the HLH was under control, the patient underwent bone marrow transplant.

General Discussion CHS is a rare autosomal recessive disorder characterized by variable bacterial infections, albinism, bleeding diathesis, and neurological deficiencies. The severity of the disease is dependent on the nature of the genetic mutation and can be sub-grouped as childhood, adolescent, or adult form. Most cases (80%-85%) are childhood CHS and present with recurrent bacterial infections before the age of 2 years, albinism, mild mucosal diathesis, neutropenia, and HLH. Most childhood CHS patients die without bone marrow transplantation. The adolescent form represents 5% of CHL and presents with recurrent bacterial infections before the age of 10 years that become less frequent with age. Adolescent CHL exhibits partial albinism and neutropenia, but neither has HLH nor develops neurologic deficiencies. The adult form represents 10%-15% of CHL and presents with neurologic symptoms after the age of 20 years, but without recurrent infections, albinism, or HLH. The neurologic symptoms include intellectual decline, tremor, ataxia, peripheral neuropathy, and white matter loss. The peripheral blood and bone marrow smears in all 3 forms of CHS have large azurophilic cytoplasmic granules in neutrophils, monocytes, eosinophils, basophils, and their precursors and in granular lymphocytes. In granulocytes and their precursors, these giant granules contain myeloperoxidase and are pathognomonic for CHS. However, enlarged vesicles are present in all cells and are composed of lysosomes, platelet dense granules, or melanosomes, depending on the cell type. Platelets show decreased to absent normal dense bodies. In most cases, the mutation in CHS is localized to the LYST gene on chromosome 1. The LYST gene, also designated CHS1, is a member of the BEACH protein family and probably regulates membrane trafficking and organelle regulation, although the exact function remains to be fully characterized. Severe childhood CHS correlates with null mutations, while missense mutations correlate with adolescent and adult CHS. Some childhood and adult forms of CHS do not have identifiable mutations in the LYST gene, suggesting mutations in other genes also cause CHS. The resulting disregulation of normal membrane trafficking and intracellular vesicle formation help explain many of the clinical symptoms. The recurrent infections result from defective cytotoxic granules in granulocytes, monocytes, cytotoxic T cells, and natural killer cells. Defective MHC peptide loading and chemotaxis further impair normal immune function. Defective melanosome formation explains the decreased pigmentation. Defective dense body formation in platelets leads to bleeding diathesis. Defective neuromelanin granules formation help explain some of the neurological symptoms. Immunoglobulins, antibody production, phagocytosis, and platelet counts remain normal. The diagnostic criteria for HLH are listed in **Table 1**.

Table 1: Diagnosis of HLH requires fulfillment of criterion 1 or 2.
1. Mutations in the genes perforin, Munc13-4, and SSX1 that are linked to familial HLH
2. Meet 5 of 8 following criteria
Fever
Splenomegaly
Cytopenias of 2 or 3 lineages
Hypertriglyceridemia and/or hypofibrogenemia
Hemophagocytosis
Low or absent NK cell activity
Ferritin >500 ng/mL
Soluble CD25 >2,400 U/mL

Niemann-Pick Disease

Imran Siddiqi, Edward Thornborrow

Patient A 3-year-old girl with abdominal distention, fever, and cough.

Clinical History Significant for developmental delay.

Family History Noncontributory.

Medications None.

Physical Examination Notable for hepatosplenomegaly.

Initial Work-Up

CBC	
WBC (×10³/μL)	59.1
RBC (×10⁶/μL)	3.8
HGB (g/dL)	11.2
HCT (%)	32.0
MCV (fL)	84.9
MCH (pg)	29.7
MCHC (g/dL)	34.9
PLT (×10³/μL)	103
RDW-CV (%)	13.5

WBC Differential	%	# (×10³/μL)
Neutrophils	76	44.9
Bands	14	8.3
Lymphocytes	8	4.7
Monocytes	2	1.2

Peripheral blood smear revealed neutrophilia with toxic changes, mild left shift, and no dysplasia or blasts. Bone marrow biopsy and clot section specimen was cellular (100%) with numerous large foamy cells and complete maturation in all lineages (**Figures 1** and **2**). Staining for CD68 confirmed these cells to be of histiocytic origin. Bone marrow aspirate smears and touch preparations: Many large cells with small, eccentric nuclei and abundant vacuolated cytoplasm were seen, both centered in marrow particles (**Figure 3**) and scattered throughout the smears. Mixed trilineage hematopoiesis with mild granulocytic hyperplasia was noted. There was no increase in blasts. Chest X-ray revealed diffuse reticular infiltrates and patchy consolidation suggestive of bronchopneumonia.

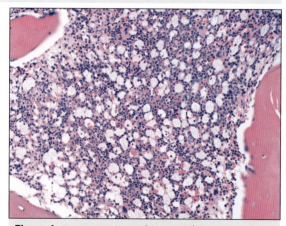

Figure 1 Bone marrow biopsy (H&E, ×200) showing many scattered foam cells interspersed with bone marrow elements.

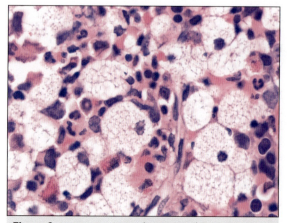

Figure 2 Bone marrow biopsy (H&E, ×1000) showing foam cells with "soap-bubble"-like cytoplasmic vacuolization.

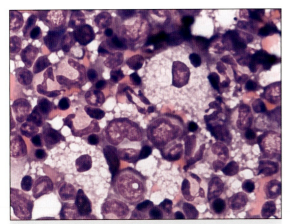

Figure 3 Bone marrow touch prep (Wright-Giemsa, ×1000) showing large cells with abundant vacuolated cytoplasm (foam cells).

Differential Diagnosis In the bone marrow, the presence of increased histiocytes is a nonspecific finding. It most frequently is a sign of increased bone marrow cellular turnover. Conditions associated with histiocytosis include lysosomal storage diseases (eg, Gaucher disease and Niemann-Pick disease), infections (eg, Whipple disease or mycobacterial), hemophagocytic syndrome (either constitutional or associated with an underlying neoplasm or viral infection) or nonspecific/reactive benign histiocytic proliferations. Neoplastic entities that can cause a proliferation of histiocytic cells include histiocytic sarcomas and certain hematopoietic neoplasms, such as monocytic leukemias and both T-cell and Hodgkin lymphomas. Neoplastic cells that can morphologically mimic histiocytes include occasional large cell lymphomas (especially anaplastic large cell lymphoma) and rare variants of myeloma.

Additional Work-Up Markedly decreased acid sphingomyelinase enzyme activity.

Final Diagnosis Marrow histiocytic infiltrate consistent with Niemann-Pick disease, or leukemoid reaction.

Management At present, no specific therapy is available and care is largely supportive. Orthotopic liver transplant has been performed to correct hepatic dysfunction, and hematopoietic progenitor cell transplantation has seen some success in Type B disease. This patient continued to demonstrate marked developmental delay with few words even by the age of 15 years. Shortly following this bone marrow biopsy the patient underwent splenectomy and orthotopic liver transplant complicated by mild acute rejection. He also developed interstitial lung disease characterized by alveolar proteinosis. However, despite the cognitive deficits, he is medically stable 12 years later.

General Discussion Niemann-Pick disease (NPD, also known as sphingomyelin lipidosis) is a heterogeneous group of autosomal recessive lysosomal storage disorders. While at least 6 types have been described, Types A and B NPD are the main subgroups. These 2 subgroups are caused by mutations in the sphingomyelin phosphodiesterase-1 gene, resulting in acid sphingomyelinase deficiency and accumulation of sphingomyelin and other lipids, primarily in cellular lysosomes of the reticuloendothelial system. This leads to varying signs and symptoms (dependent on disease subtype) including hepatosplenomegaly, failure to thrive, developmental delay, ocular abnormalities, occasional respiratory disease (including bouts of bronchopneumonia as seen in this case), and variable neurologic manifestations. Type A NPD, as compared to Type B, has an earlier age of onset and more severe disease with CNS degeneration (in general, Type B patients do not have neurologic involvement). Of note, while Type C disease shares the Niemann-Pick name (largely for historical reasons), it is a rare and distinct entity that occurs due to mutations in the NPC1 or NPC2 genes, leading to accumulation of unesterified cholesterol in cellular lysosomes. The morphologic hallmark of NPD is the presence of enlarged macrophages called storage cells (also known as "foam cells" or "Niemann-Pick cells"). These cells range in size from 20 μm-90 μm and have both eccentric nuclei and abundant cytoplasm filled with lipid droplets, which give rise to numerous crisp cytoplasmic vacuoles imparting a "soap bubble" appearance (as compared to the "crinkled tissue paper" appearance seen in Gaucher disease). In a variant of the disease referred to as sea blue histiocytosis, intermixed dark blue histiocytes may also be prominent. Foam cells are found in the viscera, spleen, bone marrow, tonsils, and lungs. Further, this process can be seen within the ganglion cells of the myenteric plexus. Immunohistochemical and special stains (eg, CD68, oil red O [on frozen sections] and luxol fast blue) can be used to highlight the cells, and a PAS stain, which is weak to negative in NPD, can be helpful in the differential with Gaucher disease (PAS positive). Electron microscopy shows secondary lysosomes that often contain concentrically lamellated, myelin-like figures and/or parallel palisaded lamellae ("zebra bodies"). Laboratory findings include increased LDL cholesterol, decreased HDL, and increased triglycerides. The finding of storage cells in tissue or bone marrow can raise the possibility of NPD, but given the morphologic overlap with other storage disorders, documentation of either decreased acid sphingomyelinase enzyme activity or molecular evidence of the genetic mutation are required for definitive diagnosis.

Mucopolysaccharidosis Type I (Hurler Syndrome)

Lakshmanan Krishnamurti, Raju K Pillai, Raymond E Felgar

Patient A 2-year-old male with recurrent respiratory tract infections and progressive abdominal distention for the past year.

Clinical History The infant was born at term without complications and demonstrated appropriate developmental milestones until 6 months of age. Motor and language development were significantly delayed. He also began developing multiple respiratory infections during the winter months.

Family History There is no history of consanguineous marriage. An older sibling, a 7-year-old sister, is asymptomatic.

Medications Antibiotics and antihistaminics.

Physical Examination Height at 5th percentile for age, head circumference at 90th percentile for age, coarse facial features, macroglossia, low hairline and short neck were noted. Crepitations were present over both lung fields. Examination of the cardiovascular system showed no abnormality. The abdomen was distended with moderate hepatosplenomegaly.

Initial Work-Up

CBC	
WBC ($\times 10^3/\mu L$)	7.8
RBC ($\times 10^6/\mu L$)	4.5
HGB (g/dL)	12.5
HCT (%)	42.0
MCV (fL)	93.3
MCH (pg)	27.8
MCHC (g/dL)	29.8
PLT ($\times 10^3/\mu L$)	189
RDW-CV (%)	15.2

WBC Differential	%	# ($\times 10^3/\mu L$)
Neutrophils	54	4.2
Lymphocytes	39	3.0
Monocytes	6	0.5
Eosinophils	1	0.1

Chest X-ray showed patchy opacities over bilateral lower lung fields. Skeletal radiographs of the limbs showed shortening and thickening of the long bones with irregular diaphyseal and metaphyseal remodeling.

CBC showed a mild normocytic normochromic anemia with a normal WBC differential. However, morphologic review of the peripheral smear revealed lymphocytes with large basophilic granules, some of which were surrounded by a clear halo. Many cytoplasmic vacuoles were seen in the monocytes (**Figure 1**).

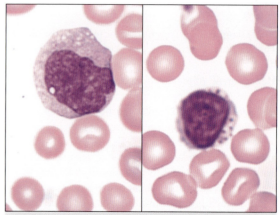

Figure 1 Blood smear (Wright-Giemsa, ×1000) showing **A** multiple vacuoles in a monocyte and **B** a lymphocyte with cytoplasmic vacuoles, many of which contain dark-staining basophilic material.

Differential Diagnosis Cytoplasmic vacuoles with or without basophilic granules in lymphocytes are seen in several constitutional storage disorders such as α mannosidosis, Chédiak-Higashi syndrome, galactosialidosis, glycogen storage disease type II (Pompe disease), mucolipidosis II (I-cell disease) and mucopolysaccharidoses (MPS), especially Hurler syndrome. These inclusions must be distinguished from the granules normally seen in large granular lymphocytes, which typically are not enclosed in a vacuole. Correlation with clinical, laboratory and radiologic studies is required for a correct diagnosis.

Additional Work-Up A skeletal survey showed the characteristic constellation of abnormalities described as dysostosis multiplex. Urinary glycosaminoglycan levels were markedly increased. Chromatographic studies showed increased levels of heparan sulphate and dermatan sulphate. Enzyme analysis of peripheral blood leukocytes showed a significant deficiency of α-L-iduronidase, confirming the diagnosis of MPS I. The patient underwent additional comprehensive skeletal, cardiac, neurologic and ophthalmologic evaluations to assess the extent of disease.

Final Diagnosis Mucopolysaccharidosis, type I (Hurler syndrome).

Management Approach Enzyme replacement therapy with Laronidase was used to stabilize the patient. Hematopoietic progenitor cell transplantation (HPCT) is currently used for treatment of MPS I. Laronidase may be used prior to transplantation as well as for a short time thereafter. HPCT is most effective when initiated before 2 years of age and before the onset of neurological symptoms. Enzyme competent donor cells in the vascular and extravascular compartments provide sufficient enzyme to improve many of the tissue abnormalities. HPCT; however, does not significantly correct skeletal defects. This patient underwent an HPCT from an HLA-matched sibling donor and made a complete hematologic recovery, but continues to have skeletal abnormalities.

General Discussion Mucopolysaccharidoses (MPS) are lysosomal storage disorders caused by deficiency of enzymes required for catabolism of glycosaminoglycans (GAGs), leading to accumulation of partially degraded GAGs in the lysosomes. The phenotype is variable and severity depends upon the quantity of residual enzyme in cells and tissues. 11 MPS disorders are recognized: Hurler syndrome (MPS I), Hunter syndrome (MPS II), Sanfilippo syndrome A-D (MPS Type III A-D), Morquio syndrome A and B (MPS IV A and B), Maroteaux-Lamy syndrome (MPS VI), Sly syndrome (MPS VII) and Natowicz syndrome (MPS IX). The estimated total incidence is 1 in 20,000 live births. Most constitutional storage disorders lead to accumulation of nondegradable material in histiocytes, which results in a foamy appearance of the cytoplasm. Other abnormalities seen in leukocytes in storage diseases include vacuolated lymphocytes and Alder-Reilly anomaly. The Alder-Reilly anomaly consists of large basophilic cytoplasmic inclusions in granulocytes and macrophages. It has been described in patients with α mannosidosis, mucopolysaccharidoses, sialic acid storage disease and multiple sulphatase deficiency. Prominent Alder-Reilly inclusions are seen in mucopolysaccharidoses, especially MPS II, MPS VI and MPS VII. The inclusions seen are not specific and it is important to recognize that these inclusions may be suspicious for the disease, if seen on smear reviews, but are not a primary diagnostic method for these diseases. Mucopolysaccharidosis type I is caused by a mutations in α-L-iduronidase (IDUA) gene located in chromosome 4p16.3, which leads to accumulation of heparan sulphate and dermatan sulphate. The disease is inherited in an autosomal recessive manner. Clinical severity varies in descending order from the most severe form, Hurler syndrome, to an intermediate form Hurler-Scheie syndrome to the least severe form, Scheie syndrome, depending on the specific causative mutations. Hurler syndrome is estimated to affect approximately 1 in 100,000 births. The affected infants do not show any dysmorphic features at birth. They usually present clinically between 9 months to 2 years of age with developmental delay and recurrent respiratory infections. Characteristic dysmorphic features (coarse facies, wide nasal bridge and flattened midface) are usually present by the first year. Other abnormalities include skeletal changes, progressive joint stiffness, hepatosplenomegaly, hydrocephalus, corneal clouding, loss of vision and hearing and cardiac abnormalities. Hematologic abnormalities include vacuoles and inclusions in lymphocytes and monocytes. Most children, despite enzyme therapy or HPCT, do not survive beyond 10 years.

Section I: Miscellaneous Hematologic Conditions

Primary Hyperoxaluria Involving Bone Marrow

Imran Siddiqi, Helen Bailey

Patient A 43-year-old Filipino woman with weakness and light-headedness.

Clinical History The patient had a history of end-stage renal disease 15 years ago secondary to staghorn calculi and obstructive nephropathy. She was status post bilateral nephrectomies and renal transplantation with transplant failure 2 years later secondary to rejection. 6 years prior, she underwent a second transplant complicated by rejection and pyelonephritis. The patient also had a history of anemia and mild pancytopenia. Bone marrow biopsy attempted at another institution was unsuccessful. Cardiac history included multiple arrhythmias, including torsade de pointes. She had pulmonary hypertension, hepatitis C, and hepatosplenomegaly thought to be due to hepatitis C or pulmonary hypertension. She was admitted to the ICU and started on amiodarone.

Family History Noncontributory.

Medications Multivitamin, dronabinol, sevelamer hydrochloride, pantoprazole.

Physical Examination She appeared ill. Her blood pressure was 80/50. Her pulse was 180 with an irregularly irregular rhythm. She had hepatosplenomegaly and surgical scars related to her renal transplants and nephrectomies.

Initial Work-Up

CBC		WBC Differential	%	# ($\times 10^3$/µL)
WBC ($\times 10^3$/µL)	6.1	Neutrophils/bands	75	4.6
RBC ($\times 10^6$/µL)	3.95	Lymphocytes	20	1.2
HGB (g/dL)	10.5	Monocytes	4.5	0.3
HCT (%)	33.2	Eosinophils	0.5	0.0
MCV (fL)	84			
MCH (pg)	26.6			
MCHC (g/dL)	31.6			
PLT ($\times 10^3$/µL)	266			
RDW-CV (%)	15.1			

Peripheral blood smear was remarkable for rare immature granulocytes, mild to moderate polychromatophilia, and minimal red cell anisopoikilocytosis.

Differential Diagnosis The patient's normocytic, normochromic anemia was attributed to renal disease/renal failure with a multifactorial etiology, including secondary to erythropoietin deficiency, anemia of chronic disease, mild iron deficiency and/or evolving vitamin B_{12} or folate deficiency. A bone marrow–specific cause, including myelodysplastic syndrome or a marrow infiltrative process, was an additional consideration.

Additional Work-Up Iron studies were suggestive of anemia of chronic disease. Vitamin B_{12} and folate levels were normal. Antinuclear antibodies (ANA), human immundeficiency virus (HIV), rheumatoid factor, antineutophil cytoplasmic antibody serologies were all negative. A faint serum IgG κ paraprotein was identified on serum electrophoresis, and raised the differential diagnosis of multiple myeloma, chronic lymphocytic leukemia, or amyloidosis. A skeletal survey was negative, and fat pad biopsy was negative. A positron emission tomography (PET) scan showed diffuse, somewhat patchy increased FDG (F18-fluro-2-deoxyglucose) uptake within the bone marrow spaces, possibly representing bone marrow hyperplasia in the setting of anemia vs marrow involvement by lymphoma. Bone marrow biopsy was performed and showed a prominent histiocytic giant cell reaction and extensive deposition of thin, needle-like and coarse, irregular crystals, occasionally in a radial pattern (**Figures 1** and **2**). These crystals were birefringent under polarized light and were consistent with oxalate crystals (**Figure 3**). A blood serum test subsequently revealed an elevated serum oxalate level of 42.8 µmol/L (normal <1.8 µmol/L). Review of slides from the previous kidney explant revealed similar crystals in the renal tubules.

Final Diagnosis Extensive marrow crystal deposition and associated histiocytic reaction, consistent with primary hyperoxaluria. This patient had no known family history of this disease, but upon being notified of the crystals seen in the bone marrow, remarked that crystals had been seen after her first nephrectomies performed in another country. The patient's history of pancytopenia and her current anemia were likely due to the oxalate deposition in the bone marrow.

Management Approach The current treatment for primary hyperoxaluria prior to the onset of renal failure includes a low-oxalate diet, maintaining adequate urinary output, and pyridoxine. For patients with renal disease, combined liver-kidney transplant is the treatment of choice. Due to her multiple medical problems, this patient was treated supportively with continued hemodialysis.

General Discussion This patient presented with multiple conditions that were likely secondary to primary hyperoxaluria. Primary hyperoxaluria is a rare autosomal recessive metabolic disorder induced by enzymatic defects that result in increased conversion of glyoxalate to poorly-soluable oxalate. There are 2 types of primary hyperoxaluria. Type 1 primary hyperoxaluria is more common, although still rare, and due to a deficiency of the liver enzyme alanine-glyoxylate aminotransferase (AGXT). Type 2 primary hyperoxaluria is due to a deficiency of the enzyme glyoxylate reductase/hydroxypyruvate reductase (GRHPR). Sequelae of oxalate accumulation in tissue include chronic renal failure and cardiac conduction defects.

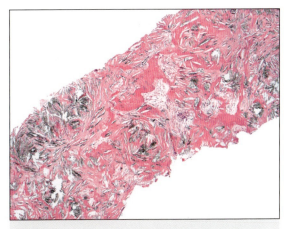

Figure 1 Bone marrow biopsy (H&E, ×40) showing marrow replacement by crystal deposition and associated giant cell reaction.

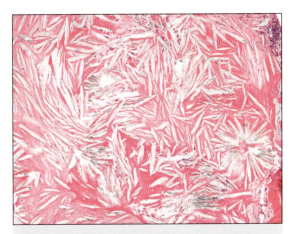

Figure 2 Bone marrow biopsy (H&E, ×100) showing thin, needle-like crystals and coarse, irregular crystals, occasionally in radial pattern.

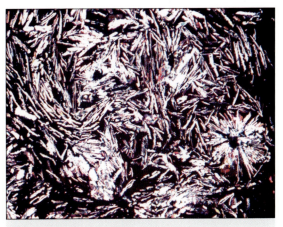

Figure 3 Bone marrow biopsy (H&E, ×100) showing birefringence of crystals under polarized light.

Factor VII Deficiency

Franklin A Bontempo

Patient A 49-year-old African-American male with gastrointestinal bleeding.

Clinical History He had presented with anemia and tarry stools, but upper endocsopy revealed no site of bleeding. The patient had a past medical history of rheumatic fever at the age of 10, a significant nosebleed at the age of 26, and had outpatient surgery for removal from his scalp of what was described as a cyst which may have been blood-filled at the age of 46. He also had a longstanding history of recurrent mild mouth bleeding. He had never been transfused with blood products. He had served in the Marines and had had mild injuries but had no major problems with bleeding.

Family History His father had a history of nosebleeds. 2 sisters were described as bleeders.

Medications Omeprazole.

Physical Examination He has a scar on scalp from prior removal of cyst. The examination of his eyes, heart, lungs, and abdomen were all normal. No bruising was noted. He had full range of motion of all his joints.

Initial Work-Up	
PT (sec)	24.4 (normal 10.5-14.0)
PTT (sec)	23.4 (normal 22-34)
PT mix (sec)	12.6 (normal 10.5-14.0)

Differential Diagnosis Typical diagnostic considerations for a prolonged PT with a normal PTT include congenital deficiency of factor VII, acquired factor VII antibody, vitamin K deficiency, and mild liver disease.

Additional Work-Up The finding of the long PT with a normal PTT isolates the patient's problem to factor VII in the clotting cascade. The normal PT mix essentially rules out the possibility of an antibody against factor VII. Factor VII activity level was 5%. The low level of factor VII in a patient with a bleeding history indicates congenital deficiency of factor VII. In addition 2 of the patient's siblings were eventually found to have a deficiency of factor VII.

Final Diagnosis Congenital deficiency of factor VII.

Management Approach Recombinant factor VIIa is the treatment of choice for congenital deficiency of factor VII. In the past, fresh frozen plasma or prothrombin complex concentrates were used but both are plasma-derived with the attendant risks of transfusion-transmitted viruses and the large volumes of fresh frozen plasma needed to replace factor VII with its relatively short half-life sometimes make its use problematic. Occasional patients who have received replacement therapy for factor VII deficiency have been reported to develop anti-factor VII antibodies, which may cause the PT mix to remain long after mixing with normal plasma and could complicate their therapy. This should be considered if a patient stops responding to factor VII replacement treatment. Patients with a higher level of factor VII and a mild bleeding history may not need to be treated with replacement therapy for minor bleeding. Deciding when to give prophylactic therapy prior to surgery should depend on the type and site of surgery, the patient's past bleeding history and factor VII level, and the relative risk of the type of replacement therapy being used. Usually factor replacement to 100% levels of factor VII is not necessary for adequate hemostasis. Replacement to 30%-40% level of factor

VII is probably adequate in many cases. This patient continued to have bleeding symptoms, including epistaxis, rectal bleeding, and dental bleeding, which have responded well to treatment with recombinant factor VIIa. For dental extractions as well as other minor surgical procedures, he has received prophylaxis with recombinant factor VIIa and has had no bleeding difficulty. He was also vaccinated for hepatitis A because of his increased risk of blood product exposure but did not receive hepatitis B vaccine since he was found to be positive for anti-HBs and anti-HBc on testing prior to vaccination.

General Discussion Congenital deficiency of factor VII is a rare autosomal recessive bleeding disorder affecting males and females equally and occurring in an estimated 1 in 500,000 individuals. More than 100 different gene mutations responsible for factor VII deficiency have been identified and many patients who are bleeders have homozygous mutations or compound heterozygous mutations. In addition several dysfunctional factor VII variants have been identified which lead to the bleeding phenotype due to factor VII molecules that are present but have reduced factor VII activity. In contrast to hemophilia A and hemophilia B, the level of factor VII in patients with congenital factor VII deficiency does not correlate well with the clinical severity of the patient's bleeding symptoms. Concern has persisted that the cause of this may be at least partially related to variability in the source of the tissue factor used in the factor VII assay. Bleeding severity is variable and ranges from asymptomatic to very mild, which is presumed to be more likely in heterozygotes, to as severe as the bleeding seen in hemophilia A or B in rare cases, which would be more likely to be expected in patients with factor VII activity <1% of normal. Common types of bleeding with factor VII deficiency include easy bruising, epistaxis, soft tissue hemorrhage, menorrhagia, bleeding with trauma, and postoperative bleeding. Postpartum and intracranial hemorrhage may be seen in severely affected patients but in general these types of hemorrhage and bleeding after abdominal and pelvic surgery appear to be less likely than bleeding after surgery on mucosal surfaces for unclear reasons. In addition, seemingly paradoxical thromboembolism has been seen in some patients with congenital deficiency of factor VII, even at low levels.

Hemophilia A (Factor VIII Deficiency)—Newborn Diagnosis

Margaret V Ragni

Patient A 3-day-old male infant with bleeding from the circumcision site.

Clinical History The infant was born at 40 weeks gestation via spontaneous vaginal delivery to a G2, P2 28-year-old mother with negative prenatal labs at an outlying hospital. APGARs were 10 and 10. Following circumcision, the child was noted to have active bleeding from the circumcision site, and the site continued to ooze despite Surgi-gel. CBC and coagulation tests were drawn. The PT was normal, APTT was elevated, and the band count was increased. Ampicillin and gentamicin were begun, and the infant was transferred to our institution for further work-up.

Family History There was no family history in any of the male relatives of the mother.

Medications Ampicillin and gentamicin.

Physical Examination On admission, physical exam revealed an alert male infant. Vital signs were stable, and there were no signs of distress, with an O_2 saturation of 99% on room air. Pupils were round, equal, and reactive to light. Extraocular movements were intact. The head was normocephalic, and the fontanelle was open and flat. Cardiovascular exam revealed regular rate and rhythm, with normal S1 and S2 and no murmurs. Lungs were clear. There was no organomegaly, lymphadenopathy or petechiae. The umbilical stump was clean, dry, and intact. A small friable clot was observed at the circumcision site. Arterial pulses were 2+. Capillary refill was within normal limits. The neurologic exam was unremarkable, with an alert child moving all extremities, with intact reflexes.

Initial Work-Up

CBC	At Birth	At Transfer
HGB (g/dL)	18.0	9.0
HCT (%)	54.0	26.4
PLT (×10³/mL)	247	
MCV (fL)	108	
PT (seconds)	12.2	(normal 10.5-14.0)
PTT (seconds)	51.0	(normal 22.0-34.0)

The peripheral smear revealed a dimorphic population with macrocytic and microcytic red cells, with occasional target cells and rare nucleated red cells, consistent with normal newborn liver dysfunction and acute blood loss anemia. White blood cell morphology was normal, and platelets were adequate.

Differential Diagnosis Circumcision bleeding is the sine qua non for hemophilia, either factor VIII deficiency (hemophilia A) or factor IX deficiency (hemophilia B). The disorders are indistinguishable clinically, although 85% of those affected have hemophilia A, and thus this is the more likely diagnosis. Other possibilities include anatomic bleeding, or mucosal bleeding due to a defect of primary hemostasis (eg, von Willebrand disease or a disorder of platelet function). Of interest, disorders of primary hemostasis generally do not present with circumcision bleeding, but are more likely to cause oral bleeding, epistaxis, or gastrointestinal bleeding.

Additional Work-Up The PTT was elevated, and because of circumcision bleeding, factor VIII and IX were drawn. The PTT was prolonged to 51 seconds, which corrected in a 1:1 mix with normal plasma to 34 seconds. The factor VIII activity level was <1 %, consistent with a diagnosis of severe hemophilia A. It should be noted that in newborns, it is not unusual to find mild decrease in liver-synthesized factors, consistent with newborn liver, which may be associated with a mildly prolonged pro time (PT). It is critical to realize this, as a factor IX activity level of 30% in a newborn may be normal and not diagnostic of hemophilia B, although a factor IX activity level of 1% or 2%, when other liver-synthesized factors are in the 30%-40% range, is entirely consistent with hemophilia B.

APTT mix	34.0 seconds	(normal 22.0-34.0)
Fibrinogen	220 mg/dL	(normal 150-350)
Factor II	60 %	(normal 60-140)
Factor V	70 %	(normal 50-150)
Factor VII	60 %	(normal 60-160)
Factor VIII	<1 %	(normal 50-150)
Factor IX	65 %	(normal 65-135)
Factor X	70 %	(normal 70-150)
Factor XI	65 %	(normal 65-140)
Factor XII	61 %	(normal 50-170)

Final Diagnosis Severe factor VIII deficiency/hemophilia A.

Management Approach A complete exam, review of the diagnosis, and counseling by the psychosocial staff followed. Information was given, and family and social history reviewed. Options for home factor supply were reviewed, and based on family choice, a home storage and factor supply program were set up. The patient was discharged after 2 hospital days, and seen in follow-up at 10 days of age at the hemophilia center at a tertiary care institution. The child was given recombinant factor VIII to stop the circumcision bleeding and given a home supply for future bleeds, as local hospitals did not carry the product. Once a diagnosis of factor VIII (hemophilia A) or factor IX (hemophilia B) is suspected, it is essential to involve a hematologist with expertise in coagulation as early as possible. This will assure the diagnosis is made quickly, that the family is involved, and that treatment is instituted early, in order to avert hemostatic complications. Failure to recognize circumcision bleeding as an early sign of hemophilia may lead to severe anemia, and even respiratory or cardiovascular compromise, and lead to severe morbidity or even mortality. The approach to management is to inform the family and iniatiate factor replacement with recombinant factor VIII to stop the bleeding. In order to maintain hemostasis, monitoring hemostasis by PTT, hematocrit, and clinical course is recommended. Treatment must be continued until bleeding stops. For circumcision, this is usually 1-2 days. In families with a history of hemophilia, an affected newborn male will have the same type and severity of hemophilia as other affected members. When women in families with hemophilia become pregnant, they are tested in the 8th month of pregnancy for factor levels to assist in delivery and given a cord blood kit to obtain a cord blood sample at delivery to ensure early testing and diagnosis. Once a diagnosis is made, the child is seen with his family within 1-2 weeks or as early as possible at the nearby hemophilia treatment center (HTC). Data from the CDC has found that patients with hemophilia who are cared for at HTCs have longer, healthier lives than those receiving care outside of HTCs.

General Discussion This case points up the problem of managing bleeding in the young infant with hemophilia A. In the absence of a family history, the diagnosis may be delayed. Up to ⅓ of hemophilia cases arise as spontaneous mutations, the defective gene occurring in the mother's X chromosome. Half of those with severe hemophilia A have a signature mutation, the factor VIII intron 22 inversion mutation, which can easily be assessed by PCR techniques. When a diagnosis is not suspected or known, potential risks during the birth process include CNS bleeding caused by vacuum extraction during delivery, which is contraindicated in children with hemophilia. Parents and pediatricians may not suspect the diagnosis until the development of hemarthroses, which usually occur as the child begins to ambulate. The typical clinical picture is that of intermittent joint hemorrhages, spontaneous or traumatic, primarily of the knees, ankles, or elbows. Optimal management is via infusion of clotting factor concentrate daily to treat joint bleeding and achieve hemostasis. The current approach; however, is to prevent joint bleeding and joint damage by the prophylactic infusion of factor VIII 3 times weekly. In very small children, intravenous infusions often require the placement of central lines, which can be complicated by infection. In up to 20% of children who receive repeated doses of clotting factor concentrate, inhibitor antibodies may form, that is alloantibodies to foreign infused factor VIII, which is not responsive to standard treatment and associated with high morbidity. In early childhood, pediatricians often avoid immunizations in children with hemophilia for fear of bleeding, but this is unfounded, and with pressure applied for 10 minutes to the immunization site, few problems arise. Recurrent hemarthroses, if inadequately prevented or not treated early enough, may lead to synovial inflammation, degeneration, pain, and disability, necessitating surgery in the early 20s. In families of a new child with hemophilia, it is also critical to provide the social services and supportive counseling to assist in optimal patient outcomes. This includes counseling regarding avoiding contact sports, early home treatment training, and counseling regarding future pregnancies and risk of hemophilia.

Hemophilia A (Factor VIII Deficiency) Carrier

Margaret V, Ragni

Patient A 45-year-old-woman, who presented to her family practice physician for preoperative clearance for carpal tunnel syndrome.

Clinical History The woman was seen by an orthopedic surgeon for painful inflammatory arthritis of the right writs with distal radioulnar joint synovitis, unresponsive to multiple injections. She also had numbness, tingling, and weakness of the 4th and 5th digits of her right hand, in the distribution of the ulnar nerve, consistent with carpal tunnel syndrome. Her past medical problems included adult-onset diabetes, lupus, autoimmune (Hashimoto) thyroiditis, restrictive pericarditis, and gastroesophageal reflux disease (GERD). Her past bleeding history was significant for longstanding bruising history and bleeding ulcers associated with use of ibuprofen. Her past surgical history included tubal ligation, ovarian cyst rupture, breast lumpectomy, and lymph node biopsy. She had been told to use DDAVP for bleeding symptoms. She was told she had von Willebrand disease and factor VIII deficiency, and was referred to the hemophilia center for treatment if bleeding was encountered in surgery.

Family History The family history was significant for a father who died from AIDS at age 40 due to hemophilia, a mother with gastric cancer, a son with an aneurysm, paternal uncle and grandfather with coronary artery disease, and a maternal aunt with breast cancer. A sister was said to have hemophilia.

Medications Furosemide, vitamin D, vitiamin B_{12}, folic acid, fish oil, and omeprazole.

Physical Examination On examination, she was a healthy appearing woman in no acute distress. Vital signs were normal. Extraocular muscles were intact, conjunctivae were clear, and pupils were equal, round and responsive to light. The neck was supple with no adenopathy. The thyroid was palpably enlarged with nodule and tenderness to palpation. The lungs were clear without wheezing, and the cardiac exam was regular rhythm with normal S1 and S2, no murmurs. Carotids were 2+ bilaterally with no bruits, and pedal pulses were 2+ and equal bilaterally. The abdomen was soft, nontender with no masses or organomegaly. The musculoskeletal exam was notable for a boggy right wrist with decreased sensation.

Initial Work-Up

PTT (seconds)	38.0	(normal 22.0-34.0)
Factor VIII activity (%)	34	(normal 50-150)

No laboratory results were available, so the hemophilia center repeated her labs, confirming a decreased factor VIII.

Differential Diagnosis The differential diagnosis of a decreased factor VIII in a woman is hemophilia A carrier or von Willebrand disease (vWD), or both. A woman may have hemophilia in the rare event she inherits 2 affected X chromosomes, ie, her mother is a hemophilia carrier and her father has hemophilia, or if she inherits an affected X chromosome, ie, if she has Turner XO syndrome. A moderately severe bleeding phenotype may be seen with hemophilia A carriers who are highly lionized carriers, and have moderately decreased factor VIII levels consistent with phenotypically mild hemophilia; or vWD with severe bleeding phenotype, eg, severe type 1 vWD, or type II or III vWD.

Additional Work-Up von Willebrand testing revealed normal vWF:RCo and normal vWF:Ag.
- vWF:RCo 89% (normal 55-160)
- vWF:Ag 117% (normal 55-160)

Final Diagnosis Mild factor VIII deficiency, consistent with hemophilia A carrier status.

Management Approach The patient underwent a right wrist fusion, with arthroplasty and hemi-replacement of the ulnar head, and carpal tunnel release, under coverage of desmopressin, tolerated the procedure well, and was discharged the following day, with arrangements for outpatient DDAVP as ordered. She saw the orthopedic surgeon in follow-up 10 days later, complaining of increased swelling, numbness, and persistently poor motion of the right wrist. Ibuprofen was recommended to decrease the inflammation, but there was no improvement in the swelling, numbness, or wrist motion, and she called the hemophilia center and was immediately begun on daily factor VIII concentrate, with slow resolution of the swelling and pain.

General Discussion Several problems developed following the otherwise straightforward diagnosis and management of this patient. Continued bleeding was not reported or recognized, and thus no treatment was provided. It is well recognized that DDAVP, which induces secretion of vWF and factor VIII from endothelial stores (Weibel Palade bodies), depletes these stores after 3 days. Thus, for ongoing bleeding, factor concentrates are required, either factor VIII concentrate for hemophilia A carriers, or vWF concentrate in those with vWD is recommended. However, the lack of recognition of the bleeding and reporting of ongoing swelling, which was caused by her ongoing bleeding, prevented early intervention with factor VIII concentrate. The recommendation by the surgeon to use ibuprofen to reduce postoperative bleeding likely actually led to its exacerbation. Concomitant use of ibuprofen in the setting of factor VIII deficiency results in 2 coagulation defects, (1) congenital factor VIII deficiency due to hemophilia A carrier status, a defect in secondary hemostasis, and (2) acquired platelet dysfunction due to ibuprofen, a defect in primary hemostasis, which together likely accounted for her severe postoperative bleeding. Drugs inhibiting platelet function are contraindicated in patients with bleeding disorders undergoing surgery, and were recommended against in the original surgical orders provided by the HTC to the hospital where she had her surgery. The fact that neither the patient nor the surgeon contacted the HTC in the face of increased swelling at the operative site in a patient with a bleeding disorder, which was due to ongoing bleeding exacerbated by ibuprofen, led to the prolonged postoperative morbidity. It is of note that families may not share information, especially with the associated stigma of AIDS. As a result, women at risk, ie, all daughters of affected males or half of the daughters of carrier females, may be unaware of their status. This patient did know of her carrier status and sought care at a hemophilia treatment center, who provided orders and postoperative management.

Hemophilia B (Factor IX Deficiency)

Franklin A Bontempo

Patient A 6-year-old Amish boy with a significant hematoma on the back of his head.

Clinical History He was working on his family's dairy farm and had fallen and hit his head on a cow stanchion (metal bar which helps keep the cow in place while being milked), which caused the hematoma. The child had a history of easy bruising but no history of significant hemorrhages, had never been hospitalized, and had no history of surgery. He had not been circumcised as a newborn and had not been seen by a dentist regularly. There was a history of bleeding in the family due to factor IX deficiency (hemophilia B) but the patient had never been tested. He was initially seen at a local hospital but because the hematoma was larger than expected and his PTT was prolonged, he was airlifted to a tertiary care center where he was found to have a subdural hematoma.

Family History There was a family history of factor IX deficiency (hemophilia B).

Medications None.

Physical Examination Hematoma on the back of head. No other bruising. He was awake and oriented and had full range of motion of all his joints.

Initial Work-Up	
PT (seconds)	12.0 (normal 10-13)
PTT (seconds)	42.5 (normal 24-34)
Platelet count (× 10^3/μL)	192

Differential Diagnosis Factor VIII deficiency (hemophilia A), factor IX deficiency (hemophilia B), von Willebrand disease, and congenital deficiency of factor XI. The patient's normal PT and prolonged PTT isolated the diagnosis of his bleeding problem to the upper part of the intrinsic clotting pathway. Factor XII deficiency was not in the differential diagnosis since the latter has not been known to be associated with bleeding. von Willebrand disease and congenital factor XI deficiency would be less likely to cause as significant a hemorrhage as this patient had at presentation although both could have been possible based on the initial PT and PTT. The family history of hemophilia B led us to measure factor IX activity level.

Additional Work-Up
- Factor IX activity 7% (normal 60-135)
- Factor IX inhibitor level 0.0 BU (normal 0.0)

Final Diagnosis Mild factor IX deficiency (hemophilia B).

Management Approach The therapy of hemophilia B has changed significantly over the past 50 years from whole blood and fresh frozen plasma to pooled plasma concentrates followed by heat-treated clotting factor concentrates with the onset of HIV infection. The current treatment of choice is recombinant factor IX concentrate which has essentially eliminated concern for transfusion-transmitted viruses or the potential allergic or immunologic consequences of plasma-derived concentrates. A small percentage of patients with hemophilia B may develop an antibody to factor IX which makes treatment with clotting factor concentrate difficult. An antibody may be suspected when the frequency of a patient's hemorrhages increases or when his usual clotting factor dose is no longer resolving his hemorrhage. Occasionally large doses of clotting factor may be tried to overwhelm the antibody or induction of immune tolerance with daily doses of clotting recombinant factor IX concentrate. Because of the possibility of the development of an antibody, inhibitor titers are usually recommended prior to any planned surgical procedures. Recent attempts in humans to use gene therapy to raise factor IX levels high enough to eliminate hemorrhages have been undertaken based on successful animal models and results of early patient trials have suggested that this therapy may have potential benefit. This patient was treated initially twice daily and then once daily with clotting factor concentrate containing factor IX for a total of 2 weeks and that led to resolution of the hematoma. He was also vaccinated for hepatitis A and hepatitis B because of concern for transfusion-transmitted viruses. He had relatively few hemorrhages in the ensuing years, about 1 per year, because the clinical severity of his hemophilia B is mild and all of the hemorrhages were associated with trauma, none was spontaneous. His knee joints were common sites of hemorrhages and he developed moderate chronic hemophilic arthropathy despite treatment with factor IX concentrate. He was also routinely treated with clotting factor prophylactically for surgical procedures after checking for the development of an anti-factor IX antibody. Initially he was treated for his hemorrhages on a PRN basis in the hospital emergency room, but as he grew older, he learned to self-administer the clotting factor at home, which allowed him to receive treatment more rapidly and prevent extension of any developing hemorrhage.

General Discussion Hemophilia A and B are sex-linked recessive disorders primarily affecting males with a relative frequency of hemophilia A to hemophilia B of 4:1. Hemophilia B or congenital factor IX deficiency is sometimes referred to as Christmas disease after the name of the first family identified with the disorder in 1952 and is found in 1 in every 25,000-30,000 male births. Women are usually carriers for the hemophilias with bleeding symptoms only occurring when a carrier female develops another, usually acquired, bleeding disorder, such as liver disease. Both hemophilia A and B patients are classified as clinically mild, moderate or severe based on the measured level of factor VIII or IX. Patients are classified as severe if the factor level is <1% of normal, moderate from 2%-5%, and mild when >5%. Hemophilia B is extremely common in Amish patients in the US due to an early Amish immigrant who had the disorder and the marked degree of inbreeding in the Amish community. As a result, occasional Amish women have 2 abnormal X chromosomes for factor IX deficiency and are clinical hemophilia B patients.

Hemophilia B (Factor IX Deficiency) Carrier

Margaret V Ragni

Patient A 23-year-old woman, who went into labor with her first child at home and was attended by a midwife.

Clinical History The woman had a 20-hour labor and an uneventful delivery of a normal 7-pound, 3-ounce girl, complicated by severe postpartum bleeding.

Family History She is a member of a large factor IX deficiency (hemophilia B) kindred. Her father was normal. Her maternal grandfather had moderately severe hemophilia B with a factor IX activity level of 4%, and experienced only traumatic bleeds. Her mother was an obligate carrier, as the daughter of an affected male with hemophilia B. Her siblings included 4 affected brothers and 1 sister who was an obligate carrier with 2 affected sons. She has been informed she had a 50/50 chance of being a carrier, depending on which of the 2 X chromosomes she inherited from her mother. Her past bleeding history was notable for occasional traumatic bruising and mouth bleeding after dental extraction. Neither she nor her mother nor sisters had menorrhagia or postpartum bleeding. The patient's factor IX activity level, obtained during routine hemophilia outreach clinic, 27% is consistent with a lionized carrier.

Medications Prenatal vitamins.

Physical Examination She was tachycardic and dizzy. Her abdomen was mildly distended and tender. She had bloody vaginal discharge. Her exam was otherwise unremarkable.

Initial Work-Up		
PTT (seconds)	42.0	(normal 22.0-34.0)
Factor IX (%)	27	(normal 50-150)

When she was 17 years old, she was tested for factor IX activity level during an outreach comprehensive hemophilia clinic during which her affected brothers and grandfather were also seen.

She was found to have a factor IX activity level of 27%, and she and her mother were counseled to notify the hemophilia treatment center (HTC) when she became pregnant and to come in for factor IX testing at the 8th month of pregnancy to assist with decisions regarding epidural anesthesia, and a cord blood testing kit to test the newborn child for hemophilia B.

Differential Diagnosis Carrier state—factor IX deficiency carrier. Given the patient's history, this is the most likely diagnosis.

Additional Work-Up In the 8th month of pregnancy, her factor IX activity level was 49%, consistent with hormonal effects of pregnancy, but persistent factor IX deficiency.

Final Diagnosis Postpartum hemorrhage in a factor IX deficiency carrier, responsive to factor IX replacement.

Management Approach Factor replacement is the general treatment of choice. Her pregnancy was complicated by postpartum bleeding. She was taken to the nearby hospital for evaluation, where she was noted to have tachycardia and shivering. The hematocrit was 21%, and hemoglobin 7 g/dL. The gynecologic exam revealed no lacerations, retained placenta, or evidence of uterine atony. The hospital and family discussed the case with the HTC physician, and she was given factor IX concentrate at 50 IU/kg daily for the next 4 days, and transfused 2 units of packed red cells. The bleeding stopped with replacement therapy and the hematocrit slowly corrected with iron replacement over the next 3 months.

General Discussion Postpartum bleeding developed in a factor IX deficient carrier following a routine delivery. The lack of menorrhagia is not unusual in hemophilia carriers, as the latter is mucosal bleeding, more typical of individuals with platelet functional defects or von Willebrand disease. Although there were no identified anatomic bleeding defects, this case represents a typical lionized carrier with postpartum bleeding. Prevention requires 4 days of factor at minimum, based on previous cases in this HTC. Dosing of recombinant factor at 50 IU/kg was chosen as this is the dose used for mild hemophilia B patients. The patient had blood loss anemia, for which she was transfused. Generally, carriers of hemophilia are counseled on the genetics of hemophilia need for levels to be drawn in the 8th month of pregnancy, to assist with decisions regarding dosing epidural anesthesia. A cord blood kit is used to determine if the newborn child is affected. Generally, midwives are discouraged in those with low factor IX levels, and factor is recommended for at minimum 4 days.

Factor V Inhibitor

James Zehnder

Patient A 73-year-old male with severe mitral regurgitation was admitted for valve replacement.

Clinical History The patient had a history of previous porcine mitral valve replacement 10 years earlier and had no other medical problems. He underwent surgery as planned. The surgery was complicated by many adhesions from the prior valve surgery and diffuse oozing of blood from the surgical site was noted. Hemostasis was achieved by packing the chest with gelfoam soaked in topical bovine thrombin. The postoperative course was uneventful until the 5th post-op day, when it was noted that the patient's PT and PTT which had previously been normal, were both increasing. On the 7th postoperative day, the PTT was 120 sec (normal 25 sec-35 sec) and PT was 60 sec (normal 11 sec-15 sec) and the patient suffered a hemothorax, requiring surgical drainage and transfusion of 4 units of red cells. He received numerous units of plasma and cryopreciptate without a significant change in his clotting times.

Family History Noncontributory.

Medications Heparin for DVT prophylaxis (discontinued on the 5th postoperative day).

Physical Examination The patient was intubated with a chest tube which continued to drain bloody fluid. He had numerous ecchymoses noted at blood draw and IV sites. The surgical dressing required changing several times/day due to saturation with blood.

Initial Work-Up

CBC		
HGB (g /dL)	11	
WBC (×10³/µL)	6	
PLT (x10³/µL)	300	
PT (sec)	43.8	(normal 11-15)
PTT (sec)	99.7	(normal 25-35)

Peripheral blood smear revealed no abnormalities. Thrombin time with human thrombin was not prolonged; however the thrombin time with bovine thrombin was >100 sec. PT, PTT and bovine TT mixing studies did not correct when mixed with normal plasma, consistent with the presence of an inhibitor.

Differential Diagnosis A common pathway inhibitor should be suspected in patients who present with prolonged PT and PTT, without correction by mixing studies. The targeted factor can be identified by specific factor assays. The TT results demonstrate that the patient has made an antibody against bovine thrombin, but not against human thrombin, so this is not likely to be the cause of bleeding. The patient has an acquired clotting factor inhibitor. As both the PT and PTT are affected, the antibody is likely to be against a common pathway factor (fibrinogen, factor II, V or X).

Additional Work-Up Specific assays of common pathway factors were performed. Factor I, II, and X were normal. However factor V was <1%, indicating a severe deficiency, which in this case was associated with significant bleeding risk. There was immunologically detectable bovine factor V contaminating the topical bovine thrombin preparation which had been used during surgery. Western blots using the patients purified IgG demonstrated reactivity with bovine and human factor V.

Final Diagnosis Acquired factor V deficiency due to contamination of the topical bovine thrombin preparation with factor V, with an immune response resulting in an IgG antibody reacting with bovine and human factor V.

Management Approach The general approach for acquired factor inhibitors is immunosuppression and preventing/controlling bleeding complications. Standard regimens would include steroids; additional considerations would include IV Ig, and various chemotherapeutic agents. Rituximab could be considered for refractory cases but will not have an immediate impact on a patient with bleeding. Plasma transfusions are unlikely to benefit an individual with a high-titer antibody and may lead to volume overload issues. Use of antifibrinolytic drugs may benefit patients with active bleeding. Plasmapheresis can rapidly decrease the titer of an inhibitor in a patient with life-threatening bleeding. However these antibodies are usually IgG with a large volume of distribution, and thus the benefit will be transient. This patient was initially treated with an immunosuppressive regimen (cyclophosphamide, vincristine, prednisone) an antifibrinolytic drug (epsilon-amino caproic acid) and platelet transfusions (which have been reported in some patients as a source of factor V in patients with inhibitors) without benefit. Because of the life-threatening nature of his bleeding the patient underwent plasmapheresis with an immediate decrease in his clotting time. His clotting times gradually became prolonged again; each time his PTT was >100 seconds, the patient experienced a bleeding complication. After a total of 3 plasmaphereses over a 70-day period, the antibody response subsided and his clotting times remained in the normal range

General Discussion Many cases of acquired factor V inhibitors developing in association with topical bovine thrombin have been reported. This has led to a FDA black box warning for topical bovine thrombin preparations. Ongoing efforts by the pharmaceutical industry to further purify bovine thrombin preparations and to develop recombinant human topical thrombin preparations may decrease the frequency of these antibodies. However, it is important to note that not all acquired factor V antibodies are related to topical bovine thrombin use. In these cases definitive causal relationships have not been made, but associations with antibiotics and other drugs have been reported. Thus factor V inhibitors remain a rare but clinically significant acquired bleeding disorder, second in frequency to acquired factor VIII inhibitors.

Factor VIII Inhibitor

Nicole Verdun, Katherine High

Patient A 2-year-old African-American male with a history of severe hemophilia A (factor VIII deficiency) was brought to the emergency room with right knee pain and swelling.

Clinical History His parents stated that he woke from a nap yesterday crying, and they noticed the swelling in his knee. There was no witnessed trauma. The parents administered 100% correction with factor VIII replacement therapy yesterday afternoon and again this morning. Despite factor infusion, the family noted a continued increase in his knee swelling, and his pain was no longer controlled with home analgesics. The patient was a passenger in a motor vehicle accident 2 months prior to presentation, and required emergent surgery for an epidural hematoma evacuation requiring intense factor VIII concentrate replacement for 10 days. He has otherwise required no treatment for bleeding and is not maintained on a prophylaxis regimen. He has had no problems with bleeding since the motor vehicle accident.

Family History The patient had an older brother with severe hemophilia A and a history of an inhibitor to factor VIII, who is now deceased.

Medications Recombinant factor VIII as needed.

Physical Examination In general, the patient was crying and pointing to his right lower extremity. He had a large fluctuant effusion over his right knee with proximal extension to his mid-thigh. He held his right lower extremity in extension. His examination was otherwise within normal limits.

Initial Work-Up	
HGB (g/dL)	10.0
PLT (x10³/μL)	250
Factor VIII activity*	<1%*

*Last treatment of 100% correction was 5 hours prior

Differential Diagnosis The differential diagnosis of persistent bleeding in a patient with severe hemophilia A despite therapy includes an inhibitor to factor VIII, incorrect mixing and administration of factor replacement, or an additional undiagnosed bleeding disorder. The assay measurement noted above indicates an inadequate response to factor replacement, making an inhibitor the most likely diagnosis.

Additional Work-Up Factor VIII inhibitor assay: 15 Bethesda units (BU).

Final Diagnosis Severe hemophilia A (factor VIII deficiency) with a high-titer inhibitor.

Management Approach The management of patients with severe hemophilia and inhibitor formation requires careful consideration of both acute and chronic therapy. The treatment used for an acute bleeding episode is dependant upon the inhibitor titer. In patients with a low-titer inhibitor, treatment of acute bleeding episodes can often be achieved with higher doses of factor VIII concentrate than traditionally used. In patients with a high-titer inhibitor, treatment with a bypassing agent, such as prothrombin complex concentrates or recombinant factor VIIa is often needed. Consultation with a hematologist is recommended. Due to the presence of a high-titer inhibitor, he was managed with recombinant factor VIIa over 3 days starting with every 2 hour dosing and increasing the interval between doses as his bleeding resolved. The patient was followed very closely as an outpatient over the next month, and his inhibitor titer dropped to 4 BU but was persistently present. Immune tolerance induction (ITI) was begun to attempt to eradicate his inhibitor completely. He received daily infusions of factor VIII at 100 IU/kg/day. His initial response to ITI was an increase in his inhibitor titer to a peak of 100 BU, but he had a subsequent decline in his titer over the next 15 months, with eradication of his inhibitor after 15 months of therapy.

General Discussion An inhibitor should be suspected in any patient with hemophilia who fails to respond to usual factor replacement. The presence of an inhibitor does not cause an increased incidence of bleeding, but does lead to difficulty in treating a bleeding episode. After a clinical suspicion is established, a Bethesda assay is performed to measure the presence of an inhibitor and its titer. In a Bethesda assay, the patient's plasma at different dilutions is mixed with equal volumes of pooled normal plasma and allowed to incubate at 37ºC for 2 hours. Residual factor VIII activity is measured in the mixed sample. The inhibitor titer is the reciprocal of the dilution of patient plasma that results in 50% factor VIII activity inhibition. A patient is further classified as having a high-titer or low-titer inhibitor if the antibody level is ≥5 Bethesda units (BU) or <5 Bethesda units, respectively. The patient above had a high titer inhibitor at diagnosis (15 BU), and a low titer inhibitor at the time of immune tolerance induction (4 BU). The incidence of inhibitor formation in those with severe hemophilia A is about 25%, and half of inhibitors seen are considered transient and disappear with no intervention and with continued exposure to factor concentrate. Patients with low-titer inhibitors at the time of initial detection are more likely to have transient inhibitors, making this less likely in our patient. The success of immune tolerance therapy (ITT) to eradicate an inhibitor is dependent upon the antibody titer at ITT onset. In the North American Immune Tolerance Registry, ITT was successful in 83% of patients with hemophilia A when the inhibitor titer prior to induction was <10 BU, vs 40% success of tolerance with titers of ≥10 BU. Regimens of immune tolerance differ both in dose and frequency, with the most success seen in regimens which include daily doses of factor VIII concentrate of 50 IU-100 IU/kg/day. As noted in our patient, many patients have an anamnestic response to immune tolerance induction, with an initial increase in their inhibitor titer followed by a progressive decrease with the continuation of therapy. Other regimens for immune tolerance include immunosuppressive agents such as corticosteroids or rituximab with mixed success rates. Some of the risk factors for inhibitor formation include mutation type, ethnicity, family history of inhibitor formation, and factor VIII polymorphisms. Large deletions, followed by nonsense mutations or inversions of intron 22 or intron 1 are overrepresented in patients with inhibitor formation. The incidence and prevalence of inhibitors is 50% in African-American patients vs 25% in Caucasian patients. Recent data suggest that differences in single nucleotide polymorphisms in the factor VIII gene may lead to these differences in inhibitor risk. Recombinant factor products correspond to haplotypes much more prevalent in Caucasian patients, and the haplotypes found to be more prevalent in African-American patients are not included. A high concordance rate among siblings has also been seen in multiple studies. In the Malmo International Brother Study the rate of inhibitor concordance between siblings (either all siblings or none of the siblings had inhibitor development) was 76%. Knowledge about risk factors for inhibitor formation continues to increase, and will inform decision-making and may lead to personalized medicine options for hemophilia in the future. Other environmental factors that have been implicated include the age of the patient at the time of initial treatment, treatment intensity, and the early use of prophylaxis regimens. Knowledge about risk factors for inhibitor formation continues to increase, and will inform decision-making and may lead to personalized medicine options for hemophilia in the future.

Acquired Factor X Deficiency

Dorothy M Adcock-Funk, Dennis Casciato

Patient A 52-year-old female with protein in her urine and elevated serum cholesterol was scheduled for renal biopsy. As a preoperative screen, a prothrombin time (PT) and an activated partial thromboplastin time (PTT) were ordered. The PT was elevated at 22.4 seconds and PTT was normal.

Clinical History The patient had undergone transabdominal hysterectomy and bilateral salpingo-oophorectomy and cystocele repair 6 years previously without any bleeding complications. She had undergone tooth extractions without bleeding and did not suffer menorrhagia, epistaxis or easy bruisability.

Family History No family history of hematologic or bleeding dyscrasias.

Medications None.

Physical Examination Unremarkable except for 2+ pitting edema of the lower extremities.

Initial Work-Up

Laboratory Test	Result	Normal
PT (sec)	22.4	10-13
PTT (sec)	31.1	23.7-37.7
Thrombin Time (sec)	14.3	9.5-14.5

Discussion Initial work-up revealed an isolated elevated PT. To discern if the prolongation was due to a factor deficiency or inhibitor, PT mixing studies, combining 1 part patient to 1 part normal plasma were performed. Mixing studies showed evidence of correction of the PT into the reference range consistent with a factor deficiency. To identify the specific factor deficiency, the assays for factors VII, X, V and II were performed. Although factor VII deficiency is often considered the sole cause of an isolated elevated PT, and may mistakenly be the only assay performed, it is important to investigate factors of the common pathway (factors II, V, and X). This is because the PT is more sensitive to abnormalities of the common pathway factors than is the APTT and therefore the PT may be prolonged with mild to moderate deficiencies of factors II, V and X while the APTT can remain in the normal reference interval. It is generally acknowledged that before a diagnosis of factor deficiency is made, the evaluation should be repeated on a new plasma sample. Factor X activity repeated on a new plasma sample at another laboratory yielded a result of 32% (normal range 65%-135%).

Laboratory Test	Result	Normal
Factor VII activity (%)	167	50-155
Factor II activity (%)	146	75-134
Factor V activity (%)	210	70-150
Factor X activity (%)	25	65-135

Differential Diagnosis Diagnostic considerations include acquired factor X deficiency, hereditary factor X deficiency, vitamin K deficiency, and liver disease.

An acquired factor X deficiency is the most likely diagnosis as the patient does not have a history of bleeding and was not known to have abnormal PTT and/or PT in the past. Isolated acquired factor X deficiency raises the possibility of amyloidosis, which is most commonly a complication of an underlying plasma cell dyscrasia. Factor X activity could also be decreased in an acquired fashion due to a factor X inhibitor although normal plasma mixing studies would typically not show evidence of correction.

An hereditary factor X deficiency seems unlikely given that the patient has no previous history of bleeding and there is no family history of such.

While factor X may be decreased with vitamin K deficiency, this would not explain an isolated deficiency of factor X. With vitamin K deficiency, all vitamin K-dependent factors, specifically factors II, VII, IX and X, decrease. Laboratory evaluation revealed that factors II and VII are normal to slightly elevated.

Although factor X may decrease with significant liver disease, this would not explain an isolated factor X deficiency. With liver disease (or vitamin K deficiency/antagonism), factor VII is usually the first factor to decrease as it has the shortest half life of all procoagulant factors produced in the liver. With significant liver disease, factor X is decreased as are all other procoagulant factors, specifically factor XI, IX, VII, V, X and II, except for factor VIII, which may be elevated.

Additional Work-Up Due to the isolated low factor X activity, especially in the presence of nephrotic syndrome, a diagnosis of amyloidosis was immediately considered. Serum protein electrophoresis revealed 1.2 g/dL of a monoclonal protein. Serum immunoelectrophoresis demonstrated an IgG λ monoclonal protein. Both monoclonal IgG-λ and free λ light chains were detected in her urine. A bone marrow biopsy demonstrated 30% plasma cells with λ restricted immunostaining, establishing the diagnosis of myeloma. Congo red stains of the bone marrow biopsy and of the aspirate of abdominal wall fat were negative for amyloidosis. Radiographic skeletal survey did not demonstrate either osteolytic lesions or osteoporosis. High-dose dexamethasone therapy resulted in a decrease in both proteinuria and serum paraprotein. The patient developed severe epigastric symptoms associated with this therapy. Esophagogastroduodenoscopy revealed no significant mucosal lesions but biopsies demonstrated amyloidosis in the mucosa of both the stomach and duodenum. At this time, she developed severe liver function test abnormalities, progressive hepatomegaly and ascites, and computerized tomography that suggested cirrhosis of the liver.

Final Diagnosis Acquired factor X deficiency in a case of multiple myeloma complicated by systemic amyloidosis (AL) resulting in nephrotic syndrome.

Management Approach Successful aggressive treatment of the underlying plasma cell dyscrasia is associated with improvement in factor X activity levels and even partial hematologic response may show improvement of factor X levels. Aggressive therapy employing high-dose chemotherapy with stem cell rescue has been used effectively to treat AL. In patients with splenomegaly, splenectomy has been reported to acutely improve factor X levels, presumably due to removal of a V large amyloid pool. In the acutely bleeding patient or in a patient requiring surgical intervention, fresh frozen plasma or recombinant activated factor VII may be of benefit. This patient was begun on dexamethasone, melphalan, bortezomib, standard therapy for multiple myeloma. Two years later she is doing exceedingly well and is totally asymptomatic, her PT has normalized, serum creatinine decreased from 1.7 mg/dL-1.0 mg/dL, total IgG decreased from 1,722 mg/dL-247 mg/dL and monoclonal protein concentration decreased from 1.17 g/dL-0.21 g/dL. Moderate proteinuria persists.

General Discussion The most common form of amyloidosis is light chain amyloidosis (AL). In this instance, the amyloid fibrils are composed of IgG light chains or light chain fragments produced by a clonal population of plasma cells. Approximately 10%-15% of patients with myeloma or Waldenström macroglobulinemia develop systemic AL. The diagnosis of AL amyloidosis requires (1) demonstration of amyloid in tissue and (2) demonstration of a plasma cell dyscrasia. Evaluation often includes investigation of serum and urine for monoclonal light chains. Systemic amyloidosis often involves the kidney, heart and bone marrow. Renal involvement usually manifests as nephrotic syndrome. Amyloid may also deposit in the gastrointestinal tract, liver and peripheral nervous system. The majority of patients with AL have 1 or 2 organs involved and about 30% have 3 or more major organ systems involved. Acquired factor X deficiency is the most common coagulation factor deficiency identified in AL amyloidosis and it occurs presumably as a result of adsorption of factor X to amyloid deposits. Decreased factor X levels in AL occurs independent of hepatic parenchymal disease and as in this case, may occur as an isolated factor deficiency. Due to the well known correlation of factor X deficiency with AL, it has been recommended that once a diagnosis of AL is made, all patients should be screened for factor X deficiency. A study of 368 new patients with AL revealed an incidence of factor X deficiency in 8.7% or 32 patients. Of these 32 patients, over half had bleeding complications and in 2, the hemorrhage proved fatal.

Section J: Bleeding Disorders
Acquired Factor X Deficiency

Bleeding severity correlated with factor X levels and those with <25% factor X activity were more likely to bleed.

Acquired isolated factor X deficiency may also occur secondary to a specific factor X inhibitor. These inhibitors are rare and may arise without provocation or may occur in association with underlying infections, such as leprosy. Laboratory evaluation typically demonstrates an elevated APTT and PT with incomplete correction in plasma mixing studies. Factor X inhibitors can be quantified using the Bethesda assay. Clinically, the majority patients with factor X inhibitors present with bleeding and factor X levels in the range of 1%-20%.

Hereditary factor X deficiency is a rare autosomal recessive, hemorrhagic disorder with a reported incidence of about 1 in 1 million. Patients with severe deficiencies (<1%) typically present with bleeding early in life, including hemarthroses, gastrointestinal bleeding, hematuria and CNS hemorrhage. Those with less severe deficiencies are often asymptomatic and may bleed only after challenged.

The diagnosis of factor X deficiency is based on measurements of factor X activity, typically using a clot-based assay, although a chromogenic factor X activity assay could be used. Typically both the APTT and PT are prolonged in patients with factor X deficiency. With less severe deficiencies, as in this case however, the PT may be prolonged while the APTT falls in the normal range as most PT reagents are more sensitive to mild deficiencies of factor X than are APTT reagents.

Factor XI Deficiency

Nicole Verdun, Katherine High

Patient A 7-year-old male with a history of recurrent prolonged epistaxis.

Clinical History For the past year, he has had intermittent episodes of bleeding from both nares, with each episode lasting 30 minutes, worse for the past 5 weeks. He has an episode of epistaxis on average 1-2 times a week, but for the past 5 weeks notes bleeding daily. His last episode of epistaxis was 2 days prior to presentation, which corresponded with his last upper airway infection. He has no history of recent trauma or surgery. His review of systems is significant for recurrent sinusitis, chronic congestion, allergies, and multiple upper airway infections. He has no bleeding with tooth brushing. He has no easy bruisability or spontaneous bruising. His past medical and surgical history are notable for a dental extraction 2 years prior with which he had "oozing" from his mouth for 2 days. He also has a history of obstructive sleep apnea. He was circumcised at birth without problems. He has no history of soft tissue bleeding or bleeding into joints, despite having suffered a fractured left ankle and deep thigh laceration while riding his bike.

Family History His parents are of Ashkenazi Jewish background. His mother and maternal aunt have a history of a prolonged bleeding time, but have never had problems with bleeding or bruising.

Medications None.

Physical Examination In general, he is well appearing. His oropharynx is clear. He nose has erythematous mucosa with swollen nasal turbinates. He has no petechiae. He has 3 2-3 cm flat ecchymoses on his shins bilaterally. His examination is otherwise within normal limits.

Initial Work-Up

PT (seconds)	11.5	(normal 11.0-13.5)
PTT (seconds)	75	(normal 21-35)
Thrombin time (seconds)	11	(normal 11-18)
Platelet count (×10^3/μL)	285	

von Willebrand factor antigen, activity, and factor VIII activity: all within normal ranges.

Differential Diagnosis The differential diagnosis of an isolated prolonged PTT in the setting of prolonged epistaxis in a male with a family history of abnormal coagulation studies includes: von Willebrand disease, hemophilia A or B, or other rare intrinsic pathway factor deficiencies. Another consideration in a child with a history of multiple viral infections is an inhibitor to an intrinsic pathway factor or an acquired lupus anticoagulant. Mucosal bleeding as the sole phenotypic expression of disease makes hemophilia A or B less likely, but should still be considered.

Additional Work-Up An isolated prolonged PTT prompted the following additional evaluation:
Inhibitor screen:
- Immediate: 28 seconds (normal 21-35)
- 1 hour: 27 seconds
- 2 hour: 27.8 seconds
- 2 additional sets of von Willebrand factor antigen, activity and factor VIII: normal
- Factor IX, factor XII activity: normal
- Factor XI activity: <1%
- Factor XI sequencing: homozygous for the E117X mutation
- Factor XI activity of father: 58%
- Factor XI activity of mother: 46%

Section J: Bleeding Disorders
Factor XI Deficiency

Final Diagnosis Severe factor XI deficiency

Management Approach Severe factor XI deficiency generally has a mild bleeding phenotype, and there is no indication for prophylactic factor replacement. Treatment options include fresh frozen plasma, antifibrinolytic agents, factor XI concentrates, and recombinant factor VIIa, which bypasses the intrinsic coagulation cascade and is not licensed for this indication. Considerations for treatment include the risk of inhibitor formation and the risk of thrombosis. Traditionally, factor XI deficiency has been treated with fresh frozen plasma (FFP) at the time of trauma or prior to surgical procedures. Antifibrinolytic agents such as aminocaproic acid are often used perioperatively with oral procedures, either in conjunction with fresh frozen plasma or as a single agent, 1 day prior to procedure and up to 7 days following the procedure. If a patient has persistent bleeding with procedures despite adequate treatment, consider the development of an inhibitor to factor XI. Patients with severe factor XI deficiency with previous exposure to plasma or concentrate are at risk for inhibitor development, and should be treated with bypassing agents if an inhibitor is detected. This patient required no treatment at the time of his clinic visit, as his bleeding had resolved.

General Discussion The additional work-up of this patient showed immediate correction of his prolonged PTT with the addition of normal pooled plasma, which is consistent with a factor deficiency. Further evaluation of the coagulation pathway factors that cause an isolated prolongation of the PTT included an evaluation of factor VIII, factor IX, factor XI, and factor XII, which were all within normal limits except for the factor XI activity level. Completion of a von Willebrand disease evaluation is prudent, as this is the most common bleeding disorder in the general population. Co-inheritance of bleeding disorders has been reported, and this patient's predilection to frequent mucosal bleeding makes this a possibility, as spontaneous mucosal bleeding is not characteristic of factor XI deficiency. In this case, his recurrent upper airway infection history and recurrent sinusitis may have led to damage of his nasal mucosa, thus leading to an increase in bleeding. Factor XI deficiency, also known as plasma thromboplastin antecedent (PTA) deficiency, is a disorder of autosomal recessive inheritance with variable penetrance. Factor XI is partially activated by thrombin generated from the extrinsic pathway, which leads to further thrombin generation. Factor XI is also thought to indirectly increase thrombin activatable fibrinolysis inhibitor (TA factor I), which reduces lysis and stabilizes clot formation. In its absence, difficulty with mucosal bleeding can arise with acquired hemostatic challenges, such as trauma or surgical procedures. Homozygotes and compound heterozygotes with factor XI deficiency are generally classified as severe, with a factor XI level of <15%-20%. Partial or mild deficiency is defined as levels between 20% and the lower limit of the normal range, which varies per institution (generally 65%-80%). The clinical phenotype is quite variable, and no genotype-phenotype correlation has been established. In addition, there is often no correlation with bleeding and baseline factor XI activity. Some patients with baseline factor XI levels of <1% never bleed, while others with levels in the mild range bleed excessively with surgery. Spontaneous bleeding is not characteristic, and most tend to have trauma and surgical related bleeding. Sites of bleeding tend to be those with dependence on high fibrinolytic activity, such as the oral and nasal mucosa, urogenital tract, and the oral cavity after dental procedures, tonsillectomy, or adenoidectomy. The prevalence of severe factor XI deficiency is 1:1,000,000 in the general population, and 1:450 in the Ashkenazi Jewish population, leading many to send a screening PTT on any person of Ashkenazi Jewish descent undergoing surgery. The factor XI gene is 23.7 kb long and is located on the long arm of chromosome 4. Factor XI is mainly expressed in hepatocytes, with trace amounts detectable in megakaryocytes and platelets. The factor XI protein has an estimated half-life of 50 hours. 180 mutations in the factor XI gene have been identified, with an even distribution of defects throughout the gene. In those of Ashkenazi Jewish descent, 2 mutations account for 95% of cases (Glu117stop and Phe283Leu). The patient described above has 2 copies of the Glu117 stop mutation. The pathogenic mechanism of disease with this mutation is thought to be premature mRNA degradation of the mutant transcripts through nonsense-mediated decay. The factor XI levels of his parents are consistent with the heterozygous state and support the pattern of inheritance described. Factor XI deficiency should be considered in any patient with isolated prolongation of the PTT and a pattern of mucosal bleeding, especially with surgical procedures involving tissues with high fibrinolytic activity. Consideration of Ashkenazi Jewish ancestry should increase suspicion of factor XI deficiency, although deficiency has been seen in people of all ethnic backgrounds. Counseling of patients with this diagnosis should include the likelihood of a mild phenotype, treatment options, and risk of inhibitor formation.

Factor XII Deficiency

Franklin A Bontempo

Patient A 17-year-old white male with abdominal pain and vomiting was found to have a prolonged activated partial thromboplastin time (PTT).

Clinical History There was initial concern for acute appendicitis. Laboratory work-up revealed a normal prothrombin time (PT) but prolonged PTT. He had a history of nose bleeds every 3 weeks since childhood, which had persisted into his teenage years. There was no history of petechiae, easy bruising, bleeding from cuts, bleeding from his gums when he brushed his teeth, or bleeding from dental procedures including primary tooth extractions. He had no history of wisdom teeth extractions or tonsillectomy. There was no history of hemoptysis, hematemesis, melena, hematochezia, hematuria, jaundice, or hemarthrosis. He had never had any other surgical procedures or stitches. He was reevaluated for abdominal pain and eventually a clinical diagnosis of a viral infection was made and he was discharged. In 3 days his symptoms resolved and he returned for repeat PT and PTT testing, which again showed a normal PT and a prolonged PTT.

Family History Neither parents (mother, 49, and father, 45) nor siblings (2 sisters, 16 and 10) had any history of bleeding symptoms.

Medications His only medication was ibuprofen, which he only took on an as-needed basis.

Physical Examination The sclerae were anicteric. The neck was negative for lymphadenopathy. There was no palpable liver or spleen. The palmar skin was very dry but there was no palmar erythema. There was no bruising.

Initial Work-Up

PT (sec)	10.6	(normal 9.0-11.0)
PTT (sec)	46.9	(normal 30.0-42.0)
PTT mix (sec)	40.7	(normal 30.0-42.0)

CBC including hemogloibin, platelets and white blood cell count were all normal. The patient's normal PT and prolonged PTT isolated the diagnosis of his bleeding problem to the upper part of the intrinsic clotting pathway. A normal result for PTT-mix ruled out an inhibitor.

Differential Diagnosis Factor VIII deficiency (hemophilia A), factor IX deficiency (hemophilia B), congenital deficiency of factor XI, congenital deficiency of factor XII, von Willebrand disease, congenital prekallikrein (Fletcher factor) deficiency, and congenital high molecular weight kininogen (Fitzgerald factor) deficiency.

Additional Work-Up
- Factor VIII activity 96% (normal 60-150)
- Factor IX activity 62% (normal 60-150)
- Factor XI activity 95% (normal 60-140)
- Factor XII activity 22% (normal 50-170)
- Ristocetin cofactor activity 131% (normal 50-150)
- vWF antigen 144% of normal (normal 50-160)
- Prekallikrein activity 66% (normal 50-150)
- HMW kininogen activity 65% (normal 50-150)

Final Diagnosis Congenital deficiency of factor XII (Hageman factor).

Management Approach Factor XII deficiency does not cause bleeding and patients do not need to be treated with clotting factor replacement regardless of the degree of elevation of the APTT or degree of depression of the factor XII level. Should a patient with factor XII deficiency have bleeding, another reason for the bleeding should be sought.

General Discussion Congenital factor XII deficiency is generally inherited in an autosomal recessive pattern. Homozygotes often have undetectable factor XII activity level, whereas heterozygotes have factor XII activity levels between 20%-60%. Low factor XII activity levels may also be seen in patients with liver disease. Factor XII deficiency does not cause bleeding even after surgical procedures or trauma. Rare cases of inhibitor against factor XII have been reported. The diagnosis of factor XII deficiency is usually not difficult since patients are asymptomatic but have the finding of a significantly elevated APTT, which corrects on mixing. Specific factor activity assay is required for the diagnosis. Testing factor XII levels in the patient's parents and siblings may be beneficial for confirming the diagnosis and alerting the relatives that they could have similar laboratory findings which could cause unnecessary concern should they need surgery or experience trauma. At least 1 of the patient's parents would be expected to have a low factor XII level, depending on whether he is heterozygously or homozygously deficient. In this patient, the clinical diagnosis was complicated by a history of epistaxis, which could have indicated von Willebrand disease, but which can be a common problem in children and young adults without von Willebrand disease. Factor VIII deficiency and factor IX deficiency are usually, but not always, associated with a family history of bleeding and are usually more severe bleeding disorders which come to attention before young adulthood. Deficiencies of prekallikrein and high molecular weight kininogen, albeit less common, can present similarly to factor XII deficiency and should be distinguished from the latter by specific factor activity assays.

Factor XIII Deficiency

Elizabeth M Van Cott

Patient A 22-year-old female with a history of intracranial hemorrhage.

Clinical History 5 months prior, after complaining of severe headache and then becoming unresponsive, she was found to have intracranial hemorrhage and intraventricular bleeding. She received 2 units of FFP in the emergency department, but no other hemostasis treatments throughout her admission. She received an external ventricular drainage device, mannitol and dexamethasone to prevent brain swelling, and levetiracetam to prevent seizures. She denied other past or present bleeding symptoms and had no other signs of bleeding (no petechiae, bruising, or other bleeding). She reported no head trauma, a toxicology screen was negative, and she had no hypertension. CT scans showed no arteriovenous malformations, aneurysms, or other sources of bleeding. Hematocrit was 33%, platelet count normal, WBC count $19 \times 10^3/\mu L$ with 90% neutrophils, which can occur with bleeding. The PTT was slightly short (attributed to elevated fibrinogen) but the PT was mildly prolonged at 14.3 seconds (normal: 10.3-13.2) with an INR of 1.3. Factor VII was normal, fibrinogen was elevated (consistent with an acute phase reaction); factors II, V and X can also prolong the PT but were not requested by the clinicians. BUN, creatinine, liver function tests, serum protein electrophoresis, light chain and immunoglobulin levels, ANA, and urinalysis were normal. von Willebrand antigen and activity (ristocetin cofactor), factor VIII, factor IX, factor XI, thrombin time, reptilase time, and antiplasmin were normal. A factor XIII screen was normal. She gradually recovered completely. Her PT became normal before she was discharged, and the temporary mild PT prolongation was attributed to mild disseminated intravascular coagulation (DIC) triggered by tissue damage caused by the intracranial bleed. Past medical history is otherwise unremarkable, including no pregnancies, miscarriages, surgeries, or major trauma.

Family History No family history of bleeding.

Medications None.

Physical Examination Unremarkable.

Initial Work-Up Repeat factor XIII screen: Positive for deficiency (**Figure 1**). Repeat von Willebrand antigen, ristocetin cofactor, factor VIII, fibrinogen: normal, blood type O.

Differential Diagnosis Bleeding disorders that have a normal PT, PTT and platelet count include factor XIII deficiency, antiplasmin deficiency, platelet dysfunction, dysfibrinogenemia (can have prolonged PT and/or PTT), von Willebrand disease (severe cases have prolonged PTT), plasminogen activator inhibitor-1 (PAI-1) deficiency, or other disorders including Marfan syndrome, Ehlers-Danlos syndrome, vitamin C deficiency, uremia, elevated immunoglobulins, and

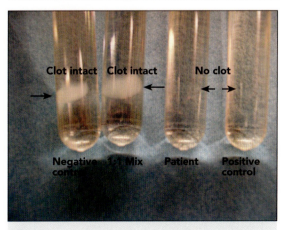

Figure 1 Arrows indicate clot.

other conditions. Bleeding disorders that present with a prolonged PT include deficiencies of factors II, V and X.

Additional Work-Up
A quantitative factor XIII activity assay was sent out, and the result was markedly low at 1.8% (normal 70-140). A quantitative factor XIII antigen assay (measuring the A subunit of factor XIII) was also markedly low at 3.5%. A factor XIII mixing study was performed to assess for a factor XIII inhibitor (see **Figure 1**). Patient plasma was mixed with normal plasma 1:1, and the factor XIII screen (urea solubility) was performed on the mix. The clot remained intact, which is not suggestive of an inhibitor. Since only a small amount of factor XIII is needed to have a normal factor XIII screen, mixing studies can also be performed using smaller amounts of patient plasma relative to normal plasma, to further exclude the possibility of a weak factor XIII inhibitor.

Final Diagnosis Factor XIII deficiency.

Management Approach Factor XIII has a very long half-life of 7 days-14 days. Therefore, treatment can usually be given infrequently (for example, once every 4 weeks-6 weeks). Factor XIII is present in FFP and cryoprecipitate. Factor XIII concentrates are available or in development in some countries. The clinical presentation is variable, therefore some patients do not require factor XIII supplementation, while other patients require prophylactic factor XIII replacement therapy.

General Discussion Hereditary factor XIII deficiency is rare (1 in 2 million) and has autosomal recessive inheritance. Factor XIII crosslinks fibrin strands with covalent bonds, stabilizing the clot. The severity of symptoms is variable, but severe deficiency of factor XIII (<1%-2%) can cause delayed bleeding, intracranial hemorrhages, delayed wound healing, and miscarriages. The incidence of intracranial hemorrhage seems to be higher than is seen with other bleeding diatheses. Umbilical stump bleeding is common in newborns. Heterozygous carriers of factor XIII deficiency are usually asymptomatic, but mild bleeding symptoms can be seen. The qualitative factor XIII screening assay evaluates clot stability. The patient sample is clotted by adding calcium (or thrombin), and then the clot is placed in 5 M urea (or 1% monochloroacetic acid). Clots are examined 24 hours later; clots formed by normal individuals remain intact, while clots from factor XIII-deficient patients dissolve. This assay detects only the most severely affected homozygous patients with <2% factor XIII activity. The key point of this case is that the 2 units of FFP that the patient received caused the first factor XIII screen to be falsely normal. Because factor XIII has a long half-life, a transfusion has the potential to cause false normal results in the screening assay for >2 months after the transfusion. If an abnormal factor XIII screen result is obtained (the clot lyses), an antiplasmin activity level should be obtained, because antiplasmin deficiency can also cause a positive factor XIII screen. Normally, factor XIII crosslinks antiplasmin to the fibrin strands, and antiplasmin protects the clot from fibrinolysis by plasmin.

von Willebrand Disease, Variant 2 Normandy

Craig Kessler

Patient A 22-year-old Caucasian male with known mild hemophilia A was admitted to the hospital after an evening of binge drinking, followed by bright red vomitus and retching.

Clinical History The patient had symptomatic acute anemia with orthostatic vertigo, decreased stamina, and tarry stools. He had a 2-year history of iron deficiency anemia. His initial hematocrit was 22% and he was treated urgently with recombinant factor VIII (recombinant factor VIII) concentrate to raise his factor VIII activity >80% from his baseline factor VIII activity level of 5%-8%. His mild hemophilia A was diagnosed after he experienced protracted bleeding with circumcision on day 2 after birth. Although he bruised easily, he had little symptomatic bleeding except following the loss of his deciduous teeth. The day after his 4 impacted wisdom teeth had been extracted uneventfully under cover of recombinant factor VIII concentrate, he awakened in a pool of blood from his mouth, requiring additional recombinant factor VIII concentrate. The only other significant bleeding episodes over his lifetime resulted from minor post sports trauma. He had never used intranasal or intravenous DDAVP to treat or prevent bleeding.

Family History There is no obvious family history pertinent for abnormal bleeding or bruising, although his sister and mother both experienced menorrhagia.

Medications Multivitamins.

Physical Examination The patient was slightly disoriented at presentation and over the next 12 hours he had another episode of hematemesis. He was hypotensive and tachycardic with a blood pressure of 105/55 supine with a pulse of 130 and regular and 90/45 when sitting. Otherwise, he had multiple small ecchymotic lesions over the extensor surfaces of all extremities and prominent telangiectasias over his face, inner lips, and nasal mucosa. His scars were well healed. Digital rectal exam was normal except for guaiac positive stool.

Initial Work-Up Coagulation lab results after the initial administration of recombinant factor VIII concentrate bleeding revealed a factor VIII activity of 80% at 1 hour but only 15% at the 12-hour point post recombinant factor VIII concentrate replacement. A factor VIII level of around 40% would be expected since the circulating half-life for recombinant factor VIII should be around 8 hours-12 hours. This rapid falloff in factor VIII activity from the established normal peak increment suggested the possible presence of an alloantibody inhibitor; however, there was no evidence for a neutralizing antibody (0 Bethesda units). The prothrombin times at baseline, 1, and 12 hours post recombinant factor VIII infusion were normal. The baseline PTT was 62 sec (normal 22 sec-35 sec), followed by 32 sec at 1 hour after recombinant factor VIII infusion, and 55 seconds at 12 hours. The comprehensive metabolic panel was unremarkable. Examination of the peripheral blood smear showed normal red cell and platelet morphology.

Differential Diagnosis Diagnostic considerations included moderate severity hemophilia A, disseminated intravascular coagulation (DIC), von Willebrand disease variant 2 Normandy, and hemophilia A with alloantibody factor VIII neutralizing inhibitor.

Additional Work-Up Mixing studies of patient plasma incubated with normal pooled plasma for up to 2 hours at 37°C demonstrated normalization of the PTT at each time point, again confirming that an alloantibody was not responsible for the rapid falloff in factor VIII activity. DIC was unlikely with normal D-dimer titers. The more rapid than expected falloff of plasma factor VIII activity after achieving the expected incremental rise in factor VIII activity immediately after infusion of recombinant factor VIII concentrate suggested the possibility of von Willebrand variant 2 Normandy. The presence of telangiectasias was also suggestive of von Willebrand disease. Subsequently, von Willebrand antigen was normal at 62% (normal 50-150) and vWF:Rco activity was 70% (normal 50-150). Multimeric analysis of the vWF protein composition by SDS polyacrylamide gel electropheresis was completely normal. A factor VIII-vWF binding assay was performed, in which patient plasma was added to recombinant factor VIII fixed to an ELISA plate. After incubation, the residual non-factor VIII bound vWF was measured and revealed 85% residual vWF activity, suggesting a defect in factor VIII-vWF binding. Since vWD 2 Normandy is characterized by defective vWF binding to factor VIII by virtue of a gene mutation at the critical binding site on vWF for factor VIII, gene sequencing studies of the exon 28 of vWF was performed. An Arg854Gln mutation was identified, confirming the presence of the vWD 2 Normandy variant.

Diagnosis von Willebrand disease variant 2 Normandy.

Management Approach Treatment for bleeding complications associated with vWD variant 2 Normandy, due to a gene mutation resulting in defective factor VIII binding to vWF, requires replacement with a source of normal vWF protein. This facilitates normal binding of endogenous factor VIII and maintains an adequate level of factor VIII activity in plasma to sustain normal hemostasis. The best commercial sources of normal vWF protein for therapeutic replacement are intermediate purity plasma derived factor VIII concentrates, as in the above case scenario.

General Discussion von Willebrand disease is the most common inherited bleeding disorder with an estimated 1% prevalence in the population and a typical autosomal dominant inheritance pattern. Subtyping of vWD is dependent on the concordance or discordance of vWF:RCo and vWF:Ag activity levels, multimeric composition of the vWF structure, inheritance pattern (type 3 variant and some type 2M are autosomal recessive), and gene mutational analysis. The vWD subtype determines the appropriate replacement therapy. In our case example, the patient presented phenotypically as mild severity hemophilia A, but the decreased factor VIII activity was due not to decreased factor VIII synthesis but to defective vWF-factor VIII binding. Thus, endogenous factor VIII loses the vWF protein chaperone capacity in plasma and leaves the circulation at an accelerated rate, with the net result phenotypically similar to mild hemophilia A. Replacement therapy is targeted to the replenishment of the host with a source of normal vWF protein. High-purity factor VIII concentrates will not accomplish this and will not provide sustained correction of the factor VIII deficiency for prolonged adequate hemostasis. The diagnosis of vWD and its variants can be somewhat elusive and often complex (**Table 1**). Clinical suspicion, often based on the results of applying a bleeding index, combined with laboratory confirmation utilizing the above mentioned assays, facilitates the diagnosis. Type 2 and 3 variants are easier to diagnose than the much more common type 1 vWD category. The ability to diagnose this latter type of vWD is often confounded by epigenetic influences on normal vWF activities in vivo, eg, pregnancy, estrogen-containing oral contraceptive use, exercise, type O red cells, hypothyroidism, etc.

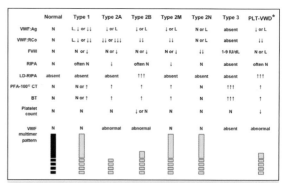

Table 1 Expected laboratory values in vWD. The symbols and values represent prototypical cases. In practice, laboratory studies in certain patients may deviate slightly from these expectations. L, 30-50 IU/dL; ↓, ↓↓, ↓↓↓, relative decrease; ↑, ↑↑, ↑↑↑, relative increase; BT, bleeding time; factor VIII, factor VIII activity; LD-RIPA, low-dose ristocetin-induced platelet aggregation (concentration of ristocetin ≤ 0.6 mg/mL); N, normal; PFA-100 CT, platelet function analyzer closure time; RIPA, ristocetin-induced platelet aggregation; vWF, von Willebrand factor; vWF:Ag, vWF antigen; vWF:RCo, vWF ristocetin cofactor activity.

Acquired von Willebrand Disease

James Zehnder

Patient An 85-year-old male with bruising and mucosal bleeding.

Clinical History The patient was in his usual state of excellent health until he presented to his primary care physician after noting a change in bowel habits. Colonoscopy revealed a large polyp which pathologically was adenocarcinoma, with muscularis invasion. The lesion was resected; 0/20 lymph nodes showed evidence of tumor; liver biopsy and imaging studies were negative. The patient recovered from surgery uneventfully; however, in the prior week he had noted spontaneous nosebleeds, easy bruising and gingival bleeding when brushing, all of which were new for him. He denied any recent use of aspirin or nonsteroidal anti-inflammatory drugs (NSAIDs) and was on no medication.

Family History Noncontributory.

Medications None.

Physical Examination Notable for numerous ecchymoses, some of which were up to 8 cm in diameter.

Initial Work-Up
- PT 12 sec (normal 11 sec-15 sec)
- PTT 80 sec (was normal prior to surgery; normal 25 sec-35 sec)
- Platelet count 300 ×10^3/μL (normal 150-400)

Differential Diagnosis Acquired bleeding disorder, the prolonged PTT with normal PT localizes the problem to the intrinsic pathway, the most common of which are acquired factor VIII inhibitors and acquired von Willebrand disease (vWD).

Additional Work-Up PTT mixing study showed correction, consistent with factor deficiency. Evaluation of intrinsic pathway factors revealed a factor VIII of 20% (normal 60-150); all other factors were normal. von Willebrand antigen was 40% (normal 60-120), ristocetin cofactor activity was 35% (normal 45-110).

Final Diagnosis Acquired von Willebrand disease.

Management Approach The general approach is immunosuppression with the goal of decreasing autoantibody production or function. Intravenous immune globulin (IV Ig) as a single agent may be sufficient for patients with mild disease; more aggressive regimens (eg, steroids, cytotoxic or anti-CD20 antibody) may be needed for patients with severe refractory disease. This patient was treated with 1 g/kg IV Ig with a prompt response, normalizing his PTT, factor VIII and von Willebrand factor (vWF) levels. His factor VIII level was monitored and when falling below 50% was given another infusion of IV Ig. After 3 infusions, his vWF parameters remained normal. He had no significant bleeding events during this time.

General Discussion Acquired von Willebrand disease should be suspected when a vWD phenotype develops in a previously healthy individual. The presentation is similar to other forms of vWD, typically presenting with bleeding from mucosal sites (gingival, epistaxis, menorrhagia, bruising). Often, acquired vWD disease occurs in the setting of another illness such as autoimmune disease or cancer. In this case, the patient has made an autoantibody which is clearing von Willebrand factor. Since the decrease in antigenic and functional activity of vWF is proportional, this antibody does not appear to be inhibiting the function of vWF. This case illustrates another important property of vWF, namely protection of circulating factor VIII. In this case the prolonged PTT and decreased factor VIII were the clues which led to the investigation of vWF status and the diagnosis of acquired vWD. Acquired vWD has been reported with many autoimmune diseases and also in association with cancers. This patient's antibody was transient and responded well to low-dose IV Ig.

Factor V Leiden

Kandice Kottke-Marchant, Bill G Richendollar

Patient A 28-year-old female with severe headache.

Clinical History She presented to her primary care physician with a sudden onset of severe headaches. Mild sinus congestion was noted and the patient was sent home on oral antibiotic therapy. By the next day, the headaches had become progressively worse and the patient went to the emergency room for further evaluation. The rest of her clinical history was unremarkable except for gastroesophageal reflux, status post Nissen fundoplication and cholecystectomy. She is a nonsmoker and denied alcohol or drug use.

Family History Unremarkable.

Medications Estrogen-based oral contraceptive therapy (5 years); levofloxacin and guaifenisen (started day of initial presentation).

Physical Examination She appeared uncomfortable. Her lung and cardiac exams were normal. Her neurologic exam was nonfocal.

Initial Work-Up PT 11.3 seconds (normal 9.9-13.0), INR 1.0 (normal 0.8-1.2), PTT 25.7 seconds (normal 24.6-34.0), Platelet count $159 \times 10^3/\mu L$ (normal 150-400).

CT and MRV Studies Dural vein thromboses involving the superior sagittal sinus and right transverse sinus.

Differential Diagnosis Diagnostic considerations included prothrombotic conditions (congenital and acquired), malignancy, vascular disease, hematologic disease, infectious disease, and trauma.

Additional Work-Up
- Chromogenic protein C 85% (normal 76-147)
- Chromogenic antithrombin 90% (normal 80-120)
- Clottable protein S 68% (normal 59-131)
- Factor VIII 164% (normal 49-134)
- Prothrombin gene G20210A PCR: normal
- Activated protein C (APC) resistance ratio: 1.24 (normal 2.00-2.81)
- Factor V Leiden PCR: homozygous for R506Q mutation; family genotyping information not available

Final Diagnosis Homozygous for factor V Leiden.

Management Approach The most common clinical management approach for venous thromboses associated with factor V Leiden is anticoagulation with heparin, followed by long-term outpatient therapy with warfarin. This patient was also started on unfractionated heparin and bridged to a vitamin K antagonist, warfarin, as an outpatient.

General Discussion Factor V Leiden is the most common cause of hereditary thrombophilia, accounting for over 40% of cases. There is considerable global variation in the reported prevalence of heterozygosity, with the highest prevalence noted in European and Eastern Mediterranean populations and the lowest prevalence noted in African and Asian populations. In the US, a study of 4,047 men and women revealed a heterozygous carrier frequency of 5.3% for Caucasians, 2.2% for Hispanic Americans, and <2% for Native Americans, African Americans and Asian Americans. Homozygous mutations are rare, accounting for only 1% of patients with factor V Leiden. It is caused by a single point mutation in the factor V gene which was identified by Rogier Bertina in 1994 and named factor V Leiden in honor of the city of discovery (Leiden, The Netherlands). The mutation at nucleotide position 1,691 results in the substitution of arginine for glutamine at codon 506, leading to a gene product which is not readily susceptible to cleavage by activated protein C (APC). Protein C is a vitamin-K dependent proenzyme which is activated by thrombin bound to thrombomodulin, an endothelial cell glycoprotein. APC (along with cofactor protein S) then acts to downregulate thrombin generation by the proteolysis of factors Va and VIIIa. The mechanism of factor V inactivation progresses as an ordered event, with cleavage occurring first at Arg506 and followed by cleavage at Arg306 and Arg679, because peptide bond cleavage at Arg506 is required for optimum exposure of the other cleavage sites. In factor V Leiden, the Arg506 cleavage site is absent, so there is resistance to the proteolytic effects of APC. The APC resistance assay is a common screening test for factor V Leiden. The test is routinely performed by running 2 aPTTs in parallel, in both the presence and absence of exogenous APC, with the result expressed as a ratio: (aPTT + APC)/aPTT. The addition of APC to the plasma of patients with factor V Leiden does not significantly prolong the clotting time, which results in a decreased APC resistance ratio. Normal patients have ratios >2.0, while factor V Leiden heterozygotes typically have ratios between 1.5 and 2.0 and factor V Leiden homozygotes typically have ratios <1.5. First generation tests used undiluted patient plasma for testing; however, these assays were found to have poor specificity and were not reliable when the baseline aPTT was elevated. Second generation assays, using dilute and factor V-depleted plasma containing a heparin-neutralizing substance, have improved both the sensitivity and specificity of the test. Other commercial methodologies for APC resistance testing include tissue factor-activated and Russell viper venom-activated clotting assays.

Genetic testing for factor V Leiden is required for a definitive diagnosis. The original method involved amplification of the factor V gene by polymerase chain reaction (PCR), restriction enzyme digestion, and analysis of the cleavage products using agarose gel electrophoresis. Since the factor V Leiden mutation eliminates an endonuclease cleavage site, loss of a digestion fragment is observed. This method is still in use, although many laboratories now perform factor V Leiden testing using commercially available real-time PCR assays. Other rare factor V mutations such as factor V Cambridge (Arg306Thr), factor V Hong Kong (Arg306Gly) and factor V Liverpool (Ile359Thr) have also been described. Factor V Cambridge and factor V Hong Kong are both associated with loss of the Arg306 APC cleavage site. While factor V Cambridge has been associated with APC resistance and increased risk of thrombosis, the clinical importance of FV Hong Kong is currently uncertain. Factor V Liverpool is not associated with loss of an APC cleavage site, but the mutation does impede APC-mediated inactivation of factor Va. Factor V gene sequencing is a useful diagnostic tool for identifying these mutations. In addition to these mutations, a group of nucleotide polymorphisms located in exons 13 and 16 of the factor V gene are associated with the factor V HR2 haplotype. The prevalence of this haplotype is reported to be similar in European, Asian and Hispanic populations, with an increased frequency in heterozygous factor V Leiden patients with the lowest APC resistance ratios. The risk of thrombosis with the HR2 haplotype in the absence of factor V Leiden is uncertain; however, and routine testing for the haplotype is not currently recommended. The most common clinical manifestation of factor V Leiden is deep venous thrombosis, alone or in conjunction with pulmonary embolism. Patients with a heterozygous factor V Leiden mutation have a 7× greater relative risk for the development of deep vein thrombosis compared to normal control populations, while patients with homozygous mutations have an 80× greater relative risk. There is also a greater risk of developing cerebral, mesenteric and portal vein thromboses and the mutation has been associated with recurrent pregnancy loss. The incidence of other thrombophilic risk factors has been reported to be higher in patients with factor V Leiden, and individuals with multiple risk factors are at a much greater risk for venous thrombosis. For example, a pooled analysis of 8 case-control studies revealed the odds ratio for venous thromboembolic disease in factor V Leiden heterozygotes increased from 4.9-20.0 when the patient was also heterozygous for the prothrombin G20210A mutation. Patients with factor V Leiden and a coexisting factor V deficiency also have an increased risk of venous thrombosis. In addition, acquired risk factors (such as oral contraceptive therapy, hormone replacement therapy and pregnancy) also substantially increase the risk for venous thromboembolic disease in factor V Leiden patients. Currently, there is no established association between arterial thrombosis and factor V Leiden.

Antiphospholipid Antibody Syndrome

James L Zehnder, Stevie Otis

Patient A 52-year-old Caucasian female with acute onset of shortness of breath followed by a syncopal episode witnessed by her husband.

Clinical History The patient, with a history of hypothyroidism secondary to Hashimoto thyroiditis, went on a month-long road trip to California, Nevada, and Utah. She felt well throughout her trip, but shortly after returning home she developed acute shortness of breath. She was unconscious for approximately 1 minute, and upon regaining consciousness remained short of breath but was not confused. The patient's husband called 911, and upon arrival of the paramedics the patient's oxygen saturation was 81%, which promptly increased to 100% with a non-rebreather mask. She had been pregnant 3 times in her life and had 3 uncomplicated deliveries. The patient had a routine mammogram 5 months prior that was normal and a colonoscopy 2 years ago that was normal. She is not a smoker.

Family History There is no family history of bleeding or thrombosis.

Medications She is not on any contraceptives or hormone replacement therapy.

Physical Examination On arrival, the patient's vital signs were within normal limits except for an increased respiratory rate of 30 and tachycardia with a heart rate of 110. Exam was remarkable for mild respiratory distress. Her lung exam was without wheezes or rales. Her cardiac exam was significant only for the tachycardia. Her left leg was minimally swollen.

Initial Work-Up An arterial blood gas analysis revealed a respiratory alkalosis and hypoxia with a PO_2 of 72% with 100% oxygen by face mask (expected PO_2 >99%). The CBC and complete metabolic panel were within normal limits. The PT and INR were normal but PTT was increased at 52 seconds (normal 25-35). A CT angiogram of the chest revealed large bilateral pulmonary emboli (PEs) extending from the main pulmonary arteries throughout multiple lobar, segmental and subsegmental branches. Bilateral lower extremity Doppler ultrasounds revealed deep vein thromboses (DVTs) in the left popliteal vein extending into the left superficial femoral vein.

Differential Diagnosis Prolonged PTT with normal PT generally points to a deficiency of one or more coagulation factors in the intrinsic pathway or an inhibitor. The inhibitor may be an antibody against one or more of these coagulation factors (usually against 1 factor) or of lupus anticoagulant type. The former is associated with bleeding, whereas the latter is usually associated with thrombosis. Clinically, this patient was diagnosed to have deep vein thrombosis and pulmonary embolism in the setting of a prolonged PTT.

Additional Work-Up A PTT mixing study demonstrated the presence of an inhibitor which corrected in the presence of excess phopholipid, consistent with a lupus anticoagulant (LA). A follow-up study performed 3 months later demonstrated the continued presence of the LA. Anticardiolipin antibody studies demonstrated high titer IgG anticardiolipin antibodies.

Final Diagnosis Antiphospholipid antibody syndrome.

Management Approach The most common management issues that arise are intensity and duration of therapy. Most experts recommend an initial target INR of 2-3. As these patients have a high risk of recurrence, indefinite anticoagulation may be indicated, depending on the risk:benefit profile of the individual. Since recurrence risk in this population is high, occasionally a patient will present with recurrent thrombosis while on therapeutic anticoagulation. Therapeutic options in this circumstance would include increasing the target INR; however this will be accompanied by an increase in bleeding risk. Alternatively a form of therapy such as low molecular weight heparin (LMWH) could be considered. Oral Xa inhibitor and thrombin inhibitors could represent another alternative. In this patient, due to the large clot burden and the syncopal episode, which is considered indicative of hemodynamic instability, the patient's PEs were initially treated with tissue plasminogen activator (t-PA) and she was started on a heparin infusion. The patient was subsequently converted to enoxaparin and bridged to warfarin with a target INR of 2-3. The patient was discharged home 4 days later.

General Discussion The salient features of antiphospholipid syndrome are a clinical presentation of idiopathic venous or arterial thrombosis, or a history of recurrent fetal loss, in the setting of a persistently positive test for antiphospholipid antibodies. These may be identified by phopholipid-sensitive coagulation tests (eg, PTT, PTT-LA, DRVVT, Kaolin) and/or anticardiolipin or anti-b2 glycoprotein 1 antibodies. When patients develop DVT or PE, certain questions should be asked. In this case, one would consider whether a hypercoagulable work-up is necessary or whether the patient's DVTs and ensuing PEs can be attributed to prolonged immobilization during her road trip. The patient's young age, high clot burden, prolonged PTT, and history of an autoimmune disorder should prompt a complete hypercoagulable work-up. If the work-up is negative for an underlying hypercoagulable disorder, then it is reasonable to call this a case of "provoked" DVT/PE. In some cases of elderly patients or patients who have undergone recent surgery or who have significant comorbidities (ie, active malignancy, connective tissue disorders, inflammatory bowel disease, myeloproliferative disorder, etc), it is reasonable to ascribe the thrombotic event to the apparent underlying risk factor without performing an extensive hypercoagulable work-up. There are certain laboratory tests which are necessary as part of this patient's initial hypercoagulable work-up. Other tests should be postponed until the acute episode has resolved and the patient is off all anticoagulation. Given this patient's history of an autoimmune disorder, she should definitely be screened for anticardiolipin antibodies and lupus anticoagulant. If these are positive, no further testing would be necessary as patients with antiphospholipid syndrome are generally anticoagulated indefinitely, and thus further testing would not impact the management. If antiphospholipid antibody tests were negative, then testing for the presence of the common mutations associated with hypercoagulable states (factor V Leiden and prothrombin 20,210) could be performed. Patients should not be tested for protein C deficiency, protein S deficiency, and antithrombin III (ATIII) deficiency as part of the initial screening labs because these factors may be falsely low in the acute setting. Furthermore, these tests cannot be done while the patient is on anticoagulation, as heparin can cause up to a 30% decline in the plasma ATIII concentration, and warfarin produces a marked reduction in the functional activity of protein C and protein S, and a lesser decline in their antigen levels. If; however, plasma levels of protein C, protein S, and ATIII are done during the initial screening process and are normal, then deficiency of these proteins is essentially ruled out. A low concentration, on the other hand, must be confirmed by repeat testing after anticoagulation has been discontinued after the initial 3 month-6 month course following the thrombotic event.

Section K: Thrombophilias

Prothrombin Gene G20210A Mutation

Ziad Peerwani, Kandice Kottke-Marchant

Patient A 41-year-old Caucasian female with worsening left lower extremity pain and erythema.

Clinical History 2 years prior to this presentation, the patient developed postpartum bilateral lower extremity superficial thrombophlebitis. This was treated with compression stockings. Oral anticoagulant therapy was not necessary at that time.

Family History The patient's mother suffered from superficial thrombophlebitis and her maternal grandmother had a history of deep vein thrombosis.

Medications None.

Physical Examination 1+ left lower extremity edema extending partially up her calf with mild erythema extending to the knee. The erythema was most prominent along the medial aspect of her left knee.

Initial Work-Up PT 11.1 seconds (normal 8.4-13), INR 1.1 (normal 0.8-1.2), PTT 31.5 seconds (normal 23-32.4) and platelet count $203 \times 10^3/\mu L$ (normal $150 \times 10^3 - 400 \times 10^3/\mu L$). An ultrasound was positive for deep venous thrombosis of the left lower extremity extending from the popliteal vein into the calf. Superficial varicose veins with evidence of a clot from the calf to the medial knee were noted.

Differential Diagnosis Diagnostic considerations included congenital vs acquired thrombophilia (factor V Leiden mutation [FVL], prothrombin gene G20210A mutation [PGM], protein C deficiency, protein S deficiency, antithrombin deficiency, hyperhomocysteinemia, and lupus anticoagulant).

Additional Work-Up
- Functional protein C 80% (normal 76-147), clottable protein S 62% (normal 59-131),
- activated protein C resistance ratio 1.74 (normal 2.14-2.74)
- Factor V Leiden R506Q PCR: heterozygous
- Prothrombin gene G20210A PCR: heterozygous

Final Diagnosis Double heterozygosity for the prothrombin gene G20210A mutation and factor V Leiden R506Q mutation.

Management Approach The majority of patients with PGM will never undergo a thrombotic event. Although current studies are equivocal, patients with PGM are at no to low risk for recurrent venous thromboembolism (VTE). Patients with this mutation should not receive anticoagulant therapy solely based on their mutational status. In general, patients with PGM who develop an isolated VTE should be treated for their VTE. This usually entails short-term, 3 months-6 months, anticoagulant therapy. Long-term anticoagulant therapy for PGM in the setting of an isolated VTE is currently not recommended. However, patients with PGM in addition to other prothrombotic risk factors, like FVL, seem to be at higher risk for isolated as well as recurrent VTE. Current clinical practice suggests that patients with PGM and one or more other prothrombotic risk factors may benefit from long-term anticoagulant therapy after an isolated VTE event. The prothrombin gene G20210A mutation and the factor V Leiden R506Q mutation act synergistically to increase the patient's thrombotic risk, including an increased risk for recurrent venous thromboembolism. This patient was started on unfractionated heparin therapy and subsequently bridged to warfarin. The clinical plan was to begin with short-term, 3 months-6 months, anticoagulant therapy to treat her acute episode. However, long-term anticoagulant therapy is being considered due to her increased risk for recurrent venous thromboembolic disease.

General Discussion In 1996, Poort et al described a point mutation in the 3′ untranslated region of the prothrombin gene, which substituted an adenine for a guanine at position 20,210. The prevalence of this mutation is essentially restricted to individuals with alleles derived from European ancestry. The gene mutation is most prevalent in southern Europe, where it is found in 2%-4% of individuals. This is approximately twice as frequent as individuals from northern Europe. The mutation is rare in Africa and far-east Asian populations. Among individuals of European ancestry who have a thrombotic event, the mutation is found in 6%-8% of patients. In families with a strong history of thrombosis, the frequency of this mutation is approximately 18%. In Poort's initial study, patients with PGM had an increased thrombotic risk (Relative risk 2.8 [95% CI, 1.4-5.6]) that was independent of other thrombophilic risk factors. Individuals with this mutation had higher levels of prothrombin compared to age-matched controls, with increasing risk of thrombotic events with higher levels of prothrombin. Subsequent studies confirmed Poort's findings, with most studies reporting odds ratios for venous thromboembolism between 2 and 4. The risk of a thrombotic event in patients with PGM is synergistic with other prothrombotic risk factors. In particular, the occurrence of double heterozygosity for PGM and FVL, which occurs in similar ethnic populations, has been extensively reported. Studies report an odds ratio for venous thromboebolism of approximately 20 in patients with combined mutations for FVL and PGM. The exact mechanism by which PGM results in a hypercoagulable state remains unclear. To date, studies reveal that PGM results in messenger ribonucleic acid (mRNA) that is more efficiently translated compared to wild type mRNA, resulting in higher levels of factor II. Although studies show increased thrombin generation secondary to increased prothrombin levels, it is unclear if this is sufficient to account for the hypercoagulability in patients with PGM. There is significant overlap between the prothrombin ranges in patients with PGM compared to those without this mutation. Therefore, prothrombin levels cannot be used as a surrogate marker for PGM. Laboratory testing for PGM uses PCR-based detection methods to identify the point mutation. The PGM mutation does not create or destroy an endonuclease cleavage site. Historically, laboratory testing utilized a PCR primer that created a second mutation only in the presence of PGM, resulting in a HindIII cleavage site in the mutated allele. This is identified as an extra band on gel electrophoresis, only seen in patients with PGM. However, alternative in-house and commercial techniques are available to identify PGM. Some laboratories use real-time PCR with melt curve analysis to identify this mutation. Fluorescent probes specific for the wild-type prothrombin gene is used. The point mutation decreases the temperature in which the probe is released from the target. The difference in temperature is significant enough to differentiate between wild-type and PGM. This assay is not as effective in identifying variant prothrombin gene mutations. Other commercial platforms are also available, including the Invader (Third Wave Technologies, Madison, Wisconsin) and the INFINITI (Autogenomics Inc, Carlsbad, California) platforms.

Section K: Thrombophilias

Hereditary Protein C Deficiency, Type I

Elizabeth M Van Cott

Patient A 26-year-old female with pain in her left calf.

Clinical History She described the pain as a "charlie horse" of 1-week duration in her left lower calf, which she had assumed was muscle soreness from a 10-mile race she had completed the day before onset while on vacation in Florida. She decided to seek medical attention because the pain persisted and her leg was beginning to appear swollen. She has no past medical history, including no pregnancies or miscarriages.

Family History Her father, 48, had an occurrence of deep vein thrombosis (DVT) after a flight to Europe 2 years ago.

Medications None.

Physical Examination The left calf was tender and warm on palpation, and appeared slightly larger in circumference than the right calf, with a faint red discoloration. She had no signs or symptoms of pulmonary embolism (PE), including no shortness of breath or chest pain. Her heart rate, blood pressure, respiratory rate, and temperature were normal. Oxygen saturation was 99% on room air.

Initial Work-Up
- PT, PTT and CBC including platelet count and differential were normal
- D-dimer positive (using an assay approved for exclusion of venous thrombosis)
- Lower extremity ultrasound identified DVT in her left popliteal and femoral vein

Differential Diagnosis Venous thromboembolism (VTE) can occur in association with specific risk factors, or it can occur spontaneously in predisposed individuals. Her risk factors for VTE were reviewed. She had never taken estrogen or progesterone medications. She does not smoke and does not use recreational drugs. She had no recent surgery, injury, illness or reduced mobility, and she was not pregnant and not obese. She lives in Florida and has not traveled in the past year. She did report frequent urinary tract infections recently. She also notes that the day of the race was unusually hot and she believes she became dehydrated. Therefore her risk factors for DVT include dehydration, infection, and family history. Certain medical conditions have an increased risk for VTE, including chronic disseminated intravascular coagulation (DIC), malignancy, polycythemia vera, essential thrombocythemia, paroxysmal nocturnal hemoglobinuria (PNH), Crohn disease, ulcerative colitis, Behcet disease, systemic lupus erythematosis (SLE), and heparin-induced thrombocytopenia (HIT). Hereditary defects in physiologic anticoagulant systems have an increased risk for VTE, including deficiencies of protein C, protein S, or antithrombin, factor V Leiden activated protein C resistance, and prothrombin G20210A. Elevated homocysteine can be hereditary or acquired, and is associated with an increased risk, although it has not yet been proven that reducing homocysteine levels reduces the risk. Antiphospholipid antibodies (lupus anticoagulant, anticardiolipin antibodies, and/or anti-β-2-glycoprotein I antibodies) are acquired antibodies that increase the risk for thrombosis.

Additional Work-Up Protein C chromogenic activity was low at 58% (normal 70-140), and the laboratory reflexively performed a protein C antigen, which was also low at 51% (normal 70-140). Normal results were obtained for protein S activity, antithrombin activity, activated protein C resistance (using an assay that essentially excludes factor V Leiden), prothrombin G20210A, lupus anticoagulant, anticardiolipin antibodies, and homocysteine. The specimen was collected prior to starting anticoagulants. To assess for acquired causes of low protein C, additional tests were performed. Albumin,

AST, ALT, alkaline phosphatase, total and direct bilirubin were normal, indicating that liver dysfunction is unlikely. Factor VII, PT and PTT were normal, indicating that there is no evidence for vitamin K deficiency or DIC. To exclude the possibility that protein C was low due to her acute thrombotic event, testing must be repeated at a later date, at least 10 days after discontinuing warfarin. The duration of time needed to wait to perform the repeat testing after an acute thrombotic event is not known, but the author suggests at least 3 months. Hereditary protein C has autosomal dominant inheritance. Therefore, identifying family member(s) with the deficiency can be helpful in confirming that a deficiency is hereditary. This patient's mother was shown to have normal protein C. Her father had low protein C activity and antigen with normal liver function tests, factor VII, D-dimer, PT and PTT, which supports the conclusion that the patient has hereditary type I protein C deficiency. Her brother, aged 15, had 57% protein C activity. However, this could be normal for age, and therefore he will need to be retested after the age of 18. Her sister, age 21, had normal protein C activity.

Final Diagnosis Hereditary protein C deficiency, type I (assuming that her protein C remains low on repeat testing, which cannot be done while on warfarin).

Management Approach She was treated with low molecular weight heparin with transition to warfarin. Current guidelines from the American College of Chest Physicians (ACCP) suggest, in general, 3 months of anticoagulation for a DVT provoked by a transient risk factor, and for unprovoked (spontaneous) proximal DVT, the guidelines suggest consideration of long-term anticoagulation. She was advised to avoid the risk factors described above, unless unavoidable (eg, surgery). If she takes long trips, she should frequently flex and stretch her calf and thigh muscles and remain well hydrated, and walk every 30 minutes-60 minutes if possible. Compression stockings help prevent and/or relieve postthrombotic syndrome.

General Discussion Acquired protein C deficiency is much more common than hereditary protein C deficiency. Therefore, causes of acquired deficiency must be assessed before making a diagnosis of hereditary deficiency. Liver dysfunction decreases protein C levels because of decreased hepatic synthesis. Protein C activity is vitamin K-dependent, therefore, oral anticoagulants or vitamin K deficiency decrease protein C. Low protein C measurements cannot be reliably interpreted during oral anticoagulant therapy, even with the use of formulas comparing the ratio of other vitamin K-dependent factors to protein C. Patients should not have received oral anticoagulants for at least 10 days prior to testing. The half-life of protein C is shorter than the half-life of protein S and antithrombin, and therefore protein C can be low with normal protein S and antithrombin during liver disease, warfarin initiation, or the onset of vitamin K deficiency, misleading the clinician into thinking that a hereditary deficiency is present (liver dysfunction can also decrease protein S and antithrombin, and warfarin/vitamin K deficiency can also decrease protein S). Factor VII has a short half-life that is similar to protein C. Therefore, if protein C is low with normal protein S and antithrombin, a factor VII assay can be considered to exclude the possibility of early liver dysfunction or vitamin K deficiency as the cause of low protein C (in which case factor VII will usually, but not always, be low as well). With warfarin initiation, protein C decreases more rapidly than does protein S, because the half-life of protein C is shorter than that for protein S. Conversely, after warfarin discontinuation, protein C increases to baseline more quickly than does protein S. Recent or current thrombosis, surgery, or DIC consume protein C and thus lower protein C levels (and usually also decrease protein S and antithrombin). At birth, protein C levels are decreased compared to normal adult values. Levels typically rise by age 6 months. However, protein C may remain below adult normal values throughout childhood. It is important to use an activity assay rather than an antigen assay for initial protein C testing, because antigen assays will not detect type II protein C deficiencies. Activity assays will detect both type I and type II deficiencies. Type I deficiency is quantitative (with reduced activity and antigen levels), whereas type II deficiency is qualitative (with reduced activity but normal antigen levels). Type I is more common than type II deficiency. Argatroban, bivalirudin, or hirudin can falsely elevate results when using clot-based activity assays. With PTT-clot-based activity assays, lupus anticoagulants can falsely elevate the results, and high factor VIII can falsely decrease the results. With chromogenic activity assays, a very rare type II variant might not be detected. Heterozygous protein C deficiency occurs in <1% of the general population, but is more common among patients with VTE. Heterozygous deficiency is associated with an increased risk for venous thrombosis. A few recent studies suggest that low protein C is also associated with arterial thrombosis such as myocardial infarction or stroke. The first thrombotic event usually presents between the ages of 10 years-50 years. Protein C deficiency also carries an increased risk for warfarin-induced skin necrosis. Homozygous protein C deficiency is very rare, with severely decreased protein C levels, presenting with purpura fulminans and DIC in the newborn period. Like other hereditary hypercoagulable conditions, the presence of a second risk factor further increases thrombotic risk.

Section K: Thrombophilias

Antithrombin Deficiency

Heesun J Rogers, Kandice Kottke-Marchant

Patient A 34-year-old Caucasian male presented with complaints of recent progressive headache, nausea and vomiting.

Clinical History The patient had experienced deep vein thrombosis (DVT) and pulmonary embolism (PE) related to a surgery for femur fracture at the age of 30 years. He was initially treated with heparin and then bridged to warfarin therapy. Warfarin was discontinued after 6 months. Four years later, he developed neck pain and dizziness about a week ago prior to presentation with progressive headache, nausea and vomiting. He was admitted for evaluation of the thrombotic event and anticoagulant therapy after finding acute thrombosis in MRI.

Family History Father died of PE at the age of 36. Sister experienced PE at the age of 23.

Medications No current medication.

Physical Examination Unremarkable.

Initial Work-Up PT 10.6 seconds (normal 9.9-13.0), INR 1.0 (normal 0.9-1.2), APTT 23.6 seconds (normal 24.6-34.0), platelet count $254 \times 10^3/\mu L$ (normal 150-400). MRI revealed acute thrombosis in right transverse and sigmoid sinus without hemorrhagic infarct.

Doppler Ultrasound Echogenic noncompressible thrombosis within popliteal vein.

Differential Diagnosis Diagnostic considerations included acquired or hereditary thrombophilia such as factor V Leiden (FVL) and prothrombin gene G20210A mutation (PGM), factor VIII activity, hyperhomocysteinemia, protein C or protein S deficiency, antithrombin (AT) deficiency, dysfibrinogenemia, hypofibrinolysis, plasminogen deficiency, and lupus anticoagulant.

Additional Work-Up Patients with venous thrombotic events (VTE) are generally screened for all inherited risk factors to identify the common and uncommon risk factors as well as co-inheritance. Screening tests, by prevalence, include DNA analysis for FVL and prothrombin gene G20210A mutation, factor VIII activity, plasma homocysteine assay, activated protein C resistance, protein C and protein S activities and antigen assays if activities are abnormal, AT activity and antigen assays if activity is abnormal. Tests for dysfibrinogenemia, hypofibrinolysis and plasminogen deficiency have a lack of consensus as a standard evaluation of thrombophilia and inclusion of the tests can be different from each institution. Lupus anticoagulant is a relatively common acquired autoantibody that shows a strong association with arterial or venous thrombosis. The results of additional tests on this patient are given in **Table 1**. With the identification of a decrease in the functional AT level, the assay was repeated using a fresh sample and AT antigen level was tested. AT antigen level was decreased to 69% (normal 80-120). After excluding possible causes of acquired AT deficiency, a family study for AT functional assay was conducted. AT activity assay performed on a 34-year-old sister with a previous history of PE yielded a result of 26%, and the activity levels for asymptomatic daughters, 6, 9 and 13 years old, were at 115%, 53% and 45%, respectively.

Table 1. Additional tests

Test	Result	Normal
Factor VIII: C assay (%)	174	50-150
Homocysteine, plasma (µmol/L)	11.6	6.4-13.7
Fibrinogen clottable (mg/dL)	346	200-400
Plasminogen assay (%)	102	68-122
Factor V Leiden R506Q PCR	Normal	Normal
Prothrombin gene for G20210A point mutation	Normal	Normal
Protein C functional assay (%)	107	70-120
Protein S clottable (%)	113	59-131
APC resistance ratio	2.33	2.00-3.00
AT functional assay (%)	65	80-120
C reactive protein (mg/dL)	0.3	0.0-2.0
β-2 glycoprotein (IgG and IgM) (SGU)	both <9	both <20
Anticardiolipin antibody (IgG, IgM and IgA)	Negative	Negative
Incubated APTT mixing study	Negative	Negative
Platelet neutralization	Negative	Negative
Dilute Russell viper venom time (DRVVT) screening and ratio	30.3, 0.99	25.0-36.9, <1.12
Hexagonal phase screening and δ (sec)	49.5, 0.0	37.7-65.8, <6.7 δ

Final Diagnosis Hereditary antithrombin deficiency, heterozygote, type 1.

Management Approach There is no recommendation for primary prophylaxis with anticoagulation therapy in asymptomatic AT deficiency, because the risk of serious hemorrhage may considerably outweigh the risk of fatal VTE event. Short-term thromboprophylaxis in high risk events is generally recommended. According to American College of Chest Physicians Evidence-Based Clinical Practice Guidelines, patients with confirmed acute DVT or PE are recommended to initiate treatment with vitamin K antagonist with concomitant low molecular weight heparin, UFH or fondaparinux for at least 5 days and until the INR is higher than 2.0 for 24 hours. If UFH is chosen, dose adjustment to maintain an APTT prolongation that corresponds to plasma heparin levels of 0.3-0.7 IU/mL anti-Xa activity is recommended. Treatment with warfarin for at least 3 months with a target INR of 2.5 (range 2.0-3.0) is suggested. After reassessing the risk-benefit ratio, patients with a second episode of unprovoked VKA require long-term treatment. For this patient, because of recurrent VTE in an unusual site in addition to strong family history, indefinite warfarin therapy with an INR target of 2.0-3.0 was recommended.

General Discussion Antithrombin (AT), a 58kD glycoprotein, is a member of the serine protease inhibitor (serpin) family. It primarily inactivates activated thrombin and factor Xa, and to a lesser extent, factors IXa, XIa, and XIIa. This serpin makes inactive forms with serpin proteases by recognizing the AT reactive site and building a covalent 1:1 complex. In the process, AT is so-called a "suicide inhibitor." Although AT is synthesized in the liver parenchyma, it is not vitamin K dependent and has a half-life of 2 days-3 days. AT deficiency can arise secondarily from various conditions, which include decreased AT synthesis in cirrhosis of the liver, increased AT loses in nephritic syndrome and protein losing enteropathy, enhanced consumption of AT in sepsis, burns, trauma, hepatic venoocclusive disease, thrombotic microangiopathies, cardiopulmonary bypass surgery, hematomas or metastatic tumors, and drug-induced AT deficiency by L-asparaginase or UFH therapy. Inherited AT deficiency is transmitted by autosomal dominant inheritance. Most cases are heterozygous because homozygosity for AT deficiency is almost fatal in utero. The prevalence rates are approximately 0.05% in the general population. Estimated annual incidence of a first episode of VTE in carriers of AT deficiency is 1.0%-2.9% per year in retrospective studies. 2 major types of inherited AT deficiency have been described. Type-1 AT deficiency is most commonly caused by a lack of gene product showing proportionately reduced functional and antigenic levels, resulting in approximately 50% AT activity and antigen levels. Type-2 AT deficiency is characterized by a qualitative defect, resulting in higher AT antigen than activity levels. Type-2 AT deficiencies are further subclassified by the site of the mutations and the performance of different AT assays: (1) Type-2a by mutations that affect AT reactive site; (2) Type-2b by an abnormality of the heparin-binding site; and (3) Type-2c by a pleiotropic effect affected by both sites. However, classification will not be clinically necessary because the initial anticoagulant therapy is the same in both types. Among the known inherited thrombophilias, AT deficiency has the highest risk for VTE. Although VTE usually occurs as DVT of the extremities and PE, it can occur in unusual sites, such as cerebral sinuses, mesenteric, portal and renal veins. It usually occurs at a young age (<50 years) with unprovoked or provoked condition although it is uncommon during the first 2 decades of life. Approximately 58% of these episodes occur spontaneously and 42% show an association with a transient and potentially preventable risk factor. Coinheritance of other defects such as FVL mutation is associated with higher risk of VTE in younger ages (median 16 years). Pregnancy related VTE and the risk of fetal loss are significantly higher in AT deficiency. The first evaluation of AT deficiency should be an AT functional assay, typically using chromogenic substrates incubating patient plasma with an excess of thrombin or factor Xa in the presence of heparin. If it is low, confirmatory functional and antigenic AT assays should be performed on the patient to determine the subtype. Screening tests for thrombophilia should include patients with unprovoked first VTE, patients younger than 50 years with provoked or recurrent VTE, VTE in unusual sites, relatives with a family history, or healthy individuals. Thrombophilia testing should be done ideally months after the VTE and at least 30 days after stopping warfarin. Some patients will develop recurrent VTE while waiting for tests with recurrent rate 7%-10% per year of unprovoked VTE. It is not appropriate to perform thrombophilia testing in the setting of an acute phase reaction, immediately after developing VTE, or on UFH therapy which can reduce the plasma AT level by about 25%. Acquired causes for AT deficiencies should be excluded and family studies may be helpful to establish a diagnosis of inherited AT deficiency.

Protein S Deficiency

Elizabeth M Van Cott

Patient A 32-year-old woman, who had had a pulmonary embolism (PE) 1 year prior.

Clinical History She had no past medical history other than the PE 1 year prior, 3 months after the birth of her first child. The evaluation at that time had included a low protein S level, with her protein S activity was 28% (normal 70-140) and protein S free antigen 32% (normal 70-140). She now presented for further evaluation.

Family History Her mother had a spontaneous lower-extremity deep vein thrombosis (DVT) in her late 30s.

Medications None at presentation. She had completed a 6-month course of warfarin 6 months prior.

Physical Examination Unremarkable.

Initial Work-Up
- PT 13.1 sec (normal 10.8-13.4)
- PTT 31 sec (normal 21-33)
- Platelet count 280 ×10^3/μL

Differential Diagnosis Acquired causes of low protein S are much more common than hereditary protein S deficiency. Protein S normally decreases during pregnancy, recovering within 3 months postpartum. Therefore, repeat testing is necessary to determine if her previously low protein S was due to the postpartum state. Protein S is consumed during thrombosis, therefore low protein S may have been due to the acute thrombotic event (however, protein C and antithrombin are usually consumed as well). Estrogen use (including oral contraceptives or hormone replacement therapy) can decrease protein S, but neither were relevant in this case. Acute phase reactions (eg. from illness, injury or stress) are a common cause of low protein S, because C4b binding protein (C4bBP) becomes elevated during acute phase reactions. C4bBP binds to protein S, which greatly reduces protein S activity. Warfarin or vitamin K deficiency decrease protein S and protein C. When warfarin is discontinued, protein S takes longer to return to the normal range than does protein C. Therefore, for up to 20 days after warfarin discontinuation, clinicians might be misled into thinking that low protein S with normal protein C indicates hereditary protein S deficiency, when it actually might be due to residual warfarin effect. Protein S can also be reduced by liver dysfunction (due to decreased hepatic synthesis) or disseminated intravascular coagulation (DIC). Protein C and antithrombin are usually also decreased if the low protein S is due to liver dysfunction or DIC. Protein S tends to be lower in women than in men. Protein S (total antigen) is low at birth but increases into adult reference range by approximately age 6 months. She did not have other risk factors for thrombosis, including no smoking, recreational drugs, obesity, and no recent surgery, injury, illness, infection, prolonged travel or reduced mobility.

Additional Work-Up Protein S activity was low at 45% (normal 70-140), and the laboratory reflexively performed a protein S free antigen which was also low at 42% (normal 70-140), as well as factor VIII and fibrinogen, which were normal. Elevated factor VIII causes falsely low protein S in PTT-based protein S activity assays. Elevated factor VIII or elevated fibrinogen occur during acute phase reactions, and acute phase reactions can decrease free protein S (and therefore protein S activity), because C4bBP becomes elevated during acute phase reactions. C4bBP binds to protein S, reducing the amount of free (unbound) protein S. Free protein S is active, whereas protein S that is bound to C4bBP is not. In this case, the normal factor VIII and fibrinogen suggest that the low protein S is not due to an acute phase reaction. Normal results were obtained for protein C activity, antithrombin activity, activated protein C resistance (using an assay that essentially excludes factor V Leiden), prothrombin G20210A, lupus anticoagulant, anticardiolipin antibodies, and homocysteine. Additional tests were performed to complete the assessment for acquired causes of low protein S. Albumin, AST, ALT, alkaline phosphatase, total and direct bilirubin were normal, indicating that liver dysfunction is unlikely (the normal protein C, PT and PTT also indicate that liver dysfunction is unlikely). The normal PT, PTT, and protein C indicate that there is no evidence for vitamin K deficiency. D-dimer was normal, which (along with the normal PT and PTT) indicate that there is no evidence for DIC. Hereditary protein S has autosomal dominant inheritance. Therefore, identifying family member(s) with the deficiency can be helpful in confirming that a deficiency is hereditary. This patient's mother was shown to have low protein S activity at 52% and free antigen at 56%, with normal factor VIII, fibrinogen, PT, PTT, D-dimer, liver function tests, and she has never been on estrogen, which supports the conclusion that the patient has hereditary protein S deficiency. Her father had normal protein S activity. Her sister, age 29, had 57% protein S activity but she is pregnant, and testing will have to be repeated at least 3 months after delivery.

Final Diagnosis Quantitative hereditary protein S deficiency. It is suggested to confirm this diagnosis by demonstrating low protein S at a later time, again in the absence of possible acquired causes of low protein S.

Management Approach Current guidelines from the American College of Chest Physicians (ACCP) suggest, in general, 3 months of anticoagulation for a PE provoked by a transient risk factor, and for unprovoked (spontaneous) PE, the guidelines suggest consideration of long-term anticoagulation. This patient was advised to avoid the risk factors described above, unless unavoidable (eg, surgery). If she takes long trips, she should frequently flex and stretch her calf and thigh muscles and remain well hydrated, and walk every 30 minutes-60 minutes if possible.

General Discussion Hereditary protein S deficiency has an increased risk for venous thrombosis. As with the other hereditary hypercoagulable conditions, the presence of additional risk factors further increases the risk for thrombosis. With heterozygous protein S deficiency, the first thrombotic event tends to present in the age range of 10 years-50 years. Homozygous protein S deficiency is rare; it can present as DIC and purpura fulminans in the newborn period, but milder phenotypes can also be seen. There are 3 types of protein S assays: activity (functional), free antigen (measures protein S that is not bound to C4bBP), and total antigen (measures both bound and unbound protein S). Activity assays detect quantitative and qualitative protein S deficiencies, but antigen assays detect only quantitative deficiencies. Thus, the major disadvantage of protein S antigen assays is that they will miss qualitative deficiencies. In addition to the potential interferences described above, activity assays have a variety of potential interferences that do not affect antigen assays. Factor V Leiden has been implicated in causing falsely low protein S in some, but not all, activity assays. Lupus anticoagulants can falsely increase protein S activity in PTT-based activity assays. Lupus anticoagulants may also interfere with PT- or Xa-based activity assays. Factor VIIa therapy can interfere with PT-based activity assays. Direct thrombin inhibitors (argatroban, hirudin, or bivalirudin) can cause falsely normal or elevated protein S in some activity assays. These potential assay interferences must be considered before excluding or diagnosing hereditary protein S deficiency. 3 types of hereditary protein S deficiency have been described. Type I is a quantitative deficiency, with low activity, free antigen, and total antigen levels. Type II is a qualitative deficiency with low activity but normal free antigen and total antigen levels. Type III deficiency may be due to excess binding of protein S to C4bBP, causing low activity and low free antigen, but normal total antigen levels.

Thrombotic Thrombocytopenic Purpura

Roy E Smith, Joseph Law

Patient A 70-year-old Caucasian male with systemic sclerosis, who developed facial drooping, confusion, and slurred speech.

Clinical History The patient's medical history was only significant for systemic sclerosis with diffuse cutaneous involvement diagnosed in January 2009. In June 2009, it was determined that his skin had significantly thickened when compared to previous measurements. He was started on D-penicillamine 250 mg/day, which he tolerated well. At that time, his platelet count and creatinine level were $240 \times 10^3/\mu L$ (normal 156-369) and 0.9 mg/dL (normal 0.5-1.4), respectively. During a follow-up visit in September 2009, the patient complained of decreased mobility of his upper and lower extremities, along with fatigue, dry eyes, and arthralgias. Physical exam revealed increased skin induration. Because of the obvious progression of his disease, his dose of D-penicillamine was increased to 500 mg/day. A few days later, he experienced worsening skin tightness, fatigue, the new onset of generalized myalgias, and transient slurring of speech and confusion. One week after the increase in dose, his platelet count was found to be $9 \times 10^3/\mu L$, and D-penicillamine was stopped. 2 days after cessation of D-penicillamine, the patient experienced right-sided facial drooping, slurring of speech, and confusion.

Family History Noncontributory.

Medications None.

Physical Examination On admission, the patient's blood pressure was 120/74 mm Hg, pulse 91/min, respiratory rate 18/min, and temperature 97.2°F. He was ill-appearing with slurring of his speech and a slight right-sided facial droop. He was anicteric, and there was no lymphadenopathy. Examination of his heart and lungs was unremarkable. His abdominal exam revealed significant induration and dilated veins on both of his flanks. His skin was hyperpigmented over his chest, arms, and legs, and he had sclerosis of his fingers and hands. He had marked induration in his arms and thighs, and limited mobility in his elbows, wrists, and hands. He had no ecchymoses or petechiae on his skin. He had poor muscle strength in his lower extremities.

Initial Work-Up An emergent MRI of the brain showed multiple punctate foci of acute infarction not conforming to a single vascular territory. His hemoglobin was 11.7 g/dL, hematocrit 33.3%, and platelet count $13 \times 10^3/\mu L$. Peripheral blood smear revealed schistocytosis (**Figure 1**). The creatinine level was within the normal range at 1.2 mg/dL. Lactate dehydrogenase was elevated at 440 U/L. Haptoglobin was decreased at 3 mg/dL (normal 36-195), and albumin was mildly decreased at 3.2 g/dL (normal 3.4-5.0). The following tests were normal: glucose, electrolytes, blood urea, white blood cells, ALT, AST, total bilirubin, and total protein. Urinalysis showed 2+ blood, 1+ ketones,

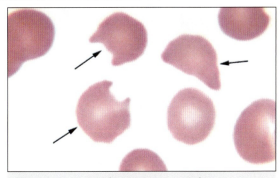

Figure 1 Blood smear (Wright-Giemsa, ×1000) showing schistocytes.

and trace protein. An ADAMTS-13 activity level was drawn, but results were not immediately available.

Differential Diagnosis Scleroderma renal crisis or thrombotic thrombocytopenic purpura (TTP).

Additional Work-Up The ADAMTS-13 activity level (using fluorescence resonance energy transfer technology) was found to be 7% (normal >68%). ADAMTS-13 autoantibodies were 44.2 AU/mL (normal <9.0 AU/mL).

Final Diagnosis Thrombotic thrombocytopenic purpura (TTP).

Management Approach Early diagnosis of TTP is important because its treatment, plasmapheresis with plasma exchange, can be life-saving if started promptly. Plasmapheresis with plasma exchange replaces the supply of ADAMTS-13 while helping to remove inhibitory antibodies This patient was thought to have either TTP or normotensive scleroderma renal crisis, and was therefore treated with daily plasmapheresis, daily plasma exchange, and captopril (as treatment for scleroderma renal crisis). After the first plasma exchange, he had significant recovery of his neurological deficits, which continued to improve until discharge. He remained normotensive and afebrile throughout his hospital stay, and his serum creatinine remained at 1.2 mg/dL or less. Captopril had to be held on several occasions because of hypotension, and corticosteroids were avoided. At discharge, his platelet count was $240 \times 10^3/\mu L$.

General Discussion In a patient with systemic sclerosis, differentiating between scleroderma renal crisis and TTP/HUS presents a diagnostic challenge. Scleroderma renal crisis often presents with a decline in renal function, rise in serum creatinine, abrupt onset of hypertension, microangiopathic hemolytic anemia (MAHA), and thrombocytopenia. Thrombocytopenia, MAHA, and renal dysfunction are also seen with TTP/HUS. Measurement of ADAMTS-13 activity levels is useful in confirming the diagnosis of TTP. ADAMTS-13 (a disintegrin and metalloproteinase with a thrombospondin type 1 motif, member 13) cleaves large multimers of von Willebrand protein. Decreased ADAMTS-13 activity leads to an accumulation of these large multimers and increased platelet adhesion to damaged endothelial surfaces. This results in microthrombi and the clinical manifestations of TTP. ADAMTS-13 activity levels are significantly decreased or absent in patients with TTP. Our patient's presentation was more consistent with TTP, but he did have features that were suggestive of scleroderma renal crisis. The patient's diffuse disease and lack of fever were more consistent with scleroderma renal crisis than TTP. Furthermore, there is a strong association between scleroderma renal crisis and ANA with speckled pattern, which had been found in our patient. The patient markedly improved after initiation of plasma exchange, suggesting TTP as his underlying disease. The diagnosis was ultimately confirmed when his ADAMTS-13 activity level was found to be severely depressed at 7%. Studies have shown a median ADAMTS-13 activity level of around 50% in scleroderma renal crisis, compared to 16% in TTP. ADAMTS-13 activity levels are thought to be decreased through 2 general mechanisms: (1) mutations leading to a congenital form of TTP, and (2) autoimmune-mediated inhibition of ADAMTS-13 function and acquired TTP. Our patient obviously had an acquired form of immune-mediated TTP, as indicated by the presence of autoantibodies to ADAMTS-13. One published study demonstrated that 97% of patients with idiopathic TTP were found to have anti-ADAMTS-13 IgG or IgM autoantibodies present. A small number of case reports in the literature have described a relationship between D-penicillamine use and TTP. One case report describes TTP occurring in a female patient with rheumatoid arthritis around 1 month after the start of D-penicillamine 250 mg daily and 8 days after an increase in dose to 250 mg twice daily. This was similar to our patient, who developed TTP around 4 months after starting D-penicillamine at 250 mg daily and around 1 week after an increase in dose to 500 mg daily. Although there is a temporal relationship between our patient's increase in D-penicillamine dose and his onset of TTP, his ADAMTS-13 level was more consistent with sporadic TTP than with drug-associated TTP. Another study found that in 95% of patients with drug-associated TTP, the ADAMTS-13 activity level was >25%. The other 5% of patients had an ADAMTS-13 activity level between 10%-25%. This is in contrast to our patient's ADAMTS-13 level of 7%. However, none of the patients in study suffered from TTP associated with D-penicillamine. Therefore, the ADAMTS-13 level in TTP associated with D-penicillamine is unknown. This patient's course was consistent with TTP and confirmed by the severe depression in ADAMTS-13 activity levels and the detection of autoantibodies to ADAMTS-13. There are approximately 10 case reports in the literature that describe the occurrence of TTP in the setting of systemic sclerosis. Since D-penicillamine is a common treatment for the disease, one must consider the possibility that some of these cases were due to D-penicillamine exposure.

Heparin-Induced Thrombocytopenia with Thrombosis

Steven E McKenzie, Douglass Drelich

Patient A 58-year-old Caucasian American male with a swollen, tender right calf 6 days after coronary artery bypass graft surgery (CABG).

Clinical History The patient was in his usual state of health until 10 days previously, when he experienced substernal chest pain while walking up steps. The pain radiated to his left arm and jaw. He presented to the emergency department, where he was evaluated for possible myocardial infarction (MI). Following admission and monitoring, MI was ruled out by cardiac enzyme and ECG evaluations, but suspicion of angina due to coronary artery atherosclerotic disease prompted cardiac catheterization. The catheterization study revealed >95% stenosis in the left main and left anterior descending arteries. On the 4th day of hospitalization he underwent CABG via median sternotomy, utilizing cardiopulmonary bypass (CPB) extracorporeal circulation and left leg saphenous vein grafts. He was extubated on the 2nd postoperative day, and was recovering with rehabilitation when he noticed a swollen, tender right calf. He denied shortness of breath, cold sensations in the right leg or foot, or parasthesias. He has a history of mild to moderate hypertension, successfully treated with diuretic therapy. His body mass index is 31. He has had a borderline glucose tolerance test, but receives no medication for Type II diabetes. His serum LDL was 150 mg/dL and HDL 45 mg/dL; he does not receive medication for dyslipidemia. He has been smoking cigarettes, 1 pack per day, for 36 years and consumes alcohol 2 times-3 times per week. He has been an automobile mechanic throughout his career.

Family History He is married and has 3 children, who are alive and well at 31, 29 and 26 years of age. His mother is alive at 79 years of age, and has osteoarthritis and hypertension. His father died at age 62 of MI. He has 2 siblings, ages 59 and 54, each with hypertension controlled by medication. There is no family history of deep vein thrombosis, pulmonary embolism, excessive hemorrhage, stroke, or cancer.

Medications On admission, he was taking hydrochlorothiazide 25 mg/day. He was placed on aspirin 325 mg/day, and received heparin (unfractionated) IV with the dose titrated for a PTT of 60 sec-80 sec. During CPB, he received high-dose heparin to prevent clotting in the extracorporeal circuit; this was reversed with protamine sulfate. He received cefazolin for the first 2 postoperative days, which was changed to vancomycin on the 3rd postoperative day when the left leg incision became suppurative.

Physical Examination The patient was in mild distress. Vital signs: pulse 78/min, blood pressure 140/88, respiration 12/min, temperature 100.2°F, and pulse oximetry 94% on room air. Chest showed a healing median sternal incision without oozing or infection evident, and lungs had scattered rhonchi, prominent at the bases. Heart showed regular rate and rhythm, S1S2 without gallop or murmur. Extremity exam showed a healing incision of the left lower leg; the right leg was red, warm, swollen and tender posteriorly from the popliteal space to the ankle, with pedal edema. There was a question of a palpable "cord." Pulses were present distally, and the foot was warm. The neurological exam was nonfocal.

Initial Work-Up
- PT on admission 12.3 sec; at time of presentation 12.7 sec (normal 10.9-13.3)
- PTT on admission 34.2 sec; at time of presentation 35.1 sec (normal 29.9-35.8)
- Platelet count on admission $195 \times 10^3/\mu L$; at time of presentation $70 \times 10^3/\mu L$

Section L: Miscellaneous Hemostasis Disorders
Heparin-Induced Thrombocytopenia with Thrombosis

Differential Diagnosis Diagnostic considerations included idiopathic deep vein thrombosis, postoperative thrombocytopenia (drug-induced or disseminated intravascular coagulation with consumption) and heparin-induced thrombocytopenia with thrombosis.

Additional Work-Up Doppler ultrasound of the lower extremities revealed a deep vein thrombosis to the level of the popliteal vein; arterial pulses were detected normally. HGB 12.2 g/dL, WBC $6.2 \times 10^3/\mu L$ with a normal differential. Comprehensive metabolic panel was notable for BUN 27 mg/dL, creatinine 1.6 mg/dL, total bilirubin 1.1 mg/dL, AST 32 IU/L, and ALT 28 IU/L. A test for anti-heparin/PF4 antibodies by ELISA was sent (PF4 stands for platelet factor 4), as was a test for the serotonin release assay.

Final Diagnosis A clinical diagnosis of heparin-induced thrombocytopenia with thrombosis was made. Therapy was initiated while final laboratory confirmation was pending.

Management Approach All sources and forms of heparin were discontinued. Anticoagulation therapy with a direct thrombin inhibitor was initiated, in this case argatroban intravenously. Argotroban was chosen because of the presence of adequate hepatic function. The major FDA-approved alternative is lepirudin, which is sensitive to impaired renal function. The patient was monitored closely for signs or symptoms of pulmonary embolism, other deep vein thrombi, arterial thrombi, or hemorrhage. The CBC was performed daily and it showed a stable HGB and a return over 4 days to a platelet count of $155 \times 10^3/\mu L$. On the 2nd day of argatroban therapy, the anti-heparin/PF4 antibody titer was reported as positive at optical density 1.1 (top normal 0.4) in an ELISA that measured IgG, A, and M antibodies to heparin/PF4. 2 days later, the serotonin release assay was reported as positive with 78% serotonin release at 0.5 U/mL of added heparin, and 8% and 9% serotonin release at 0 U/mL and 100 U/mL of added heparin, respectively. After recovery of the platelet count, oral warfarin was added with argatroban as bridging therapy for 4 days, until the INR met the conversion nomogram criteria for adequate warfarin effect while on concurrent argatroban. He received warfarin with a goal INR of 2.0-3.0 for 120 days, with resolution of the DVT. He was instructed to inform any future medical personnel that he had been diagnosed with heparin-induced thrombocytopenia.

General Discussion Heparin-induced thrombocytopenia (HIT) is one of the most common drug-induced thrombocytopenias. It is a thrombotic disorder, with the paradox that thrombi develop in the setting of low platelet counts and concurrent anticoagulant (heparin) therapy. Patients can present with thrombocytopenia, often moderate (50×10^3-$125 \times 10^3/\mu L$) and ~30%-50% below baseline, on the 5th to 10th day of heparin therapy. Patients could also present with concurrent thrombosis. Earlier drops in the platelet count occur in those exposed previously to heparin in the prior 120 days. Clinical suspicion is necessary, as treatment decisions are necessary before definitive lab tests are generally available. Several investigators have proposed pretest clinical probability scores to aid in decision-making. The disorder is due to platelet-activating IgG antibodies directed against the complex of heparin and platelet chemokine PF4. The ELISA test shows whether such antibodies are present. Unfortunately, this test currently has good sensitivity but poor specificity, as many patients show detectable antibodies without manifesting HIT. The serotonin release assay is the gold standard for confirmatory diagnosis, showing heparin-dependent antibodies in the serum of affected patients which activate donor platelets in the test tube to release serotonin. Both unfractionated heparins and low molecular weight heparins have been shown to cause the disorder. The pentasaccharide fondaparinux has shown cross-reactivity with HIT antibodies, and is not approved by the FDA for HIT therapy. All sources and forms of heparin must be discontinued, and treatment with alternative anticoagulation instituted, such as the direct thrombin inhibitors. Initiation of therapy with a vitamin K antagonist such as warfarin is contraindicated, as it can deplete essential natural vitamin K-dependent anticoagulants such as Proteins C and S. Approximately 35%-40% of patients with HIT have clinically detected thrombosis; of those, ~70% are venous, and the remainder arterial. HIT has a high morbidity, eg, from limb loss, and mortality, eg, from thrombotic stroke or M.I. Anticoagulant therapy should continue during the 30 days-120 days following diagnosis, with the duration based on the clinical presentation, such as the presence of clinically evident thrombosis and the risks and benefits of anticoagulation for the individual.

Disseminated Intravascular Coagulation (DIC)

Roy E Smith, An Tran

Patient A 69-year-old woman with dyspnea on exertion and low-grade fever for 2 weeks.

Clinical History The patient had been receiving total parenteral nutrition (TPN) for the prior 11 months after total colectomy and ileostomy for ischemic colitis. She had low-grade fever without mental status changes or seizures. She had a remote history of epistaxis and denied bloody or black stools from the ileostomy, rash, pruritus, or lower extremity edema. Because of her deteriorating condition, she was referred to a large medical facility for specialty care. Upon arrival, blood cultures were obtained from her tunneled central venous catheter and from peripheral venous sites which subsequently were positive for yeast. She had a normal complete blood count and platelet count at this time. A transthoracic echocardiogram was suspicious for the presence of a tricuspid valve vegetation. 4 days after the onset of symptoms she was noted to have a platelet count of $44 \times 10^3/\mu L$.

Family History Noncontributory.

Medications Caspofungin, loperamide, acetaminophen as needed, tiotropium bromide inhalation, ondansetron as needed, total parenteral nutrition. It was uncertain if she had been exposed to heparin products recently.

Physical Examination The patient was alert and oriented to time, person, and place and comfortable. Her vital signs were normal. There were no petechiae or rashes. There was a grade 3/6 systolic murmur heard best along the right sternal border. There were no stigmata of liver dysfunction and no other remarkable findings.

Initial Work-Up

Date	Platelet ($\times 10^3/\mu L$)	HGB (g/dL)	WBC ($\times 10^3/\mu L$)	PTT (sec)	PT (sec)	INR
On admission	169	11.9	8.9	35.4	16.3	1.3
2 days prior to evaluation	124	11.4	6.3	31.2	16.7	1.3
1 day prior to evaluation	78	12.5	5.0	35.0	18.0	1.5
Day of evaluation	44	12.1	4.3	33.7	17.5	1.4

Transthoracic echocardiogram showed multiple large tricuspid valve masses consistent with vegetations; the largest mass measured 1.8 × 0.9 cm; the left ventricle size and function were normal

Differential Diagnosis Disseminated intravascular coagulation (DIC), heparin-induced thrombocytopenia (HIT), thrombotic thrombocytopenic purpura (TTP), and liver dysfunction.

Additional Work-Up D-dimer was positive at 6.18 µg/mL (normal <0.45), fibrin degradation products >20 µg/mL (normal is <20), antithrombin III activity was at 49% (normal 80-120), and fibrinogen activity at 123 mg/dL (normal 205-508). Heparin-PF4 antibody ELISA assay and heparin-associated platelet aggregation tests were negative. There were no schistocytes seen in the peripheral blood smear.

Final Diagnosis Disseminated intravascular coagulation.

Management Approach Disseminated intravascular coagulation (DIC) is always secondary to a triggering event (usually infection, malignancy or trauma). The appropriate treatment is to address the underlying cause of the coagulopathy. When complicated by bleeding or thrombosis, or a high risk of either, measures to arrest or otherwise modify the consequences of this process characterized as activated coagulation ± fibrinolysis are often undertaken. For patients at risk of bleeding, the target platelet count is $20 \times 10^3/\mu L$ or greater. For patients actively bleeding, the platelet count should be kept at $50 \times 10^3/\mu L$ or greater. The efficacy of platelet replacement may be detrimentally affected by elevation of the products of fibrin(ogen) degradation which impairs platelet function. Patients with DIC often have a multiple coagulation defects, including decreases in coagulation factors due to consumption or fibrinolysis or liver synthetic defects. Since almost all of the patients receive antibiotics for presumed infection and these antibiotics may reduce gut bacteria or interfere with vitamin K metabolism, vitamin K replacement is always indicated. In addition to platelet replacement therapy, bleeding patients may require the administration of frequent, large doses of fresh frozen plasma (FFP) until the process is controlled. Fibrinogen levels should be kept ≥100 mg/dL with either FFP or cryoprecipitate or both if the severity of the coagulopathy so indicates. The use of heparin either subcutaneously or intravenously to counteract the thrombotic propensity in DIC has been reported; however, there is little evidence that this is a worthwhile treatment strategy in most patients. In patients with low antithrombin levels, replacement with FFP or antithrombin III concentrates may be required either alone or as an adjunct to heparin therapy. Recombinant activated protein C (rAPC) has been shown to be effective in some patients with severe sepsis complicated by DIC. Since rAPC inhibits the forward reactions of coagulation, its use may increase bleeding risk. The patient reported here was treated with supportive care and antibiotics. She did not have thrombotic or bleeding complications from DIC, although her fibrinogen and platelet count were decreased. Her fungemia was treated with caspofungin which was later switched to fluconazole. Her platelet count decreased to $39 \times 10^3/\mu L$ the day after, but it increased to $44 \times 10^3/\mu L$ and continued to increase thereafter. The patient's condition deteriorated 1 week after the initial evaluation and she subsequently died from the infection.

General Discussion DIC is characterized by the systemic activation of the forward and reverse reactions of coagulation and the associated consumption of key procoagulants, natural inhibitors, and platelets. Proinflammatory mediators such as endotoxin, exotoxin, interleukin-6 and TNFα are thought to cause endothelial cell injury triggering activation of the contact factors, the release of tissue factor, and the direct enzymatic activation of prothrombin. Septic episodes are often associated with liver hypoperfusion resulting in decreased liver-mediated plasma clearance of activated coagulation factors and tissue plasminogen activator, urokinase and fibrin(ogen) degradation platelets triggering further exacerbation of the coagulopathy. Characterized by excessive fibrin formation and dissolution, and the increased consumption of both platelets and fibrinogen, there is no single diagnostic test. Static parameters of the forward and reverse reactions of coagulation are often helpful, but nevertheless the diagnosis can be challenging (especially when liver dysfunction is present). Since many patients have additional confounding comorbidities, the existence of lesser degrees of activation of coagulation and fibrinolysis may be difficult to ascertain.

The key laboratory findings are elevated D-dimers or fibrin(ogen) degradation products, prolonged PT (seen in 70% of cases) and/or PTT (seen in 50% of cases), and decreased platelets and fibrinogen (seen in 50% of cases). The examination of the peripheral blood smear can be helpful since the formation of fibrin strands in the small vessels may cause microangiopathic hemolysis as evidenced by the presence of schistocytes (seen in 50% of the cases) and a decrease or absence of platelets. The physiologic response of anticoagulation ultimately results in the consumption of various anticoagulant factors such as protein C and S and antithrombin, and the appearance of excessive antithrombin:thrombin complexes. It should be noted that D-dimers and fibrin(ogen) degradation products can be elevated with physiologic clot lysis, inflammation and in the presence of liver dysfunction. In addition, fibrinogen, an acute phase reactant, may be normal or elevated in early or low-grade DIC. In this situation the measurement of serial fibrinogen levels and platelet counts can be used to establish the presence of increased consumption of both, a finding consistent with the presence of DIC.

HELLP Syndrome (Hemolysis, Elevated Liver Enzymes, Low Platelets Syndrome)

Craig Kessler

Patient A 32-year-old African-American primagravida female presented to the emergency department in labor in her 35th week of gestation.

Clinical History The patient had a 3-day history of severe occipital headache, associated with nausea and intermittent blurred vision. She has been healthy all her life. Her pregnancy had been uneventful up to the day before admission when she noted easy bruising and darkened urine. She denied changes in mental status although her husband had observed that she was unable to remember her telephone number, address, and social security number when she was being registered.

Family History Noncontributory.

Medications Prenatal multivitamins and supplemental oral ferrous sulfate.

Physical Examination The patient appeared slightly disoriented and complained of increasing intensity of her headache. Her blurred vision persisted. She had a blood pressure of 155/105 with a regular pulse rate of 110. She was afebrile. Her examination was remarkable for a gravid uterus, multiple ecchymotic lesions over her extensor surfaces, trace of bipedal edema, and +3 knee jerk reflexes bilaterally. The fetal heart sounds were normal and ultrasound of the placenta appeared normal.

Initial Work-Up

CBC

WBC (×10³/μL)	3.5
RBC (×10⁶/μL)	3.39
HGB (g/dL)	10.3
HCT (%)	29.5
MCV (fL)	87.1
MCH (pg)	30.4
MCHC (g/dL)	34.9
PLT (×10³/μL)	60
RDW-CV (%)	14.5
Reticulocyte count (%)	5.9
Absolute neutrophil count (×10³/μL)	2.2

The comprehensive metabolic panel was remarkable for BUN of 43 mg/dL and serum creatinine of 1.8 mg/dL. Her urine was dark pink in color and positive for blood by dipstix, but no red cells were seen in the sediment. PT 16.5 sec (normal 12.5-14.0); PTT 62 sec (normal 22-35); thrombin time 26 sec (normal 10-15); fibrinogen 295 mg/dL.

Peripheral blood smear showed aniso and poikilocytosis with scattered schistocytes, microspherocytes, and occasional Howell-Jolly bodies, features associated with hemolysis (**Figure 1**). Occasional giant platelets were present.

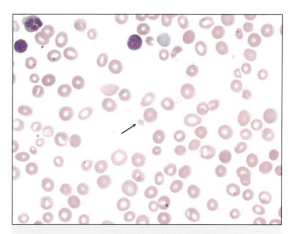

Figure 1 Blood smear (Wright-Giemsa, ×1000) showing scattered schistocytes, Howell-Jolly bodies and occasional microspherocytes.

Section L: Miscellaneous Hemostasis Disorders
HELLP Syndrome (Hemolysis, Elevated Liver Enzymes, Low Platelets Syndrome)

Differential Diagnosis Diagnostic considerations included disseminated intravascular coagulation (DIC), immune thrombocytopenic purpura (ITP), thrombotic thrombocytopenic purpura (TTP)/hemolytic uremic syndrome (HUS), antiphospholipid antibody syndrome, HELLP syndrome with preeclampsia, malignant hypertension and acute fatty liver syndrome.

Additional Work-Up LDH 685 U/L, AST 628 U/L, ALT 1,040 U/L, Total bilirubin 2.3 mg/dL. Mixing studies of patient with normal pooled plasma did not correct the abnormal tests. D-dimers were increased to >10,000 ng/mL (normal 0-200). Antiphospholipid antibodies were negative. The presence of proteinuria would be more consistent with preeclampsia than TTP. Pre-eclampsia associated with significantly elevated D-dimers is more likely to progress to HELLP. The increased D-dimers and lower than expected fibrinogen concentration for the stage of pregnancy are also compatible with DIC. Significantly high D-dimers do not occur usually with TTP. Increased serum soluble endoglin/CD105 levels are considerably higher in HELLP than preeclampsia and may offer another laboratory discrimination between the 2 diagnoses.

Final Diagnosis HELLP syndrome.

Management Approach For this case of HELLP superimposed on preeclampsia, the initial treatment should be focused on normalization of the BP, prevention of seizures, and then evacuation of the uterus. The increased liver function tests should normalize within 4 days postpartum. The use of platelet transfusions is controversial and should be reserved primarily for active bleeding. The aggressive use of dexamethasone (10 mg IV bid) early in the course of HELLP may reduce the need for subsequent platelet transfusions. Plasmapheresis and intravenous γ-globulin may also be helpful in symptomatic refractory thrombocytopenic patients. No specific treatment for DIC should be initiated other than attempting to eradicate its cause, eg, evacuate the uterus. Placental abruption is not uncommon in HELLP and usually requires C-section delivery. The platelet count should be >50,000/μL for C-section and platelet support to achieve or maintain that level is not unreasonable. Women with HELLP with one pregnancy are at risk for recurrence with subsequent pregnancies. This patient was stabilized following administration of magnesium and labatelol, and absent active bleeding, she was taken immediately to C-section delivery as ultrasound showed some evidence of placental abruption. The delivery was uneventful but her liver function test results continued to rise along with increased abdominal pain. Ultrasound of the abdomen ruled out a ruptured liver capsule. Dexamethasone was prescribed and the liver function tests and platelet counts normalized over the next 4 days.

General Discussion HELLP syndrome occurs far less frequently as a pregnancy complication than preeclampsia (approximately 0.5% vs 5%); however, HELLP occurs in 4%-18% of preeclampsia cases. Up to 30% of HELLP cases may not become apparent until 24 hrs-48 hrs postpartum. When preeclampsia is not present, the diagnosis of isolated HELLP syndrome is often delayed. The basic pathophysiology is related to microvascular endothelial cell damage, associated with accelerated intravascular platelet consumption and subsequent DIC. The presence of the fetus is considered necessary and there may be a decidual cell contribution to maternal endothelial damage and vasoconstriction. HELLP is associated with up to 35% maternal mortality and morbidity. Fetal demise is not uncommon. The coagulation mixing studies suggest the presence of a circulating inhibitor, in this case, the very elevated D-dimers. The presence of an elevated thrombin time, elevated D-dimers, absolute decreases in fibrinogen levels, and decreased platelet count are consistent with DIC, as is the presence of schistocytes on peripheral smear. Microspherocytes, darkened urine, and increased LDH are consistent with intravascular hemolysis, a component requisite for the diagnosis of the HELLP syndrome (Coombs test-negative hemolysis; elevated liver function with LDH>600 U/L, AST >70 U/L; total bilirubin>1.2 mg/dL; and low platelets<100,000/μL). Sometimes the differential diagnosis is challenging; however, the acute rise in liver function studies sets this syndrome apart. This may actually be a moot point since some consider HELLP to be a variant of severe preeclampsia or eclampsia.

Thrombotic Thrombocytopenic Purpura in a Patient with Sickle Cell Crisis

Cordelia Sever

Patient A 56-year-old African-American woman with back pain and hip pain.

Clinical History She had recently traveled from sea level to a high altitude, and then developed back and hip pain. The patient was discharged with narcotic pain medication but was brought back to the hospital a day later because she had become unarousable and was in respiratory failure. After naloxone administration, she had a brief period of regaining consciousness, albeit with confusion and episodic combativeness; nevertheless she became obtunded again. Past medical history included sickle cell trait, hypertension, autoimmune thyroiditis (Graves disease) treated with radioactive iodine, and a hysterectomy for uterine fibroids accompanied by excessive bleeding which required transfusion postoperatively.

Family History Hypertension.

Medications Thyroid hormone replacement.

Physical Examination A well nourished female, intubated, sedated, but with spontaneous movements, temperature 100.4°F, BP 151/74, heart rate 81/minute. She had no adenopathy and no petechiae.

Initial Work-Up

CBC

WBC (×10³/μL)	17.9
RBC (×10⁶/μL)	3.66
HGB (g/dL)	8.5
HCT (%)	27
MCV (fL)	73.0
MCHC (g/dL)	32.2
PLT (×10³/μL)	117
RDW-CV (%)	17.6

WBC Differential	%	# (×10³/μL)
Neutrophils	85	15.5
Bands	0	
Lymphocytes	12	2.1
Monocytes	1	0.2
Eosinophils	0	
Basophils	1	0.2
NRBC (#/100 WBC)	40	

Peripheral blood smear revealed microcytic hypochromic red cells, target cells, sickle cells, polychromasia, and probable schistocytes (**Figures 1** and **2**).

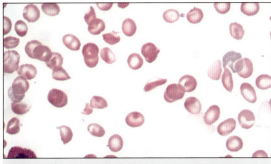

Figure 1 Blood smear (Wright-Giemsa, ×1000) showing microcytic hypochromic red cells, target cells, sickle cells, polychromasia, and probable schistocytes.

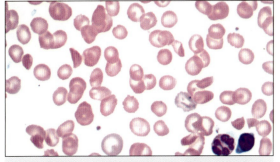

Figure 2 Blood smear (Wright-Giemsa, ×1000) showing microcytic hypochromic red cells, target cells, sickle cells, polychromasia, and a Howell-Jolly body.

Differential Diagnosis The presence of sickle cells and clinical presentation were compatible with a sickle cell crisis, most likely precipitated by travel to high altitude. Since homozygous sickle cell disease would in all likelihood have manifested much earlier with more severe anemia and recurrent sickle cell crises, the patient was suspected to have hemoglobin S with either concurrent hemoglobin C trait or β-thalassemia trait. The differential diagnosis for her CNS symptoms included narcotic overdose vs CNS symptoms of sickle cell crisis.

Additional Work-Up

On the day of admission:
- Hemoglobin electrophoresis: A_1 17.4%, A_2 6.2%, F 5.7%, and S 70.7%
- CT scan showed a hypodense cerebellar lesion consistent with a subacute cerebellar infarct

After red cell exchange on day 2 of admission:
- Hemoglobin electrophoresis: A_1 77.4%, A_2 3.7%, F 0.5%, and S 18.4%
- WBC $17.6 \times 10^3/\mu L$, HGB 9.2 g/dL, PLT $66 \times 10^3/\mu L$
- Peripheral blood smear: target cells, a few schistocytes, and occasional spherocytes (**Figure 3**)
- LDH 5,100 U/dL (normal 300-650)
- There was no initial clinical explanation for the mild thrombocytopenia, which; however, worsened after red cell exchange. The additional finding of high serum LDH with some peripheral blood spherocytes and occasional schistocytes raised the question of a superimposed thrombotic thrombocytopenic purpura (TTP)

Final Diagnosis Thrombotic thrombocytopenic purpura in a patient with sickle cell crisis secondary to sickle-β+ thalassemia disease.

Management Approach The patient was treated with therapeutic plasma exchange daily, starting on the third day of admission. Within 24 hours her respiratory failure improved; within 48 hours her mental status changes completely resolved and she could be weaned from the ventilator and extubated. 10 days after admission she was receiving plasma exchanged every other day with platelet counts improving; she was well enough to be discharged in order to transfer her care to her home town at sea level.

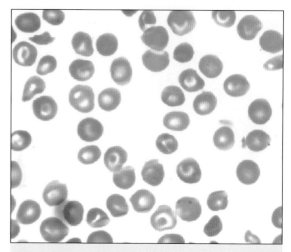

Figure 3 Blood smear (Wright-Giemsa, ×1000) showing target cells, schistocytes and occasional spherocytes.

General Discussion The first event in the patient's disease course was a sickle cell crisis precipitated by travel to high altitude. She presented with classic sickle cell crisis symptoms including lumbosacral ("back") pain, followed by a relatively mild manifestation of acute chest syndrome and evidence of central nervous system infarcts (cerebellum). The mild initial thrombocytopenia would raise the question of an acute sequestration crisis; however, there was no splenic enlargement. The lack of response to red cell exchange which usually is very effective in improving clinical symptoms led to consideration of thrombotic thrombocytopenic purpura (TTP). There are many case reports on patients with TTP-like disease manifestations in sickle cell crisis, documenting the effectiveness of plasma exchange in patients with multiorgan failure. The cases are characterized by severe thrombocytopenia, which is not a feature of usual sickle cell crisis, and evidence of hemolysis. When measured, there was no evidence of decreased ADAMTS13 activity, suggesting a different mechanism of disturbance of the platelet-endothelial interactions. Likewise, peripheral blood findings of schistocytes and spherocytes are more subtle than in typical TTP. A small case series of critically ill patients with multiorgan failure and sickle cell vaso-occlusive episodes showed similar favorable response to plasma exchange, suggesting that, at least in a subset of patients, factors other than sickling may contribute to the severity of clinical symptoms.

Coagulopathy Associated with Cirrhosis

Nancy Rosenthal

Patient A 49-year-old male admitted for liver transplantation due to end-stage liver disease.

Clinical History The patient has cirrhosis due to a variety of underlying causes including α-1-antitrypsin deficiency, alcoholism, and hepatitis C. He has had several episodes of gastrointestinal bleeding in the past due to esophageal varices, which have been banded. He has also had several episodes of spontaneous bacterial peritonitis.

Family History Unremarkable.

Medications Furosemide, lactulose, spironolactone, cholestyramine, ferrous sulfate.

Physical Examination Patient appeared older than his stated age with severe jaundice and numerous spider angiomas. His abdomen was grossly distended with a marked fluid wave. Further examination of the abdomen was precluded by the ascites. 1+ pedal edema was present.

Initial Work-Up

PT (sec)	36	(normal 9-12)
INR	4.1	(normal 0.9-1.1)
PTT (sec)	64	(normal 23-31)
Fibrinogen (mg/dL)	145	(normal 180-350)
Platelet Count (×10^3/μL)	70	(normal 150-400)

Differential Diagnosis This case is rather straightforward, but the differential diagnosis of a patient with a prolonged PT and PTT would include heparin contamination, a dysfibrinogenemia, vitamin K deficiency which may be due to warfarin or superwarfarin poisoning, disseminated intravascular coagulation, multiple factor deficiencies and a lupus anticoagulant which on rare occasions may prolong both the PT and the PTT.

Additional Work-Up

Total protein (g/dL)	5.4	(normal 6-8)
Albumin (g/dL)	2.1	(normal 3.4-4.8)
Total bilirubin (mg/dL)	7.4	(normal 0.2-1.0)
Alanine aminotransferase U/L	56	(normal 0-35)
Aspartate aminotransferase (U/L)	107	(normal 0-37)
GGT (U/L)	32	(normal 8-61)
Alkaline phosphatase (U/L)	112	(normal 40-129)

These findings are consistent with the patients liver disease. No further coagulation studies were done on this patient.

Final Diagnosis Coagulopathy due to cirrhosis.

Management Approach In patients with liver disease who are actively bleeding, treatment is often aimed at correcting the underlying lesions which are causing the bleeding such as banding esophageal varices, as was done in this patient. Therapeutic agents for a bleeding patient include vitamin K, if a deficiency is suspected, platelet transfusions, plasma replacement and cryoprecipitate. The volume expansion that these preparations provide should be taken into account in patients with vascular compromise. The use of recombinant activated factor VIIa has been suggested as it can provide a thrombin burst and jump-start the coagulation cascade; however, this use is controversial and a recent randomized controlled trial did not show benefit in patients with esophageal varices. In this case the treatment was an orthotopic liver transplant which was successful and led to the normalization of his coagulation studies soon after surgery.

General Discussion Chronic liver disease is associated with defects that affect all aspects of hemostasis including platelets, coagulation factors, and fibrinolysis. As many of the proteins in the coagulation cascade are made in the liver, severe hepatic dysfunction has long been associated with a hemorrhagic diathesis. Patients with severe liver disease often have impaired production of the coagulation factors with the exception of factor VIII, which is typically increased. The presence of a concomitant decrease in natural anticoagulants such as protein C, protein S, and antithrombin may balance out the bleeding tendency caused by the decrease in the factors of the coagulation cascade. Platelets are often decreased due to hypersplenism. In addition, platelet function defects have been proposed due to endothelial dysfunction leading to increased levels of nitric oxide and prostacyclin which impair platelet attachment. These defects may be balanced by increased levels of von Willebrand factor which aid in platelet adhesion to the subendothelium. However it has been shown that thrombin generation in patients with liver disease is similar to normal controls if the platelet count does not fall below $56 \times 10^3/\mu L$. Decreased levels of both activators and inhibitors of fibrinolysis including plasminogen, α-1 antiplasmin, factor XIII and thrombin-activatable fibrinolysis inhibitor (TAFI) have been found in patients with cirrhosis; the latter may be associated with hyperfibrinolysis. But again the interplay between the positive and negative controls of fibrinolysis are not well understood. It is unclear whether fibrinolysis is increased in patients with cirrhosis. The degree to which the typical coagulation studies correlate with a bleeding diathesis has been brought into question recently. The decrease in coagulation factors leads to a prolongation of first the prothrombin time (PT) and then the partial thromboplastin time. These tests are not affected by the decreased in the natural anticoagulants and may not accurately predict the bleeding tendency in these patients. PT, and specifically in INR, is also used as a screening test to determine the severity of liver disease as part of the work-up for possible liver transplant. The PT-INR is included as part of the model end-stage liver disease (MELD) score. Again, the conventional wisdom of using an INR that was validated based on patients receiving anticoagulation has not been deemed useful by some authors. Re-evaluation of the INR based on patients with liver disease, the so-called INRliver, validated in patients with liver disease has been called for to decrease the variation in results from center to center as in the PT-INR. It is also unclear to what extent prolonged PT-INRs need to be corrected in a patient with liver disease prior to an invasive procedure such as a liver biopsy. Most clinicians will give prophylactic replacement therapy when the INR is greater that 1.5, despite the fact that this test may not be a good predictor of bleeding. Finally, it should be remembered that the bleeding tendency in patients with liver disease may be compounded by other medical problems common in these patients. Renal insufficiency with uremia may cause platelet dysfunction and bacterial infections such as spontaneous bacterial peritonitis may cause endotoxin release which triggers the coagulation cascade. Fluid and pressure imbalances caused by portal hypertension leading to esophageal varices may also lead to increased bleeding in these patients.

Plasminogen Deficiency, Type 1

Craig M Kessler

Patient A 28-year-old Japanese female with a swollen and painful left leg.

Clinical History She had presented 4 weeks earlier with a fracture of her left lower extremity and had been placed in a knee-high plaster cast for immobilization. The leg was now swollen and painful. She had no pleuritic pain, dyspnea, palpitations, or hemoptysis, and her arterial blood gases were completely normal. Duplex Doppler ultrasound was positive for a left lower extremity deep venous thrombosis extending from the mid-superficial femoral vein to the mid-peroneal vein. Of note is the fact that she had been on estrogen-containing oral contraceptives for 4 years and had a family medical history of a remote venous thromboembolism in her maternal grandmother. She was discharged on a therapeutic dose of a low molecular weight heparin preparation and bridged to warfarin therapy as an outpatient. She did well until 1 year later, when she developed symptoms of pain and swelling in her right lower extremity reminiscent of the DVT she had experienced previously. Duplex Doppler ultrasound confirmed the presence of right lower extremity DVT.

Family History Her family was asymptomatic for any arterial or thrombotic complications except for a sister with low plasma plasminogen level and heterozygosity for the factor V Leiden gene mutation, discovered after a spontaneous miscarriage and accompanying proximal DVT of the right lower extremity.

Medications Oral estrogen-containing contraceptive pills and warfarin.

Physical Examination Her physical examination revealed evidence of local right lower extremity tenderness, warmth, and erythema, left lower extremity swelling with prominent venous vasculature dilatation and cyanotic discoloration (consistent with post thrombotic syndrome). Gingival hyperplasia and a right "sticky" eye with crusting around the lid margin and a "fleshy" mass under the upper eye lid, encroaching on the cornea was noted. This was consistent with the diagnosis of ligneous conjunctivitis.

Initial Work-Up Laboratory data in the emergency department revealed a significantly increased titer of D-dimers. CBC and complete metabolic panel results were within normal limits.

Differential Diagnosis Diagnostic considerations based on clinical presentation and family history included thrombophilia with factor V Leiden gene mutation and plasminogen deficiency.

Additional Work-Up Hypercoagulability evaluation after completing 3 months of oral anticoagulation for this provoked VTE was remarkable for the concurrent presence of the heterozygous factor V Leiden polymorphism by PCR; plasma plasminogen activity level of 15% of normal with plasminogen antigen level of 21%.

Final Diagnosis Plasminogen deficiency, Type 1, factor V Leiden gene mutation, and ligneous conjunctivitis.

Management Approach Treatment of plasminogen deficiency can be accomplished by administering exogenous sources of plasminogen to replace the deficient zymogen or by the enhancement of plasminogen levels by preventing its natural degradation in vivo or by stimulating the release of endogenous plasminogen from storage sites. The former strategy involves the IV transfusion of fresh frozen plasma or commercial concentrates of lys-plasminogen (not available in the US). The latter strategy employs oral estrogen contraceptives or androgen analogs, eg, stanazol, etc. Local surgical extirpation of pseudomembranes or topical medications, eg, plasminogen eye drops, FFP, etc, to promote local lysis of those membranes may also be tried. Systemic or topical heparin or oral warfarin therapy has limited usefulness although those with hypercoagulability complications will certainly benefit from acute and chronic anticoagulation regimens. This patient was placed on lifelong anticoagulant therapy and was prescribed with plasminogen eye drops.

General Discussion Plasminogen is the pivotal zymogen in the fibrinolytic pathway. It is synthesized predominantly in the liver and circulates in the plasma as a Glu or Lys isoform. Plasminogen can be proteolytically cleaved to form plasmin by tissue plasminogen activator (t-PA), synthesized and released from endothelial cells lining normal blood vessels, or by urokinase type-plasminogen activator (u-PA), synthesized in and secreted from monocytes/macrophages or from glomerular and renal tubular epithelial cells. It is believed that the bulk of plasmin generated for fibrinolysis is derived from fibrin-bound plasminogen activated by t-PA, which has very high fibrin binding affinity. Lys-plasminogen is more susceptible than the Glu isoform to t-PA cleavage. Once formed, plasmin functions as a critical serine protease to dissolve fibrin into D-dimer degradation fragments (fibrinolysis). Plasmin also lyses factor VIII and von Willebrand factor protein, which downregulates thrombin formation and impedes overall coagulation; and degrades matrix metalloproteinases and fibronectin to interfere with the wound healing process. Systemic fibrinolysis is broadly modulated by complex formation of plasminogen activator inhibitors (PAI-1 and 2) with t-PA and u-PA and by specific α-2-antiplasmin inhibition of circulating free, non-fibrin bound plasmin. α-1-macroglobulin "scavenges" residual circulating plasmin to reinforce the inhibition of fibrinolysis. Thus, intuitively, plasminogen/plasmin deficiency, whether inherited or acquired, should be associated with a hypercoagulable state and the unregulated and excessive accumulation of fibrin. However, the older studies of etiological association of hypoplasminogenemia (both type I and type II) with hypercoagulabilty have been questioned by relatively newer studies. The 36th College of American Pathologists Consensus Conference (2001) has recommended against the inclusion of plasminogen activity or antigen measurements in thrombophilia evaluations. The development of so-called fibrin-rich pseudomembranes is a unique clinical complication of hypoplasminogenemia, noted in over 80% of affected individuals. This phenomenon likely results from the disordered wound healing arising secondary to plasmin deficiency and the overgrowth of fibrinous granulation tissue and predominantly occurs on mucous membranes. Ligneous conjunctivitis represents the prototypical example of hypoplasminogenemia. It appears to be triggered by chronic infection, trauma, or surgery; involves the upper eyelid more than the lower lid; may cause corneal damage and blindness; and is observed almost exclusively in type I quantitative plasminogen deficiency states. Thus, our clinical case example of type II qualitative plasminogen deficiency did not experience similar clinical signs or symptoms. From the etiological perspective, a homozygous plasminogen knock-out mouse model has been reported to develop ligneous conjunctivitis, which is indistinguishable from the human histology. The pivotal role of plasminogen/plasmin was also corroborated by studies that described the development of ligneous conjunctivitis in an individual treated with the antifibrinolytic agent tranexamic acid, which impedes plasmin generation by interfering with t-PA proteolysis of plasminogen. The pseudomembrane resolved with the withdrawal of tranexamic acid and recurred with rechallenge. Ligneous pseudomembranes can also form on gingival surfaces, skin, upper respiratory tract and larynx, genitourinary tract, and in the brain in plasminogen deficient patients and can lead to dramatic complications, such as infertility, hydrocephalus, and loss of teeth. The laboratory diagnosis of plasminogen deficiency is very straightforward. Plasminogen is measured by functional assays, based on plasmin proteolysis of chromogenic substrates, or by immunological assays, which quantitate antigen levels in ELISA assays. Commercial assay kits are widely available for both. Activity assays are most helpful from a clinical perspective, whereas the antigen level is reserved primarily to classify the deficiency state as type I (hypoplasminogenemia) or type II (dysplasminogenemia). Plasminogen activity is increased in association with the use of estrogen containing medications and hyperlipidemic states and is decreased by end-stage liver disease and DIC.

Congenital Dysfibrinogenemia

Nancy S Rosenthal, Adam M Bell

Patient A 6-year-old girl for preoperative evaluation prior to tonsillectomy and adenoidectomy.

Clinical History No history of bleeding or thrombosis.

Family History The patient's mother and a maternal aunt both experienced bleeding requiring transfusion during childbirth. The patient's father and a younger brother are healthy without history of bleeding or thrombosis.

Medications None.

Physical Examination Unremarkable.

Initial Work-Up

CBC	All values within normal limits	
Liver function tests	All values within normal limits	
PTT (sec)	36	(normal 23-30)
PT (sec)	24	(normal 9-12)
INR	2.5	(normal 0.9-1.1)
1:1 mixing study (PTT)	Corrected	
1:1 mixing study (PT)	Corrected	
TT (sec)	56	(normal 16-19)

Differential Diagnosis Prolongation of both the prothrombin time (PT) and activated partial thromboplastin time (PTT) suggests an abnormality within the common pathway. Full correction of both PT and aPTT with 1:1 mixing studies, as in this case, excludes a factor inhibitor. The differential diagnosis of prolonged PT and aPTT with correction includes dilutional coagulopathy, drugs (warfarin), liver disease, vitamin K deficiency, disseminated intravascular coagulation (DIC), factor deficiency (II, V, X), fibrinogen deficiency, and dysfibrinogenemia. As there is no evidence of recent bleeding and transfusion, a dilutional coagulopathy is not a concern. In addition, there is no history of warfarin therapy or evidence of liver disease. Vitamin K deficiency sufficient to cause prolonged PT and aPTT is unusual, and is confirmed by low levels of the vitamin K-dependent clotting factors (II, VII, IX, X). Disseminated intravascular coagulation (DIC), most commonly caused by a severe underlying illness, is characterized by elevated fibrin degradation products and D-dimers with thrombocytopenia. The thrombin time (TT) is a direct measure of the fibrinogen conversion to fibrin, and its prolongation is seen most frequently in cases of exposure to heparin or direct thrombin inhibitors, DIC, and qualitative or quantitative abnormalities of fibrinogen. Again, there is no history of anticoagulation therapy, excluding drug exposure as a possible diagnosis. Given the lack of significant history the likely diagnosis is a dysfibrinogenemia; however, vitamin K deficiency and common pathway factor deficiencies should be excluded.

Section L: Miscellaneous Hemostasis Disorders
Congenital Dysfibrinogenemia

Additional Work-Up

TT 1:1 mix	Corrected	
FDP (µg/mL)	<10	(normal <10)
D-dimer (µg/mL)	<0.50	(normal <0.50)
Factor VII activity level (%)	120	(normal >50)
Factor IX activity level (%)	105	(normal >50)
Factor X activity level (%)	100	(normal >50)
Reptilase time (sec)	49	(normal 13-15)
Fibrinogen level (mg/dL)	304	(normal 180-350)
Fibrinogen activity (mg/dL)	105	(normal 200-420)

The full correction of the TT, as well as normal platelet count and levels of FDP and D-dimer, combined with no apparent underlying cause makes DIC very unlikely. Severe vitamin K deficiency is excluded on the basis of normal levels of the vitamin K-dependent clotting factors. The reptilase time is used as a specific test for abnormalities of fibrinogen, and it is prolonged in this case. Fibrinogen abnormalities can be either congenital or acquired. Most cases of acquired fibrinogen deficiency are due to liver or biliary tract disease, which are excluded by history and normal liver function testing. The normal fibrinogen level with decreased activity is consistent with a qualitative deficiency of fibrinogen. The overall laboratory findings, in conjunction with the family history of bleeding, strongly support a diagnosis of congenital dysfibrinogenemia.

Diagnosis Congenital dysfibrinogenemia.

Management Medical treatment is often not necessary as most patients are asymptomatic. Bleeding complications may be managed by fibrinogen replacement with fresh frozen plasma or cryoprecipitate. Continuous anticoagulation with warfarin is recommended in patients with thrombotic complications. Thrombophilic patients may also require preoperative plasmapheresis with replacement of fresh frozen plasma to remove the abnormal fibrinogen and restore normal fibrinogen temporarily before surgical intervention. In this patient, tonsillectomy was performed without bleeding complications. Cryoprecipitate was available during surgery, and would have been the treatment of choice in the event of significant hemorrhage.

Discussion Congenital dysfibrinogenemia is an uncommon disorder characterized by an abnormal fibrinogen resulting in impaired cleavage into fibrin as the final step in the coagulation cascade. This abnormality results in prolongation of PT and PTT, due to disruption within the common pathway, and prolongation of TT as a direct measure of fibrinogen conversion to fibrin. Dysfibrinogenemia may manifest clinically with bleeding or thrombosis, though a significant proportion of patients are asymptomatic. The TT is also prolonged by heparin; therefore, the reptilase time is used as a more specific test for abnormalities of fibrinogen, as reptilase is not inhibited by heparin. The fibrinogen activity:antigen ratio is important for distinction between dysfunction due to quantitative (ratio approximates 1:1) and qualitative (ratio decreased) causes. Fibrinogen gene sequencing may be used to identify a specific mutation, though molecular testing was not performed in this case. Congenital dysfibrinogenemia is usually inherited as a dominant trait, and the most common mechanism is a missense mutation in any of the 3 fibrinogen genes, Aα (FGA), Bβ (FGB) or γ (FGG). Point mutations at 2 specific gene locations account for almost half of all dysfibrinogenemia cases; residue FGA Arg35 (Arg16) in the Aα chain, and residue FGG Arg301 (Arg275) in the γ chain. Certain mutations, specifically a single amino acid substitution at position 275 of the fibrinogen γ-chain, have been associated with increased incidence of thrombosis. Inheritance of an independent risk factor for hypercoagulability, most commonly a factor V Leiden mutation, also significantly increases the likelihood of developing a blood clot. Therefore, while thrombosis is relatively uncommon in cases of dysfibrinogenemia, molecular testing for specific fibrinogen gene mutations as well as other common causes of thrombophilia may be useful to identify the subset of patients at increased risk for a thromboembolic event.

Ischemic Stroke, Secondary to Atherosclerosis From Elevated Lp(a) Levels

Roy E Smith and Joseph Law

Patient A 29-year-old morbidly obese Caucasian male with right-sided weakness and aphasia.

Clinical History On the morning of admission, the patient's wife heard him fall while in the shower and discovered that he was unable to move his right side and could not speak. An emergent noncontrast CT scan demonstrated early ischemic changes in the left middle cerebral artery (MCA) territory. He was given intravenous tissue plasminogen activator (TPA) in the emergency department and rapidly transferred to a larger facility for specialized care. The patient had no significant past medical history, was never a smoker, and did not use illicit drugs.

Family History No family history of early strokes or clotting disorders.

Medications None on admission.

Physical Examination Blood pressure was 147/78, pulse rate was 78 beats/min, pupils were symmetric and reactive to light bilaterally. Heart and lung examinations were unremarkable. Abdomen was obese and there were no masses or organomegaly. He had no clubbing, cyanosis or edema of his extremities. He was obtunded, aphasic, had a leftward deviation of gaze, and intermittently followed commands. A right hemiparesis was present. He had no spontaneous movement, minimal withdrawal to noxious stimuli, and a positive Babinki response in his right lower extremity. Muscle strength and movement in his left extremities remained intact.

Initial Work-Up An MRI of the brain demonstrated infarction in the left anterior cerebral artery (ACA) and MCA distributions with a marked mass effect and a thrombus in the left internal carotid artery and carotid terminus.
- HGB was 14.1g/dL, HCT 40.4 %, WBC count $10.7 \times 10^3/\mu L$, and platelets $235 \times 10^3/\mu L$
- PT was 12.9 sec (normal 11.6-14.3), INR 1.0 (normal 0.9-1.1), PTT 26.6 sec (normal 22.7-35.6) LDL-cholesterol was elevated at 138 mg/dL (normal <129)

Differential Diagnosis Ischemic stroke secondary to hypercoagulable state, thromboembolism, or atherosclerotic disease.

Additional Work-Up Lipoprotein(a) (Lp(a)) was found to be >225 nmol/L (normal <75). Tissue thromboplastin inhibition tests (TTI) were 1.5 and 1.6 (normal 0.7-1.3) at 1:50 and 1:500 dilutions, respectively. He was found to be homozygous for the methylenetetrahydrofolate reductase (MTHFR) A1298C gene variant. Total homocysteine was normal at 11.4 µmol/L (normal 5.5-13.8).

Normal protein C activity, protein S activity, factor V mutation, ATIII kinetics, hexagonal lipid neutralization, dilute Russel viper venom time (dRVVT), B2 glycoprotein IgG, IgM, IgA, anticardiolipin IgA, activated protein C resistance, platelet glycoprotein IIIa PLA1/A2 polymorphism. A transesophageal echocardiogram demonstrated a small right-to-left shunt consistent with a patent foramen ovale (PFO), with no evidence of a cardiac thrombus. A venous duplex of the lower extremities showed no evidence of DVT. A Doppler analysis of the carotid arteries revealed minimal atherosclerotic disease at the carotid bifurcations, but was otherwise normal.

Final Diagnosis Ischemic stroke, likely secondary to atherosclerosis from elevated Lp(a) levels.

Section L: Miscellaneous Hemostasis Disorders
Ischemic Stroke, Secondary to Atherosclerosis From Elevated Lp(a) Levels

Management Approach Thrombolytic therapy should be considered in patients suffering from an acute ischemic stroke. Inclusion criteria for intravenous thrombolysis include the diagnosis of ischemic stroke causing neurological deficit with symptom onset <3.0 hours prior to treatment. For patients with stroke onset >3 hours but <4.5 hours, intravenous thrombolysis is relatively contraindicated. When onset is >4.5 hours intravenous thrombolysis is not indicated. If the exact time of the onset of stroke is unknown, it is assumed to be the last time that the patient was known to be normal. There are numerous exclusion criteria for thrombolytic therapy. Other recommended therapies include antithrombotic medications started within 48 hours of stroke onset, DVT and PE prophylaxis, antithrombotic therapy at discharge, lipid lowering therapy, blood pressure reduction after the acute phase of ischemic stroke, and smoking cessation. Pharmacologic therapy for elevated Lp(a) levels is directed toward lowering LDL levels to target levels based on risk factors. If the LDL concentration cannot be reduced to the patient's target level, medications that specifically lower Lp(a) may be initiated. Extended-release nicotinic acid (2 g-4 g/day) ± omega-3-ethyl esters (4 g/day) is the most effective therapy for reducing Lp(a) levels. It has the additional benefit of raising HDL levels and reducing levels of LDL cholesterol, apo B-100, and triglycerides. Other therapies include (1) the fibric acid derivative bezafibrate, currently not approved for use in the United States, which can lower Lp(a) levels by up to 39%; (2) estrogen replacement therapy, which can reduce Lp(a) levels by up to 50%, although its clinical role is uncertain; and (3) neomycin, which can lower Lp(a) by as much as 24% but has numerous side effects. Statins, bile acid sequestrates, and most fibric acid derivatives do not lower Lp(a) levels. Furthermore, lifestyle modifications, such as aerobic exercise and changes in diet, generally do not significantly lower Lp(a) levels. Although treatment exists for lowering Lp(a) levels in patients, clinical trials have not yet evaluated their efficacy in preventing coronary heart disease, ischemic stroke, or venous thrombosis. Our patient was treated with thrombolytic therapy at an outside hospital. After being transferred to our facility, he underwent a left frontotemporoparietal hemicraniectomy with duraplasty for impending uncal herniation. The patient had a long hospital course complicated by respiratory failure, requiring mechanical ventilation. He was started on atorvastatin for elevated LDL levels, aspirin, and heparin. After additional work-up revealed an elevated Lp(a) level, he was started on nicotinic acid 500 mg/day, which was eventually increased to 2 g/day. Within 3 months his markedly elevated Lp(a) fell to normal levels (<75 nmol/L).

General Discussion Due to the patient's age, the cause of his ischemic stroke was initially thought to have been due to either a cardioembolic event or a hypercoagulable state. Although an echocardiogram demonstrated a small right-to-left shunt, there was no evidence of a cardiac thrombus. Initial testing showed weak evidence for a lupus anticoagulant with slightly elevated TTI values, though subsequent testing did not support the diagnosis of a hypercoagulable state. Because both a cardioembolic event and a hypercoagulable state had been ruled out, we concluded that the patient's markedly elevated Lp(a) level was the most likely underlying cause for the patient's stroke. Lp(a) has been reported to be an acute phase reactant and can be elevated after a stroke, but this patient's Lp(a) level was measured around 2 months after the event. Lp(a) is a low-density lipoprotein in which apolipoprotein B-100 is covalently bound to apoprotein(a) by a disulfide bridge. One domain of the apo(a) chain is homologous with the fibrin-binding domain of plasminogen. Lp(a) levels are genetically determined and vary between racial groups. Lp(a) levels are normally distributed in African-American populations and skewed toward lower levels in Caucasian, eastern Asian, and Asian Indian populations. African Americans tend to have higher levels than Caucasians. Elevated Lp(a) levels have been associated with cardiovascular and cerebrovascular disease and perhaps venous thrombosis. A 2009 meta-analysis of over 126,000 patient records found a continuous association between Lp(a) levels and coronary heart disease risk. The risk ratio for coronary heart disease, adjusted for age, sex, and conventional risk factors, was 1.13 (95% CI, 1.09-1.18) per 3.5-fold higher usual Lp(a) concentration. The same study also found an adjusted risk ratio of 1.10 (95% CI, 1.02-1.18) for ischemic stroke. Another meta-analysis of over 56,000 patients also found that elevated Lp(a) was a risk factor for stroke. The association of elevated Lp(a) levels with venous thrombosis remains in dispute. Several mechanisms have been proposed to explain the association between elevated Lp(a) and vascular disease:
(1) Because of structural similarity between apoprotein(a) and plasminogen, Lp(a) may compete with and inhibit the thrombolytic activity of tissue plasminogen.
(2) Studies have suggested that Lp(a) has a role in the initiation, progression, and rupture of atherosclerotic plaque.
(3) Lp(a) has been associated with endothelial dysfunction.
(4) Lp(a) activates monocytes, colocalizes with plaque macrophages, stimulates smooth-muscle cells, and may induce inflammation.

CYP2C9 Genotyping for Management of Coumadin Therapy

Domnita Crisan, Wendy Wiesend

Patient A 67-year-old male with acute myocardial infarction.

Clinical History Significant for hyperlipidemia.

Family History Noncontributory.

Medications Patient's only medication prior to admission was atorvastatin. Patient was started on IV heparin and clopidogrel in the hospital, and was subsequently started on coumadin therapy.

Physical Examination Unremarkable.

Initial Work-Up When started on coumadin therapy (5 mg/day), patient had a baseline INR of 1.2. He reached a therapeutic INR of 2.6 after 3 days of therapy. On the 4th day of treatment, the INR reached a supratherapeutic level of 8.1, and coumadin therapy was stopped. INR values decreased to a normal level with discontinuation of treatment. coumadin therapy was again restarted, and the INR increased to 3.5 after a single dose.

Differential Diagnosis Differential diagnosis of supratherapeutic INR levels following coumadin therapy is broad and includes (but not limited to) drug interactions, liver disease, vitamin K deficiency, malabsorption, diarrhea, fever, heart failure, lab error (falsely elevated INR), and genetic susceptibility. The main differential diagnoses in our patient, due to the recurrent supratherapeutic INR, included drug interaction (atorvastatin, an HMG-CoA reductase inhibitor, may inhibit coumadin metabolism) and genetic susceptibility for coumadin hyperresponsiveness.

Additional Work-Up Due to suspected diagnosis of genetic risk for coumadin hyperresponsiveness, CYP2C9 genotyping was ordered. DNA from the patient's peripheral blood sample was extracted, followed by PCR-based amplification of the CYP2C9 gene, allele-specific restriction digestion, and agarose gel electrophoresis. The wild-type allele of the CYP2C9

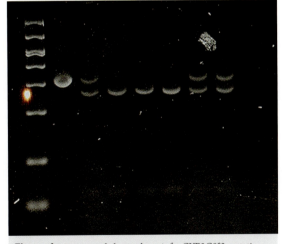

Figure 1 Agarose gel electrophoresis for CYP2C9*2 mutation and CYP2C9*3 mutation.

gene is designated CYP2C9*1. 2 variant alleles, *2 and *3 have been reported to be associated with decreased enzymatic activities. The patients genotype was determined to be CYP2C9*1/*2 (**Figure 1**).

Final Diagnosis Genetic hyperresponsiveness to coumadin therapy due to CYP2C9 mutation (CYP2C9 genotype *1/*2).

Management Approach Patients found to have mutations in their CYP2C9 genes have increased responsiveness to standard coumadin doses. Web-based resources to help clinicians initiate coumadin dosing for patients based on genotype and clinical factors are now available. The individualized initial coumadin dosing strategy for this patient was determined to be 4.2 mg/day (lower than standard dose of 5 mg/day) using the algorithm at www.warfarindosing.org.

General Discussion Coumadin is the most commonly prescribed anticoagulant, with well-established efficacy in prevention and therapy of thrombosis. Bleeding complications are seen at significant rates, making coumadin second, behind digoxin, in adverse drug events. Coumadin has a narrow therapeutic window, and often wide, unpredictable therapeutic dose. Due to the risks in coumadin therapy, the FDA issued a black box warning on the coumadin label in October 2006, to highlight the serious bleeding risks and importance for regular therapeutic INR monitoring. Coumadin metabolism is under genetic control. The drug is metabolized in the liver into inactive metabolites by the cytochrome P450 system (mainly the CYP2C9 enzyme). Several polymorphisms have been identified in the CYP2C9 gene, which are associated with decreased enzyme activity. The wild-type form of the allele is designated CYP2C9*1. Point mutations in the CYP2C9 gene generate variant alleles. The most common variants include the CYP2C9*2 and CYP2C9*3 alleles. The CYP2C9*2 and CYP2C9*3 alleles have been reported to be associated with decreased enzymatic activities (12% and 5% of wild-type activity respectively). Carriers of these mutant alleles require lower coumadin doses to achieve therapeutic effect, and are at increased risk for adverse bleeding events. CYP2C9 mutations can be identified using genotyping methods. In August 2007, the FDA approved updated labeling for coumadin to highlight the importance of genetic testing and to encourage physicians to use the data in initial dosing of patients to decrease adverse drug events. Multiple studies are underway to reveal the clinical utility of CYP2C9 genotyping, suggest initial coumadin doses depending on genotype, and to develop personalized coumadin dosing strategies.

Self-Study Case 1 with Questions

Discussion on page 468

Patient A 16-year-old Cambodian boy with fever, abdominal pain, nausea, vomiting, headache and sore throat of several days duration.

Clinical History The family came to the United States about 2 months before the onset of the present illness. The patient never had a similar episode in the past. He had no history of malarial infection and no history of anemia or blood transfusion.

Family History Mother is known to have "mental problems," the exact nature of which is unknown. A sister and a brother have no medical problems.

Medications None.

Physical Examination Very lethargic but arousable. Temperature was 101°F, pulse 120/min and regular, respiratory rate 30/min, blood pressure 120/80 mmHg, weight 41.2 kg, and height 165 cm. Sclerae were icteric. He had dry mucus membranes. His lungs were clear. His heart exam included a grade IV/VI systolic ejection murmur over entire precordium. His liver edge was just palpable below the costal margin and his spleen was markedly enlarged to about 5 cm in left midcostal line. He had no lymphadenopathy.

Initial Work-Up

CBC

WBC (×10³/μL)	15.6
RBC (×10⁶/μL)	4.22
HGB (g/dL)	7.7
HCT (%)	24.9
MCV (fL)	59
MCH (pg)	18.2
MCHC (g/dL)	30.9
PLT (×10³/μL)	425
RDW-CV (%)	17.9

WBC Differential	%	# (×10³/μL)
Neutrophils	74	11.5
Bands	5	0.8
Lymphocytes	10	1.6
Monocytes	11	1.7
Eosinophils	0	
Basophils	0	

Serum ferritin was 550 ng/mL. Total serum bilirubin was 5.3 mg/dL, LDH 380 IU/L, alkaline phosphatase 179 IU/L and the rest of the biochemical profile was unremarkable. Liver enzymes were within normal limits. Hepatitis B surface antigen was negative but Hep B core Ab was positive. Peripheral blood smear revealed anisocytosis, poikilocytosis, occasional polychromasia, microcytic hypochromic red cells, and occasional target cells (**Figure 1**).

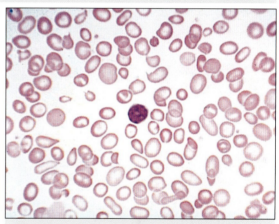

Figure 1 Blood smear (Wright-Giemsa, ×1000) showing anisocytosis, poikilocytosis, microcytic hypochromic red cells and occasional target cells.

Question 1. Given the initial presentation findings, name a minimum of 3 clinical conditions that you will include in the differential diagnosis of this case.

Question 2. What additional work-up will help you arrive at the final diagnosis?

Question 3. What is the most likely diagnosis?

Question 4. Outline the course of management for this patient and/or the condition.

Question 5. Describe the salient features of the case and/or the condition.

Self-Study Case 2 with Questions

Discussion on page 469

Patient A 24-year-old woman in her 4th month of pregnancy with the complaint of nausea.

Clinical History The patient had been unable to maintain a proper diet due to extreme nausea for past several days.

Family History Noncontributory.

Medications Oral ferrous sulfate pills.

Physical Examination Findings consistent with pregnancy of 4 months.

Initial Work-Up		
CBC		
WBC (×10³/µL)	8.4	
RBC (×10⁶/µL)	1.84	
Hgb (g/dL)	8.7	
Hct (%)	27.6	
MCV (fL)	149.6	
MCH (pg)	47.2	
MCHC (g/dL)	31.5	
PLT (×10³/µL)	136	
RDW-CV (%)	31.5	
MPV (fL)	8.8	
WBC Differential	**%**	**# (×10³/µL)**
Neutrophils	71	6.0
Bands	7	0.6
Lymphocytes	13	1.1
Monocytes	7	0.6
Eosinophils	2	0.2
Basophils	0	

*Peripheral blood smear revealed macroovalocytes and hypersegmented neutrophils (**Figure 1**).*

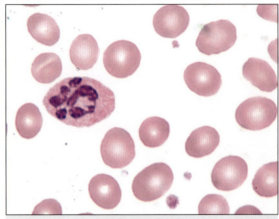

Figure 1 Blood smear (Wright, ×1000) showing macroovalocytes and a hypersegmented neutrophil.

Question 1. Given the initial presentation findings, name a minimum of 2 clinical conditions that you will include in the differential diagnosis of this case.

Question 2. What additional work-up will help you arrive at the final diagnosis?

Question 3. What is the most likely diagnosis?

Question 4. Outline the course of management for this patient and/or the condition.

Question 5. Describe the salient features of the case and/or the condition.

Self-Study Case 3 with Questions

Discussion on page 471

Patient A 2-year-old male child of Mediterranean descent with malaise, irritability, yellowish discoloration of the eyes and brown urine.

Clinical History The mother noticed the discoloration of the eyes and urine 1 day following eating freshly-made red cabbage and fava beans.

Family History An older brother passed away from presumably severe anemia following an acute urinary tract infection for which he was treated with trimethoprim-sulfamethoxazole.

Medications None.

Physical Examination An irritable child who was pale and jaundiced with no hepatosplenomegaly.

Initial Work-Up

CBC	
WBC (×10³/μL)	18.0
RBC (×10⁶/μL)	1.70
HGB (g/dL)	3.9
HCT (%)	11.7
MCV (fL)	72
MCH (pg)	27.0
MCHC (g/dL)	29.0
PLT (×10³/μL)	320
RDW-CV (%)	18.0
MPV (fL)	11.0

WBC Differential	%	# (×10³/μL)
Neutrophils	60	10.8
Bands	10	1.8
Lymphocytes	22	4.0
Monocytes	6	1.1
Eosinophils	2	0.4
Basophils	0	
Reticulocyte count	5.3	

Peripheral blood smear revealed anisocytosis, polychromasia, bite cells and other red cell fragments (schistocytes), and eccentrocytes (red cells with irregularly contracted hemoglobin)/blister cells (**Figure 1**).

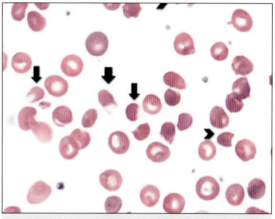

Figure 1 Blood smear (Wright, ×1000) showing red cells with asymmetrically distributed hemoglobin, bite and blister cells following an oxidative challenge.

Question 1. Given the initial presentation findings, name a minimum of 2 clinical conditions that you will include in the differential diagnosis of this case.

Question 2. What additional work-up will help you arrive at the final diagnosis?

Question 3. What is the most likely diagnosis?

Question 4. Outline the course of management for this patient and/or the condition.

Question 5. Describe the salient features of the case and/or the condition.

Self-Study Case 4 with Questions

Discussion on page 473

Patient A 26-year-old African-American man with history of sickle cell disease with severe pain secondary to what the patient claimed to be "typical crisis pain."

Clinical History Pain awoke the patient at 3:00 AM on the day of hospital admission. Pain started in his low back and then radiated to the chest and sternum. The pain was constant and sharp/throbbing in nature in his low back and chest and tight over the sternum. Pain intensity was 10/10 on a scale of 0, no pain, to 10, most severe pain. He also complained of mild dyspnea due to limited inspiration from the pain. He did not recall any triggers or activity that precipitated the pain. No history of fever, chills, cough, nausea, vomiting or headache. Past medical history is significant for frequent painful crises that required hospital admission, the last being about 2 weeks prior. During the previous 8 months, he was treated in the emergency room 11 times, 6 of which required hospital admission. Moreover he was treated in other emergency rooms in the area at least 2 or 3 times. Other past complications included acute chest syndrome, open cholecystectomy, priapism and avascular necrosis of both hip joints. He was transfused occasionally in the past.

Family History Father has sickle cell disease but its exact nature is not known, mother had sickle cell trait and diabetes mellitus type 2. A brother has sickle cell disease of unknown specific type.

Medications Folic acid, hydroxyurea, hydromorphone and extended release morphine.

Physical Examination Vital signs including pulse oximetry on room air were within normal limits. He had poor dentition, tenderness over the low back and a grade II/VI systolic murmur over the precordium.

Initial Work-Up

CBC

WBC ($\times 10^3/\mu L$)	27.2	
RBC ($\times 10^6/\mu L$)	3.18	
HGB (g/dL)	7.6	
HCT (%)	23.2	
MCV (fL)	73	
MCH (pg)	23.8	
MCHC (g/dL)	32.8	
PLT ($\times 10^3/\mu L$)	330	
RDW-CV (%)	16.7	
Reticulocyte count	11.6%	

Hemoglobin electrophoresis results from the time of original diagnosis: hemoglobins S 83.2%, F 11.6%, and A_2 5.2% (confirmed by column microchromatography). Serum ferritin done during a previous admission was 983 ng/mL.

WBC Differential

	%	# ($\times 10^3/\mu L$)
Neutrophils	69	18.7
Bands	5	1.4
Lymphocytes	14	3.8
Monocytes	5	1.4
Metamyelocytes	3	0.8
Myelocytes	4	1.1
Nucleated red cells	23/100 WBC	

Chest X-ray on admission was clear.

Peripheral blood smear showed anisopoikilocytosis with numerous target cells, polychromasia, microcytic and hypochromic red cells, nucleated red cells and occasional Howell-Jolly bodies (**Figure 1**).

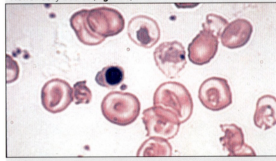

Figure 1 Blood smear (Wright-Giemsa, ×1000) target cells, hypochromic red cells, a Howell-Jolly body and a nucleated red cell.

Question 1. Given the initial presentation findings, name a minimum of 2 clinical conditions that you will include in the differential diagnosis of this case.

Question 2. What additional work-up will help you arrive at the final diagnosis?

Question 3. What is the most likely diagnosis?

Question 4. Outline the course of management for this patient and/or the condition.

Question 5. Describe the salient features of the case and/or the condition.

Self-Study Case 5 with Questions

Discussion on page 474

Patient A 57-year-old woman, who was admitted to a local hospital for altered mental status.

Clinical History The patient's caregivers reported progressive decline in her energy over the prior 3 months and confusion in the prior 2 weeks. The patient had severe anemia (hemoglobin 3 g/dL) and received red blood cell transfusions. Additional abnormalities on the peripheral blood smear (see below) prompted transfer to a tertiary care hospital.

Family History Noncontributory.

Medications Temazepam, zolpidem, amoxicillin, clonazepam.

Physical Examination Vital signs were normal except for a temperature of 99.3°F and the heart rate of 106 beats/minute. The patient was somnolent but arousable with stimulation. She was oriented to self and year but not place. Rest of the examination was unremarkable.

Initial Work-Up

CBC

WBC ($\times 10^3/\mu L$)	20.3
RBC ($\times 10^6/\mu L$)	2.69
HGB (g/dL)	9.3
HCT (%)	25.8
MCV (fL)	96
MCH (pg)	34.6
MCHC (g/dL)	36.0
PLT ($\times 10^3/\mu L$)	123

WBC Differential

	%	# ($\times 10^3/\mu L$)
Neutrophils	9	1.8
Bands	0	
Lymphocytes	13	2.6
Monocytes/promonocytes	55	11.2
Eosinophils	0	
Basophils	0	
Blasts	23	4.7

Peripheral blood smear revealed that blasts and promonocytes (blast equivalents) accounted for 41% of cells.

Question 1. Given the initial presentation findings, name a minimum of 2 clinical conditions that you will include in the differential diagnosis of this case.

Question 2. What additional work-up will help you arrive at the final diagnosis?

Question 3. What is the most likely diagnosis?

Question 4. Outline the course of management for this patient and/or the condition.

Question 5. Describe the salient features of the case and/or the condition.

Section M: Self-Study

Self-Study Case 6 with Questions

Discussion on page 476

Patient A 48-year-old man with lower extremity weakness and low back pain.

Clinical History The patient had no past medical history. He had developed a sore back over the last week or so, which he presumed was due to heavy lifting. On the day he presented, he had also developed weakness in both legs and was having trouble walking. He had not had any fevers or sweats. He had no problems with bowel or bladder control.

Family History Noncontributory.

Medications None, other than acetaminophen as needed for the back pain.

Physical Examination His vital signs were all normal. He had no palpable liver, spleen or lymph nodes. He had tenderness over his lumbar spine and weakness (3+/5) on testing of plantar flexion and dorsiflexion of the ankles, flexion and extension of both knees. He had normal sphincter tone on rectal examination.

Initial Work-Up			
CBC			
WBC (×10³/μL)	8.6		
RBC (×10⁶/μL)	3.8		
HGB (g/dL)	11.1		
HCT (%)	32.0		
MCV (fL)	85.1		
MCH (pg)	29.4		
MCHC (g/dL)	34.6		
PLT (×10³/μL)	178		
RDW-CV (%)	13.1		
MPV (fL)	9.0		
WBC Differential	**%**		**# (×10³/μL)**
Neutrophils	73		6.3
Lymphocytes	20		1.7
Monocytes	6		0.5
Eosinophils	1		0.1
Basophils	0		

Peripheral blood smear did not reveal any morphologic abnormality; no circulating immature myeloid cells were seen. The results of chemistry panel including LDH, uric acid, liver panel and kidney function were normal. Imaging revealed a paraspinal mass (L4, L5, S1), which was biopsied during emergent spinal decompression. Sections of the paraspinal mass were similar and showed a monotonous infiltrate of intermediate-to-large cells with high nuclear-to-cytoplasmic ratio and fine chromatin (**Figures 1- 3**). There was abundant crush artifact.

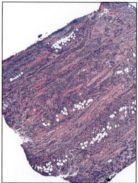

Figure 1 Paraspinal mass biopsy (H&E, ×20) showed an infiltrate of medium to large cells involving the paraspinal skeletal muscle and adipose tissue.

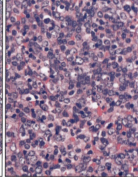

Figure 2 Paraspinal mass biopsy (H&E, ×400) showed an infiltrate of medium to large cells with immature blast-like chromatin.

Question 1. Given the initial presentation findings, name a minimum of 3 clinical conditions that you will include in the differential diagnosis of this case.

Question 2. What additional work-up will help you arrive at the final diagnosis?

Question 3. What is the most likely diagnosis?

Question 4. Outline the course of management for this patient and/or the condition.

Question 5. Describe the salient features of the case and/or the condition.

Self-Study Case 7 with Questions

Discussion on page 477

Patient A 51-year-old female, who presented with fatigue, fever and shortness of breath.

Clinical History The patient was in good health until she developed low-grade fevers, dyspnea on exertion and a left molar infection. Her primary care physician was concerned for the possibility of endocarditis. An echocardiogram was normal; however, a CBC demonstrated an elevated white blood cell count of $65.0 \times 10^3/\mu L$ with blasts seen on the peripheral smear. The patient was admitted to the hospital for further evaluation.

Family History Noncontributory.

Medications None.

Physical Examination She had fever of 100.4°F, mild tachycardia with pulse of 110, and left molar swelling and tenderness. She had no adenopathy, splenomegaly or petechiae.

Initial Work-Up

CBC	
WBC ($\times 10^3/\mu L$)	43.4
RBC ($\times 10^6/\mu L$)	2.70
HGB (g/dL)	9.0
HCT (%)	25.6
MCV (fL)	94.6
MCH (pg)	33.4
MCHC (g/dL)	35.2
PLT ($\times 10^3/\mu L$)	54
RDW-CV (%)	18.2

WBC Differential	%	# ($\times 10^3/\mu L$)
Neutrophils	4	1.7
Bands	0	
Lymphocytes	18	7.8
Monocytes	23	10.0
Eosinophils	1	0.4
Basophils	1	0.4
Blasts	53	23.0

Peripheral blood smear revealed many blasts and an absolute monocytosis (**Figure 1**).

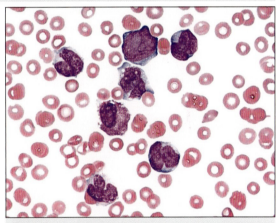

Figure 1 Blood smear (Wright-Giemsa, ×500) showing blasts and promonocytes.

Question 1. Given the initial presentation findings, name a minimum of 2 clinical conditions that you will include in the differential diagnosis of this case.

Question 2. What additional work-up will help you arrive at the final diagnosis?

Question 3. What is the most likely diagnosis?

Question 4. Outline the course of management for this patient and/or the condition.

Question 5. Describe the salient features of the case and/or the condition.

Self-Study Case 8 with Questions

Discussion on page 479

Patient A 72-year-old male with fever, chills and dizziness.

Clinical History The patient had had a low-grade fever and upper respiratory tract infection 2 weeks prior. He had a 58-year history of smoking (1/2 pack a day).

Family History Noncontributory

Medications Azithromycin, guaifenesin, and multivitamin

Physical Examination Other than a general "ill appearance," his exam was unremarkable.

Initial Work-Up

CBC		WBC Differential	%	# (×10³/μL)
WBC (×10³/μL)	27.0	Neutrophils	18	4.9
RBC (×10⁶/μL)	3.83	Bands	3	0.8
HGB (g/dL)	11.0	Lymphocytes	3	0.8
HCT (%)	33.7	Monocytes	3	0.8
MCV (fL)	88	Eosinophils	2	0.5
MCH (pg)	28.7	Basophils	1	0.3
MCHC (g/dL)	32.6	Atypical cells	70	18.9
PLT (×10³/μL)	19			
RDW-CV (%)	15.9			

Peripheral blood smear revealed many large and small atypical cells (**Figure 1**).

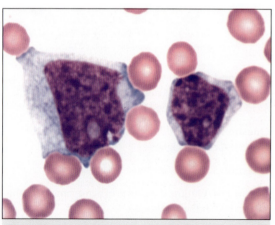

Figure 1 Blood smear (Wright-Giemsa, ×1000) showing large and small atypical cells.

Question 1. Given the initial presentation findings, name a minimum of 2 clinical conditions that you will include in the differential diagnosis of this case.

Question 2. What additional work-up will help you arrive at the final diagnosis?

Question 3. What is the most likely diagnosis?

Question 4. Outline the course of management for this patient and/or the condition.

Question 5. Describe the salient features of the case and/or the condition.

Self-Study Case 9 with Questions

Discussion on page 481

Patient A 65-year-old woman with abdominal pain.

Clinical History The patient also complained of diarrhea and fever of 3 days duration.

Family History Noncontributory.

Medications None.

Physical Examination The patient appeared ill and in moderate distress. He weighed 75 kg. The rest of the physical examination was unremarkable except for a mildly distended abdomen with tenderness to palpation in the lower quadrants and voluntary guarding. Blood pressure was 138/87, pulse 110/min, temperature 98.1°F, respiratory rate 25× min, pulse oximetry on room air 94%.

Initial Work-Up

CBC			
WBC (×10³/μL)	136.0		
RBC (×10⁶/μL)	3.23		
HGB (g/dL)	9.4		
HCT (%)	29.5		
MCV (fL)	91.3		
MCH (pg)	29.1		
MCHC (g/dL)	31.9		
PLT (×10³/μL)	75		
RDW-CV (%)	17.2		
WBC Differential	**%**	**# (×10³/μL)**	
Neutrophils	1	1.4	
Lymphocytes	7	9.5	
Blasts	92	125.1	
LDH (U/L)	613		
AST (U/L)	37		
Alkaline phosphatase (U/L)	40		
Albumin (g/L)	2.2		
Calcium (mg/dL)	5.2		
Total bilirubin (mg/dL)	0.4		
Direct bilirubin (mg/dL)	0.4		
BUN (mg/dL)	17		
Creatinine (mg/dL)	1.2		
PT (sec)	26.6	(normal 12.5-14.3)	
INR	2.4	(normal 0.9-1.1)	
PTT (sec)	42	(normal 23-35)	
Fibrinogen (mg/dL)	263	(normal 165-455)	
D-dimer (μg/mL)	5.51	(normal <0.5)	

Peripheral blood smear review revealed monotonous population of blasts, which were small to medium in size and had round nuclei with fine chromatin, high N:C ratio, and small amount of basophilic cytoplasm (**Figure 1**).

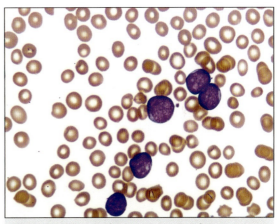

Figure 1 Blood smear (Wright-Giemsa, ×1000) showing several blasts.

Question 1. Given the initial presentation findings, name a minimum of 2 clinical conditions that you will include in the differential diagnosis of this case.

Question 2. What additional work-up will help you arrive at the final diagnosis?

Question 3. What is the most likely diagnosis?

Question 4. Outline the course of management for this patient and/or the condition.

Question 5. Describe the salient features of the case and/or the condition.

Self-Study Case 10 with Questions

Discussion on page 482

Patient A 61-year-old man with easy bruising and occasional night sweats.

Clinical History He has had a biopsy of a right neck basal cell carcinoma with postoperative "oozing," 6 months prior. At that time he was found to have a WBC of $151.9 \times 10^3/\mu L$ comprised mostly of mature neutrophils. A bone marrow biopsy had been performed, with reported findings suggestive of a BCR-ABL1– myeloproliferative neoplasm, and the patient was started on hydroxyurea. The patient presented for further evaluation and treatment 6 months later, with history of easy bruising and occasional night sweats; but no fevers, chills, weight loss, body pains, bone aches, or bleeding.

Family History Brother with lymphoma, father with bladder cancer, mother with recurrent skin lesions/cancers.

Medications Allopurinol, hydroxyurea.

Physical Examination Afebrile, no lymphadenopathy, spleen tip palpated slightly below the costophrenic angle.

Initial Work-Up

CBC	
WBC ($\times 10^3/\mu L$)	51.0
RBC ($\times 10^6/\mu L$)	3.84
HGB (g/dL)	13.6
HCT (%)	39.8
MCV (fL)	100
MCH (pg)	35.4
MCHC (g/dL)	34.2
PLT ($\times 10^3/\mu L$)	115
RDW-CV (%)	16.0

WBC Differential	%	# ($\times 10^3/\mu L$)
Neutrophils	94	47.9
Lymphocytes	4	2.0
Monocytes	1	0.5
Eosinophils	1	0.5

Peripheral blood smear revealed leukocytosis comprised almost entirely of mature neutrophils without toxic changes (**Figure 1**). Only rare immature granulocytes were present (<1%), and no dysplasia or blasts were found. Monocytes, basophils, and eosinophils were not increased. Bone marrow core biopsy was hypercellular (>95%) with granulocyte predominance (**Figure 2**). The bone marrow aspirate smear was comprised predominantly of maturing granulocyte elements with a myeloid/erythroid ratio of 9:1 (**Figure 3**) and minimal left-shift. Blasts were not increased (<5%) and no significant granulocytic or erythroid dysplasia was noted. Rare megakaryocytes were noted with hypolobation or nuclear lobe separation, but a majority of forms were unremarkable. Plasma cells and lymphocytes were not increased.

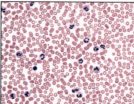

Figure 1 Peripheral blood smear (Wright-Giemsa, ×200) showing elevated WBCs with predominance of mature neutrophils; no blasts present.

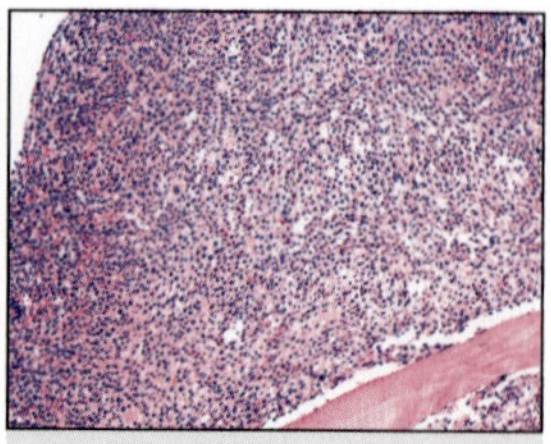

Figure 2 Bone marrow biopsy (H&E, ×100) showing markedly hypercellular marrow.

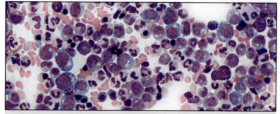

Figure 3 Bone marrow aspirate smear (Wright-Giemsa, ×200) showing granulocytic hyperplasia, with a full maturation spectrum.

Question 1. Given the initial presentation findings, name a minimum of 3 clinical conditions that you will include in the differential diagnosis of this case.

Question 2. What additional work-up will help you arrive at the final diagnosis?

Question 3. What is the most likely diagnosis?

Question 4. Outline the course of management for this patient and/or the condition.

Question 5. Describe the salient features of the case and/or the condition.

Self-Study Case 11 with Questions

Discussion on page 484

Patient A 47-year-old male with persistent peripheral blood eosinophilia.

Clinical History An elevated peripheral blood eosinophil count ($8.5 \times 10^3/\mu L$) was noted on routine CBC with differential performed as part of the routine physical examination at the office of the primary care physician (PCP) approximately 7 months prior. A second CBC with differential performed also at the PCP office at 4 months interval revealed an eosinophil count of $9.9 \times 10^3/\mu L$.

Family History Noncontributory.

Medications The patient was on no medications or over-the-counter supplements.

Physical Examination Unremarkable. No palpable lymphadenopathy or hepatosplenomegaly.

Initial Work-Up

CBC	
WBC ($\times 10^3/\mu L$)	17.4
RBC ($\times 10^6/\mu L$)	4.12
HGB (g/dL)	12.7
HCT (%)	37
MCV (fL)	90
MCH (pg)	31
MCHC (g/dL)	34
PLT ($\times 10^3/\mu L$)	262
RDW-CV (%)	13.8

WBC Differential	%	# ($\times 10^3/\mu L$)
Neutrophils	25	4.4
Bands	2	0.3
Lymphocytes	3	0.5
Monocytes	2	0.3
Eosinophils	67	11.7
Basophils	1	0.2

Peripheral blood smear revealed increased number of morphologically normal eosinophils (**Figure 1**).

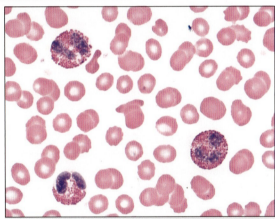

Figure 1 Blood smear (Wright-Giemsa, ×500) showing several eosinophils.

Question 1. Given the initial presentation findings, name a minimum of 4 clinical conditions that you will include in the differential diagnosis of this case.

Question 2. What additional work-up will help you arrive at the final diagnosis?

Question 3. What is the most likely diagnosis?

Question 4. Outline the course of management for this patient and/or the condition.

Question 5. Describe the salient features of the case and/or the condition.

Self-Study Case 12 with Questions

Discussion on page 486

Patient A 3-year-old boy with multiple previous health problems was evaluated for a high white blood cell count and monocytosis.

Clinical History The patient was a full-term baby delivered by spontaneous vaginal delivery. His mother was 43 at the time and on phenytoin due to epilepsy. The patient has had numerous health problems starting around 2 months of age when he was hospitalized due to jaundice and hepatic failure. He was diagnosed with autoimmune hepatitis and was treated with azathioprine. Around 1 year of age he developed hypersplenism with thrombocytopenia which required splenectomy. About that time the patient developed a subdural hematoma, presumed secondary to thrombocytopenia, that required evacuation. In his second year of life, the patient was diagnosed with hyper-IgD syndrome to explain periodic fevers. He also fractured his tibia due to brittle bones and has a history of asthma. The patient remained under the care of his hepatologist and infectious disease specialists. He subsequently was noted to have an elevated white blood cell count and underwent further evaluation.

Family History The patient's mother has epilepsy and was treated with phenytoin during the pregnancy. There are histories of a brain tumor in his maternal grandfather, breast cancer in a maternal aunt and liver cancer in a paternal aunt.

Medications Erythromycin, penicillin, albuterol and azathioprine.

Physical Examination The patient was at the 10th percentile for height, and in the 25-50th percentile range for weight. The exam was notable for a saddle bridge nose, slightly low set ears, a right tympanostomy tube, abdominal scars status post splenectomy and liver biopsy, candidal diaper rash, all digits clubbing, clinodactyly and a café-au-lait spot.

Initial Work-Up

CBC		
WBC (×10³/μL)	50.3	
RBC (×10⁶/μL)	4.23	
HGB (g/dL)	11.8	
HCT (%)	35.7	
MCV (fL)	84	
MCH (pg)	28.0	
MCHC (g/dL)	33.2	
PLT (×10³/μL)	97.0	
RDW-CV (%)	16.9	
MPV (fL)	9.3	
WBC Differential	**%**	**# (×10³/μL)**
Neutrophils+bands	73	36.7
Lymphocytes	9	4.5
Monocytes	12	6.0
Eosinophils	5	2.5
Basophils	0	
Metamyelocytes+myelocytes	1	0.5

Peripheral blood smear demonstrated an absolute monocytosis and dyspoietic changes in the granulocytes (**Figure 1**).

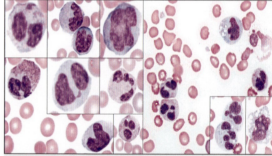

Figure 1 Composites of peripheral blood smear cells from when patient was 12 months and 13.5 months, respectively (Wright-Giemsa, ×1000) showing monocytosis and hypogranular neutrophils.

Question 1. Given the initial presentation findings, name a minimum of 2 clinical conditions that you will include in the differential diagnosis of this case.

Question 2. What additional work-up will help you arrive at the final diagnosis?

Question 3. What is the most likely diagnosis?

Question 4. Outline the course of management for this patient and/or the condition.

Question 5. Describe the salient features of the case and/or the condition.

Self-Study Case 13 with Questions

Discussion on page 487

Patient A 62-year-old male, who was recently diagnosed with chronic lymphocytic leukemia (CLL), came to our institution for a second opinion.

Clinical History The patient's WBC count had risen from $47 \times 10^3/\mu L$ to $72 \times 10^3/\mu L$ with approximately 80% lymphocytes over a period of 4 months. He was told he has chronic lymphocytic leukemia and "no need to worry about it since you're asymptomatic." He had remained asymptomatic all this time and had no symptoms other than mild fatigue at presentation. Past medical history includes sleep apnea, gastroesophageal reflux disease, depression, and an enlarged prostate. He used to smoke a pack per day, but had quit 20 years ago. He drinks on a social basis, and denied recreational drug use. He lives with his wife and works as a machinist.

Family History There is no known history of malignancy in his family.

Medications Desomeprazole, escitalopram.

Physical Examination Unremarkable. In particular, he had no palpable adenopathy or hepatosplenomegaly.

Initial Work-Up

CBC

WBC ($\times 10^3/\mu L$)	94.0
RBC ($\times 10^6/\mu L$)	4.78
HGB (g/dL)	15.5
HCT (%)	47.4
MCV (fL)	99.2
MCH (pg)	32.4
MCHC (g/dL)	32.7
PLT ($\times 10^3/\mu L$)	264
RDW-CV (%)	14.5

WBC Differential	%	# ($\times 10^3/\mu L$)
Neutrophils	3	2.8
Bands	0	
Lymphocytes	94	88.4
Monocytes	0	
Eosinophils	1	0.9
Basophils	0	
Prolymphocytes	2	1.9

Results of routine coagulation studies (PT and PTT) were normal as were those of comprehensive metabolic panel. Peripheral blood smear revealed preponderance of lymphocytes, many of which, though counted in the differential as lymphocytes, had prominent nucleoli, 1 per cell, suggestive of prolymphocytic morphology (**Figure 1**). A few smudge cells were also noted.

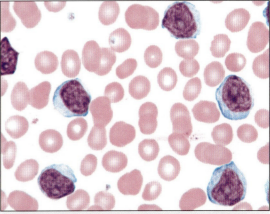

Figure 1 Peripheral blood smear (Wright-Giemsa, ×1000) showing several lymphocytes with prominent mucleoli (1 per cell).

Question 1. Given the initial presentation findings, name a minimum of 3 clinical conditions that you will include in the differential diagnosis of this case.

Question 2. What additional work-up will help you arrive at the final diagnosis?

Question 3. What is the most likely diagnosis?

Question 4. Outline the course of management for this patient and/or the condition.

Question 5. Describe the salient features of the case and/or the condition.

Self-Study Case 14 with Questions

Discussion on page 488

Patient A 45-year-old woman with groin discomfort.

Clinical History The patient was previously healthy and noticed a lima-bean size mass in the right groin 3 months before seeking medical attention. She had fever but no weight loss.

Family History Noncontributory.

Medications None.

Physical Examination Bilateral inguinal lymphadenopathy and fullness in the right pelvic region. No hepatosplenomegaly.

Initial Work-Up		
CBC		
WBC ($\times 10^3/\mu L$)	15.7	
RBC ($\times 10^6/\mu L$)	4.19	
HGB (g/dL)	11.3	
HCT (%)	34.3	
MCV (fL)	82	
MCH (pg)	26.9	
MCHC (g/dL)	32.8	
PLT ($\times 10^3/\mu L$)	255	
RDW-CV (%)	15.8	
WBC Differential	**%**	**# ($\times 10^3/\mu L$)**
Neutrophils	80	12.6
Bands	0	
Lymphocytes	13	2.0
Monocytes	7	1.1
Eosinophils	0	
Basophils	0	

CT scan showed bilateral inguinal lymphadenopathy, and a right pelvic mass (7cm) encroaching on the bladder and involving the anterior abdominal wall musculature. Pelvic ultrasound showed a normal uterus with a mass in the right pelvis encroaching on the uterus. The ovaries were poorly visualized. Pelvic tumor excision with inguinal lymph node biopsy, and hysterectomy were performed. The mass was 6.5cm in greatest dimension and lymph nodes (7) ranged in size from 2.5 cm to 0.6 cm in greatest dimension. Histologic sections of the mass showed a tumor composed of cohesive clusters of large cells (**Figure 1**) associated with extensive necrosis. Tumor was present in para-aortic and inguinal lymph nodes (**Figure 2**) as well as a portion of skin attached to the mass. The uterus and ovaries were normal.

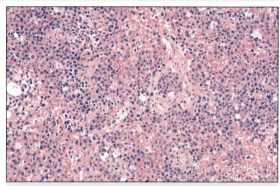

Figure 1 Pelvic mass (H&E, ×100) showing large cells in cohesive clusters.

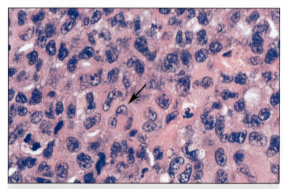

Figure 2 Lymph node (H&E, ×400) showing large cells with an ample amount of cytoplasm and visible nucleoli. The arrow points to a hallmark cell.

Question 1. Given the initial presentation findings, name a minimum of 2 clinical conditions that you will include in the differential diagnosis of this case.

Question 2. What additional work-up will help you arrive at the final diagnosis?

Question 3. What is the most likely diagnosis?

Question 4. Outline the course of management for this patient and/or the condition.

Question 5. Describe the salient features of the case and/or the condition.

Self-Study Case 15 with Questions
Discussion on page 490

Patient A 61-year-old male with a history of "chronic lymphocytic leukemia" (CLL) and an increasing white blood cell count.

Clinical History The patient was diagnosed with "CLL" 8 months prior when he was found to have a WBC of $37 \times 10^3/\mu L$ comprised mostly of small lymphocytes. The phenotype reportedly showed monoclonal B cells with CD5, partial CD23 and equivocal FMC7. The patient was felt to have stable disease, and was not treated until 3 months later when his WBC rose to $51 \times 10^3/\mu L$. He received Rituximab, but with little effect. He was transferred for suspected "transformation" when his count suddenly rose to $283 \times 10^3/\mu L$.

Family History No pertinent family history.

Physical Examination Generalized lymphadenopathy, including cervical and axillary.

Initial Work-Up

CBC

WBC ($\times 10^3/\mu L$)	283.0
RBC ($\times 10^6/\mu L$)	3.02
HGB (g/dL)	9.0
HCT (%)	28.6
MCV (fL)	94.7
MCH (pg)	29.8
MCHC (g/dL)	31.5
PLT ($\times 10^3/\mu L$)	83
RDW-CV (%)	13.9

WBC Differential	%	# ($\times 10^3/\mu L$)
Neutrophils	0	
Bands	0	
Lymphocytes	60	169.8
Monocytes	0	
Eosinophils	0	
Basophils	0	
Others (blastoid)	40	113.2

Peripheral blood smear revealed 60% smaller abnormal lymphoid cells and 40% larger cells with fine chromatin and scant cytoplasm (**Figures 1** and **2**).

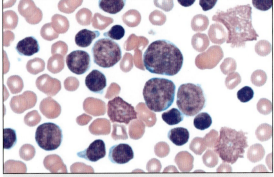

Figure 1 Peripheral blood smear (Wright, ×200) showing marked lymphocytosis.

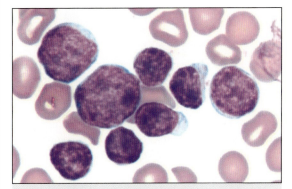

Figure 2 Peripheral blood smear (Wright, ×500) showing a mix of smaller atypical cells and larger blastoid cells.

Question 1. Given the initial presentation findings, name a minimum of 3 clinical conditions that you will include in the differential diagnosis of this case.

Question 2. What additional work-up will help you arrive at the final diagnosis?

Question 3. What is the most likely diagnosis?

Question 4. Outline the course of management for this patient and/or the condition.

Question 5. Describe the salient features of the case and/or the condition.

Section M: Self-Study

Self-Study Case 16 with Questions
Discussion on page 492

Patient A 59-year-old white male, who was noted to be anemic as an incidental finding.

Clinical History The patient has a history of osteoarthritis of the neck and hips and had received bilateral hip replacements in the recent past.

Family History Noncontributory.

Medications Meloxicam (nonsteroidal anti-inflammatory agent).

Physical Examination He was alert, cooperative, oriented with appropriate mood and affect and appeared well nourished. There were no petechiae or purpura and no palpable lymphadenopathy was noted.

Initial Work-Up CBC was significant for anemia with hemoglobin of 11.0 g/dL; WBC differential was normal, but peripheral blood smear review revealed red cell rouleaux. Total protein was elevated (10.6 g/dL) with normal IgA and IgG levels. IgM was elevated (5,080 mg/dL); serum protein electrophoresis with immunofixation showed an M spike of IgM κ paraprotein (**Figures 1** and **2**).

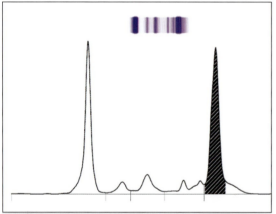

Figure 1 Serum protein electrophoresis and tracing show an M spike in the γ region, which is highlighted.

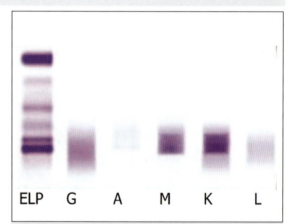

Figure 2 Serum immunofixation electrophoresis showing monoclonal IgM κ paraprotein.

Question 1. Given the initial presentation findings, name a minimum of 3 clinical conditions that you will include in the differential diagnosis of this case.

Question 2. What additional work-up will help you arrive at the final diagnosis?

Question 3. What is the most likely diagnosis?

Question 4. Outline the course of management for this patient and/or the condition.

Question 5. Describe the salient features of the case and/or the condition.

Self-Study Case 17 with Questions
Discussion on page 494

Patient A 38-year-old obese female with lower extremity edema that had worsened over the prior 2 months.

Clinical History The patient had multiple complaints related to chronic joint pains and more recent onset of abdominal fullness and both right and left upper quadrant discomfort. She noted decreased appetite and early satiety over the last month. Most troublesome was the recent onset of lower extremity edema and pain. She had first noted ankle swelling 2 months prior, and thought it was related to increased salt intake. It had gotten worse and now included swelling and discomfort to her mid thigh. Her past history includes hypertension, arthritis, anxiety, gastroesophageal reflux disease and a distant past history of recreational drug use.

Family History Her mother is alive at 60 years of age with hypertension and diabetes. Her father's history is unknown. Both of her sisters have hypertension.

Medications Alprazolam, omeprazole, amlodipine, fluoxetine, multivitamins.

Physical Examination Blood pressure was 105/60; pulse was 80 and regular. Her hair was thinning. The tongue appeared a little enlarged. She had no palpable adenopathy. The spleen tip was palpable 2 cm below the costal margin on the left and was mildly tender. The liver was palpable 1 cm below the costal margin on the right. She also had mid epigastric tenderness. Her legs had pitting edema to the thighs. Range of motion of her knees and ankle was severely limited by the edema. She had no rash.

Initial Work-Up

CBC						Normal
WBC (×10³/μL)	8.1	Although serum protein electrophoresis revealed no discrete abnormalities, a faint IgG λ band was detected by immunofixation. Urine sp gravity 1.036, 3+ protein, otherwise unremarkable. 24-hour urine sample showed 11.8 g of protein, primarily albumin. UPEP and immunofixation showed a very faint band consistent with λ light chains.	Protein (mg/dL)	5.7	(6.0-8.5)
RBC (×10⁶/μL)	3.26		Albumin (g/dL)	2.5	(3.2-4.9)
HGB (g/dL)	10.6		Cholesterol (mg/dL)	658	(<200)
HCT (%)	31.6		Protein, Total (g/dL)	6.7	(6.0-8.5)
MCV (fL)	97		Albumin, Fract Elect (g/dL)	4.0	(3.3-5.2)
MCH (pg)	32.7		α-1 globulin (g/dL)	0.2	(0.1-0.3)
MCHC (g/dL)	33.7		α-2 globulin (g/dL)	0.8	(0.5-0.9)
PLT (×10³/μL)	183		β globulin (g/dL)	0.9	(0.5-1.2)
RDW-CV (%)	15.8		γ globulin (g/dL)	0.8	(0.5-1.6)
WBC Differential	**%**	**# (×10³/μL)**	IgG (mg/dL)	1,220	(723-1,685)
Neutrophils	61.2	5.0	IgA (mg/dL)	232	(69-382)
Lymphocytes	28.2	2.3	IgM (mg/dL)	71	(63-277)
Monocytes	9.0	0.7	Free κ (mg/dL)	1.44	(0.33-1.94)
Eosinophils	1.2	0.1	Free λ (mg/dL)	1.16	(0.57-2.63)
Basophils	0.4	0.0	κ/λ ratio	1.24	(0.26-1.65)

Question 1. Given the initial presentation findings, name a minimum of 2 clinical conditions that you will include in the differential diagnosis of this case.

Question 2. What additional work-up will help you arrive at the final diagnosis?

Question 3. What is the most likely diagnosis?

Question 4. Outline the course of management for this patient and/or the condition.

Question 5. Describe the salient features of the case and/or the condition.

Section M: Self-Study

Self-Study Case 18 with Questions
Discussion on page 496

Patient A 58-year-old woman with fatigue.

Clinical History The patient had joint pains and "aches all over," which she attributed to arthritis.

Family History Noncontributory.

Medications Ibuprofen, as needed for pain.

Physical Examination Notable for hepatosplenomegaly. There was no papable peripheral lymphadenopathy. Neurological exam was unremarkable.

Initial Work-Up

CBC	
WBC (×10^3/μL)	3.8
RBC (×10^6/μL)	4.3
HGB (g/dL)	9.8
HCT (%)	30.8
MCV (fL)	71
MCH (pg)	22.7
MCHC (g/dL)	32.0
PLT (×10^3/μL)	133

WBC Differential	%	# (×10^3/μL)
Neutrophils	84	3.2
Bands	0	
Lymphocytes	7.6	0.3
Monocytes	4.4	0.2
Eosinophils	3.7	0.1
Basophils	0.3	0.0

Peripheral blood smear examination did not reveal any morphologic abnormality other than microcytic red cells. Bone marrow biopsy and clot section: Extensive marrow replacement by pale eosinophilic histiocytic cells. Decreased residual hematopoiesis (**Figures 1** and **2**).

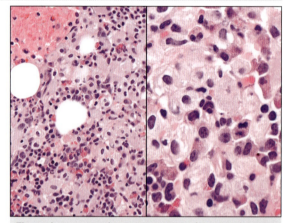

Figure 1 Clot section (H&E, ×400 and ×1000) showing histiocytic cell infiltrate and many cells with linear cytoplasmic striations.

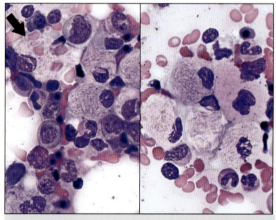

Figure 2 Bone marrow aspirate smear (Wright-Giemsa, ×1000) showing histiocytic cells with low nuclear:cytoplasmic ratios, eccentric nuclei, mature chromatin, and voluminous pale, basophilic cytoplasm with striated, "crinkled tissue paper" appearance.

Question 1. Given the initial presentation findings, name a minimum of 2 clinical conditions that you will include in the differential diagnosis of this case.

Question 2. What additional work-up will help you arrive at the final diagnosis?

Question 3. What is the most likely diagnosis?

Question 4. Outline the course of management for this patient and/or the condition.

Question 5. Describe the salient features of the case and/or the condition.

Self-Study Case 19 with Questions

Discussion on page 498

Patient A 4-month-old female infant with continuous fever up to a maximum of 103.5°F (rectal) and irritability since her vaccination 3 days prior to hospitalization.

Clinical History The child was irritable with poor oral intake. The abdomen was distended. There was no history of diarrhea or vomiting, bleeding, bruising or abnormal behaviors. Her only known sick contact was her 4-year-old sister, who had upper respiratory tract infection.

Family History Unremarkable.

Medications None.

Physical Examination Well-nourished infant, very irritable, intermittently consolable, abdominal distension, diffuse petechiae, no lymphadenopathy or icterus, massive hepatosplenomegaly.

Initial Work-Up

CBC		WBC Differential	%	# (×10³/μL)
WBC (×10³/μL)	2.4	Neutrophils	10	0.2
RBC (×10⁶/μL)	2.74	Bands	0	
HGB (g/dL)	7.6	Lymphocytes	64	1.5
HCT (%)	21.2	Monocytes	3	0.1
MCV (fL)	77.4	Eosinophils	0	
MCH (pg)	27.9	Basophils	0	
MCHC (g/dL)	36.1	Atypical lymphs	23	0.6
PLT (×10³/μL)	7			
RDW-CV (%)	13.2			

CT scan revealed hepatosplenomegaly, ascites, and anasarca. No other masses in the chest or abdomen were seen.

Question 1. Given the initial presentation findings, name a minimum of 2 clinical conditions that you will include in the differential diagnosis of this case.

Question 2. What additional work-up will help you arrive at the final diagnosis?

Question 3. What is the most likely diagnosis?

Question 4. Outline the course of management for this patient and/or the condition.

Question 5. Describe the salient features of the case and/or the condition.

Self-Study Case 20 with Questions

Discussion on page 500

Patient A 14-year-old previously healthy male presented to the hospital with a 2-month history of increasing weakness, complaints of diffuse pain in his extremities, fevers, night sweats, 30-lb weight loss, and a growing mass on the foot.

Clinical History The patient had been evaluated a few days earlier. At that time, his ESR, CRP, CPK, and LDH were elevated and IgG for CMV and EBV infections was positive. He was discharged from a hospital with diagnosis of plantar fasciitis and possible viral infection. He returned to the hospital few days later due to progression of symptoms.

Family History Niece was recently diagnosed with acute myeloid leukemia.

Medications Oxycodone for pain.

Physical Examination The patient was markedly obese. Lower extremities appeared proportionately smaller than his size and had a somewhat shiny and smooth appearance. Diffuse pain on light touch and deep palpation in lower extremities was present as well as pain on deep palpation of the back. There was a 5 × 5 cm round, firm, tender, nonerythematous mass on the lateral aspect of the foot.

Initial Work-Up

CBC		WBC Differential	%	# (×10³/µL)
WBC (×10³/µL)	7.5	Neutrophils	56	4.2
RBC (×10⁶/µL)	4.87	Lymphocytes	30	2.3
HGB (g/dL)	14.2	Monocytes	6	0.5
HCT (%)	41	Eosinophils	1	0.1
MCV (fL)	83	Variant lymphocytes	1	0.1
MCHC (g/dL)	35	Metamyelocytes	1	0.1
PLT (×10³/µL)	150	Myelocytes	2	0.2
RDW-CV (%)	12.5	Blasts	3	0.2
		NRBC (#/100WBC)	5	

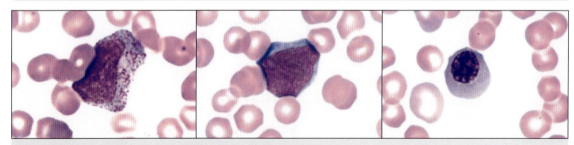

Figure 1 Blood smear (Wright-Giemsa, ×1000) showing leukoerythroblastosis.

Question 1. Given the initial presentation findings, name a minimum of 3 clinical conditions that you will include in the differential diagnosis of this case.

Question 2. What additional work-up will help you arrive at the final diagnosis?

Question 3. What is the most likely diagnosis?

Question 4. Outline the course of management for this patient and/or the condition.

Question 5. Describe the salient features of the case and/or the condition.

Self-Study Case 21 with Questions

Discussion on page 502

Patient A 54-year-old male, who presented with 1-week history of fatigue, fevers, myalgias and diarrhea.

Clinical History The patient was 3 months status post renal transplant.

Family History Noncontributory.

Medications He had recently been prescribed ciprofloxacin by his primary care physician. He was taking routine mycophenolate mofetil and tacrolimus to prevent transplant rejection.

Physical Examination Unremarkable with chest clear to auscultation and no fever upon admission. He had no palpable adenopathy. He had a well healed surgical scar in the right lower quadrant with the transplanted kidney palpable.

Initial Work-Up

CBC		WBC Differential	%	# (×10³/µL)
WBC (×10³/µL)	1.1	Neutrophils	36	0.4
RBC (×10⁶/µL)	3.21	Bands	3	0.0
HGB (g/dL)	8.4	Lymphocytes	41	0.5
HCT (%)	24.3	Monocytes	19	0.2
MCV (fL)	75.6	Eosinophils	0	
MCH (pg)	26.1	Basophils	0	
MCHC (g/dL)	34.5	Metamyelocytes	1	0.0
PLT (×10³/µL)	28			
RDW-CV (%)	19			
MPV (fL)	8.0			

Question 1. Given the initial presentation findings, name a minimum of 2 clinical conditions that you will include in the differential diagnosis of this case.

Question 2. What additional work-up will help you arrive at the final diagnosis?

Question 3. What is the most likely diagnosis?

Question 4. Outline the course of management for this patient and/or the condition.

Question 5. Describe the salient features of the case and/or the condition.

Self-Study Case 22 with Questions

Discussion on page 503

Patient A 30-year-old Caucasian American male with severe factor VIII deficiency and a chief complaint of right hip and low back pain.

Clinical History The patient was in his usual state of health when he awoke in the morning with right hip and low back pain. He recalled no specific traumatic event. He did not notice fever, fatigue, nausea, vomiting, diarrhea, change in urination, right leg weakness or paresthesia. The pain felt by the patient was of grade 6 severity on a scale of 10 (1 = least, 10 = most). He took ibuprofen 600 mg and traveled by subway to his job in an insurance office. By mid-morning the pain had intensified, and so after calling his hemophilia treatment center (HTC), he presented there for evaluation. His past medical history was notable for the diagnosis of severe factor VIII deficiency shortly after birth, as his maternal uncle was affected. Throughout early childhood he received intravenous factor VIII replacement therapy on demand for hemorrhagic episodes, using plasma-derived factor VIII. Bleeding occurred in his elbows and ankles most often, and his right elbow had been considered a target joint. Starting at the age of 12, he began prophylactic factor VIII replacement therapy 3 times per week, using recombinant factor VIII. He occasionally used additional factor VIII therapy for breakthrough traumatic bleeding or as preparation for invasive dental work. He was immunized for hepatitis A and B, and has remained negative for HIV. At the age of 18 he was found to be positive for antibody to hepatitis C. Subsequent studies showed persistent hepatitis C viral load in the peripheral blood, of genotype 1, with normal ALT and AST tests. He underwent treatment for the hepatitis C with pegylated interferon α and ribavirin at the age of 25. Despite initial reduction in viral load, he did not clear his viremia. Starting at age 27, he discontinued prophylactic therapy and now is treated for bleeding episodes. He has not undergone any orthopedic procedures. He has a history of mild iron deficiency, responsive to a multivitamin supplement.

Family History He is an only child. His mother and father are alive and well at ages 53 and 55. His maternal uncle with severe factor VIII deficiency died of AIDS in 1989.

Medications He uses factor VIII replacement therapy episodically, most recently 10 days previously for a spontaneous left ankle bleed; he uses ibuprofen occasionally, and takes a daily multivitamin. He denied use of aspirin, fish oil or herbal supplements.

Physical Examination The patient appeared pale and in moderate distress. Pulse 78/min, blood pressure 140/80, temperature 98.6°F, respirations 16/min. Physical exam was notable only for tenderness of the right hip anteriorly, with decreased range of motion in flexion and extension and tenderness of the upper medial right thigh.

Initial Work-Up

PT (sec)	13.5	(normal 10.9-13.3)
PTT (sec)	130	(normal 29.9-35.8)
HGB (g/dL)	11.6	
PLT (×10^3/μL)	355	

Question 1. Given the initial presentation findings, name a minimum of 2 clinical conditions that you will include in the differential diagnosis of this case.

Question 2. What additional work-up will help you arrive at the final diagnosis?

Question 3. What is the most likely diagnosis?

Question 4. Outline the course of management for this patient and/or the condition.

Question 5. Describe the salient features of the case and/or the condition.

Self-Study Case 23 with Questions
Discussion on page 504

Patient A 75-year-old African-American female with progressive mental status decline, weakness and several falls over the past few weeks.

Clinical History Past medical history failed to reveal any prior bleeding problems.

Family History Noncontributory.

Medications Acetaminophen.

Physical Examination The patient was found to be febrile with a temperature of 101°F. Her pupils were equal, round and reactive to light. The remainder of the neurologic exam was unremarkable. Swelling of the right wrist and forearm, lower extremity edema (1+), bony deformities of the hands, feet and left wrist and right axillary lymphadenopathy were noted.

Initial Work-Up

CBC

WBC (×10^3/μL)	3.8
HGB (g/dL)	7.8
PLT (×10^3/μL)	185
WBC differential was unremarkable	
PT (seconds)	14.6 (normal 12.6-14.4)
PTT (seconds)	105 (normal 24-34)
PTT-mix (1:1)	96 seconds

X-ray examination of the right forearm and right wrist demonstrated factures of the right radial styloid and scaphoid and a head CT scan demonstrated a focal area of acute parenchymal hemorrhage in the anterior right frontal lobe. 2 years previously the PT was 15.8 seconds and PTT 40 seconds.

Question 1. Given the initial presentation findings, name a minimum of 2 clinical conditions that you will include in the differential diagnosis of this case.

Question 2. What additional work-up will help you arrive at the final diagnosis?

Question 3. What is the most likely diagnosis?

Question 4. Outline the course of management for this patient and/or the condition.

Question 5. Describe the salient features of the case and/or the condition.

Section M: Self-Study

Self-Study Case 24 with Questions

Discussion on page 506

Patient A 38-year-old male with a gastrointestinal bleed.

Clinical History The patient was diagnosed with von Willebrand disease (VWD) after work-up for a facial hematoma noted at birth. Throughout life he has developed multiple episodes of major bleeds, primarily gastrointestinal, requiring recombinant factor VIII.

Family History There is a family history of VWD. He is the youngest of 7 children. A sisters suffers from severe VWD and a brother has mild VWD. His other 3 siblings are unaffected. His father has mild VWD and his mother is unaffected.

Medications None.

Initial Work-Up

The laboratory work-up performed shortly after birth showed a normal prothrombin time (PT), PTT >100 seconds (normal 22.7-35.6), and unmeasurable factor VIII activity (FVIII:C), von Willebrand ristocetin cofactor activity (VWF:RCo) and factor VIII antigen level (FVIII:Ag).

Question 1. Given the initial presentation findings, name a minimum of 2 clinical conditions that you will include in the differential diagnosis of this case.

Question 2. What additional work-up will help you arrive at the final diagnosis?

Question 3. What is the most likely diagnosis?

Question 4. Outline the course of management for this patient and/or the condition.

Question 5. Describe the salient features of the case and/or the condition.

Self-Study Case 25 with Questions

Discussion on page 508

Patient A 45-year-old woman, who was referred for presurgical evaluation of an elevated PTT.

Clinical History The patient, a relatively healthy woman, has suffered from menorrhagia for the past 1 year. She has had a pelvic ultrasound which demonstrated a 4 cm × 6 cm uterine fibroid. She had been scheduled for a hysterectomy. However, pre-admission testing revealed an elevated PTT. She denied easy bruising to trivial injury and has had no epistaxis or gum bleeding. There was no history of hemarthrosis or deep tissue bleeding. Her menses lasted for 8 days-10 days and she used 10 pads-12 pads per day. Occasionly she even had midcycle breakthrough bleeding. She had not been placed on hormonal therapy to control this because of past history of a deep venous thrombosis (DVT). The DVT occurred approximately 3 years prior and had been attributed to a car trip of approximately 1 hour in length that she took 2 days prior to the diagnosis. At that time she was admitted to a local hospital for evaluation of left lower extremity pain and swelling. She was treated with low molecular weight heparin (LMWH) and transitioned to coumadin. She completed 6 months of therapy with coumadin without incident.

Family History She is married and has a daughter who is age 28. She had a miscarriage at 12 weeks and another miscarriage at 18 weeks. There is no known family history of a bleeding diathesis. No family members are known to have had a pulmonary embolism (PE), deep venous thrombosis (DVT), myocardial infarction (MI), or cerebrovascular accident (CVA).

Medications A multivitamin daily.

Physical Examination Notable only for substantial varicosity of the veins on the lower extremities, greater on the left than on the right. Pulse 74/min, respiration 14/min, blood pressure 128/78, and temperature 98.8°F.

Initial Work-Up

Preadmission Testing:

PT (sec)	11.6	(normal 11.0-13.4)
PTT (sec)	58	(normal 28.4-36.4)
WBC (×10^3/μL)	5.4	
HGB (g/dL)	13.1	
HCT (%)	39	
PLT (×10^3/μL)	164	

Question 1. Given the initial presentation findings, name a minimum of 3 clinical conditions that you will include in the differential diagnosis of this case.

Question 2. What additional work-up will help you arrive at the final diagnosis?

Question 3. What is the most likely diagnosis?

Question 4. Outline the course of management for this patient and/or the condition.

Question 5. Describe the salient features of the case and/or the condition.

Self-Study Case 26 with Questions

Discussion on page 510

Patient A 66-year-old male with severe abdominal pain was transferred from an outside facility.

Clinical History It was determined that the patient had an acute abdomen secondary to a perforated viscus and was immediately taken to surgery. 2 weeks later the platelet count began to drop. Hematology was consulted when the platelet count was $105 \times 10^3/\mu L$.

Family History Noncontributory.

Medications Patient had been receiving intravenous heparin which had been switched to argatroban when the platelet count began to drop.

Physical Examination Vital signs were all normal. He had a healing surgical scar on his abdomen. There was no active bleeding.

Initial Work-Up

CBC		WBC Differential	%	# ($\times 10^3/\mu L$)
WBC ($\times 10^3/\mu L$)	25.7	Neutrophils	77	19.8
RBC ($\times 10^6/\mu L$)	2.96	Bands	18	4.6
HGB (g/dL)	8.8	Lymphocytes	1	0.3
HCT (%)	25.9	Monocytes	4	1.0
MCV (fL)	87.4	Eosinophils		
MCH (pg)	29.6	Basophils		
MCHC (g/dL)	33.8			
PLT ($\times 10^3/\mu L$)	115			
RDW-CV (%)	17.4			
MPV (fL)	10.7			

Question 1. Given the initial presentation findings, name a minimum of 2 clinical conditions that you will include in the differential diagnosis of this case.

Question 2. What additional work-up will help you arrive at the final diagnosis?

Question 3. What is the most likely diagnosis?

Question 4. Outline the course of management for this patient and/or the condition.

Question 5. Describe the salient features of the case and/or the condition.

Self-Study Case 27 with Questions

Discussion on page 514

Patient A 33-year-old female, 35 weeks pregnant with vaginal bleeding starting <1 day prior.

Clinical History This is patient's first pregnancy. She has no prior history of bleeding, including no menorrhagia, but she has had no prior surgery and no dental extractions. She has had no prior coagulation testing for comparison. She is known to have placenta previa according to prior ultrasounds, showing posterior low-lying placenta approximately 1 cm from the internal os. Her bleeding has been intermittent over the last 24 hours and is described by the patient as "a little less than with a menstrual period."

Family History No family history of bleeding.

Medications Prenatal vitamins.

Physical Examination Unremarkable, with gravid abdomen.

Initial Work-Up

PT (sec)	12	(normal 10.8-13.4)
PTT (sec)	83.1	(normal 21-33)
Platelet count (×10^3/μL)	231	

Question 1. Given the initial presentation findings, name a minimum of 4 clinical conditions that you will include in the differential diagnosis of this case.

Question 2. What additional work-up will help you arrive at the final diagnosis?

Question 3. What is the most likely diagnosis?

Question 4. Outline the course of management for this patient and/or the condition.

Question 5. Describe the salient features of the case and/or the condition.

Case 1: Hemoglobin H Disease

Samir Ballas

Differential Diagnosis Malaria, autoimmune hemolytic anemia, iron deficiency anemia, β-thalassemia syndrome, α-thalassemia (Asian type), and hepatitis B.

Additional Work-Up Examination of thin and thick blood smears was negative for malaria. Direct and indirect antiglobulin (Coombs) tests were negative thus ruling out autoimmune hemolytic anemia. Hemoglobin electrophoresis showed the presence of hemoglobin A (81.7%) and a fast-moving hemoglobin suggestive of hemoglobin H (15%). Hemoglobin A_2 was 1.3%, HbF 2.0% and sickle cell preparation was negative. The presence of hemoglobin H (b4) was confirmed by positive brilliant cresyl blue (BCB) test (**Figure 1**) and positive methyl violet and Heinz bodies preparations. Molecular diagnostic studies using DNA isolated from peripheral leukocytes showed that his α genotype was (––/–α) consistent with Hb H disease. The α genotype of his mother was (––/αα). The father was not available for testing. Accordingly the patient inherited the –α gene from his father and the –– gene from his mother. Examination of a stool sample taken on admission showed the presence of *Yersinia enterocolitica*, thus explaining the cause of the febrile gastrointestinal upset with decompensation of hemoglobin H disease.

Final Diagnosis Hb H disease (––/–α) with *Yersinia* enterocolitis and hepatitis B.

Management Approach With the general approach to management, which consists of symptomatic and supportive therapy, he continued to improve gradually. His fever subsided and his hemoglobin was raised with transfusion of 2 units of blood.

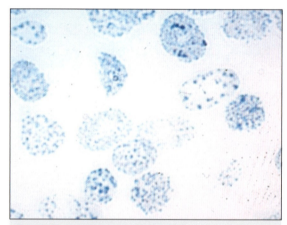

Figure 1 Hemoglobin H preparation (brilliant cresyl blue, ×1000) showing golf-ball appearance of hemoglobin H inclusions.

General Discussion The α gene is normally duplicated and, hence, we normally inherit 2 α genes from each parent. This duplication seems to be necessary to maintain adequate hemoglobin levels in the fetus. The γ gene is also duplicated in order to maintain an adequate hemoglobin F level that is essential for fetal life. Patients with hemoglobin H disease, and patients with other types of hemoglobinopathies, decompensate in the presence of other morbidities with worsening of the anemia and the clinical signs and symptoms. α-thalassemia trait and β-thalassemia trait are often confused with each other since they are often prevalent in the same populations and ethnic groups. Study of family members and molecular diagnostics can differentiate them.

Case 2: Macrocytic Anemia Associated with Folate Deficiency

John R Krause, Gene Gulati, Joanne Filicko O'Hara

Differential Diagnosis Macrocytic anemia with right shift of neutrophils can be due to megaloblastic anemia such as caused by vitamin B_{12} deficiency or folate deficiency or nonmegaloblastic anemia such as myelodysplastic syndrome, AIDS and/or associated therapy, and liver disease. Nutritional deficiency of folate and/or B_{12} was considered the most likely in this case based on clinical presentation and peripheral blood findings.

Additional Work-Up Serum B_{12} level 300 pg/mL (normal 200-900); serum folate 0.6 ng/mL (normal 2 ng-18 ng/mL); red cell folate 40 ng/mL of packed red cells (normal 170-705).

Final Diagnosis Macrocytic (megaloblastic) anemia associated with folate deficiency.

Management Approach Recommendations for proper diet and folate supplementation are the treatment of choice. Oral dose of 1 mg-5 mg/day is usually sufficient. Parenteral preparations of folate are also available. Prenatal vitamins generally include 400-1,000 μg of folate, although some studies have recommended doses as high as 4 mg in early pregnancy to prevent neural tube defects in the baby. This patient was started on a folate supplement and given instructions for a proper diet.

General Discussion Folic acid deficiency is associated with dietary deficiencies and/or increased requirements as may be found during pregnancy. Other causes include chronic hemolytic anemia, alcoholism, malabsorption conditions, intestinal resections (jejunum), various drug or medication induced folate deficiencies and rare inherited disorders of DNA metabolism. The underlying defect in megaloblastic anemia is abnormal purine or pyramidine metabolism resulting in a decline of DNA synthesis that leads to a delay in cell division in all proliferating cells. The resulting morphologic changes are similar in both folate and vitamin B_{12} deficiencies. The most valuable findings on examination of the peripheral blood smear for differentiating megaloblastic from macrocytic anemia are hypersegmentation of neutrophils (>5 lobes) and the presence of oval macrocytes. Howell-Jolly bodies and basophilic stippling may be present and in severe cases neutropenia and thrombocytopenia may be present. Cabot rings and ring-shaped nuclei in neutrophils are occasionally seen. The bone marrow examination is not necessary to make a diagnosis but if performed it will show erythroid hyperplasia and megaloblastic changes (**Figure 1**) in all proliferating cell lineages. Megaloblastic changes refer to the increased size of the hematopoietic precursors with enlarged nuclei showing poorly condensed chromatin which persists into the late stages of cell maturation. Leukopoiesis

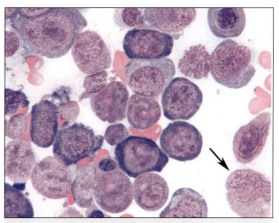

Figure 1 Bone marrow aspirate smear (Wright, ×1000) showing megaloblastic changes in red cell precursors and a giant band (arrow).

is also abnormal, resulting in large leukocytes, mainly giant metamyelocytes and bands. Megakaryopoiesis is less disturbed but abnormalities in nuclear chromatin and increased numbers of large nuclei may occur (**Figure 2**). In the core biopsy, immature erythroid precursors predominate (**Figure 3**) and care must be taken to not mistake the core biopsy as an acute leukemia particularly if examination of the aspirate smear is not performed.

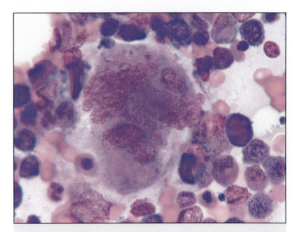

Figure 3 Bone marrow aspirate smear (Wright, ×1000) showing hyperlobated megakaryocyte with fine nuclear chromatin (megaloblastic change).

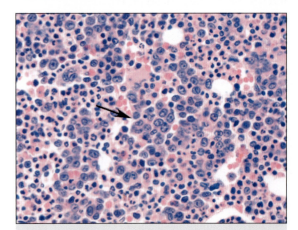

Figure 4 Bone marrow biopsy (H&E, ×400) showing hypercellular marrow, erythroid hyperplasia, and clusters of promegaloblasts (arrow).

Case 3: Glucose-6-Phosphate Dehydrogenase Deficiency-Associated Hemolytic Anemia

Sherrie L Perkins, Hassan M Yaish, Mohamed E Salama

Differential Diagnosis The severe hemolytic anemia (HA) following ingestion of fava beans and family history raised suspicion for the presence of glucose-6-phosphate dehydrogenase (G6PD) deficiency. However, other considerations included paroxysmal nocturnal hemoglobinuria and unstable hemoglobins.

Additional Work-Up	
Coombs test was negative	
PT and PTT were normal	
Bilirubin, total (mg/dL)	5.4
Bilirubin, direct (mg/dL)	0.6
Bilirubin, indirect (mg/dL)	4.5
Serum LDH (U/L)	2,110
Haptoglobin (mg/dL)	<8
Erythrocytic G6PD activity (IU/g HGB)	0.6 (normal 3.8-5.9)

A supravital stain preparation revealed large numbers of red cells with Heinz body inclusions (**Figure 1**).

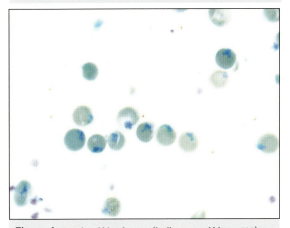

Figure 1 Peripheral blood smear (brilliant cresyl blue, ×500) showing Heinz bodies as multiple deposits of precipitated denatured hemoglobin following an oxidative challenge.

Final Diagnosis G6PD deficiency-associated hemolytic anemia.

Management Infants with G6PD deficiency and severe neonatal hyperbilirubinemia may require exchange transfusions. Adult patients with G6PD deficiency should avoid the ingestion of fava beans and oxidative drugs. Splenectomy is not usually useful. Our patient was hydrated and transfused with 5 × 3 mL/kg packed red cells, increasing the levels of hemoglobin to 9.1 g/dL. Parents were instructed to avoid the ingestion of fava beans and oxidative drugs.

General Discussion G6PD catalyzes the first step of the hexose monophosphate shunt, which protects cells against oxidative injury. G6PD deficient red cells are unable to deal with oxidative stress, resulting in hemoglobin denaturation and precipitation in the form of Heinz bodies with premature splenic red cell lysis. G6PD deficiency usually manifests as an episodic acute HA following infection or ingestion of an oxidant agent in an otherwise apparently healthy person. Hemolysis is often severe, leading to hemoglobinemia (pink to brown plasma), hemoglobinuria, and jaundice. The length of the hemolytic episode and its severity are variable and dependent on the degree of the oxidative stress as well as the type of G6PD mutation. In patients with G6PD A–, hemolysis is usually self-limited while in other types of G6PD deficiency may cause severe, prolonged hemolysis, which could be fatal if not managed by blood transfusions. The severe clinical course described in this family is characteristic of the Mediterranean type of the enzyme deficiency (G6PDMED). Due to the polymorphic nature of the enzyme mutations and resultant effects on enzymatic activity, the World Health Organization (WHO) classified different G6PD variants based on the degree of enzyme deficiency and severity of hemolysis. Only the Class I, II, and III variant groups are clinically significant, with Class I disease being very rare. Class IV and V disease have no significant clinical manifestations and are associated with normal to supranormal enzymatic activity levels. Screening test for G6PD, including dye decolorization test, the methemoglobin reduction test and the fluorescent spot test, may not be useful in the posthemolytic period when reticulocyte counts are high or in heterozygous females and should be confirmed with quantitative NADPH production test. Quantitative NADPH test is highly reliable for the detection of both severe and mild types of G6PD deficiency in men not experiencing an active episode of hemolysis. NADPH may be detected fluorescently but NAPD+ does not fluoresce. Normal samples show a bright fluorescence after 5 or 10 minutes of incubation, whereas deficient samples show no fluorescence. In ongoing or acute hemolysis the younger red cells and reticulocytes have normal or near-normal G6PD activity, and most of the older enzyme-deficient cells may have been lysed. Diagnosis under these circumstances requires repeating the test in 2 or 3 weeks or by modifying the test using reticulocyte-poor fractions. Quantitative enzyme/cytochemical assays may be useful in identifying deficiencies in patients who have had an episode of hemolysis, women with heterozygous disease or in confirming a screening test. Although not necessary for clinical management, precise identification of the G6PD variants requires electrophoresis, kinetic studies, and other biochemical techniques that are also performed in specialized laboratories. G6PD-deficient cells, as well as those with other rare enzyme deficiencies, or unstable hemoglobin types show increased formation of Heinz bodies upon oxidative challenge. The Heinz body test may be used as a screening test and a positive result in association with episodic hemolysis supports the diagnosis of drug/oxidative-induced hemolysis due to G6PD deficiency; however, it is not diagnostically specific.

Case 4: Sickle-β-Thalassemia

Samir Ballas

Differential Diagnosis Iron deficiency anemia, sickle cell anemia, sickle thalassemia, and sickle cell disease. Iron deficiency is unlikely in view of the clinical history and the high serum ferritin level during a previous admission.

Sickle cell anemia (SS) This is the most common type of sickle cell disease in the USA. Except for the microcytic hypochromic red cells and the high hemoglobin A_2, the clinical picture and the CBC are consistent with sickle cell anemia. The coexistence of α- or β-thalassemia with SS may explain the red cell indices and the hemoglobin A_2 level.

Sickle-β+-thalassemia The anemia, the red cell indices and the target cells are strongly in favor of this diagnosis. One would expect; however, milder anemia than a HGB of 7.6 g/dL and the absence of hemoglobin A by hemoglobin electrophoresis is against this diagnosis.

Sickle-β⁰-thalassemia This is a probable diagnosis.

Hb SC disease This diagnosis is easily ruled out by the findings of the initial hemoglobin electrophoresis.

Additional Work-Up The high hemoglobin F level was due to hydroxyurea therapy. The absence of hemoglobin A and the high level of hemoglobin A_2 are consistent with the diagnosis of sickle-β⁰-thalassemia or sickle cell anemia with 2 α gene deletions. His α genotype; however, was normal with 4 α genes present thus confirming the diagnosis of sickle-β⁰-thalassemia. In order to determine the nature of the thalassemia, mutation molecular diagnostics were performed. To that end DNA was extracted from peripheral leukocytes by PCR and tested by reverse dot hybridization. His DNA mutation was at the IVSI-I level with G→A mutation that is known to be associated with sickle-β⁰-thalassemia.

Final Diagnosis Sickle-β⁰-thalassemia with acute sickle cell painful crisis, avascular necrosis and priapism.

Management Approach He was placed on intravenous fluids and hydromorphone by patient controlled analgesia (PCA) pump. Folic acid and hydroxyurea were given. He had a transient episode of priapism overnight that resolved without medical intervention. His condition was stable until the 3rd hospital day when he suddenly became febrile with temperature 101.1°F, pulse 148/min, respiratory rate 30/min and he desaturated to SpO_2 = 79% on room air that increased to 95% on 100% non-rebreather mask Repeat chest X-ray showed new bilateral infiltrates indicating the onset of acute chest syndrome. He developed acute mental status changes, urinary and fecal incontinence and had a cardiac arrest. Code Blue was called and he was successfully intubated, resuscitated with epinephrine and atropine and moved into the intensive care unit. His HGB dropped to 3.2 g/dL and his platelet count decreased to $42 \times 10^3/\mu L$. Examination of the peripheral smear showed blister-like cells that are often seen in acute chest syndrome. He was started on 2 antibiotics, ceftriaxone and azithromycin, and transfused with a total of 6 units of red cells that brought his HGB up to 9.2 and decreased his hemoglobin S level to 18%. The antibiotics were later replaced with levofloxacin for fear that they may have caused thrombocytopenia. The patient improved gradually and was finally discharged after 27 days of hospitalization.

General Discussion The type of sickle cell disease a patient has must be confirmed on new patients and made obvious on the records of old patients. Responders to hydroxyurea do get crises and acute chest syndrome, albeit less frequently. A high adjusted WBC count is a bad sign especially in a patient on hydroxyurea that is known to decrease the WBC count. A high WBC in a patient in crisis is enough reason to consider hospital admission. Thrombocytopenia occurs in acute chest syndrome and should be considered in the differential diagnosis; in this patient heparin induced thrombocytopenia and drug-induced thrombocytopenia were rightly considered but not the acute chest syndrome.

Case 5: Acute Myeloid Leukemia with FLT3/ITD+

Joan E Etzell, Ellen F Krasik

Differential Diagnosis Based on the blast percentage, the peripheral smear findings are diagnostic of acute leukemia. The presence of increased promonocytes favors acute myeloid leukemia (AML). Possible morphologic subcategories of AML include AML with or without maturation (if marrow monocytes <20%), acute myelomonocytic leukemia (if marrow monocytes and granulocytes are each ≥20%), and acute monoblastic/monocytic leukemia (if marrow monocytes ≥80%), as well as AML with a recurrent genetic abnormality. Recurrent genetic abnormalities associated with monocytic differentiation include 11q23 translocation, inv(16) (with associated abnormal eosinophils), and NPM1 mutations (in adults); although other mutations, including FLT3, can show varying morphology/differentiation.

Additional Work-Up The bone marrow biopsy was hypercellular (95% cellularity) with diffuse infiltration by blasts/promonocytes (80% of marrow nucleated elements) (**Figures 1** and **2**). Flow cytometric immunophenotyping showed myeloid blasts (34% of events) expressing weak CD11c, CD13, weak CD33, CD34, weak CD117, HLA-DR, and TdT without coexpression of MPO, CD61, or CD64. A second population, 46% of events, expressed CD4, CD11c, CD13, variable CD14, variable CD15, CD33, and HLA-DR, consistent with monocytic precursors. Cytogenetics revealed a normal female karyotype, 46, XX. Molecular testing showed the FLT3-ITD mutation but lacked mutation of NPM1.

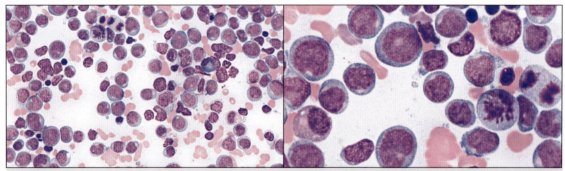

Figure 1 Bone marrow aspirate smear (Wright-Giemsa × 400 [left] and ×1000 [right]) showing that blasts, including monoblasts/promonocytes, comprise the majority of cells.

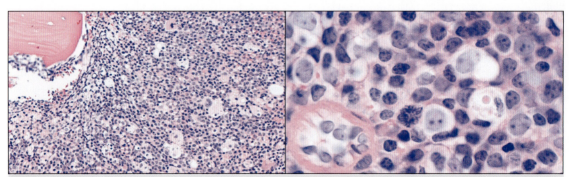

Figure 2 Bone marrow biopsy (H&E, left [×200] and right [×1000]) showing hypercellular marrow comprised of a relatively monotonous population of immature cells with fine chromatin and small nucleoli. Occasional tingible body macrophages (left) and a mitotic figure (right) are also noted.

Final Diagnosis Acute myeloid leukemia with myelomonocytic features, normal cytogenetics and FLT3-ITD+, NPM1–.

Management Approach Standard induction chemotherapy includes continuous infusion cytarabine over 7 days along with an anthracycline such as daunorubicin or idarubicin for 3 days (7+3 regimen). High-dose cytarabine or addition of other agents such as etoposide, fludarabine, or cladribine may be included as part of a clinical investigation. Consolidation therapy generally includes high-dose cytarabine. Patients with "good risk" disease usually receive 3 cycles-4 cycles of high-dose cytarabine, whereas those with "high risk" disease are usually offered hematopoietic progenitor cell transplantation (HPCT) in first remission if a donor is available. Risk is stratified based on cytogenetics, with normal cytogenetics in the intermediate risk category. More recently, the FT3-ITD has been shown to also be associated with poor prognosis, and thus, HPCT is the treatment of choice in normal karyotype AML with FLT3-ITD. This patient underwent induction chemotherapy with daunorubicin, etoposide ansd AraC. Bone marrow biopsy on day 14 of the chemotherapy cycle showed persistent leukemia, and a biopsy on day 28 could not exclude minimal residual disease. Comorbid medical conditions precluded HPCT. She underwent consolidation therapy with high-dose cytarabine but relapsed 8 months after initial diagnosis.

General Discussion Karyotypic abnormalities in AML can provide prognostic information but are identified in only 55%-60% of cases. If cytogenetics are normal, testing for mutations of FLT3, NPM1, and CEBPA can provide prognostic information. FLT3 encodes fms-related tyrosine kinase 3, a receptor tyrosine kinase involved in hematopoietic stem cell differentiation and proliferation. FLT3 is expressed on normal progenitor cells and in AML and ALL. FLT3 mutations occur in all AML subtypes (30% of all AML) and in myelodysplastic syndromes (MDS). Cup-like nuclear invaginations have been reported with FLT3-ITD and NPM1 abnormalities (**Figure 3**). The 2 main types of FLT3 mutations render the kinase constitutively active. The more common mutation, comprising 75%-80% of FLT3 mutations and present in 15%-34% of all AML, is an internal tandem duplication (FLT-ITD) within the juxtamembrane domain, leading to in frame protein elongation. FLT-TKD mutation, present in 8%-12% of AML, results from point mutations within the "activation loop" or tyrosine kinase domain. AML with normal karyotype and FLT3-ITD is associated with adverse outcomes, including reduced complete remission rates and shorter disease-free and overall survival. Some studies suggest shorter disease free survival in patients with normal karyotype AML and FLT3-TKD mutation; although there is presently no clear consensus. Despite intensive induction chemotherapy, 20%-40% of AML patients do not achieve complete remission, and of those who do achieve remission, 50%-70% relapse within 3 years. Small molecule inhibitors of FLT3 are in development, and early clinical trials are underway to investigate drugs including lestaurtinib, midostaurin, and tandutinib. Sorafenib, an oral small molecule, originally designed to target the Raf-1 kinase, is also being investigated. When used as single agents, these inhibitors have produced partial and transient therapeutic responses. The inhibitors have proven to be synergistic when given concurrently with or after chemotherapy. Resistance develops from point mutations in FLT3 or acquired mutations downstream of FLT3 in the signaling pathway.

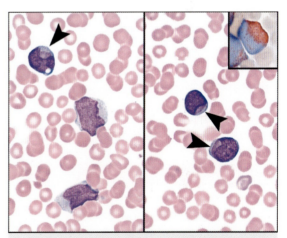

Figure 3 Blood smear from another patient with AML who had a normal karyotype and was FLT3-ITD+ and NPM1+, (Wright-Giemsa, ×1000) showing cup-like nuclear inclusions within blasts that have been described in AML with FLT3 and/or NPM1 abnormalities. The inset in the right upper corner shows cytochemical staining for myeloperoxidase with positivity in a blast.

Case 6: Myeloid Sarcoma

Imran Siddiqi, Ryan M Gill, Stefania Pittaluga

Differential Diagnosis Lymphoma (Burkitt, lymphoblastic, and blastic mantle cell), acute myeloid leukemia (AML), a myeloproliferative neoplasm, blastic plasmacytoid dendritic cell neoplasm, and myeloid sarcoma.

Additional Work-Up By immunohistochemical staining, the neoplastic cells were positive for MPO (**Figure 1**), CD117 (**Figure 2**), CD34 (**Figure 3**), CD56, TdT (focal), PAX5 (weak), CD68/KP-1 (focal), CD4, lysozyme, and CD33 and were negative for CD3, CD79a, CD123, CD20, and CD14. Immunophenotyping by flow cytometry demonstrated expression of CD34, CD33, CD38, CD117, CD11b, and HLA-DR on 73% of cells. A subsequent bone marrow biopsy and aspirate were performed which showed no marrow involvement.

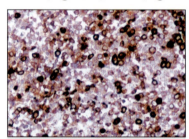

Figure 1 Paraspinal mass biopsy (MPO, ×200) showing positivity for MPO.

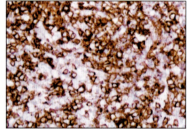

Figure 2 Paraspinal mass biopsy (CD117, ×200) showing positivity for CD117.

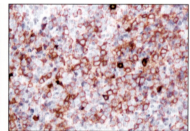

Figure 3 Paraspinal mass biopsy (CD34, ×200) showing positivity for CD34.

Final Diagnosis Myeloid sarcoma.

Management Approach Although myeloid sarcoma can occur in association with acute or chronic myelogenous leukemia, the absence of circulating blasts, a subsequent normal bone marrow, and imaging findings argue for presentation as a solitary mass in this case. Nonetheless, most patients will develop evidence of leukemia on follow-up and the management approach is similar to AML. Consequently, this patient received an anthracycline and cytarabine (ARA-C)-based induction, followed by consolidation therapy and an allogeneic hematopoietic progenitor cell transplant.

General Discussion Myeloid sarcoma is currently defined as a tissue-based mass outside the bone marrow consisting of myeloid blasts. Patients with concurrent leukemia may still be classified as having myeloid sarcoma if the cells form a tumor that effaces underlying architecture, as opposed to focal involvement of various tissues with blasts that do not efface tissue architecture. A diagnosis of myeloid sarcoma is clinically equivalent to a diagnosis of acute myeloid leukemia (AML). Myeloid sarcoma can occur prior to manifestation of AML (or relapse) or present concurrently with AML. Myeloid sarcoma occurs over a wide age range and has slight male predilection. The areas most commonly affected include skin, lymph node, GI tract (in particular the intestine), and bone. Myeloid sarcoma consists of myeloblasts with a wide morphologic spectrum, as in AML, most commonly with evidence of monocytic and/or granulocytic maturation, and rarely with erythroid and/or megakaryocytic differentiation. Immunohistochemical evaluation is useful in the diagnosis and allows distinction from other entities in the differential diagnosis. Aberrant expression of lymphoid markers (eg, Pax5, TdT) can be seen in some myeloid sarcomas, such as those carrying the t(8;21) RUNX1/RUNX1T1 fusion.

Section N: Discussion of Self-Study Cases

Case 7: Acute Myeloid Leukemia with inv(16)(p13.1q22)

Lydia Contis

Differential Diagnosis Acute myelomonocytic leukemia, acute monocytic leukemia, and acute monoblastic leukemia.

Additional Work-Up Bone marrow biopsy was hypercellular for age (90% cellularity). The marrow aspirate demonstrated the following: blasts 40.5%; promyelocytes 3%; myelocytes 1%; metamyelocytes 1%; bands 1%; neutrophils 3.3%; eosinophilic myelocytes/metamyelocytes 8.5%; eosinophilic bands 3.0%; eosinophil segmented 10.5%; basophils 0.3%; monocytes 14.8%; normoblasts 3.3%; lymphocytes 5.3%; plasma cells 4.8%. Blasts demonstrated rounded or convoluted nuclear contours with scant to moderate amounts of cytoplasm. Increased eosinophils and precursors were present and a number of eosinophils contained basophilic granules (**Figures 1** and **2**). Mature monocytes were also noted, some with atypical nuclear features. Flow cytometry studies performed on the bone marrow demonstrated the following phenotype of the blasts (40.3% of all events): dim CD45+, CD34+, CD13+, dim CD4+, CD33+, CD117+, HLA-DR+, myeloperoxidase +. A myelomonocytic component was also present (18% of total events) with the following phenotype: CD14+, CD64+, partial CD36+, HLA-DR+, CD15+, CD13+, CD11b+, CD33+ and CD34–. Dual esterase cytochemical staining performed on the aspirate smear demonstrated chloroacetate esterase positive myeloid cells and α-naphthyl acetate esterase positive monocytic cells with fluoride inhibition (**Figure 3**). Cytogenetic studies performed on the bone marrow: 46, XX, inv(16)(p13.1q22). FISH studies were positive for the CBFβ gene rearrangement in 184 of 201 interphase cells examined (91.5%).

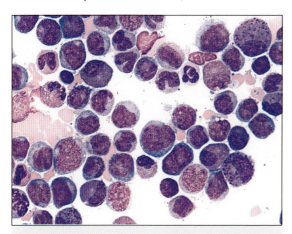

Figure 1 Bone marrow aspirate (Wright-Giemsa, ×500) showing blasts, promonocytes, and eosinophils with basophilic granules.

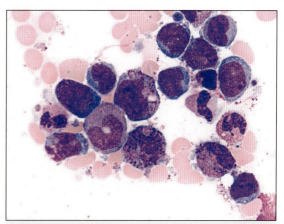

Figure 2 Bone marrow aspirate (Wright-Giemsa, ×1000) showing blasts, promonocytes, and eosinophils with basophilic granules.

Section N: Discussion of Self-Study Cases
Acute Myeloid Leukemia with inv(16)(p13.1q22)

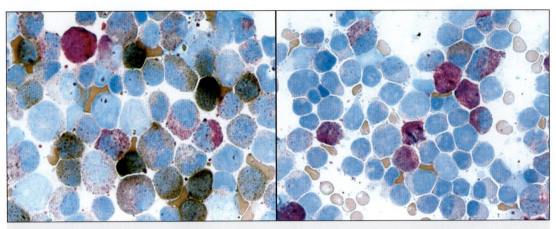

Figure 3 Bone marrow aspirate smear (×1000). Chloroacetate esterase (red) and α-naphthyl acetate esterase (brown) stain without (left) and with (right) fluoride inhibition.

Final Diagnosis Acute myeloid leukemia with inv(16)(p13.1q22); CBFB-MYH11.

Management Approach Most patients achieve complete remission after standard induction chemotherapy with anthracycline and high-dose cytarabine-based protocols and long-term remission rates of 60%-70% have been reported. Up to 30% of patients relapse and benefit from stem cell transplantation. Monitoring of minimal residual disease can be achieved by conventional cytogenetic and FISH studies. RT-PCR for CBFβ/MYH11 detection can be of benefit, especially in those cases with normal cytogenetic and morphologic findings. This patient underwent induction therapy with idarubicin and cytarabine and achieved morphologic and cytogenetic remission. This was followed by 4 cycles of consolidation therapy with high-dose ARA-C. She currently remains in remission 10 months after diagnosis.

General Discussion Acute myeloid leukemia (AML) with inv(16)(p13.1q22), or less commonly t(16;16)(p13.1;q22), CBFB-MYH11 is a distinct subtype of acute myeloid leukemia characterized by monocytosis and eosinophilia in the bone marrow along with abnormal eosinophils which contain large basophilic granules. This type of leukemia is associated with a good prognosis and accounts for 5%-8% of all cases of AML. It occurs mostly in children or young adults. Inv(16)(p13q22) results in the fusion of 2 genes: the core binding factor gene (CBFβ) at 16q22, which encodes the β subunit of core binding factor (CBF), and the MYH11 gene at 16p13, which encodes the smooth muscle myosin heavy chain. CBFβ is necessary for the generation of hematopoietic progenitor and stem cells, and CBFβ-MYH11 blocks embryonic hematopoiesis at the stem-progenitor cell stage. The role of this chimeric gene in leukemogenesis remains unknown. Secondary cytogenetic abnormalities can also be seen and include +8, +22, del (7q) or +21. Eosinophils are often not increased in the peripheral blood and if present, do not typically demonstrate abnormal granulation. Blasts, including promonocytes, are typically increased in the peripheral blood. The bone marrow demonstrates blasts with monocytoid features, myeloblasts as well as abnormal eosinophils. The eosinophils associated with this type of leukemia often contain eosinophilic as well as large basophilic granules which, unlike normal eosinophils, are periodic acid-Schiff and faintly chloroacetate esterase positive. The abnormal basophilic granules are myeloperoxidase and toluidine blue negative, a feature helpful in distinguishing them from basophils. The presence of increased eosinophils without abnormal granulation can be seen in other types of AML and would not be suggestive of this subtype of AML. The monoblasts and promonocytes demonstrate nonspecific esterase reactivity, but this can also be absent. Neutrophils are decreased in the marrow while the number of eosinophils in the peripheral blood are not typically increased. Dyspoietic hematopoiesis can be prominent. Flow cytometry studies may demonstrate a myeloblast population with expression of myeloid antigens, including CD13, CD33, CD15 as well as CD34 and CD117. The monocytoid population can demonstrate expression of CD14, CD4, CD11b, CD11c and CD64. CD2 expression has also been reported in this type of AML but is not specific and does not appear to affect clinical outcome. Complete remission rates are high (approximately 90%) after standard induction therapy. Mutations in the KIT gene have been associated with a higher risk of relapse.

Case 8: Blastic Plasmacytoid Dendritic Cell Neoplasm

Kathryn Foucar, Jordan M Hall

Differential Diagnosis Acute leukemia of B-, T-, or myeloid lineage and other less common precursor neoplasms (eg, NK-cell and plasmacytoid dendritic cell lineages).

Additional Work-Up Bone marrow examination revealed complete effacement of the marrow by atypical cells (**Figure 1**). The aspirate smear showed intermediate to large atypical cells with patchy or dotted nuclear chromatin (**Figure 2**). By flow cytometry, the atypical cells were positive for CD45, CD56, CD4, CD2, cytoplasmic CD3, CD7 and HLA-DR, and negative for surface CD3, CD1a, CD8, CD57, CD10, CD19, CD20, CD13, CD33, CD117, CD34, and TdT. By immunohistochemical stains, the atypical cells were positive for CD123 and TCL-1 and negative for CD68 and TIA-1. A high proliferative index (80%) was evident with Ki-67 immunostaining. Epstein-Barr virus encoded small nuclear RNA (EBER) was not detected by in situ hybridization. T-cell receptor γ (TCRg) genes were germline. Cytogenetic analysis revealed a complex karyotype including del(6q), add(12p), and loss of chromosomes 9, 13, 17, 20, and 22.

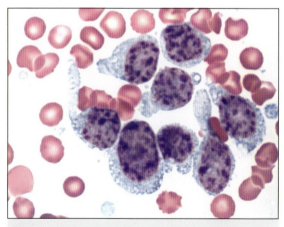

Figure 1 Bone marrow aspirate smear (Wright-Giemsa, ×1000) showing many atypical cells.

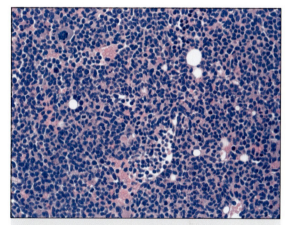

Figure 2 Clot section (H&E, ×200) showing diffuse involvement of the marrow by atypical cells.

Section N: Discussion of Self-Study Cases
Blastic Plasmacytoid Dendritic Cell Neoplasm

Final Diagnosis Blastic plasmacytoid dendritic cell neoplasm.

Management Approach While an initial satisfactory response is often seen with aggressive systemic chemotherapy (80%-90% of cases), relapse regularly occurs within a relatively short period of time. In some cases hematopoietic progenitor cell transplantation (HPCT) in first remission has shown improved results. This patient received 3 cycles of induction chemotherapy (cyclophosphamide, vincristine, doxorubicin and dexamethasone [hyper-CVAD]) with attainment of morphologic remission; however, 4 months later, a follow-up bone marrow examination revealed focal CD3+/CD123+ aggregates suspicious for recurrent/residual disease, and 2 months later the patient was deceased.

General Discussion Blastic plasmacytoid dendritic cell neoplasms (BPDCN) are rare and aggressive hematopoietic tumors derived from precursors of plasmacytoid dendritic cells (pDC), a specialized subset of immune regulatory dendritic cells. There is a predilection for elderly men, although any age group may be affected. Patients often present with asymptomatic skin lesions (eg, nodules, plaques or bruise-like lesions) and otherwise good health. Peripheral blood involvement may be minimal at the outset, and cytopenias, particularly thrombocytopenia, are not uncommon, although widespread dissemination with bone marrow, peripheral blood, splenic, and/or lymph node involvement is frequently seen at presentation or early on in the course of the disease. Occasionally, patients may have an acute leukemic presentation in the absence of cutaneous lesions. In general, the prognosis is poor, and the overall survival is in the order of 12 months-16 months. Morphologically, the neoplastic cells often have a lymphoblastic appearance with scant to moderate, pale blue, agranular cytoplasm; round to irregular nuclei with "blastic" chromatin; and variably conspicuous nucleoli. Characteristically, though inconstant, cytoplasmic microvacuoles arranged in a "pearl necklace-like" fashion and/or polarized pseudopod-like cytoplasmic projections can be seen (**Figure 1**). In cases with cutaneous involvement, tumor cells diffusely infiltrate the dermis with characteristic sparing of the overlying epidermis. The typical immunophenotype includes positivity for CD4, CD56, CD43, HLA-DR, CD45RA, and pDC-associated antigens (eg, CD123, TCL1, and/or BDCA2), and negativity for CD3, myeloperoxidase, CD13, CD19, and CD34. Of note, variable expression of markers such as TdT, CD7, CD2, CD33, and CD68 can also be observed; and in exceptional cases, cytoplasmic CD3 may be detected; in such cases, caution is advised, and the presence of germline TCRg genes and the absence of tumor-associated EBV are especially helpful in establishing the diagnosis. Last, while no specific cytogenetic abnormality has been reported, a complex karyotype is often revealed, particularly with abnormalities of 5q, 12p, 13q, 6q, 15q, and/or chromosome 9 being more common. As illustrated by this case, careful integration of clinical, morphologic, immunophenotypic, and genetic features is often required to definitively establish a diagnosis of BPDCN.

Case 9: Acute T-Cell Lymphoblastic Leukemia in an Adult

R Patrick Dorion

Differential Diagnosis Presence of many blasts in the peripheral blood narrowed the differential diagnosis to acute leukemia (myeloid vs lymphoid vs biphenotypic), and peripheralizing lymphoma.

Additional Work-Up Bone marrow was hypercellular (70%) and mostly replaced by blasts (**Figure 1**). The aspirate smear examination yielded 80% blasts, which were characterized by medium size, high N/C ratio, fine chromatin, slightly irregular nuclear contours and a small amount of light basophilic cytoplasm with no granules (**Figure 2**). By immunohistochemstry, the blasts stained positive for CD3 (**Figure 3**), CD7, CD34 and focally positive for TDT. By flow cytometry the blasts expressed cytoplasmic CD3, CD5, surface CD7, CD11b(partial), CD33(partial), CD34 and CD38. Cytoplasmic TDT and CD79a were partially positive. CD13, CD15, CD117, MPO, HLA-DR, CD2, CD4, CD8, CD10, CD16 and CD56 were negative. The majority of the blasts were of medium size based on forward scatter. Cytogenetically no abnormal chromosomes were found. Likewise, FISH studies revealed no chromosomal abnormalities.

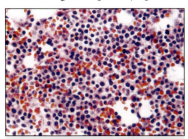

Figure 1 Bone marrow biopsy (H&E, ×200) showing hypercellular marrow with monotonous population of blasts.

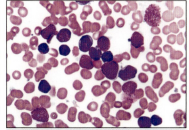

Figure 2 Bone marrow aspirate smear (Wright-Giemsa, ×1000) showing monotonous population of blasts.

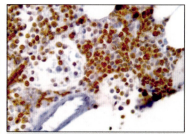

Figure 3 Bone marrow biopsy (CD3, ×100) showing that blasts are positive.

Final Diagnosis Acute T-cell lymphoblastic leukemia.

Management Approach Without therapy, survival of patients with acute adult T-cell leukemia is measured in days to weeks. Combination chemotherapy gives the best chance of survival. The optimal combination of agents is unclear. Multiple regimens have been utilized. Patients may initially respond but relapses are frequent. Medium survival with multiagent chemotherapy ranges from 5 months-13 months. All patients require central nervous system (CNS) prophylaxis with intrathecal chemotherapy, since there is a 10%-25% risk of CNS involvement. In elderly patients (70 years or more) less intensive therapy with cyclophosphamide, doxorubicin, vincristine and prednisone (CHOP) has been suggested as it is tolerated better; however, only short remissions are obtained. Patients with T-cell ALL are immunocompromised and are at risk for opportunistic infections with organisms such as candida, fungi, cytomegalovirus and *Pneumocystis*. Hypercalcemia can be severe and monitoring is recommended. Therapeutic leukapheresis was started in an attempt to reduce the number of white cells in this patient. Following the initiation of vigorous intravenous hydration and allopurinol prophylaxis, chemotherapy with cyclophosphamide, vincristine, doxorubicin and dexamethasone (hyper-CVAD) was begun. She expired 1 month after admission.

General discussion T-cell lymphoblastic leukemia in adults is a rare form of leukemia accounting for 15% of all adult lymphoid leukemias. B-cell leukemias are relatively more common in adults, especially the Philadelphia chromosome positive (Ph1+) type in young adults. The patients usually present with a high blast count and can have a large mediastinal mass or other tissue mass. The disease carries a poor prognosis although it has been reported that T-cell ALL in adults has a better prognosis than B-cell ALL. It carries a 5-year survival of 40% for children. Some adult T-cell leukemias are associated with the HTLV 1 virus and have a higher incidence in Japan, Africa and the Caribbean. The majority of T-cell leukemias have an unknown etiology. As seen in this case, T-cell lymphoblastic leukemias in adults have a very poor prognosis despite aggressive therapy.

Case 10: Chronic Neutrophilic Leukemia

Imran Siddiqi, Ari B Molofsky, Babis Andreadis

Differential Diagnosis Leukemoid reactions: reactive neutrophilia secondary to infections, drugs/cytokines, malignancies. Myeloproliferative neoplasms (MPN): chronic myelogenous leukemia BCR-ABL1 positive (CML), polycythemia vera (PV), primary myelofibrosis (PMF), chronic neutrophilic leukemia (CNL). Myelodysplastic/myeloproliferative neoplasms (MDS/MPN): chronic myelomonocytic leukemia (CMML) and atypical chronic myelogenous leukemia, BCR-ABL negative (aCML) and myeloid neoplasms with PDGFR-α, PDGFR-β, or FGFR1 abnormalities.

Additional Work-Up This patient had a sustained peripheral blood and bone marrow neutrophilia despite hydroxyurea treatment. The absence of monocytosis or significant dysplasia excludes an MDS/MPN overlap such as CMML or aCML. Eosinophilia, a finding typically associated with PDGFRA, PDGFRB, and FGFR1 abnormalities, is not present. Finally, the patient had no known chronic infection, underlying malignancy, or drug/cytokine that would result in a chronic reactive neutrophilia. Thus, a myeloproliferative neoplasm (MPN) was considered most likely. Reticulin and trichrome stains performed on bone marrow biopsy sections were essentially negative for fibrosis. CD138 staining revealed 2%-3% marrow plasma cells, which were mixed for κ and λ light chains. Cytogenetics revealed a normal male karyotype; 46, XY[20]. PCR was negative for the JAK2 V617F and JAK2 exon 12 mutations. Testing for the BCR-ABL1 t(9;22) translocation was negative by both PCR and FISH. Serum protein electrophoresis/immunofixation was negative and a serum free light chain ratio was normal.

Final Diagnosis Myeloproliferative neoplasm (MPN), most consistent with chronic neutrophilic leukemia (CNL).

Management Approach CNL is a MPN with variable course (6 months-20 years), although it may progress with increasing thrombocytopenia, anemia, and/or development of a MDS or acute myeloid leukemia (AML). Symptomatic control can be achieved with hydroxyurea or other mild chemotherapeutics. There is a case report of a patient with a t(15;19) translocation that responded to imatinib. Splenomegaly can be controlled with splenectomy. This patient had a modest response to hydroxyurea. He has remained stable with persistent neutrophilic leukocytosis.

General Discussion Chronic neutrophilic leukemia (CNL) is an exceedingly rare myeloproliferative neoplasm (MPN) that results in the clonal proliferation of mature neutrophils. It is likely a heterogeneous disorder, as no single causative molecular abnormality has been identified, and its morphology overlaps with causes of chronic reactive neutrophilia. Approximately 150 cases of CNL are reported in the literature, with an apparent predilection for the elderly. Patients often present with hepatosplenomegaly. In a minority of patients, a history of GI bleeding, gout, and pruritus can be elicited. CNL is a diagnosis of exclusion and should only be rarely applied. Per WHO 2008 criteria, CNL is defined by a sustained peripheral blood WBC count of $>25 \times 10^3/\mu L$ with >80% mature neutrophils/bands, <10% immature granulocytes, and <1% myeloid blasts. Although neutrophil toxic changes (granulation, Döhle bodies) may be present, they are often not prominent. The bone marrow is hypercellular with relatively increased mature myeloid forms. Physiological neutrophilia, as well as alternate MPN or MDS/MPN overlap syndromes, must be ruled out. As such, blasts are not increased (<5%) and there is no significant dysplasia or monocytosis. Reticulin fibrosis is minimal, and polycythemia and thrombocytosis are typically absent. Additionally, BCR-ABL1, PDGFRA, PDGFRB, and FGFR1 rearrangements must be absent. Finally, hepatosplenomegaly should be present. Unfortunately, clonal cytogenetic abnormalities are only detected in a minority of CNL cases (10%), including trisomy 8, 9, 21, deletion 20q, 11q, or 12p, and are generally not helpful in diagnosing CNL. Rare cases with the JAK2 V617F mutation in heterozygous or homozygous form are reported. Of note, up to 20% of patients diagnosed with CNL have concurrent multiple myeloma (plasma cell myeloma), and neutrophil clonality has not been established in such cases, suggesting a cytokine-driven neutrophilia. Therefore, plasma cell neoplasms should be specifically considered when diagnosing CNL, and if found, a diagnosis of CNL should be questioned. Among the myeloproliferative neoplasms (MPN), there is significant morphologic overlap, with the common feature of increased effective hematopoiesis. As CNL is the rarest form of MPN, more common etiologies must be ruled out. Chronic myelogenous leukemia, BCR-ABL1 positive (CML) is the most common MPN, often presenting with peripheral blood granulocytosis, but with a more pronounced immature granulocyte component ("myelocyte bulge") and frequent basophilia. A rare variant of CML with a BCR/ABL p230 transcript can present with isolated blood neutrophilia, similar to CNL. Polycythemia vera (PV) is another common MPN, often presenting with elevated RBC mass and bone marrow panmyelosis, quite distinctive from CNL. However, early phase PV can include a nonpolycythemic phase. Primary myelofibrosis (PMF) is an MPN that usually presents as marrow fibrosis, distinctive from CNL. However, a prefibrotic cellular phase often occurs, which can include blood neutrophilia. PMF will typically progress over time to marrow fibrosis. Additionally, even in early PMF, megakaryocyte atypia is usually pronounced. In summary, CNL should be diagnosed sparingly, and only after extensive testing to rule out other more common myeloid neoplasms and reactive causes of neutrophilia. Even in this case, given the lack of established clonality and the relatively limited 6-month period of neutrophilia, a diagnosis of CNL is suggested but not definitive.

Case 11: Chronic Eosinophilic Leukemia Associated with PDGFRA Rearrangement

Mehmet I Goral

Differential Diagnosis Primary (clonal) as well as secondary (reactive) causes of eosinophilia were considered in the differential diagnosis. Primary conditions include chronic myeloproliferative neoplasms, acute myeloid and lymphoblastic leukemias and idiopathic hypereosinophilic syndrome (HES). Secondary eosinophilia is much more common and may be related to drug reactions, toxins, allergic reactions, autoimmune conditions, infections (specifically tissue invasive parasitosis), malignancies and other conditions.

Additional Work-Up The bone marrow was moderately to markedly hypercellular (**Figure 1**) with myeloid hyperplasia showing a prominent, morphologically normal, eosinophilic population (**Figure 2**). No increase in number of blasts, lymphocytes or plasma cells was detected. There was no evidence of myelodysplasia. The number of mast cells was within normal range. Flow cytometry studies did not show an increase in number of blasts; an abnormal B- or T-cell population was not identified. RT-PCR studies for FIP1L1-PDGFRA were positive. FISH studies for BCR-ABL and pyrosequencing for JAK-2 mutations were negative. Cytogenetic studies revealed a normal male karyotype.

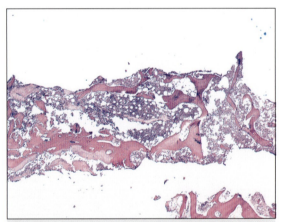

Figure 1 Bone marrow biopsy (H&E, ×40) showing hypercellular marrow.

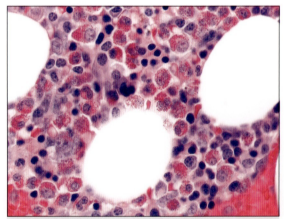

Figure 2 Bone marrow biopsy (H&E, ×400) showing increased number of eosinophils and eosinophilic precursors.

Final Diagnosis Chronic eosinophilic leukemia with FIP1L1-PDGFRA (WHO classification: chronic myeloproliferative neoplasm with eosinophilia and PDGFRA abnormality).

Management Approach Neoplasms associated with PDGFRA and PDGFRB mutations respond well to treatment with imatinib. This patient was started on imatinib and his response to the treatment will be monitored by RT-PCR based evaluation of FIP1L1-PDGFRA transcript suppression.

General Discussion According to the 2008 WHO classification, chronic eosinophilic leukemia (CEL) is defined as a clonal proliferation of eosinophilic precursors with peripheral blood, bone marrow and tissue eosinophilia. Eosinophilia associated with PDGFRA, PDGFRB and FGFR1 rearrangements with aberrant tyrosine kinase activity are grouped in a new entity in the 2008 WHO classification "myeloid and lymphoid neoplasms with eosinophilia and abnormalities of PDGFRA, PDGFRB or FGFR1." The FIP1L1-PDGFRA fusion is the most common abnormality observed in cases of CEL with PDGRA rearrangement and is produced by an interstitial deletion at chromosome 4q12. This deletion is cryptic and is not detectable by conventional cytogenetic banding techniques. The result of this rearrangement is a constitutively active tyrosine kinase, which is highly sensitive to inhibition by imatinib. Most patients with this rearrangement present as CEL, but cases presenting with eosinophilia and acute myeloid leukemia or T-lymphoblastic leukemia have also been reported. Transformation to acute leukemia may be seen in patients who present initially with CEL. CEL with PDGFRA rearrangements is a rare disease with substantial male predominance; most patients are between ages of 25 and 55 years at presentation, with a range of 7 years-77 years. Clinical features are variable and are related to extent of leukemic involvement of the bone marrow and/or tissue damage related to eosinophil infiltration. Most common presenting symptoms are fatigue and pruritus. Splenomegaly is common but hepatomegaly is rare. Serum tryptase and vitamin B_{12} levels may be elevated. The most significant morphologic feature of CEL with PDGFRA is eosinophilia in peripheral blood and bone marrow. The bone marrow is usually hypercellular with eosinophilic and myeloid hyperplasia. Occasionally, the number of blasts in bone marrow is increased, but peripheral blood involvement with blasts is rare. The eosinophils and their precursors may be morphologically normal or may show a scope of changes including variation in amount, size and maturation of granules. The number of mast cells is increased in most of the cases. Clinical manifestations of primary and secondary eosinophilia may be indistinguishable, so prompt diagnosis and treatment is critical to prevent tissue damage, which may be life threatening.

Case 12: Juvenile Myelomonocytic Leukemia

Cheryl Hirsch-Ginsberg, Sara Szabo

Differential Diagnosis Diagnostic considerations included juvenile myelomonocytic leukemia (JMML), persistent Epstein-Barr virus infection, combined immunodeficiency and congenital viral infections.

Additional Work-Up Bone marrow was 99% cellular and showed monocytosis with no increase in blasts (**Figure 1**). Monocytic lineage was confirmed by nonspecific (butyrate) esterase as well as CD68 immunohstochemical staining (**Figures 2** and **3**). Review of spleen section revealed monocytic infiltrate in the red pulp (**Figure 4**). Reports of other findings included normal karyotype, absence of BCR-ABL fusion gene, and monocytic infiltrate in the liver.

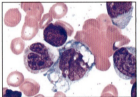

Figure 1 Bone marrow aspirate smear (Wright-Giemsa, ×1000) showing monocytosis.

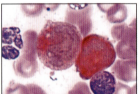

Figure 2 Bone marrow aspirate smear (butyrate esterase, ×1000) showing positivity in monocytes.

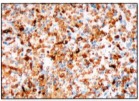

Figure 3 Bone marrow biopsy (CD68, ×200) showing positivity in monocytic cells.

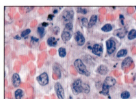

Figure 4 Spleen (H&E, ×400) showing monocytic infiltrate in the red pulp.

Final Diagnosis JMML, possibly present as early as the time of the splenectomy.

Management Approach General management of patients with JMML includes intensive chemotherapy, which may prolong survival. Allogeneic hematopoietic progenitor cell transplantation (HPCT) is recommended for long-term remission. This patient was started on hydroxyurea and etanercept. He never achieved remission.

General Discussion JMML was previously known as juvenile chronic myelogenous leukemia. It is analogous to chronic myelomonocytic leukemia (CMML), the adult counterpart, with significant overlap both in diagnostic criteria and associated genetic abnormalities. Patients typically present with fever, persistent infections, organomegaly, skin rash (eczematoid or xanthomatoid), bleeding and failure to thrive. Lymphadenopathy is more common than in acute myelomonocytic leukemia, although splenomegaly tends to be less common. JMML may also be seen in patients with neurofibromatosis. Diagnostic criteria include (1) monocytosis in the peripheral blood (PB) >1 × 10^3/μL, (2) blasts with promonocytes comprising <20% of leukocytes in the PB and of the nucleated bone marrow (BM) cells, (3) lack of Ph chromosome or *BCR-ABL1* fusion gene, and (4) 2 or more of the following findings: (a) hemoglobin F increased for age, (b) immature granulocytes in the PB, (c) WBC count >10 × 10^3/μL, (d) clonal chromosomal abnormality (eg, monosomy 7) and (e) GM-CSF hypersensitiviy of myeloid progenitors in vitro. Dysplastic granulocytic features may be seen, including abnormal segmentation (eg, pseudo-Pelger-Huët forms), hypogranularity, or persistence of primary granules. The BM is typically hypercellular, and trilinage dysplastic features may be seen. Polyclonal hyperγ-globulinemia is present in the majority of patients. Genetic abnormalities overlapping with CMML include −7/del(7q) seen in 25% of JMML patients, and abnormal signal transduction secondary to mutations in the RAS/MAPK pathway. The latter include mutations in *PTPN11* (effect via SHP2 phosphatase activation, in 35% of JMML patients), in NRAS and KRAS2 (via Ras activation, in 20% of patients), and in *NF1* (via neurofibromin deregulation, in 20% of patients). These are also consistent with syndromic associations with neurofibromatosis type 1 (about 10% of JMML cases) and rarely with Noonan syndrome. In addition to evidence of myelomonocytic proliferation in the PB and BM, virtually all cases present with organ infiltration, (at least liver and spleen, and often skin, lymph nodes and respiratory tract). Progression to BM failure is common.

Case 13: T-Prolymphocytic Leukemia

Margaret Kasner, Jascha Rubin

Differential Diagnosis Lymphocytosis may be associated with a number of benign conditions (eg, persistent polyclonal B-lymphocytosis, viral infections, etc) as well as malignant conditions (eg, chronic lymphocytic leukemia (CLL), prolymphocytic leukemia (PLL), chronic lymphocytic leukemia in prolymphocytic transformation (CLL/PLL), and leukemic phase of non-Hodgkin lymphoma.

Additional Work-Up Peripheral blood flow cytometry demonstrated an atypical population of T-lymphoid cells which constituted 79% of all analyzed cells (95% of the lymphoid cells) and had the following antigenic pattern: CD2+, cytoplasmic CD3+, CD4+, CD5+, CD7+, CD52+, CD38±, dim surface CD3−/+, CD1a−, CD8−, α-β TCR−, γ-δ TCR−, CD34−, HLA−DR−, and TDT−. No blast population was identified. Flow cytometry performed on a bone marrow aspirate sample duplicated the immunophenotypic profile seen in blood. Bone marrow biopsy was hypercellular and showed diffuse infiltration by medium and large lymphoid cells with prominent nucleoli (**Figure 1**). A differential performed on the aspirate smear yielded a lymphocyte count of 50%. A majority of the lymphoid cells had clumped chromatin and prominent nucleoli.

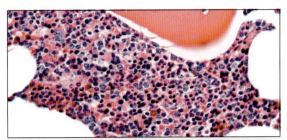

Figure 2 Bone marrow biopsy (H&E, ×400) showing hypercellular marrow with diffuse infiltration by medium and large immature cells (prolymphocytes).

Final Diagnosis T-cell prolymphocytic leukemia (T-PLL).

Management Approach T-cell prolymphocytic leukemia (T-PLL) is a rare malignancy associated with a poor prognosis. There is currently no standard therapy. Limited success has been achieved using various chemotherapies including purine analogues, chlorambucil, and combination chemotherapy using cyclophosphamide and anthracyclines. Better success has been seen with alemtuzumab, a monoclonal antibody directed against the CD52 antigen of lymphocytes. Consolidation therapy with stem-cell transplant does help to prolong survival. Therapy should be initiated shortly after diagnosis, given the aggressive nature of the disease. This patient was treated with combination chemotherapy with cyclophosphamide, vincristine, doxorubicin and prednisone. His family was HLA typed for possible allogeneic stem-cell transplant donation.

Discussion T-PLL represents approximately 1%-2% of adult lymphocytic leukemias. Its origin is that of a mature, postthymic T-cell, though slightly more naïve than that of CLL. This can be appreciated morphologically by a predominance of prolymphocytes which have generous cytoplasm and prominent nucleoli. Most patients present with generalized lymphadenopathy, hepatosplenomegaly, anemia, and thrombocytopenia. In this regard, this patient represented an exception to the rule by presenting with neither adenopathy/organomegaly nor cytopenias. The WBC count, particularly the lymphocyte count is generally markedly increased to over $100 \times 10^3/\mu L$. The diagnosis is generally based on morphology and immunophenotypic profile of the lymphoid population along with clinical presentation findings. T-PLL cells usually express CD2, CD3, CD7, and CD52 but are negative for TdT and CD1a. In 60% of cases the leukemic cells are CD4+CD8−, consistent with helper-cell immunophenotype. The CD4+CD8+ and CD4−CD8+ variants make up 25% and 15% of cases respectively. The most common cytogenetic abnormalities involve chromosome 14. T-PLL carries a very poor prognosis, with a median survival of 7.5 months from the time of diagnosis.

Case 14: Anaplastic Large Cell Lymphoma

Beverly P Nelson

Differential Diagnosis Carcinoma, sarcoma, and lymphoma.

Additional Work-Up By immunohistochemical stains tumor cells were CD45–, CD30+ (**Figure 1**), ALK+ (**Figure 2**), CD20–, CD3–, CD4+, CD8–, TIA1+, cytokeratin –, desmin–, actin–, inhibin–, melaninA–, HMB45–, and calretinin–.

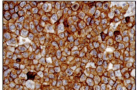

Figure 1 Lymph node (CD30, ×400); lymphoma cells show uniform, strong membrane staining for CD30.

Figure 2 Lymph node (ALK, ×500); there is both cytoplasmic and nuclear staining indicating presence of t(2;5)(p23;q35).

Final Diagnosis Systemic anaplastic large cell lymphoma, ALK+.

Management Approach Systemic anaplastic large cell lymphoma (ALCL) is an aggressive lymphoma that requires chemotherapy. Treatment is not standardized but is usually CHOP-based. Hematopoietic progenitor cell transplantation may be an option for selected patients with refractory or relapsed disease. This patient was treated with 6 cycles of hyperfractionated cyclophosphamide, vincristine, doxorubicin and dexamethasone (hyper-CVAD) alternating with high-dose methotrexate and cytarabine (MTX/AraC), and she had complete resolution of disease.

General Discussion ALCL is a peripheral T-cell lymphoma that was first recognized because of its strong uniform staining with CD30 and large bizarre tumor cells with abundant cytoplasm. ALCL shows a wide morphologic spectrum varying from tumors rich in small lymphocytes that resemble peripheral T-cell lymphomas (the small cell variant) to tumors composed of uniformly large cells with bizarre nuclei (giant cell variant). Some variants contain many reactive cells and only rare tumor cells. ALK+ tumor cells aids in recognition of these variants. However, some ALCL are ALK–; thus an ALK stain is not always helpful for diagnosis. For example, primary cutaneous ALCL that by definition is confined to the skin at initial diagnosis is uniformly ALK negative. Similarly, up to 40% of systemic ALCL (that by definition involves non-cutaneous sites such as lymph nodes at diagnosis) are ALK negative (**Figure 3**). The characteristic strong CD30 staining (**Figure 4**) in every tumor cell is helpful to distinguish ALK– ALCL from other CD30+ lymphomas. However, CD30 is often weak/– on the small cell variant ALCL lymphoma cells, but rare large lymphoma cells, including hallmark cells are typically located around blood vessels and are brightly CD30+. In addition, small cell ALCL is virtually always ALK+. Distinction between ALK+ and ALK– ALCL is worthwhile because of their different clinical behavior. ALK+ ALCL is more common in children (20% of childhood lymphomas vs. 3% of adults) and generally has a better survival (70% vs. 49% at 5 years). However, despite being consistently ALK negative, primary cutaneous ALCL has an excellent prognosis with 5-year

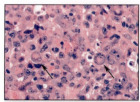 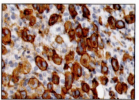

Figure 3 Lymph node from a different case of ALK– anaplastic large cell lymphoma (H&E, ×40); lymphoma cells display similar morphology as the ALK positive variant. The arrows point to hallmark cells.

Figure 4 Lymph node from a different case of ALK– anaplastic large cell lymphoma (CD30, ×400) in which lymphoma cells are uniformly, brightly positive for CD30.

survival of over 90%, and may spontaneously regress. ALK protein is present in lymphoma cells that harbor aberration of the anaplastic lymphoma kinase gene located on chromosome 2 band p23. The most common aberration, t(2;5)(p23;q35), results in fusion of ALK with the nuclophosmin gene on chromosome 5q35 causing constant transcription of the NPM-ALK hybrid gene. Several other translocations involve the ALK gene, and location of ALK staining in the ALCL cells (nucleus, cytoplasm, membrane) correlates with the type of translocation. Nuclear staining ± cytoplasmic staining indicates t(2;5)(p23;q35). Cytoplasmic staining is present in the other translocations except for 1 involving the X chromosome that shows membranous staining. ALCL may resemble carcinomas on H&E sections because of its cohesive growth pattern. However, large tumor cells with horseshoe-shaped nuclei, abundant cytoplasm, and eosinophilic areas adjacent to the nucleus (hallmark cells) indicate ALCL. In addition, ALCL are uniformly cytokeratin–. Inflammatory myofibroblastic tumors (IMTs) and some diffuse large B-cell lymphomas (DLBCL) are ALK+. IMTs lack hallmark cells and are usually EBV+ while ALCL are EBV–. ALK+ DLBCL are CD20+, PAX5+, and CD30–.

Case 15: Blastoid Variant of Mantle Cell Lymphoma

John Anastasi

Differential Diagnosis CLL in transformation, mantle cell lymphoma (blastoid variant), leukemic phase of large cell lymphoma, or other lymphoid malignancy.

Additional Work-Up Flow cytometry (blood): the small and larger cells had a similar phenotype. The cells were monoclonal B cells that expressed CD19, CD20, CD5 and bright sIg with κ restriction. CD23 was variable; FMC7 was weak. CD10 and TdT were negative. Immunohistochemical stains performed on a cell block prepared from the peripheral blood showed Cyclin D1 expression in the cell nuclei (**Figure 1**). The bone marrow biopsy was hypercellular with a preponderance of blastoid cells associated with a high mitotic rate (**Figure 2**). Cervical lymph node biopsy: diffuse effacement with small cells with features of mantle cells and larger cells consistent with the blastoid cells (**Figure 3**). Cytogenetic analysis: clone 1: 46XY, t(11;14)(p13;q32) clone 2: 46XY, t(11;14)(p13;q32),t(2;8)(p12;q24), del(17p).

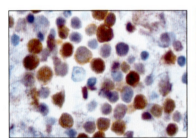

Figure 1 Cell block of peripheral blood cells (cyclin D1, ×400) showing nuclear reactivity indicates overexpression of cyclin D1.

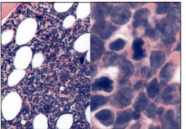

Figure 2 Bone marrow biopsy (H&E, left ×200; right, ×500) in which marrow is markedly hypercellular and extensively involved by MCL. On higher power blastoid features of the cells and the associated high mitotic rate are evident.

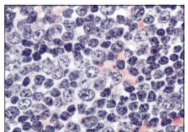

Figure 3 Cervical lymph node biopsy (H&E, ×400) showing the architecture is effaced by the lymphoma cells, which include the typical smaller mantle cell lymphoma cells and the larger blastoid cells.

Final Diagnosis Mantle cell lymphoma, blastoid variant with t(11;14)(q13;q32) and associated Burkitt translocation t(2;8)(p12;q24).

Management Approach The blastoid variant of mantle cell lymphoma is an aggressive lymphoma and those with t(11;14) and MYC rearrangements have a rapidly fatal course. Therapy is aggressive. Chemotherapy usually includes rituximab, cyclophosphamide, doxorubicin, vincristine and steroids, in alternating cycles with high-dose methotrexate and cytarabine (Hyper CVAD/AraC-Methotrexate), or similar therapy. Most patients will relapse quickly. Autologous stem cell transplant has not been shown to provide any real survival benefit, but allogeneic stem cell transplantation has been promising in some studies. This patient was given aggressive hydration and allopurinol to prevent complications related to tumor lysis syndrome. He received chemotherapy with cyclophosphamide, vincristine, doxorubicin and dexamethasone. His WBC dropped quickly over the first 5 days. His course was complicated by febrile neutropenia, sepsis and a need for intensive care unit monitoring. He received growth factor and transfusion support and recovered a normal WBC and platelet count about 3 weeks after starting chemotherapy. He was able to be discharged to home and subsequently returned to the hospital for several cycles of inpatient chemotherapy. He subsequently underwent reduced intensity allogeneic stem cell transplantation from his HLA identical brother. He remains in complete remission 18 months following transplant.

General Discussion MCL is an aggressive lymphoma. When it is in leukemic phase it must be distinguished from CLL. The clues to MCL include the presence of cells with irregular nuclear contours and more open chromatin than CLL cells, and lack of the distinctive prolymphocytes which are seen in CLL. The distinction based on morphology can be difficult and unreliable, and flow should be employed. Absence of CD23 and intense sIg help distinguish MCL. Sometimes, equivocal staining can make the flow findings less than accurate, so the expression of cyclinD1 and the presence of t(11;14)(q13;q32) should be evaluated to confirm MCL. In the absence of a tissue specimen, one can take peripheral blood and produce a cell block for cyclin D1 analysis. FISH analysis or conventional cytogenetics can be used to detect BCL2-IGH or t(11;14). In some cases of blastoid variant of MCL, the t(11;14) is associated with complex additional abnormalities whereas in others the t(11;14) may be seen with 1 of the 3 Burkitt translocations involving the MYC gene (ie, t(8;14), t(2;8) and t(8;22). The few reports of cases of the blastoid variant of MCL associated with a MYC translocation show that patients have a very aggressive course and very poor prognosis.

Case 16: Lymphoplasmacytic Lymphoma (Waldenström Macroglobulinemia)

Bernard Greenberg, Mehmet I Goral

Differential Diagnosis Monoclonal gammopathy of undetermined significance (MGUS), lymphoplasmacytic lymphoma/Waldenström macroglobulinemia (LPL/WM), other B-cell lymphomas, and multiple myeloma (MM).

Additional Work-Up The bone marrow biopsy showed markedly hypercellular marrow (**Figure 1**) with a diffuse infiltrate of small lymphocytes, plasmacytoid lymphocytes and plasma cells (**Figures 2** and **3**). There was no evidence of myelodysplasia, granulomas, or metastatic neoplasm. Flow cytometry studies performed on bone marrow aspirate showed a monoclonal IgM positive B-cell population (CD19 and CD20+) with a small population of clonally related plasma cell component. Neoplastic lymphocytes were positive for CD23 and were negative for CD5 and CD10. The monoclonal plasma cells showed bright CD38 expression. Cytogenetic studies demonstrated 6q– and an interstitial deletion of long arm of chromosome 16. Urine immunoelectrophoresis revealed free κ light chains. Serum viscosity was increased to 3.1 relative viscosity (normal 1.4-1.8). Serum calcium and creatinine levels were within normal limits. β-2 microglobulin was 2.8 mg/dL (normal 1.1-2.4). Skeletal bone survey was negative. CT studies of chest, abdomen and pelvis did not show any evidence of lymphadenopathy.

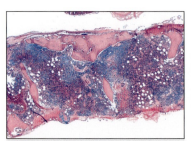

Figure 1 Bone marrow biopsy, (H&E, ×100) showing hypercellular marrow.

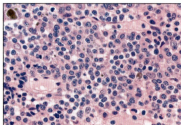

Figure 2 Bone marrow biopsy (H&E, ×400) showing sheets of small lymphocytes with varying degree of plasmacytic differentiation.

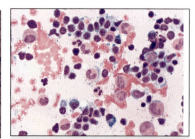

Figure 3 Bone marrow aspirate smear (Wright-Giemsa, ×1000) showing numerous small lymphocytes, plasmacytoid lymphocytes and few plasma cells.

Final Diagnosis Lymphoplasmacytic lymphoma/Waldenström macroglobulinemia.

Management Approach While asymptomatic patients may be followed with close observation, patients with cytopenias, bulky adenopathy, organomegaly, symptomatic hyperviscosity, severe neuropathy, amyloidosis, cryoglobulinemia or transformation to more aggressive histopathology require immediate treatment. The management is usually individualized based on symptoms and extent of disease. This symptomatic patient was treated with cyclophosphamide, vincristine, and prednisone (CVP).

Rituximab administration was delayed until serum IgM levels were normalized in order to avoid paradoxical increase in serum viscosity. The patient responded to treatment well with significant decrease in paraprotein levels and improvement of anemia at his most recent follow-up, 6 months after the diagnosis.

General Discussion Lymphoplasmacytic lymphoma (LPL) is a low-grade neoplasm of small B lymphocytes, plasmacytoid lymphocytes and plasma cells. LPL does not have specific immunophenotype or genetic abnormalities; other small cell lymphomas with plasmacytic differentiation should be excluded before reaching the diagnosis. Most cases of LPL are associated with IgM monoclonal gammopathy; rare cases may produce IgG or IgA class paraprotein. Waldenström macroglobulinemia (WM) is associated with most cases of LPL and is defined as LPL with bone marrow involvement and any level of IgM monoclonal gammopathy. Other common sites of involvement include liver and spleen; peripheral blood may also be involved, but significant lymphocytosis is usually not present. LPL/WM is a rare disease of older adults with median age of 65 years; males are more commonly affected. Approximately a quarter of patients are asymptomatic at diagnosis; most common presenting symptoms are fatigue and weakness related to anemia. The etiologies of symptoms observed in LPL/WM are multifactorial and are related to tumor infiltration of bone marrow and/or effects of circulating and/or deposits of IgM. Replacement of bone marrow with neoplastic cells may cause cytopenias and related clinical symptoms. The effects of IgM monoclonal protein include hyperviscosity, cryoglobulin activity, autoimmune function, deposition to tissues and interaction with coagulation factors that result in a variety of clinical manifestations, including but not limited to, headaches, blurred vision, bleeding disorders, anemia, diarrhea, malabsorption, proteinuria, renal failure and neuropathies. The immunophenotype of neoplastic cells in LPL/WM may differ based on the level of plasmacytic differentiation. The neoplastic lymphocytes are positive for surface immunoglobulin, IgM class in majority of cases, and express B-cell markers (CD20, CD19, CD22), and are negative for T-cell markers. In most cases morphologic features with immunophenotype allow to differentiate LPL from other B-cell lymphomas. Differentiation of marginal zone lymphoma (MZL) from LPL can be difficult, if not impossible in some cases, both of these lymphomas may show plasmacytic differentiation and they do not have a distinct immunophenotype or genetic abnormality. There are no chromosomal abnormalities that are specific for LPL. LPL/WM has an indolent course with median survival of 5 years-10 years and is incurable with conventional treatment modalities. The adverse prognostic indicators are older age, presence of B symptoms, anemia, high β-2-macroglobulin levels and elevated liver function tests. A small number of cases transform to diffuse large B-cell lymphoma; cases that developed Hodgkin lymphoma have also been described.

Case 17: Amyloidosis

Joanne Filicko-O'Hara, Ryan Gentzler, Gene Gulati

Differential Diagnosis Diagnostic considerations included multiple myeloma, monoclonal gammopathy of undetermined significance (MGUS), primary amyloidosis, and light chain deposition disease.

Additional Work-Up Bone marrow: normocellular with approximately 5% CD38+ plasma cells (**Figure 1**), without clear evidence of light chain restriction. Perivascular deposits of amorphous, eosinophilic acellular material were noted (**Figure 2**).

The deposits were Congo red+. Skeletal survey was negative for fractures or lytic lesions. Kidney biopsy revealed prominent mesangial expansion with accumulation of amorphous eosinophilic material (**Figure 3**) that was PAS+ and Congo red+ (**Figure 4**) was noted. Echocardiogram showed normal left ventricular systolic function without segmental wall motion abnormalities and suggested abnormal diastolic function.

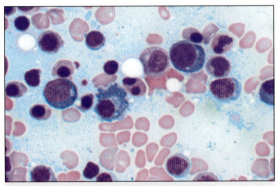

Figure 1 Bone marrow aspirate smear (Wright-Giemsa, ×1000) showing normal hematopoietic elements with a plasma cell. A bilobed neutrophil is also present.

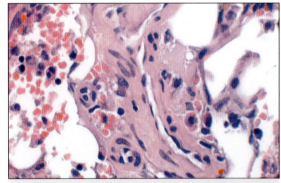

Figure 2 Bone marrow biopsy (H&E, ×400) showing perivascular, pale and waxy amorphous deposits.

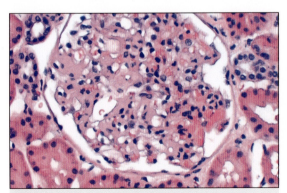

Figure 3 Kidney biopsy (H&E, ×200) showing glomerular mesangial expansion due to accumulation of amorphous eosinophilic material.

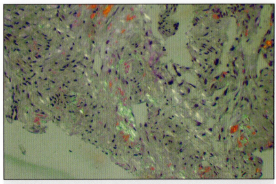

Figure 4 Kidney biopsy (Congo red, ×200) showing apple green birefringence of AL amyloid.

Final Diagnosis Systemic AL amyloidosis involving the kidney, soft tissue, and likely the heart.

Management Approach Historically, patients with light chain (AL) amyloidosis have had a poor prognosis with a median survival of 12 months-18 months. However, recent advances over the last 10 years have led to some improvements. In patients who are diagnosed early enough and have few comorbidities, autologous stem cell transplantation using high-dose melphalan is a treatment which can provide long-term remissions. While the risk of death related to transplantation is higher than in other patients with plasma cell dyscrasias (10%), 5-year survival after transplant is as high as 60%. Contraindications for autologous stem cell transplantation include >2 organs affected by light chain deposition, severe cardiac involvement, creatinine >2mg/dL or age >65. For those patients ineligible for transplant, some studies have shown that treatment with oral melphalan in combination with high-dose dexamethasone daily for 4 days every 28 days has been shown to increase survival and improve organ function in half of patients receiving the regimen after a median time of 4.5 months of therapy. Treatment is often difficult given the propensity for multisystem organ involvement. Newer agents such as bortezomib and lenalidomide are showing promise, although it is unclear what long-term survival will be. As is usual in cases of primary amyloidosis, the therapy is aimed at the underlying clonal plasma cell disorder, not the destruction of the amyloid protein. Thus it may be many months before the signs or symptoms of the disease improve even when therapy is successful. This patient was diagnosed 13 years ago and had minimal response to the nontransplant-based therapies available at that time. She underwent autologous transplant 1 year following diagnosis, using high-dose melphalan and stem cell rescue. 18 months following that she finally had resolution of her nephrotic range proteinuria. She did well until 11 years later, when she was found to have proteinuria again and renal biopsy revealed amyloid. She has continued on lenalidomide for over 1 year with no obvious evidence of disease following 18 months of therapy.

General Discussion Amyloidosis is a group of disorders charactereized by misfolding of extracellular proteins which are then deposited in tissue as b-sheets. There are many different types of amyloid which are differentiated by their precursor protein, distribution, and whether they are acquired or hereditary. This case is an example of AL amyloidosis caused by deposition of immunoglobulin light chains, and is a plasma cell dyscrasia. AL amyloidosis may present alone or in conjunction with multiple myeloma. The association may be linked to the particular λ idiotype of the immunoglobulins produced by the clonal plasma cells. AL amyloid deposits can be found in any organ with the kidney, heart, and liver being the most common. Diagnosis is made by identification of apple-green birefringence (Congo red stain) on polarized light microscopy of biopsied tissue.

Section N: Discussion of Self-Study Cases

Case 18: Gaucher Disease

Imran Siddiqi, Edward Thornborrow, Joan Etzell

Differential Diagnosis The presence of increased number of histiocytes in the bone marrow is a nonspecific finding that can be seen in a number of congenital, reactive, and neoplastic conditions, and is often reflective of increased bone marrow cellular turnover. The differential diagnosis includes constitutional lysosomal storage diseases (including Gaucher disease), infections (eg, Whipple disease or mycobacterial), hemophagocytic syndrome (either constitutional or associated with an underlying neoplasm or viral infection) or nonspecific/reactive benign histiocytic proliferations. Neoplastic entities that can cause a proliferation of histiocytic cells include histiocytic sarcomas and certain hematopoietic neoplasms, such as monocytic leukemias and both T-cell and Hodgkin lymphomas. Neoplastic cells that can morphologically mimic histiocytes include occasional large cell lymphomas (especially anaplastic large cell lymphoma) and rare variants of myeloma. The morphology of histiocytes seen in the bone marrow led us to consider Gaucher disease as the most likely diagnosis.

Additional Work-Up Testing on peripheral blood leukocytes confirmed decreased glucocerebrosidase levels.

Final Diagnosis Gaucher disease, extensive marrow involvement.

Management Approach The mainstay of therapy for Gaucher disease, particularly in symptomatic children and patients with severe disease, is enzyme replacement with recombinant glucocerebrosidases (imiglucerase). The effectiveness of enzyme replacement therapy is questionable in neuronopathic disease (ie, types 2 and 3 disease), as the recombinant enzyme does not cross the blood-brain barrier. Small studies; however, suggest stabilization of neurologic disease with therapy. In patients unable or unwilling to receive enzyme replacement therapy, substrate reduction therapy with miglustat (decreases the synthesis of glucocerebroside) is an option. Additional supportive measures are typically necessary to manage bone disease, cytopenias, and other complications. This patient was treated with enzyme replacement therapy, which led to some reduction in the splenic volume and subjective improvement in symptoms.

General Discussion Gaucher disease is the most common lysosomal storage disease. It is an autosomal recessive disorder caused by a variety of mutations in the gene encoding the β-glucocerebrosidase enzyme (GBA gene), leading to defective breakdown of glucocerebroside, and its consequent accumulation in the lysosomes of mononuclear phagocytic cells. These abnormal histiocytic cells, termed Gaucher cells, deposit in multiple organs, including spleen, liver, bone marrow, lymph nodes, and bones. These histiocytes with a characteristic "crinkled tissue paper" appearance of the cytoplasm and an eccentric lobulated nucleus represent Gaucher cells and are helpful in the distinction from other histiocytic proliferations. Still, this appearance is not completely specific for Gaucher disease, as abnormal histiocytes with similar morphology (pseudo-Gaucher cells) can be seen in a variety of other disease processes, such as chronic myelogenous leukemia, lymphoid malignancies, myeloma, thalassemia, and mycobacterial infections. While there is morphologic overlap, true Gaucher cells show distinct ultrastructural features with a fibrillar pattern rather than the tubular inclusions seen in pseudo-Gaucher cells. An association with Gaucher disease and various neoplasms, particularly multiple myeloma, has been described and, therefore, in these settings one may need to distinguish between pseudo-Gaucher cells and "true" Gaucher disease. Given the relative lack of specificity for the finding of Gaucher-like cells in the bone marrow, it is imperative that a suspected diagnosis of Gaucher disease be confirmed by measuring glucocerebrosidase levels/production in either peripheral blood leukocytes or cultured fibroblasts. Alternatively, molecular testing for germline mutations in the GBA gene also is available. Gaucher disease shows a clinical spectrum of severity, ranging from major multiorgan manifestations to asymptomatic patients who are incidentally diagnosed in late adulthood. Three main subtypes are recognized. Type I (non-neuronopathic), the most common form of Gaucher disease, has a highly variable clinical phenotype and lacks primary central nervous system involvement. This type is most prevalent in patients of Ashkenazi Jewish descent. Common presenting symptoms include painless splenomegaly, thrombocytopenia, anemia, leukopenia, and excessive bleeding later progressing to liver involvement. Ocular and skin manifestations can be seen, and Erlenmeyer flask deformity of the distal femur is considered highly characteristic. Types II and III Gaucher disease have a more aggressive course, with central nervous system involvement and neurologic manifestations; disease occurs early in life and is rapidly progressive in type II, and usually begins in later childhood in type III. Gaucher disease has a variable clinical spectrum of manifestations, depending on the particular mutation. While most commonly diagnosed in childhood, it is important to bear in mind that a significant minority of patients with type I disease present during late adulthood, as seen in this patient.

Section N: Discussion of Self-Study Cases

Case 19: Hemophagocytic Lymphohistiocytosis

Lakshmanan Krishnamurti, Idhi Aggarwal, Raymond E Felgar

Differential Diagnosis Fever with pancytopenia and hepatosplenomegaly in an irritable infant is suspicious for acute viral infectious processes such as acute Epstein-Barr virus and cytomegalovirus infections, infiltration of bone marrow and reticuloendothelial system by acute leukemia, juvenile myelomonocytic leukemia, neuroblastoma and hemophagocytic lymphohistiocytosis.

Additional Work-Up Bone marrow biopsy and aspirate revealed trilineage hematopoiesis with an increase in the number of histiocytes (**Figure 1**), which stained positive with CD163 on biopsy (**Figure 2**). Aspirate smears of the bone marrow showed readily identifiable histiocytes with erythrophagocytosis and lymphophagocytosis (**Figure 3**). Blasts were not increased. Cytogenetic studies revealed a normal female karyotype, 46, XX. Other pertinent laboratory findings included: elevated LDH: 380 IU/L (normal 105-333), markedly elevated ferritin: 9,729 ng/mL (normal 10-95), slightly increased total bilirubin: 2.8 mg/dL (conjugated bilirubin: 2.2 mg/dL), ALP: 155 IU/L (normal <360), ALT: 146 IU/L (normal 14-54), AST: 247 IU/L (normal 15-41), triglycerides: 177 mg/dL (normal <150), PTT: 67 sec (normal 27.0-39.4), PT: 30 sec (normal 11.5-16.1), INR: 2 2.7 (0.9-1.3), elevated D-dimers and decreased fibrinogen. Tests for HHV6 and HIV were negative. Diagnostic lumbar puncture revealed numerous histiocytes. NK cell lytic function was found to be absent by chromium release assay and soluble IL-2 receptor (sIL2R) levels were found to be increased as determined by a solid-phase, 2-site chemiluminescent immunometric assay. Cytoplasmic perforin expression was absent in peripheral blood when stained with both surface and intracellular mono clonal antibodies and analyzed using 4-color flow cytometry.

Final Diagnosis Familial hemophagocytic lymphohistiocytosis.

Management Approach According to the protocol of the second international HLH study (HLH 2004)

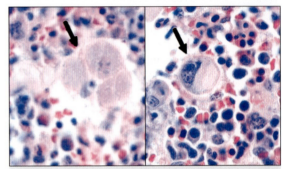

Figure 1 Bone marrow biopsy (H&E, ×500) showing large histiocytes (arrows) in the midst of normal hematopoeisis.

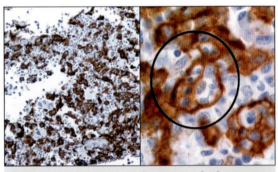

Figure 2 Bone marrow biopsy (CD163, ×200 [left] and ×1000 [right]) showing that numerous histiocytes are highlighted, some of which have phagocytosed hematopoietic cells (circle).

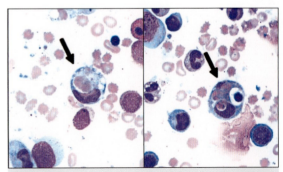

Figure 3 Bone marrow aspirate smear (Wright-Giemsa, ×500) showing histiocytes with phagocytosed red cells and lymphocytes (arrows).

patients are given a combination therapy with dexamethasone, cyclosporine A, and etoposide for the first 8 weeks. Children younger than 1 year in whom genetic HLH is likely, patients with severe signs and symptoms and patients with relapse are candidates for maintenance therapy until hematopoietic progenitor cell transplantation (HPCT). This is irrespective of the identification of an infectious organism (exception: leishmaniasis). In nonfamilial disease, treatment is discontinued after 8 weeks if the disease responds (marked by normalization of blood counts and other lab parameters and absence of fever). Children have to be followed for signs of progression, which include new CNS symptoms. Intrathecal therapy with methotrexate is recommended in patients with a persistent involvement of CSF after 2 weeks. Antithymocyte globulin, drugs directed at TNF-α, anti-CD25 antibody daclizumab, and anti-CD52 antibody alemtuzumab have been tried for nonresponders. Before these therapies the median survival was <2 months in 1980s. Etoposide and allogeneic HPCT have improved the prognosis to an estimated 3-year survival of 55%. This patient was treated with dexamethasone, cyclosporine A and etoposide as well as intrathecal therapy with methotrexate. This was followed by HPCT from an unrelated donor. She has made a complete hematologic recovery.

General Discussion HLH is caused by a variety of etiologies. The common denominator appears to be a resultant functional or inherited defect in cytotoxic lymphocyte function. This may be related to viral infections, rheumatic diseases or other malignancies (such as certain T-cell lymphomas), and inherited defects in perforin and other cytotoxic T and NK cell associated proteins. While erythrophagocytosis and/or lymphophagocytosis are present on bone marrow and/or tissue biopsy evaluations, its presence is neither required nor sufficient alone for establishing a diagnosis. Specific diagnosis is established by meeting a number of established laboratory criteria in the right clinical setting as listed below, with diagnosis usually made if 5 of these 8 criteria are met
– Fever
– Splenomegaly
– Cytopenias ≥2 cell lines (hemoglobin <9.0 g/dL [below 4 weeks <12.0 g/dL], platelet <100 × 10^3/μL, neutrophils <1 × 10^3/μL)
– Hypertriglyceridemia (fasting level ≥3 mmol/L) and/or hypofibrinogenemia (<150 mg/dL)
– Ferritin ≥500 ng/mL
– Soluble IL2 receptor (sCD 25) ≥2,400 U/mL
– Decreased or absent NK-cell activity
– Hemophagocytosis in bone marrow, CSF, or lymph nodes

In addition, diagnosis may be established if a known hereditary or familial form is present in the family. Prolonged fever and hepatosplenomegaly are usual findings at presentation. Less frequently lymphadenopathy or icterus is seen. Neurological signs are seen in up to a third of the patients. Chest radiographs may show interstitial opacities, pulmonary edema and pleural effusions. Ascites, thickening of the gall bladder wall and enlargement of kidneys are frequent findings on abdominal ultrasonography. Anemia and thrombocytopenia are early signs. Leukopenia is seen in about ⅓ and leukocytosis in about ¼ of the children. Elevated bilirubin (mostly conjugated) and lactate dehydrogenase can also be seen. CSF reveals slight pleocytosis and/or moderately increased protein content in more than half of the patients, including 40% of those who do not have neurological features clinically. The histological picture is indistinguishable in genetic and acquired forms. Characteristic histologic findings include diffuse infiltration with T-lymphocytes and cytologically bland histiocytes. Hemophagocytosis may be seen in biopsies of the liver, spleen, lymph nodes, bone marrow, and central nervous system. Practically no organ is spared, but not all tissues may show hemophagocytosis in all patients and the amount of hemophagocytosis is not directly related to symptoms or disease severity. Atrophy of the lymphoid tissues may be seen. The histiocytes express typical markers for macrophages (CD68, CD163), and CD1a and S 100. Bone marrow is usually normocellular to hypercellular; with marked increase in erythropoiesis, and moderate reticulocytosis indicative of ineffective erythropoiesis. Liver involvement is in the form of a chronic hepatitis-like pattern with portal lymphohistiocytic infiltrates. A prominent loss of intrahepatic bile ducts may be seen. The hallmark of HLH is impaired or absent function of natural killer (NK) cells and cytotoxic T lymphocytes (CTL). HLH is characterized by high levels of cytokines such as interferon γ (INF-γ), interleukin (IL)-6, IL-8, IL-10, IL-12, IL-18, tumor necrosis factor α (TNF-α) and macrophage inflammatory protein (MIP 1-α). These cytokines are most likely secreted by activated T lymphocytes, monocytes/macrophages and endothelial cells. Other good markers for disease activity include the α chain of the soluble IL-2 receptor (sCD25), soluble CD95- ligand (sCD95-L) and β-2 microglobulin.

Case 20: Alveolar Rhabdomyosarcoma

Kathryn Foucar, Bakhirev A

Differential Diagnosis Neoplasm primary in the foot or metastatic with paraneoplastic inflammatory syndrome (eg, acute myeloid or lymphoblastic leukemia, lymphoma, sarcoma), systemic inflammatory process (ie, polymyositis), osseous tuberculosis or environmental fungal infection (ie, *Coccidioides immitis*).

Additional Work-Up X-ray and MRI of the foot: soft tissue mass in the foot encircling metatarsal bone with abnormal signal from bone marrow of metatarsal and middle cuneiform bones, suspicious of neoplastic process. Histologic examination of the foot mass biopsy revealed large aggregates and nests of neoplastic cells separated by fibrovascular septa (**Figure 1A**). The neoplastic cells stained negative with CD45 (**Figure 1B**) but positive with desmin (**Figure 1C**) and myogenin (**Figure 1D**). Bone marrow biopsy examination revealed effacement of architecture with extensive infiltration by neoplastic cells (**Figures 2A** and **2B**). A loose clustering of neoplastic cells was noted on the touch preparations and aspirate smears. Morphologically, the neoplastic cells had hyperchromatic nuclei and high N:C ratio and some had cytoplasmic vacuoles (**Figures 2C** and **2D**).

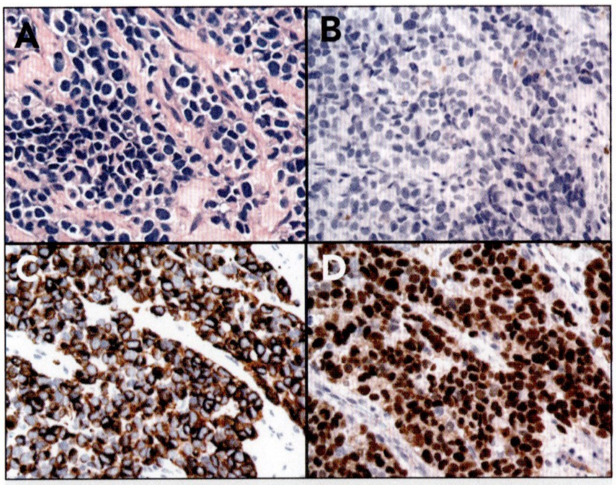

Figure 1 Foot mass biopsy **A** (H&E, ×400) showing neoplastic cells in aggregates and nests separated by fibrovascular septa; **B** (CD45, ×400) showing a negative reaction; **C** (desmin, ×400) showing positivity; **D** (myogenin, ×400) showing positivity.

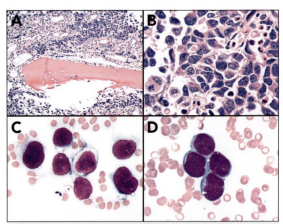

Figure 2 Bone marrow biopsy **A** (H&E, ×200) and **B** (H&E, ×1000) showing neoplastic cells extensively infiltrating and effacing bone marrow. **C** Touch preparation and **D** aspirate smear (Wright, ×1000) showing mononuclear "blast" cells with occasional cytoplasmic vacuoles. On high magnification the neoplastic cells exhibit loose clustering, hyperchromatic round to irregular nuclei with high nuclearcytoplasmic ratio, moderate amount of cytoplasm, and little evidence of differentiation.

Final Diagnosis Extensive bone marrow involvement by metastatic tumor, morphologically compatible with alveolar rhabdomyosarcoma.

Management Approach Management is often a multidisciplinary approach in these patients and dictated by an anatomical site of the primary tumor and risk category based on staging and histology. Therapy options include local surgical excision, radiation, and a main treatment modality—chemotherapy. Combination of vincristine and dactinomycin (VA protocol) or addition of cyclophosphamide (VAC protocol) has often been used. This patient was enrolled in a high-risk group rhabdomyosarcoma treatment protocol with intensive multiagent therapy (ifosfamide/etoposide [IE] and vincristine/doxorubicin/cyclophosphamide [VDC]) and radiation to the primary foot and metastatic sites. A follow-up bone marrow biopsy demonstrated no residual malignancy in the bone marrow space and primary and metastatic sites have shown reduction in size during treatment.

General Discussion Alveolar rhabdomyosarcoma (ARMS) mostly occurs in children, generally before 10 years of age. Although infrequent, these tumors can present in a manner resembling leukemia due to an extensive involvement of the bone marrow at presentation, if the primary lesion is clinically occult. Similarly, involved lymph nodes can closely mimic malignant lymphoma. Differentiation between metastatic ARMS and hematopoietic malignancy is crucial because they have different treatment modalities. When available, a timely flow cytometric analysis displaying an absence of hematopoietic markers can help in directing to a correct work-up, although reported expression of CD56 in some cases may be misleading for the diagnostician. A search of the literature in the past 2 decades revealed a number of cases where metastatic ARMS has been misdiagnosed as acute myeloid or lymphoblastic leukemia, undifferentiated leukemia, and non-Hodgkin lymphoma. Immunohistochemistry is invaluable in distinguishing primary hematolymphoid neoplasms from ARMS. In addition, ARMS often displays its characteristic cytogenetic translocation (ie, t(2;13)(q35;q14)), which can be shown with conventional karyotyping on fresh tissue or fluorescence in situ hybridization (FISH) on fresh and paraffin-embedded tissues. Although less common, t(1;13)(p21;q14) has been reported in small percent of ARMS cases. Prognosis depends on multiple factors, including age at presentation, anatomic site of involvement, systemic spread of the disease, and morphologic subtype, and given this patient's presentation, prognosis is relatively poor in this case.

Case 21: Human Granulocytic Ehrlichiosis

Amy Gewirtz

Differential Diagnosis Based on clinical presentation and the finding of pancytopenia, diagnostic considerations included active infection and myelosuppression secondary to immunosuppression medication. The immunosuppression medications were temporarily discontinued while an infectious disease consultation was obtained.

Additional Work-Up Review of the blood smear at admission demonstrated intracellular inclusions within the granulocytes suggestive of *Ehrlichia* species (**Figure 1**). Additional clinical history obtained at this time revealed that 3 weeks prior to clinical presentation the patient found a tick on the back of his neck. Antibody studies for *Ehrlichia* were negative. PCR studies were positive for *Ehrlichia ewingii/canis* and negative for *Ehrlichia chaffeensis* and *Anaplasma phagocytophilum*.

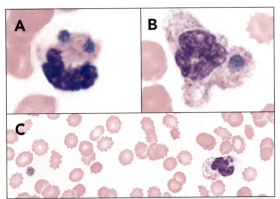

Figure 1 Blood smear (Wright, ×1000) demonstrating the classic intracytoplasmic inclusions of *Ehrlichia*. Compare the morphology of the morula in **C** to the platelet present to the left.

Final Diagnosis Human granulocytic ehrlichiosis.

Management Approach Treatment is doxycycline (100 mg twice a day for 10-14 days). Typically defervescence of fever is noted within 24 hours of the initiation of therapy and resolution of the cytopenias within 2-3 days. This patient was started on doxycycline. Within 5 days his white count had reached $7.1 \times 10^3/\mu L$ with filgrastim support and platelets increased to $65.0 \times 10^3/\mu L$. The immunocompromised status of this patient likely contributed to the marked leukopenia and clinical decision to administer filgrastim.

General Discussion This patient's history is typical for infection by human granulocytic ehrlichiosis. Ehrlichiosis is a tick-borne illness caused by obligate intracellular gram-negative bacteria. They are coccobacilli and have tropism for infecting leukocytes (lymphocytes, monocytes or granulocytes depending on the species) as they propagate most efficiently within cytoplasmic vacuoles. Microcolonies consisting of clusters of the organism which are termed morulae then form within the vacuoles. The leukocytes then undergo lysis allowing the release of bacteria to infect other cells within the body. The typical clinical presentation of a case of acute human ehrlichiosis is 1 of fever, headache and myalgias. The median incubation time is 9 days. Gastrointestinal disturbances as was noted in this patient are uncommon. The laboratory findings include cytopenias, particularly leukopenia and thrombocytopenia as well as increased levels of hepatic enzymes such as AST and ALT and occasionally a mild bilirubinemia. Morphologic identification of the organism on blood smear review typically reveals the characteristic cytoplasmic leukocyte inclusions. Depending on the ehrlichial species typically only granulocytes or mononuclear cells (lymphocytes and monocytes) are infected in a given patient. The morulae appear dark blue and may show purplish granules (representing individual organisms) on Wright-stained samples. By gram stain they are pink. The morphologic differential diagnosis includes a platelet overlying the white blood cell and Döhle bodies. Definitive laboratory diagnosis rests on the ability to detect ehrlichial DNA or RNA utilizing PCR on a blood sample. While serologic studies can also be used, both acute and convalescent titers must be drawn with demonstration of a 4-fold rise in antibody production to establish serologic evidence of infection. Immunocompromised patients may not be able to mount an antibody response rendering serologic testing much less sensitive and valuable as a confirmatory test compared to molecular diagnostic methods (as occurred in this case).

Case 22: Factor VIII Deficiency

Steven E McKenzie, Douglass Drelich

Differential Diagnosis Diagnostic considerations from clinical standpoint included hip hemorrhage, thigh hemorrhage, other soft tissue hemorrhage, appendicitis, and a tumor.

Additional Work-Up The WBC count was $6.8 \times 10^3/\mu L$, with normal differential. A factor VIII level drawn before infusion of factor VIII was <1 IU/dL and no inhibitor was detected. ALT 66 IU/L, AST 58 IU/L, and total bilirubin 1.4 mg/dL.

An ultrasound exam of the right lower quadrant, hip and thigh showed no evidence of appendicitis or hip joint hemorrhage. A $5 \times 3 \times 4$ cm mass in the right iliopsoas muscle was identified, with characteristics consistent with hemorrhage.

Final Diagnosis (1) Severe Factor VIII deficiency with right iliopsoas muscle hemorrhage. (2) Hepatitis C, chronic active, failed antiviral therapy.

Management Approach The patient received recombinant factor VIII product IV at a dose of 40 U/kg, with a goal peak factor VIII level of 80 IU-100 IU/dL. Treatment was repeated 8 hours later, and then at 25 U/kg every 12 hours thereafter for 7 days. After the 4th dose, trough and peak factor VIII values were measured at 50 IU/dL and 102 IU/dL, respectively. He also received analgesia with opiate medication, transitioned to ibuprofen. Initially he was placed on bed rest, which was liberalized to walking with crutches as the pain improved and his HGB (measured daily) dropped only slightly to 11.2 g/dL. Physical examination showed reduction in tenderness and improved range of motion. Follow-up at the Hemophilia Treatment Center, for consideration of resumption of prophylactic factor replacement, and with hepatology for imaging of the liver and evaluation of AFP levels, was arranged pre-discharge home. He was counseled to use an initial dose of factor replacement treatment at home by self-infusion in the event of new onset pain in or near a joint, or with trauma.

General Discussion Severe factor VIII deficiency (Hemophilia A) and severe factor IX deficiency (Hemophilia B) are X-linked disorders in which the affected patient has no detectable factor protein, reported as <1 IU/dL. Patients are at risk for spontaneous hemorrhage, traumatic hemorrhage, and excessive hemorrhage with invasive medical/surgical procedures. The PTT is markedly prolonged and specific factor assays are necessary. Up to 30% of patients may develop an IgG antibody inhibitor of the missing factor and its replacement product, necessitating approaches to bypass the inhibitor with activated prothrombin complex concentrates or recombinant factor VIIa. The inhibitors can also be approached with immune tolerance induction regimens. While severe hemophiliacs can bleed at mucosal surfaces such as the mouth and GI tract and into vital organs such as the brain, there is also a marked tendency for joint and muscle bleeding events. The hip/thigh area and the lower abdominal quadrants along with the retroperitoneum can be very challenging to diagnose and treat. Bleeding into large muscles such as the iliopsoas or thigh can cause massive loss of blood internally that can cause severe anemia and shock, unless the correct diagnosis is made and appropriate therapy initiated. This case also illustrates 2 points about hemophilia: (a) following the patient response and monitoring factor levels during therapy are essential for major bleeding episodes, and (b) much of modern hemophilia care has been influenced by the occurrence of blood-borne infections such as HIV and hepatitis C. Current approaches are to find long-acting forms of recombinant factors, possibly administered subcutaneously or intranasally; to explore novel gene therapy approaches, many of which have been or are in clinical trials; and to find better tolerated and more effective treatments for HIV and hepatitis C while we await vaccines.

Case 23: Factor VIII Inhibitor

Amy Gewirtz

Differential Diagnosis A prolonged PTT, which did not correct with PTT-mix suggests the presence of an inhibitor, which may be factor-specific or lupus-like.

Additional Work-Up
- Fibrinogen 263 mg/dL (normal 220-410)
- Thrombin time (seconds) 15.1 (normal 13-20)
- DRVVT (seconds) 34.4 (normal 30-42)
- StaClot LA negative
- Anticardiolipin IgG (GPL units) 12.6 (normal 0-15)
- Anticardiolipin IgM (MPL units) 8.1 (normal 0-12)
- Factor VIII activity (%) <1
- Factor VIII inhibitor (Bethesda units [BU]) 12,800

Lymph node biopsy demonstrated reactive lymphoid hyperplasia with changes most consistent with Castleman disease, hyaline vascular type.

Final Diagnosis Acquired factor VIII inhibitor in association with Castleman disease.

Management Approach Treatment is initially aimed to stop ongoing bleeding utilizing therapeutic agents that bypass the need for factor VIII and contain factors VIIa, II, IX and X (prothrombin complex concentrates). At the same time immunosuppression to stop the production of the autoantibody is initiated. In cases which are idiopathic, approximately 1/3 will have spontaneous disappearance of the antibody over a period of many months or even years. This patient was initially placed on oral prednisone while the work-up was being completed and then placed on recombinant factor VIIa and prednisone. At discharge the recombinant factor VIIa was replaced with anti-inhibitor coagulant complex (FEIBA) as needed for control on hemorrhagic episodes. The patient had minimal response to the prednisone so approximately 1 month later cyclophosphamide was added. 2 months later, due to lack of response, the prednisone and cyclophosphamide were discontinued and rituximab therapy was initiated. Due to continued difficulty in reducing the factor VIII inhibitor, different immunosuppressive agents have been used over time, including the reinitiation of prednisone, cyclophosphamide and the addition of cyclosporine and azathioprine. Over the next year, the lowest titer of factor VIII inhibitor present was 1,442 Bethesda units, with the most recent being 3,700 Bethesda units. She has continued to suffer several deep tissue acute bleeding episodes in various locations, including her arm, breast and most recently the right thigh.

General Discussion Acquired factor inhibitors are uncommon. They most commonly occur secondary to repeated exposure to factor supplementation in association with therapy for a hereditary factor deficiency such as hemophilia as an alloantibody. The spontaneous development of a factor VIII inhibitor (also termed acquired hemophilia A) occurs usually in previously healthy elderly individuals but may be associated with pregnancy/postpartum, and the presence of other autoimmune disorders. Rarely their development is associated with a lymphoproliferative disorder as noted in this case. The bleeding presentation in cases due to the spontaneous development of a factor VIII inhibitor is different than that in association with factor VIII antibodies that occur in individuals with hemophilia A. Hereditary factor VIII deficiency classically presents with hemarthroses. In patients with acquired factor VIII deficiency due to a factor inhibitor, the bleeding presentation is typically deep seated tissue bleeds, ecchymoses, gastrointestinal bleeding and intracerebral bleeding. Most coagulation factor antibodies are IgG in nature and are termed neutralizing antibodies as they interfere with the procoagulant activity of the factor. Infrequently factor-specific antibodies simply bind to the factor and result in clearance of that specific factor through the spleen in a manner similar to other antigen-antibody complexes. Most patients with factor specific inhibitors present with bleeding. The laboratory work-up for the bleeding patient includes PT, PTT and platelet count along with a thorough history. The presence of an unexplained prolongation of the PT or PTT warrants a mixing study with normal plasma to be performed. If the mixing study corrects the previously abnormal value, a factor(s) deficiency is favored. Typically the PTT for the mixing study is read immediately and following incubation for an hour at 37°C. In the absence of a correction, the presence of a circulating inhibitor is favored. Most commonly the inhibitor is of a lupus type, which typically is an antiphospholipid antibody. Lupus inhibitors do not have to occur in association with lupus and paradoxically these individuals do not bleed but are at risk for thrombosis. If a factor specific inhibitor is suspected appropriate factor assays are performed based on whether the PT, PTT or both are prolonged. Once the factor specificity of the inhibitor is determined, the amount of inhibitor is expressed in Bethesda units. A Bethesda unit is the amount of antibody that will inhibit 50% of the factor activity. The patient plasma is diluted to demonstrate a residual activity of between 25% and 75% and then multiplied by that dilution to determine the Bethesda units.

Case 24: von Willebrand Disease, Type 3

Roy Smith, Rushir Choksi

Differential Diagnosis Initial presentation with a facial hematoma and a family history of VWD, placed the presence of a deficiency of von Willebrand factor (VWF) at the top of our differential diagnosis for this patient. Another possibility would be hemophilia A.

Additional Work-Up Factor VIII collagen binding assay (FVIII:CB) showed a level of 0.02 units/mL (normal 0.5-0.2 U/mL).

Final Diagnosis von Willebrand disease, type 3.

Management Approach Patients with VWD, type 3 lack VWF and need replacement with a factor VIII concentrate which contain VWF. In the case of VWD type 3 patients with known inhibitors, recombinant factor VIII (rFVIIIa) concentrate, which does not contain VWF or recombinant FVIIa (rFVIIa) concentrate is indicated. This patient did receive additional factor VIII concentrate upon presentation of his gastrointestinal bleed and he responded very well. His gastrointestinal bleeding subsided and he was placed on a maintenance dose of factor VIII concentrate.

General Discussion von Willebrand factor is a multimeric protein which has 2 primary properties: (1) it serves as the carrier protein for factor VIII procoagulant (FVIII:C) and (2) it mediates adhesion of platelets to sites of vascular injury. There are 3 major types of VWD: type 1, which is a partial quantitative deficiency of VWF, type 2, which is a qualitative defect of VWF and can be divided into 4 subtypes (2A, 2B, 2M, and 2N), and type 3, which is a total deficiency of VWF and its apparent characteristics (FVIII:C; VWF:RCo; VWF:Ag). VWD type 1 is a partial deficiency of VWF. It usually has an autosomal dominant inheritance pattern with variable penetrance, and is the most common type of VWD accounting for approximately 70% of the reported cases. The prevalence is not known precisely as many people have asymptomatic VWD, but is thought to be approximately 1%. Patients usually present with mild bleeding, most commonly epistaxis, prolonged bleeding from trivial wounds, oral cavity bleeding and excessive menstrual bleeding. Some of the tests specific for VWD include functional tests such as VWF:RCo or the less commonly available VWF:collagen binding (CB). VWF:Ag and FVIII:C levels are also measured. The extreme range of normal VWF levels can complicate the diagnosis of VWD type 1 and the diagnosis should incorporate the patient's clinical picture. FVIII:C, VWF:RCo (or VWF:CB) and VWF:Ag should be proportionally decreased in VWF type 1. Patients with blood type O inherently have lower levels of VWF:Ag and VWF:RCo at baseline and may be mislabeled as VWD if that is not taken into account. VWD type 1 can be caused by nonsense mutations, deletions or frameshifts. There is also evidence that quantitative VWD can be caused by mutations that result in an increased clearance of VWF from the blood. Treatment is usually desmopressin (1-desamino-8-D-arginine vasopressin; DDAVP) and if patients don't respond appropriately then a concentrate of plasma-derived FVIII concentrate containing a large amount of VWF, such as Humate-P Alphanate or Koate DVI, may be needed. In the United States, only Humate-P and Alphanate are FDA approved for the treatment of patients with VWD. The hemostatic properties of VWF include its propensity to assemble into large multimeric configurations and the presence of functional binding sites to surface ligands on connective tissue and platelets. Mutations that disrupt any of these functions lead to VWD type 2, which accounts for 7%-30% of all VWD. Decreased function of VWF with preserved VWF:Ag quantity leads to discrepancies between the level of VWF:Ag and functional assays such as VWF:RCo or VWF:CB. A ratio of VWF:RCo or VWF:CB to VWF:Ag <0.6 or 0.7 (depending on the study) is considered abnormal and VWD type 2 should be considered. There are 4 different subtypes of VWD type 2 depending on the defect: type 2A, 2B, 2M, and 2N. The VWD type 2A occurs when there is a disruption of the normal assembly of large VWF multimers. There is a disproportionately low VWF:RCo or VWF:CB relative to

VWF:Ag. VWD type 2A accounts for most of the reported cases categorized as VWD type 2. It occurs with single amino acid substitutions resulting in the absence of large VWF multimers by impairing intracellular assembly of multimers or by increasing proteolysis of VWF. A disintegrin and metalloprotease with thrombospondin type 1 motif 13 (ADAMTS13) normally cleaves plasma VWF. A pathological increase in its activity can cause acquired VWD type 2A characterized by loss of the large VWF multimers in plasma. Platelet VWF multimers are physiologically protected from the effect of ADAMTS 13. The decrease in large molecular weight VWF multimers on the platelet surface in VWD type 2A may be caused by either impaired assembly or ADAMTS13-mediated proteolysis. The different etiologies of VWD type 2A cannot be distinguished clinically and are treated the same. Some patients respond to DDAVP and using a test dose can identify these patients. If they do not respond, Humate-P (or an alternative factor VIII concentrate which contains a large amount of VWF) may be required for the treatment of bleeding or in preparation for invasive procedures. Another property of VWF multimers is that they bind to platelets and have an increased affinity for platelets. VWD type 2B is characterized by the spontaneous binding of large VWF multimers to platelets, followed by destruction of these multimers with a variable decrease in platelet count. The remaining multimers are small and are not as effective in hemostasis leading to discordance between the amount of bleeding and the VWF:RCo or VWF:CB activities. The initial laboratory tests can be confusing in that they can be similar to those found with other types of VWD. VWF:RCo can be disproportionately more decreased than VWF:Ag, which can look like VWD type 2A. Also, although less common, a decrease in both VWF:RCo and VWF:Ag may suggest VWD type 1. Electrophoresis gels multimeric analysis cannot distinguish between VWD type 2A and 2B since both subtypes lack large multimers of VWF. However, a ristocetin-induced platelet aggregation (RIPA) test is useful for this purpose. When ristocetin is added to normal platelet-rich plasma (PRP), there is a dose response effect of ristocetin on the degree of platelet aggregation as detected in a platelet aggregometer. In contrast, when low concentrations of ristocetin are added to PRP from patients with VWD type 2B, the platelet aggregation response is enhanced relative to that seen in control PRP. In patients with VWD type 2A, high concentrations of ristocetin are needed to achieve an aggregatory response. Intermittent mild thrombocytopenia is also characteristic of VWD type 2B and can be worsened if patients are given DDAVP. Only in rare circumstances, is DDAVP effective. Platelet transfusions are not usually helpful. These patients should receive Humate-P in most incidences. VWD type 2M ("M" for multimer) is a disorder where the VWF multimers are preserved, but there is impaired binding of the multimers to platelets or connective tissue. For example, there are many reports of impaired binding of VWF multimers to platelet GP1b. In laboratory assays, the results look similar to VWD type 2A, but VWF multimer gel electrophoresis shows that the large multimers are preserved. These patients are treated similarly to patients with VWD type 2A. A disruption of the binding of FVIII:C to VWF is characteristic of VWD type 2N, an autosomal recessive disorder. This is caused by missense mutations that inactivate the FVIII:C binding site on the von Willebrand protein. FVIII:C levels are usually <10 IU per dL. The clinical laboratory findings often mimic hemophilia A. The other properties of VWF are preserved and therefore the patient will have normal VWF:RCo (or VWF:CB), VWF:Ag, RIPA and multimeric analysis. The diagnosis is made by establishing decreased binding for FVIII:C in a VWF:FVIII binding assay. In contrast to patients with hemophilia A, patients with VWD type 2N do not benefit from rFVIII concentrates. (They do not contain VWF). Also, these patients usually will not benefit from DDAVP. Humate-P (or other factor VIII concentrate which contains large amounts of VWF, such as Alphanate or Koate-DVI) is needed. VWD type 3 is a recessive disorder in which the VWF protein is almost absent. These patients have a combined defect of both platelet adhesion and blood clotting. FVIII:C, VWF:RCo (or VWF:CB) and VWF:Ag are undetectable (<10%). There is also an elevated PTT as a result of the secondary deficiency of FVIII:C. Heterozygous patients usually are phenotypically normal, but can also have mild bleeding and can be confused with VWD type 1. VWD type 3 is caused by nonsense, deletion, and frameshift mutations with a prevalence in the United States and Canada of approximately 1.5 per million people. DDAVP has no effect in patients with VWD type 3 and Humate-P or alternative VWF containing factor VIII concentrates should be used. Transfusion of platelets from a normal donor pool can be considered in patients who are actively bleeding since it is presumed that normal platelets carry a substantial concentration of VWF. 3%-10% of patients with VWF type 3 may develop alloantibody inhibitors to VWF. If VWD type 3 patients with these inhibitors are transfused with FVIII concentrations containing VWF, severe allergic reactions can occur (anaphylaxis, abdominal pain or hypotension). These patients should be treated with rFVIII concentrate (which do not contain VWF) or FVIIa concentrate.

Section N: Discussion of Self-Study Cases

Case 25: Antiphospholipid Antibody Syndrome

Douglass A Drelich, Steven McKenzie

Differential Diagnosis Diagnostic considerations included factor deficiency (VIII, IX, XI, or XII), von Willebrand disease, lupus anticoagulant, and an artifactual error.

Additional Work-Up Repeat PT was 11.2 seconds and repeat PTT was 54.3 seconds. Coagulation tests are extremely sensitive to underfilling of the test tube leading to an excess of anticoagulant to blood in the tube. However, the normal PT and repeatedly abnormal PTT argue against this. PTT mix was 46 seconds. The failure of the PTT to correct on 1:1 mix with normal plasma suggested an inhibitor rather than a factor deficiency. The possibility of a lupus anticoagulant was considered. The lupus anticoagulant may or may not be associated with the antiphospholipid antibody syndrome. Dilute Russell viper venom test (DRVVT) was prolonged at 52.4 sec (normal 27.1-39.7). DRVVT mix was 48.4 sec. The addition of excess phospholipid to the DRVVT showed a confirmatory time of 38.4 sec. Assays for anti-cardiolipin antibodies were negative. However, antibodies to b2-glycoprotein showed an IgM of 94 units (upper limit of normal is 17).

Final Diagnosis Likely antiphospholipid antibody syndrome (APS).

Management Approach Menorrhagia in the setting of a prolonged PTT can suggest a work-up for a bleeding disorder. However, in this patient there was a defined anatomic abnormality suggesting an etiology of the menorrhagia. In addition to this there were no signs or symptoms in other areas suggestive of a systemic bleeding disorder. Of additional note, she has a history of DVT and had previously tolerated 6 months of therapy with coumadin without excessive bleeding. In this case the patient does not represent an increased risk of surgical bleeding. In fact, she may paradoxically represent an increased risk of perioperative thrombosis. The brief car trip she had undertaken previously was not of adequate length to confidently consider that a "provoked" event. In addition she has had 2 pregnancy losses after 10 weeks of gestation. Either of these would be adequate to fulfill the diagnostic criteria of antiphospholipid antibody syndrome. If the laboratory evidence of APS was repeatedly present 12 weeks later the diagnosis would be confirmed. In this patient, a strong argument could be made for indefinite duration of anticoagulation as the recurrence rate for thrombotic events can be as high as 20%-30%. In the setting of surgery she should have meticulous attention to DVT prophylaxis optimally with the use of a low molecular weight heparin (LMWH).

General Discussion The antiphospholipid antibody syndrome is a clinical entity defined as the presence of a thrombotic event or pregnancy morbidity coupled with the persistent presence of laboratory evidence of either a lupus anticoagulant or anticardiolipin antibodies or antibodies to b2-glycoprotein in moderate to high titers. The presence of a lupus anticoagulant is a functional determination and requires 3 criteria to be met. The first is the prolongation of a phospholipid dependent clotting time such as the activated partial thromboplastin time (PTT), the dilute Russell viper venom time (DRVVT), the kaolin clotting time (KCT), or uncommonly, the prothrombin time (PT). Secondly, this prolongation should fail to correct in a 1:1 mix with normal plasma. Thirdly, this prolongation should correct on the addition of excess phospholipid. The laboratory criteria should be present on testing greater then 12 weeks apart. Persons with APS have a high rate of recurrent events. Intriguingly, people with arterial events tend to have arterial recurrence and people with venous events tend to have venous recurrence. Due to the high rate of recurrence the standard approach in patients diagnosed with APS is anticoagulation with a vitamin K antagonist of indefinite duration.

Clinical and Laboratory Criteria for APS

Antiphospholipid antibody syndrome (APS) is present if at least 1 of the clinical criteria and 1 of the laboratory criteria that follow are met.

Clinical criteria

- Vascular thrombosis. One or more episodes of arterial, venous, or small vessel thrombosis, in any tissue or organ. Thrombosis must be confirmed by objective validated criteria
- Pregnancy morbidity, includes any of the following: (a) one or more unexplained deaths of a morphologically normal fetus at or beyond the 10th week of gestation, with normal fetal morphology; (b) one or more premature births of a morphologically normal neonate before the 34th week of gestation because of eclampsia or severe preeclampsia defined according to standard definitions or recognized features of placental insufficiency; (c) 3 or more unexplained consecutive spontaneous abortions before the 10th week of gestation, with maternal anatomic or hormonal abnormalities and paternal and maternal chromosomal causes excluded

Laboratory criteria

- Lupus anticoagulant (LA) present in plasma, on 2 or more occasions at least 12 weeks apart
- Anticardiolipin (ACL) antibody of IgG and/or IgM isotype in serum or plasma, present in medium or high titer (ie, >40 GPL or MPL, or >the 99th percentile), on 2 or more occasions, at least 12 weeks apart
- Anti-b2 glycoprotein-I antibody of IgG and/or IgM isotype in serum or plasma (in titer >the 99th percentile), present on 2 or more occasions, at least 12 weeks apart

Case 26: Heparin-Induced Thrombocytopenia, Type II

Amy Gewirtz

Differential Diagnosis Sepsis vs heparin-induced thrombocytopenia, type II.

Additional Work-Up Heparin-induced thrombocytopenia platelet aggregation studies were positive (**Figures 1**, **2**, and **3**).

Final Diagnosis Heparin-induced-thrombocytopenia (HIT), type II.

Management Approach In cases of suspected heparin-induced thrombocytopenia the first and most critical step is to discontinue all sources of heparin, including heparin flushes, and list heparin as an "allergy" for the patient. In patients where the clinical need for anticoagulation is still felt necessary, an alternative form of anticoagulation such as a direct thrombin inhibitor should be considered. This patient received argatoban and the platelet count began to rise back to normal levels 2 days following cessation of heparin therapy (**Table**).

Day	Platelet Count (×10/μL)
Day of Admission	437
10 days later	393
11 days later	175
12 days later	173
13 days later	118
14 days later – heparin discontinued	103
15 days later	105
16 days later	154
17 days later	250
18 days later	294
19 days later	414

General Discussion Heparin therapy is associated with thrombocytopenia through 2 distinct mechanisms: HIT type I (nonimmune) and HIT type II (immune). The nonimmune thrombocytopenia is idiopathic and typically occurs within the first few days of heparin therapy, and platelet levels typically do not reach below $100 \times 10^3/\mu L$. The immune form of HIT typically begins 5-10 days following heparin exposure with platelet counts typically falling below $100 \times 10^3/\mu L$. This form of HIT may or may not be associated with thrombosis and thromboembolic complications. The thrombocytopenia is secondary to the formation of IgG antibodies which bind to the heparin-platelet factor 4 (PF4) complex on the surface of the platelet. These antibody coated platelets undergo activation and aggregation and are then cleared by the spleen similar to other circulating antibody-antigen complexes. The incidence of HIT is reported in up to 5% of all patients receiving bovine, unfractionated heparin. This complication is lower with porcine heparin and much lower when fractionated low molecular heparin is used (0.6%). The risk is directly related to higher heparin dosing and longer duration of the heparin therapy. When a clinical suspicion of HIT is present all forms of heparin, including heparin flushes and if possible the removal of heparin-coated catheters is recommended. If indicated an alternative form of anticoagulation should be implemented. It is important to realize that not all patients with a falling platelet count have HIT. In 2003, the "4T score" was introduced to help determine which patients could safely continue to receive heparin therapy in association with a decrease in platelet count. This algorithm takes into account the degree and timing of the thrombocytopenia, the presence of thrombosis, skin necrosis or a system reaction and the possibility of an alternative cause being the etiology of the thrombocytopenia. Laboratory testing for the presence of heparin-PF4 antibodies can then be ordered if clinically indicated. The gold standard laboratory test for the diagnosis of HIT is the serotonin release assay. In this assay the release of 14C-serotonin from normal

Section N: Discussion of Self-Study Cases
Heparin-Induced Thrombocytopenia, Type II

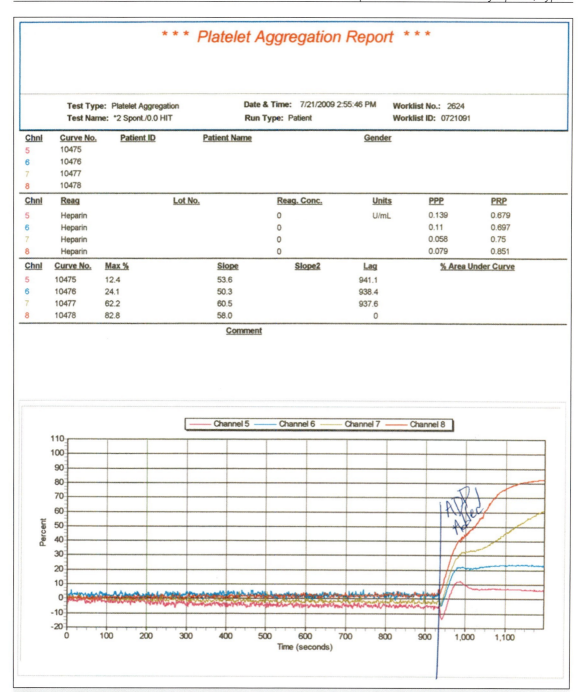

Figure 1 Saline control (0 units of heparin added). Tube 5 (fuchsia line) contains donor 1 plasma and donor 1 platelets. Tube 6 (aqua line) contains patient plasma and donor 1 platelets. Tube 7 (tan line) contains donor 2 plasma and donor 2 platelets. Tube 8 (red line) contains patient plasma and donor 2 platelets. There is no evidence of aggregation; this is a negative control. The additional of ADP at the end demonstrates that the platelets remain viable.

donor platelets that have been incubated with patient plasma and heparin is measured. This is a very specific assay in that a positive assay confirms the presence of HIT although a negative assay does not exclude that diagnostic possibility (high positive predictive value but low negative predictive value due to low sensitivity). As this assay requires the use of a radioisotope it is rarely performed today. Two laboratory tests are more available for the diagnosis of HIT. The first is an ELISA test for the presence of heparin-PF4 antibodies. This test

Section N: Discussion of Self-Study Cases
Heparin-Induced Thrombocytopenia, Type II

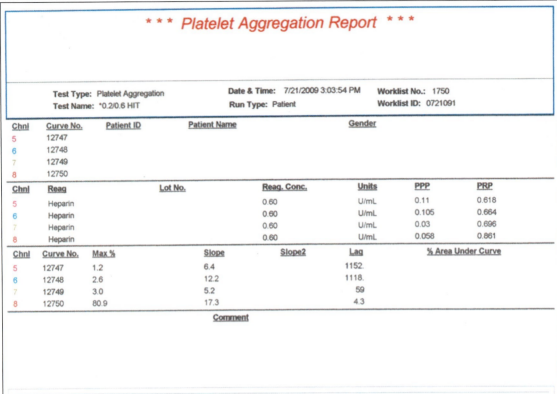

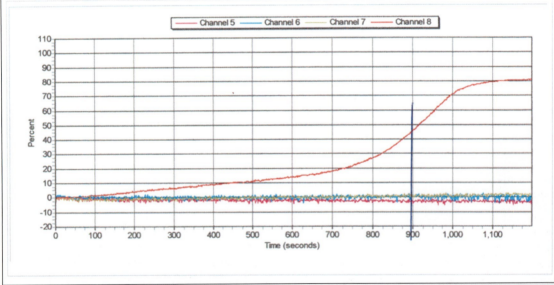

Figure 2 0.8 units of heparin. Tube 5 (fuchsia line) contain donor 1 plasma and donor 1 platelets. Tube 6 (aqua line) contains patient plasma and donor 1 platelets. Tube 7 (tan line) contains donor 2 plasma and donor 2 platelets. Tube 8 (red line) contains patient plasma and donor 2 platelets. 0.8 units of heparin (saline) have been added to each tube. Aggregation is noted in tube 8 with >20% change compared to tube 7.

is often used as a screening test as it is reported to have a relatively higher rate of false positives (due to the ability to detect the formation of heparin-PF4 antibodies secondary to any etiology) compared to the standard confirmatory test for HIT, which is a functional assay that is based on the presence of platelet aggregation in the presence of heparin. This assay may be slightly less sensitive to the ELISA method but is more specific.

Section N: Discussion of Self-Study Cases
Heparin-Induced Thrombocytopenia, Type II

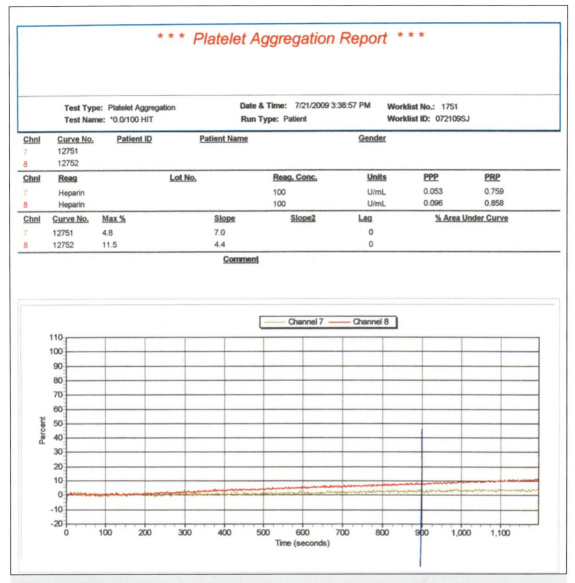

Figure 2 Confirmatory testing with 100 units of heparin added.

The platelet aggregometry testing is performed by creating a platelet-rich sample from donors shown to be reactive to the heparin-PF4 antibodies. Comparison tubes are made from donor platelets and patient plasma suspected to contain heparin-PF4 antibodies as well as donor platelets and donor plasma (devoid of heparin-PF4 antibodies). Heparin is then added to the tubes and an increase in light transmission >20% (reflective of aggregation) is considered to be a positive test in comparing patient to donor plasma. All positive tests are confirmed by adding an excessive amount of heparin (100 μL) to induce a prozone effect, resulting in disappearance of the aggregation previously noted. ADP is added at the end of the assay to ensure that the donor platelets are viable. **Figures 1**, **2** and **3** demonstrate the tracings from a platelet aggregometer utilized in HIT testing. Utilizing the same donor sample that was positive for aggregation with 0.8 units of heparin, there is absence of aggregation and demonstrating the specificity of the reaction to the presence of heparin. Patients who are demonstrated to be HIT positive by laboratory testing or in whom there had been a high clinical suspicion of HIT with a normalization of the platelet count following the cessation of heparin therapy should be told that they should avoid all forms of heparin in the future.

Case 27: Prekallikrein Deficiency

Elizabeth M Van Cott

Differential Diagnosis Heparin prolongs the PTT. The normal PT (and clinical history) excludes other anticoagulants such as warfarin, argatroban, bivalirudin, and hirudin. Deficiencies (or less often, an inhibitor) of factors VIII, IX, XI, XII, prekallikrein, or high-molecular weight kininogen prolong the PTT but not the PT. Lupus anticoagulants sometimes prolong the PTT and, much less often, the PT. If factor VIII is low, possibilities include von Willebrand disease, hemophilia A (factor VIII deficiency) carrier (or for males, hemophilia A), or a factor VIII inhibitor.

Additional Work-Up The PTT was prolonged on repeat testing. The PTT remained prolonged after treating the specimen with heparinase, which degrades heparin. The 2-hour PTT mixing study corrected to normal (24.0 seconds at time 0, and 26.0 seconds at 2 hours), which excluded the possibility of a PTT factor inhibitor. Fibrinogen at 629 mg/dL (normal 150-400) and factor VIII at 266% (normal 50-200) were elevated, which occurs during normal pregnancy. Factors IX at 134% (normal 60-140), XI at 83% (normal 60-140) and XII at 140% (normal 60-140) were normal.

The PTT screening assay (a lupus anticoagulant-sensitive PTT called PTT-LA) was prolonged at 136.9 seconds, correcting to normal in a mixing study. The confirmatory lupus anticoagulant assay (a commercial hexagonal phase phospholipid neutralization assay) was negative, indicating that the laboratory tests are negative for a lupus anticoagulant. Since no explanation for the prolonged PTT had been found, a prekallikrein screen was performed. To perform the prekallikrein screen, the PTT incubation time is extended to 10 minutes, and the result is compared to a PTT performed in the usual manner (3- or 5-minute incubation). A usual PTT is performed by combining the PTT reagent and patient plasma, followed by a 3- or 5-minute incubation at 37°C, followed by addition of calcium. Clotting cannot proceed until calcium is added. The modified PTT is performed by extending the incubation to 10 minutes. If the PTT prolongation is due to prekallikrein, the clotting time shortens to normal or near-normal when the incubation time is extended. The results for this patient are as follows:

Incubation time	5 min	10 min
Normal control	26.3	24.1
Prolonged PTT control	40.5	38.0
Patient	50.4	38.8

The patient's PTT shortened from 50.4 seconds to 38.8 seconds with the prolonged incubation, which was suspicious for prekallikrein deficiency. Therefore, a quantitative prekallikrein activity assay was sent out to a specialized reference laboratory, and the result was low at 15% (normal 65-135). In the meantime, the patient's clinician requested additional assays to assess for possible causes of bleeding. von Willebrand factor antigen and ristocetin cofactor activity were both elevated >200%, which can occur during normal pregnancy, and is not suggestive of von Willebrand disease. She has blood type O. Factors IX and XI activities were normal. A factor XIII screening assay (urea clot solubility) revealed no evidence for a severe factor XIII deficiency. In this case, her bleeding episode was ultimately attributed to placenta previa, with no underlying bleeding diathesis.

Final Diagnosis Prekallikrein deficiency.

Management Approach Prekallikrein deficiency is rare, does not cause bleeding, and does not require treatment. However, knowledge of the diagnosis is essential, because if the cause of the PTT remains unknown, clinicians might transfuse her unnecessarily to correct her prolonged PTT, or they might unnecessarily cancel or delay medically-indicated procedures due to the prolonged PTT.

General Discussion (1) If the PTT is performed with ellagic acid as the intrinsic pathway activator, the PTT will usually be normal in prekallikrein deficiencies.

(2) Another approach to screening for prekallikrein deficiency: Patient plasma is mixed 1:1 with prekallikrein-deficient plasma. The PTT in the mix will remain prolonged if the PTT prolongation is due to prekallikrein deficiency. If the PTT in the mix is normal, then the PTT prolongation is due to something other than prekallikrein deficiency.

(3) With prekallikrein deficiency, sometimes the PTT might correct only partially with the prolonged incubation. For example, a 59-year-old woman was incidentally found to have a prolonged PTT (107 seconds) preoperatively prior to shoulder surgery. Her PTT with 5-minute incubation was 129 seconds, vs 85 seconds after a 10-minute incubation. The quantitative prekallikrein activity assay revealed 6% prekallikrein. The patient also had mildly low factor XII (45%), which apparently explains why the PTT did not correct fully in the 10-minute incubation. The PTT mixing study corrected, factors VIII, IX, XI, high-molecular-weight kininogen, PT, and lupus anticoagulant tests were normal, heparin was not detected, and the patient was not on anticoagulant therapy.

Index

Pages in *italics* represent self-study presentations; pages in ***bold italics*** represent self-study case discussions.

A

Abnormal myelopoiesis, transient, 351
Acanthocytosis, 74
Acquired platelet function defect, 313
Acute graft-vs-host disease, 342
Acute leukemia of ambiguous lineage, 144
Acute lymphoblastic leukemia, 130-141
    B-cell, Ph–, 130
    precursor B, Ph+, in an adult, 141
    precursor B, pediatric, 133
    precursor T, pediatric, 136
    T-cell, in an adult, 139
B-cell acute lymphoblastic leukemia in an adult with t(9;22), 141
Acute myeloid leukemia, 95-125, 445-448/474-479
    blastic plasmacytoid dendritic cell neoplasm, 125, *448*/***479***
    with FLT3/ITD+, *445*/***474***
    with inv(3), 113
    with inv(16), *447*/***477***
    with mutated NPM1, 98
    with t(8;21), 95
    megakaryoblastic leukemia, 116
    monoblastic leukemia, 110
    myeloid sarcoma, *446*/***476***
    myeloid/lymphoid neoplasm with eosinophilia and PDGFRA abnormality, 128
    myelomonocytic leukemia, 104
    panmyelosis with myelofibrosis subtype, 122
    promyelocytic, 101
    therapy-related, 119
    with myelodysplasia-related changes, 107
Acute megakaryoblastic leukemia, 116
Acute monoblastic leukemia, 110
Acute myeloid leukemia, therapy-related, 119
Acute myeloid leukemia, with FLT3/ITD+, *445*/***474***
Acute myeloid leukemia, with inv(3), 113
Acute myeloid leukemia, with inv(16), *447*/***477***
Acute myeloid leukemia with myelodysplasia-related changes, 107
Acute myeloid leukemia, with mutated NPM1, 98
Acute myeloid leukemia, with t(8;21), 95
Acute myelomonocytic leukemia, 104
Acute panmyelosis with myelofibrosis, 122
Acute Ph– lymphoblastic leukemia, 130
Acute Ph+ lymphoblastic leukemia, 141
Acute promyelocytic leukemia, 101

Index

Acute T-lymphoblastic leukemia, 449/481
Acquired factor V inhibitor, 392
Acquired factor X deficiency, 396
Acquired von Willebrand disease, 407
Adult T-cell lymphoma/leukemia, 210
Alloimmune neonatal neutropenia, 334
Alveolar rhabdomyosarcoma involving the bone marrow, 364, 460/**500**
Amyloidosis, primary, 291, 457, **494**
Anaplasmosis, 318, *461,* **502**
Anaplastic large cell lymphoma, *454,* **488**
Anemia, 1-92, 441, 468-444, 473
    aplastic, 76
    associated with acanthocytosis, 74
    associated with B_{12} deficiency, 25
    associated with chronic renal insufficiency, 72
    associated with copper deficiency, 15
    associated with iron deficiency, 1
    associated with fetomaternal hemorrhage, 42
    associated with folate deficiency, 22, *442*/**469**
    associated with G6PD deficiency, 34, *443*/**471**
    associated with hemochromatosis, HFE-associated, 89
    associated with hemochromatosis, non-HFE-associated, 92
    associated with hemoglobin E disease, 17
    associated with hemoglobin H disease, *441*/**468**
    associated with hemoglobin SC disease, 53
    associated with hemolytic disease of the newborn, 39
    associated with hereditary elliptocytosis, 60
    associated with hereditary spherocytosis, 55
    associated with hereditary pyropoikilocytosis, 65
    associated with hypotransferrinemia, 6
    associated with lead poisoning, 10
    associated with liver disease, 68
    associated with methemoglobinemia, 31
    associated with pyruvate kinase deficiency, 36
    associated with renal disease, 72
    associated with sickle-α-thalassemia, 62
    associated with sickle-β-thalassemia, *444*/**473**
    associated with sickle cell anemia, 57, 70
    associated with thalassemia intermedia, 12
    associated with thalassemia major, 8
    associated with thalassemia minor, 4
    autoimmune hemolytic anemia, cold-reactive, 48
    autoimmune hemolytic anemia, warm-reactive, 45
    congenital dyserythropoietic, type II, 82
    congenital sideroblastic anemia, 19
    Diamond-Blackfan anemia, 79
    Donath-Landsteiner hemolytic anemia, 50
    Fanconi anemia with myelodysplastic syndrome, 84
    macrocytic, associated with B_{12} deficiency, 25
    macrocytic, associated with folate deficiency, 22, *442*/**469**
    megaloblastic anemia due to B_{12} deficiency, 25
    pernicious anemia, 28
    pure red cell aplasia, 87

Angioimmunoblastic T-cell lymphoma, 249
Antiphospholipid antibody syndrome, 410, *465*/**508**
Antithrombin deficiency, 416
Aplastic anemia, 76
Atypical chronic myelogenous leukemia, 152
Autoimmune hemolytic anemia, cold-reactive, 48
Autoimmune hemolytic anemia, warm-reactive, 45
Autoimmune thrombocytopenic purpura (immune thrombocytopenic purpura), 300
Autoimmune lymphoproliferative syndrome, 213
Autoimmune neutropenia of childhood, 339

B

B_{12} deficiency-associated macrocytic anemia, 25
Babesiosis, 315
B-acute lymphoblastic leukemia with t(9;22), 141
B-cell acute lymphoblastic leukemia, Ph– in an adult, 130
B-cell prolymphocytic leukemia, 197
β-thalassemia major, 8
Blast phase of chronic myelogenous leukemia, 146
Blastic plasmacytoid dendritic cell neoplasm, 125, *448*, **479**
Blastoid variant of mantle cell lymphoma, *455*/**490**
Borreliosis, 323
Burkitt lymphoma, 236

C

Carcinoma, metastatic, involving bone marrow (primary breast), 367
Castleman disease, 277
Chédiak-Higashi syndrome, 373
Chronic benign neutropenia of childhood, 339
Chronic eosinophilic leukemia, *451*, **484**
    associated with PGFRA rearrangement, *451*/**484**
Chronic graft-vs-host disease, 346
Chronic lymphocytic leukemia (CLL), 192
Chronic lymphoproliferative disorders, 192-213, 453, 487
    adult T-cell lymphoma/leukemia, 210
    autoimmune lymphoproliferative syndrome, 213
    B-prolymphocytic leukemia, 197
    chronic lymphocytic leukemia, 192
    hairy cell leukemia, 199
    post transplant lymphoproliferative disorder, 202
    T-large granular lymphocytic leukemia, 208
    T prolymphocytic leukemia, 205, *453*/**487**
    Richter transformation in CLL, 195
Chronic myelogenous leukemia (CML), 149
Chronic myelogenous leukemia, atypical, 152
Chronic myelogenous leukemia in blast phase, T-cell type, 146

Chronic myelomonocytic leukemia, 189
Chronic myeloproliferative neoplasms, 149,152, 155-162, 168, 170, 450, 451, 482/484
    chronic eosinophilic leukemia, *451*/**484**
    chronic myelogenous leukemia, case 149
    chronic neutrophilic leukemia, 155, *450*/**482**
    essential thrombocythemia, 160
    mastocytosis, systemic 165
    polycythemia, congenital, 168
    polycythemia vera, 158,
    primary myelofibrosis, 162
    unclassifiable (MPN, U), 170
Chronic neutrophilic leukemia, 155, *450*/**482**
Coagulopathy due to cirrhosis, 431
Congenital dyserythropoetic anemia, type II, 82
Congenital dysfibrinogenemia, 435
Congenital polycythemia, 168
Congenital sideroblastic anemia, 19
Copper deficiency associated anemia, 15
Cutaneous T-cell lymphoma, primary, γ/δ type, 255
CYP2C9 genotyping for management of coumadin therapy, 439

D

δ storage pool deficiency, platelet, 309
Diamond-Blackfan anemia, 79
Diffuse large B-cell lymphoma, 239
Disseminated *Histoplasma capsulatum*, 325
Disseminated intravascular coagulation, 425
Donath-Landsteiner hemolytic anemia, 50
Donor lymphocyte infusion therapy, 348
Double-hit high-grade B-cell lymphoma, 241
Dyserythropoetic anemia, type II, congenital, 82
Dysfibrinogenemia, congenital, 435

E

Ehrlichiosis, human granulocytic, 318, *461*, **502**
Elliptocytosis, hereditary, 60
Essential thrombocythemia, 160

F

Factor V inhibitor, 392
Factor V Leiden, 408
Factor VII deficiency, 382
Factor VIII deficiency, 384, *462*, **503**
Factor VIII deficiency carrier, 386
Factor IX deficiency, 388
Factor IX deficiency carrier, 390

Factor VIII inhibitor, 394, *463/**504***
Factor X deficiency, acquired, 396
Factor XI deficiency, 399
Factor XII deficiency, 401
Fanconi anemia with myelodysplastic syndrome, 84
Fetomaternal hemorrhage associated anemia, 42
Folate deficiency associated anemia, 22, *442/**469***
Follicular hyperplasia, 266
Follicular lymphoma, 227, 261

G

G6PD deficiency associated hemolytic anemia, 34, *443/**471***
Gastric MALT lymphoma, 233
Gaucher disease, *458/**496***
Genotyping (CYP2C9) for management of coumadin therapy, 439
Glanzmann thrombasthenia, 303
Gray platelet syndrome, 305
Gray zone lymphoma (double-hit high-grade C-cell lymphoma), 241
Graft-vs-host disease, acute, 342
Graft-vs-host disease, chronic, 346
Growth factor therapy-associated leukemoid reaction, 337

H

Hairy cell leukemia, 199
HELLP syndrome, 427
Hemochromatosis, HFE-associated, 89
Hemochromatosis, non-HFE-associated, 92
Hemoglobin E disease, 17
Hemoglobin H disease, *441,* ***468***
Hemoglobin SC disease, 53
Hemoglobin SS disease, 57, 70
Hemoglobinopathies, 17, 53, 57, 62, 70, 441, 444, 468, 473
    hemoglobin E disease, 17
    hemoglobin H disease, *441/**468***
    hemoglobin SC disease, 53
    hemoglobin SS disease, 57, 70
    sickle α thalassemia, 62
    sickle β thalassemia, *444/**473***
    sickle cell anemia, 57, 70
Hemolytic anemia associated with G6PD deficiency, 34, *443/**471***
Hemolytic anemia associated with pyruvate kinase deficiency, 36
Hemolytic disease of the newborn, 39
Hemophagocytic lymphohistiocytosis, 361, *459/**498***
Hemophagocytic syndrome (hemophagocytic lymphohistiocytosis), 361, *459/**498***

Hemophilia A
    carrier, 386
    in a newborn, 384
Hemophilia B, 388
    carrier, 390
Heparin-induced thrombocytopenia, type II, 466, **510**
Heparin-induced thrombocytopenia with thrombosis, 423
Hepatosplenic T-cell lymphoma, 252
Hereditary elliptocytosis, 60
Hereditary pyropoikilocytosis, 65
Hereditary spherocytosis, 55
Hermansky-Pudlak syndrome, 309
High grade B-cell lymphoma, 241
Histiocytic necrotizing lymhadenitis, 271
Histoplasmosis, 325
HIV and/or HIV therapy-related myelodysplasia, 359
Hodgkin lymphoma, 216-225
    nodular sclerosis, classical, 216
    lymphocyte-rich, classical, 222
    mixed cellularity, classical, 225
    nodular lymphocyte predominant, 219
Human granulocytic ehrlichiosis, 318, *461*/**502**
Hurler syndrome, 378
Hyperoxaluria involving bone marrow, 380
Hypotransferrinemia, 6

I

Idiopathic thrombocytopenic purpura, 300
IgM secreting myeloma, 286
Immune thrombocytopenic purpura, 300
Infectious mononucleosis, 331
inherited platelet secretion defect, 311
Iron deficiency anemia, 1
Ischemic stroke secondary to atherosclerosis from elevated Lp(a) levels, 437

J

Juvenile myelomonocytic leukemia, *452*/**486**

K

Kikuchi-Fujimoto disease, 271

L

Large B-cell lymphoma in chronic lymphocytic leukemia, 195
Large granular lymphocytic leukemia, T-cell, 208

Lead poisoning associated anemia, 10
Leukemoid reaction associated with growth factor therapy, 337
Light chain deposition disease, 294
Liver disease associated anemia, 68
Liver disease associated coagulopathy, 431
Lobular carcinoma of the breast, metastatic to the bone marrow, 367
Lymphocyte-rich classic Hodgkin lymphoma, 222
Lymphocytosis, persistent polyclonal, 328
Lymphohistiocytosis, hemophagocytic, 361, *459/**498***
Lymphomas, 216-264, 454-456, 488-492
    anaplastic large cell, *454/**488***
    angioimmunoblastic T-cell, 249
    Burkitt lymphoma, 236
    Cutaneous T-cell, 255
    diffuse large B-cell, 239
    double-hit, 241
    extranodal NK/T cell, 246
    follicular, 227, 261
    gray zone, 241
    hepatosplenic T-cell, 252
    high-grade B-cell, 241
    Hodgkin, classic, 216
    lymphocyte-rich classic Hodgkin, 222
    lymphoplasmacytic, *456/**492***
    maltoma, gastric, 233
    mantle cell, 230
    mantle cell, blastic variant , *455/**490***
    marginal zone, nodal, 258
    mixed cellularity classic Hodgkin, 225
    nodal, marginal zone, 258
    nodular lymphocyte predominant Hodgkin, 219
    NK-cell, extranodal 246
    primary cutaneous T-cell, 255
    Sézary syndrome, 264
    T-cell lymphoma/leukemia, adult, 210
    T-lymphoblastic, 244
Lymphoplasmacytic lymphoma, *456/**492***
Lymphoproliferative disorders, chronic, 192-213, 453, 456, 487, 492
    adult T-cell lymphoma/leukemia, 210
    autoimmune lymphoproliferative syndrome, 213
    B- cell prolymphocytic leukemia, 197
    chronic lymphocytic leukemia, 192
    hairy cell leukemia, 199
    large B-cell lymphoma in chronic lymphocytic leukemia, 195
    lymphoplasmacytic lymphoma, *456/**492***
    post transplant lymphoproliferative disorder, 202
    Richter transformation in chronic lymphocytic leukemia, 195
    T-prolymphocytic leukemia, 205, *453/**487***
    T-large granular lymphocytic leukemia, 208

M

Macrocytic anemia associated with B$_{12}$ deficiency, 25
Macrocytic anemia associated with folate deficiency, 22, *442*, **469**
Malaria (*Plasmodium vivax*), 320
Maltoma, gastric, 233
Mantle cell lymphoma, 230
Mantle cell lymphoma, blastoid variant, *455*, **490**
Marginal zone lymphoma, nodal, 258
Mastocytosis, systemic 165
May-Hegglin anomaly, 357
Megaloblastic anemia due to B$_{12}$ deficiency, 25
Megaloblastic anemia due to folate deficiency, 22, 442/**469**
Metastatic carcinoma involving bone marrow (primary, breast carcinoma), 367
Methemoglobinemia, 31
Mixed cellularity classic Hodgkin lymphoma, 225
Monoclonal gammopathy of undetermined significance, 280
Mucopolysaccharidosis type I, 378
Multiple myeloma, 284, 286
Multiple myeloma and acquired von Willebrand disease, 297
Mycosis fungoides/Sézary syndrome, 264
Myelodysplasia, HIV/therapy-related, 359
Myelodysplastic syndromes, 173-187
    with isolated del(5q), 184
    refractory anemia with excess blasts-2, 181
    refractory anemia with ring sideroblasts, 173
    refractory anemia with ring sideroblasts and marked thrombocytosis, 176
    refractory cytopenia with multilineage dysplasia, 178
    unclassifiable (MDS-U), 187
Myelodysplastic/myeloproliferative neoplasms, 152, 189, 452, 486
    chronic myelogenous leukemia, atypical, 152
    chronic myelomonocytic leukemia, 189
    juvenile myelomonocytic leukemia, 452/**486**
Myelofibrosis, 162
Myeloid sarcoma, 446/**476**
Myeloid/lymphoid neoplasms with eosinophilia and PDGFRA rearrangement, 128
Myeloma, IgM secreting, 286
Myelomonocytic leukemia, chronic, 189
Myelomonocytic leukemia, juvenile, *452*, **486**
Myeloproliferative disorder, transient, 351
Myeloproliferative neoplasms, 149, 152, 155-162, 168, 170, 450, 451, 482, 484
    chronic eosinophilic leukemia, *451*/**484**
    chronic myelogenous leukemia, case 149
    chronic neutrophilic leukemia, 155, 450/**82**
    essential thrombocythemia, 160
    mastocytosis, systemic 165
    polycythemia, congenital, 168
    polycythemia vera, 158,
    primary myelofibrosis, 162
    unclassifiable (MPN,U) , 170

N

Neonatal neutropenia, alloimmune, 334
Neutropenia, alloimmune, neonatal, 334
Neutropenia of childhood, chronic, 339
Neutrophilic leukemia, chronic, 155, *450/**482***
Niemann-Pick disease, 376
NK-cell lymphoma, extranodal, 246
Nodal marginal zone lymphoma, 258
Nodular lymphocyte predominant Hodgkin lymphoma, 219
Nodular sclerosis, Hodgkin lymphoma, classic, 216

O

Organisms, 315-325, 461, 502
    anaplasmosis, 318, *461/**502***
    babesiosis, 315
    borreliosis, 323
    histoplasmosis, 325
    plasmodium vivax, 320
Oxaluria involving bone marrow, 380

P

Pancytopenia associated with copper deficiency, 15
Paroxysmal nocturnal hemoglobinuria, 370
Parvovirus B-19 associated pure red cell aplasia, 87
Pelger-Huët anomaly, 354
Peripheralization of follicular lymphoma, 261
Pernicious anemia, 28
Persistent polyclonal B-lymphocytosis, 328
Plasma cell disorders, 280-297, 457, 494
    amyloidosis, primary, 291, *457/**494***
    IgM secreting myeloma, 286
    light chain deposition disease, 294
    monoclonal gammopathy of undetermined significance, 280
    multiple myeloma, 284, 286
    multiple myeloma and acquired von Willebrand disease, 297
    plasmacytoma, 282
    POEMS syndrome, 288
Plasmacytoma, 282
Plasminogen deficiency, Type 1, 433
Plasmodium vivax, 320

Platelet disorders, 300-313
    acquired platelet function defect, 313
    Glanzman thrombasthenia, 303
    gray platelet syndrome, 305
    Hermansky-Pudlak syndrome, 309
    immune thrombocytopenic purpura, 300
    inherited platelet secretion defect, 311
    storage pool deficiency, platelet, 309
    Wiskott-Aldrich syndrome, 307
Platelet function defect, acquired, 313
Platelet function defect induced by selective serotonin-reuptake inhibitor, 313
Platelet secretion defect/signal transduction defect, inherited, 311
Platelet storage pool deficiency, 309
POEMS syndrome, 288
Polycythemia, congenital, 168
Polycythemia vera, 158
Post transplant lymphoproliferative disorder, 202
Precursor B acute lymphoblastic leukemia, pediatric, 133
Precursor T acute lymphoblastic leukemia, pediatric, 136
Prekallikrein deficiency, 467/**514**
Primary amyloidosis, 291, 457/**494**
Primary cutaneous T-cell lymphoma, γ/δ type, 255
Primary hyperoxaluria involving bone marrow, 380
Primary myelofibrosis, 162
Progrssive transformation of germinal centers, 274
Prolymphocytic leukemia, 197, 205, 453, 487
    B-cell, 197
    T-cell, 205, 453/**487**
Promyelocytic leukemia, acute, 101
Protein C deficiency, 414
Protein S deficiency, 419
Prothrombin gene G20210A mutation, 412
Pure red cell aplasia associated with parvovirus B-19 infection, 87
Pyropoikilocytosis, hereditary, 65
Pyruvate kinase deficiency associated anemia, 36

R

Red cell aplasia, associated with parvovirus B-19 infection, 87
Refractory anemia with excess blasts-2, 181
Refractory anemia with ring sideroblasts, 173
Refractory anemia with ring sideroblasts and marked thrombocytosis, 176
Refractory cytopenia with multilineage dysplasia, 178
Relapsing fever secondary to *Borrelia hermsii*, 323
Renal disease associated anemia, 72
Rhabdomyosarcoma involving the bone marrow, 364, *460,* **500**
Richter syndrome, 195

Richter transformation in chronic lymphocytic leukemia, 195
Rosai-Dorfman disease, 269
rosebud, 527

S

Sézary syndrome, 264
Sickle-α-thalassemia, 62
Sickle-β-thalassemia, 444, **473**
Sickle cell anemia in a newborn, 57
Sickle cell anemia with leg ulcer, 70
Sickle-thalassemia, 62, 444, **473**
Spherocytosis, hereditary, 55
Storage pool deficiency, platelet, 309
Systemic mastocytosis, 165

T

T-acute lymphoblastic leukemia in an adult, 139, 449, **481**
T-large granular lymphocytic leukemia, 208
T-lymphoblastic phase in chronic myelogenous leukemia, 146
T-lymphoblastic leukemia, 139, 449, **481**
T-lymphoblastic lymphoma, 139
T-prolymphocytic leukemia, 205, 453, **487**
Thalassemias, 4, 8, 12
    intermedia, 12
    major, 8
    minor, 4
Therapy-related acute myeloid leukemia, 119
Thrombocytopenia, heparin-induced, type II, 466, **510**
Thrombocytopenia, heparin-induced with thrombosis, 423
Thrombotic thrombocytopenic purpura, 421
Thrombotic thrombocytopenic purpura (TTP) in a patient with sickle cell crisis, 429
Transient abnormal myelopoiesis, 351
Transient myeloproliferative disorder, 351

V

von Willebrand disease, variant 2 Normandy, 405
von Willebrand disease, acquired, 407
von Willebrand disease, type 3, 464, **506**

W

Waldenström macroglobulinemia, 456, **492**
Wiskott-Aldrich syndrome, 307

Abbreviations Used in this Publication

Abbreviation	Explanation
α	alpha
ABL	Abelson gene
AIDS	acquired immunodeficiency syndrome
AL	amyloidosis, light chain
ALK	anaplastic lymphoma kinase
Alk Phos	alkaline phosphatase
ANA	antinuclear antibody
ALT	alanine aminotransferase
APOB	apolipoprotein B
AST	aspartate aminotransferase
Baso	basophils
BCL	B-cell lymphoma
BCR	breakpoint cluster region gene
β	beta
Bili	bilirubin
BM	bone marrow
BMI	body mass index
BMP	basic metabolic panel
BP	blood pressure (mmHg)
BPM	beats per minute
BRCA	breast cancer (gene)
BUN	blood urea nitrogen
°C	degree centigrade
Ca	calcium
C-ANCA	anti-neutrophil cytoplasmic antibody
CBC	complete blood cell (count)
CCND	cyclin D gene
CD	cluster designation
CK	creatine kinase
Cl⁻	chloride
cm	centimeter
CMP	comprehensive metabolic panel
CMV	cytomegalovirus
CNS	central nervous system
CO_2	carbon dioxide
CR	creatinine
CSF	colony stimulating factor

Abbreviation	Explanation
CT	computed tomography
DAT	direct antiglobulin test
dL	deciliter
δ	delta
DNA	deoxyribonucleic acid
DRVVT	dilute Russel viper venom time
DVT	deep vein thrombosis
EBER	EBV-encoded RNA
EBV	Epstein-Barr virus
EKG	electrocardiogram
Eos	eosinophils
EM	electron microscopy
°F	degree Fahrenheit
FAB	French, American, British (classification)
FGFR	fibroblast growth factor receptor
FIPIL1	filamine-A-interacting protein 1
FISH	fluorescence in-situ hybridization
fL	femtoliter
FLT3	fms-related tyrosine kinase 3
γ	gamma
G6PD	glucose-6-phosphate dehydrogenase
GM-CSF	granulocyte/macrophage colony stimulating factor
H&E	hematoxylin and eosin (stain)
HARP	hypobetalipoproteinemia, acanthocytosis, retinitis pigmentosa, and pallidal degeneration
HGB	hemoglobin
HCT	hematocrit
HIV	human immunodeficiency virus
HLA	human leukocyte antigen
HMWK	high-molecular-weight kininogen
h	hour
HR	heart rate (beats per minute)
IgA	immunoglobulin A
IgD	immunoglobulin D
IgG	immunoglobulin G